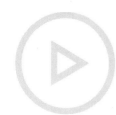

IMPORTANT:

HERE IS YOUR REGISTRATION CODE TO ACCESS YOUR PREMIUM McGRAW-HILL ONLINE RESOURCES.

For key premium online resources you need THIS CODE to gain access. Once the code is entered, you will be able to use the Web resources for the length of your course.

If your course is using **WebCT** or **Blackboard**, you'll be able to use this code to access the McGraw-Hill content within your instructor's online course.

Access is provided if you have purchased a new book. If the registration code is missing from this book, the registration screen on our Website, and within your WebCT or Blackboard course, will tell you how to obtain your new code.

Registering for McGraw-Hill Online Resources

TO gain access to your McGraw-Hill web resources simply follow the steps below:

1. USE YOUR WEB BROWSER TO GO TO: **www.mhhe.com/lewisgenetics6**
2. CLICK ON **FIRST TIME USER**.
3. ENTER THE REGISTRATION CODE* PRINTED ON THE TEAR-OFF BOOKMARK ON THE RIGHT.
4. AFTER YOU HAVE ENTERED YOUR REGISTRATION CODE, CLICK **REGISTER**.
5. FOLLOW THE INSTRUCTIONS TO SET-UP YOUR PERSONAL UserID AND PASSWORD.
6. WRITE YOUR UserID AND PASSWORD DOWN FOR FUTURE REFERENCE. KEEP IT IN A SAFE PLACE.

TO GAIN ACCESS to the McGraw-Hill content in your instructor's **WebCT** or **Blackboard** course simply log in to the course with the UserID and Password provided by your instructor. Enter the registration code exactly as it appears in the box to the right when prompted by the system. You will only need to use the code the first time you click on McGraw-Hill content.

REGISTRATION CODE

NPVN-OYAD-IE6K-WCOU-RJLI

Thank you, and welcome to your McGraw-Hill online Resources!

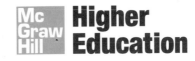

YOUR REGISTRATION CODE CAN BE USED ONLY ONCE TO ESTABLISH ACCESS. IT IS NOT TRANSFERABLE.

0-07-294728-4 T/A LEWIS: HUMAN GENETICS, 6/E

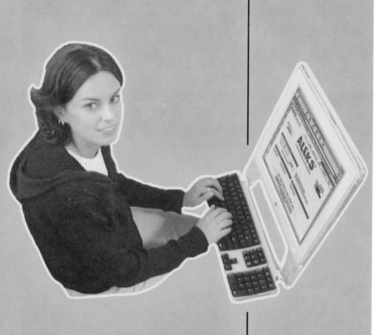

Human Genetics

Concepts and Applications

Sixth Edition

Ricki Lewis

CareNet Medical Group,
Schenectady, New York

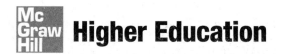

Boston   Burr Ridge, IL   Dubuque, IA   Madison, WI   New York   San Francisco   St. Louis
Bangkok   Bogotá   Caracas   Kuala Lumpur   Lisbon   London   Madrid   Mexico City
Milan   Montreal   New Delhi   Santiago   Seoul   Singapore   Sydney   Taipei   Toronto

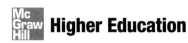

Higher Education

HUMAN GENETICS: CONCEPTS AND APPLICATIONS, SIXTH EDITION

Published by McGraw-Hill, a business unit of The McGraw-Hill Companies, Inc., 1221 Avenue of the Americas, New York, NY 10020.
Copyright © 2005, 2003, 2001, 1999, 1997 by The McGraw-Hill Companies, Inc. All rights reserved. No part of this publication may be reproduced or distributed in any form or by any means, or stored in a database or retrieval system, without the prior written consent of The McGraw-Hill Companies, Inc., including, but not limited to, in any network or other electronic storage or transmission, or broadcast for distance learning.

Some ancillaries, including electronic and print components, may not be available to customers outside the United States.

This book is printed on recyled, acid-free paper containing 10% postconsumer waste.

1 2 3 4 5 6 7 8 9 0 VNH/VNH 0 9 8 7 6 5 4

ISBN 0–07–287735–9 (hardcover)
ISBN 0–07–284605–4 (soft cover)

Publisher: *Martin J. Lange*
Senior sponsoring editor: *Patrick E. Reidy*
Senior developmental editor: *Deborah Allen*
Managing developmental editor: *Patricia Hesse*
Director of development: *Kristine Tibbetts*
Marketing manager: *Tami Petsche*
Senior project manager: *Rose Koos*
Production supervisor: *Kara Kudronowicz*
Senior media project manager: *Jodi K. Banowetz*
Media technology producer: *Renee Russian*
Senior coordinator of freelance design: *Michelle D. Whitaker*
Cover/interior designer: *John Rokusek*
Cover image composite: Woman's profile: © *Getty Images;* DNA Text Strings: © *Daisuke Morita/Getty Images*
Lead photo research coordinator: *Carrie K. Burger*
Photo research: *Chris Hammond/PhotoFind, LLC*
Supplement producer: *Brenda A. Ernzen*
Compositor: *Precision Graphics*
Typeface: *10/12 Minion*
Printer: *Von Hoffmann Corporation*

The credits section for this book begins on page C-1 and is considered an extension of the copyright page.

Library of Congress Cataloging-in-Publication Data

Lewis, Ricki,
    Human genetics : concepts and applications / Ricki Lewis. — 6th ed.
        p. cm.
    Includes index.
    ISBN 0–07–287735–9 (hard copy : alk. paper)
    1. Human genetics. I. Title.

QH431.L41855   2005
599.93'5—dc22   2003026153
                                                 CIP

www.mhhe.com

About the Author

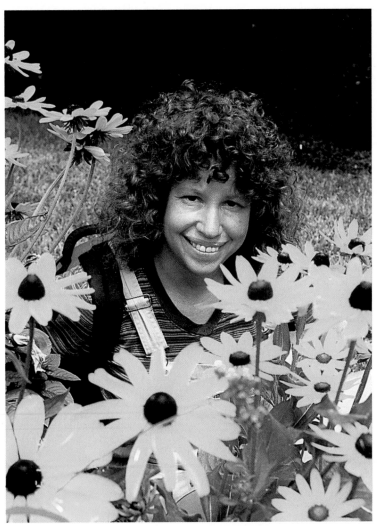

Photo credit: Barry Palevitz

Ricki Lewis has built a multifaceted career around communicating the excitement of life science, especially genetics and biotechnology. She earned her Ph.D. in genetics in 1980 from Indiana University, working with homeotic mutations in *Drosophila melanogaster.*

Ricki is the original author of *Life,* an introductory biology text; co-author of two human anatomy and physiology textbooks; and author of *Discovery: Windows on the Life Sciences,* an essay collection about research and the nature of scientific investigation. She writes frequently on research and news in genetics, cell biology, biotechnology and other areas for *The Scientist* (www.the-scientist.com). Since 1980, Ricki has published widely, including one of the first stories on DNA fingerprinting in *Discover* magazine. She has taught a variety of life science courses at Miami University, the University at Albany, Empire State College, and community colleges. She brought science experiments to grade school classrooms for three years as part of a traveling science museum, for which she obtained a Howard Hughes Medical Institute grant. Ricki has been a genetic counselor for a large private medical practice in Schenectady, NY, since 1984. She enjoys travel, often to give talks on the human genome, stem cell biology, or how the media reports on science.

Ricki lives in upstate New York with chemist husband Larry, one daughter, and two others away at college, and many cats.

Dedicated to
Shirley Epstein
Aaronson, who
encouraged an
inquisitive child
to become a
scientist.

Brief Contents

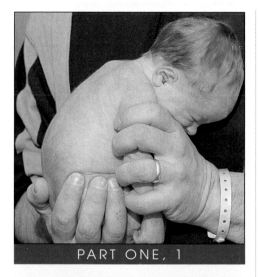

PART ONE, 1

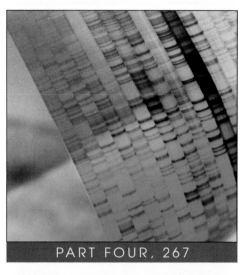

PART FOUR, 267

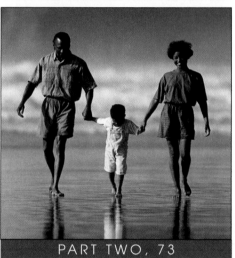

PART TWO, 73

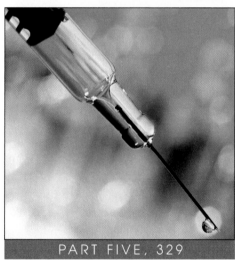

PART FIVE, 329

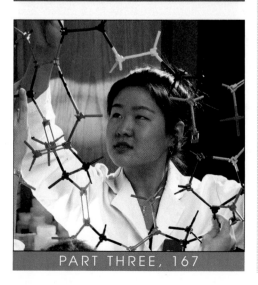

PART THREE, 167

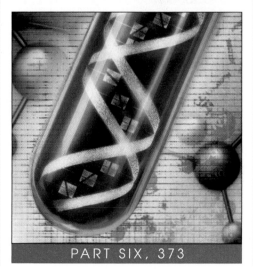

PART SIX, 373

v

List of Boxes

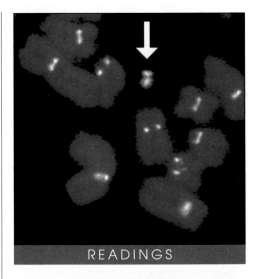

READINGS

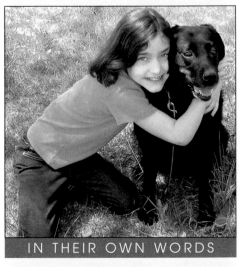

IN THEIR OWN WORDS

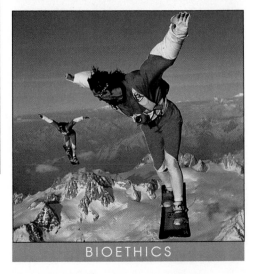

BIOETHICS

Clinical Coverage

Case Studies

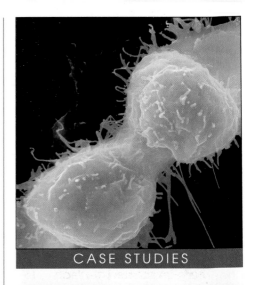

CASE STUDIES

Solving a Problem

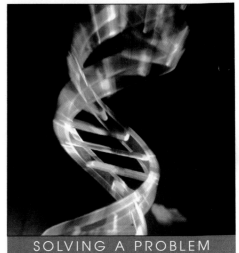

SOLVING A PROBLEM

Contents

PART FOUR

Population
Genetics   267

PART FIVE

Immunity
and Cancer   329

Preface

Genomics Comes of Age

The transformation of genetics into genomics is finally happening.

Human Genetics: Concepts and Applications has evolved along with the field it covers. In the decade since the first edition was published, genetics has grown from a focus on the rarest of the rare to a field so familiar that the world watched Saddam Hussein have his DNA sampled shortly after his capture. In the first edition, the human genome project was little more than a footnote and table.

By the fourth edition, genomics had earned its own chapter. By the fifth edition, genomic explanations began to permeate the other chapters, as recognition of many genes increasingly explained the actions of single genes. In this new sixth edition, that trend continues, with genomic information seamlessly integrated with the basic concepts it explains:

- genetic testing of college roommates that has gone from fiction to fact over the editions (chapter 1, "Overview of Genetics")
- scrutinizing the genomes of healthy 100+-year-olds (chapter 3, "Development")
- how the chimp and human genomes differ (chapter 16, "Human Origins and Evolution")
- immunity from the point of view of the pathogen, courtesy of sequenced genomes (chapter 17, "Immunity")
- a new form of leukemia revealed through gene expression DNA microarray analysis (chapter 18, "Cancer")
- accounting for redundant gene function in planning gene therapies (chapter 20, "Gene Therapy and Genetic Counseling").

Audiences Enjoy a Unique Writing Style

From the beginning, the clarity, flavor, and immediacy of *Human Genetics: Concepts and Applications* has been uniquely interesting and accessible to non-scientist readers. Into the book flows my 25 years of experience as a journalist, 20 years as a genetic counselor, and my PhD background in genetics. As a frequent contributor to the magazine *The Scientist* for 15 years, I have had access to scientific meetings and researchers that are simply not available to the average professor-turned-textbook author. I speak regularly to the people in the labs and clinics, to patients, to family members and doctors, and combine their words with my own into articles. From my network of sources, I learn of new research results before they are published, thus avoiding the built-in obsolescence that is the bane of textbooks. *Human Genetics: Concepts and Applications* is and always has been ahead of its time—and that's vital for a scientific field that is racing ahead as fast as genetics/genomics.

My approach is straightforward: present the essential concepts in clear language, then demonstrate them with the very best, sometimes quirky, examples. Tables, illustrations, and pedagogical aids reinforce the main points. Consider chapter 15, "Changing Allele Frequencies," which covers the five ways that genes defy Hardy-Weinberg equilibrium. The cast of characters providing examples includes Genghis Khan, Bulgarian gypsies, a young physician helping Amish children, and the blind Pingelapese of Micronesia. The five mechanisms that form the chapter's core are all wrapped up in figure 15.10, which also summarizes Hardy-Weinberg equilibrium from the previous chapter. A student who masters this illustration will be well prepared for an exam—and more importantly, will understand the intimate relationship between genetics and evolution.

Instructional Art Program Provides Dynamic Examples

The art program is not only spectacular in appearance, but remarkably easy to follow. Often all a reader needs to do is follow the arrows. In this manner, figures 2.19 and 2.20 reduce two complex cellular processes—cell death and signal transduction—to their essentials, fostering instant understanding. Other illustrations provide a size perspective. Figure 9.12, for example, shows how DNA is condensed, and also how it winds into a chromosome, which fits into a nucleus inside a cell. Two photographs bring the illustration to life. Similarly, figure 4.10 depicts Mendel's second law at the level of genes, chromosomes, and peas, all at once—a perspective essential for understanding how gametes connect generations. Figure 14.7 is perhaps the best example of putting molecular information into a familiar context: A man lying in an alley has his DNA analyzed to establish the identities of victim and attacker.

Extraordinary Learning Aids Assist Students

Pedagogical aids ensure that students can identify the basic concepts presented and exemplified within each chapter. Chapters open with an **annotated outline** previewing the chapter contents. At the end of each major section, **key concepts** are summarized to reinforce important core material. **Chapter summaries** review the contents of the chapter, calling attention to important new vocabulary.

Each chapter ends with a great variety of **review questions** to measure content knowledge and **applied questions** to provide practice using that knowledge. Both sets of questions are written to engage students in understanding the mechanisms of genetics and enable them to master content from a basic to a more advanced level. **Answers** to all questions are provided at the end of the book.

At the end of each chapter, a list of **suggested readings** provides further information and includes the sources used to write the chapter. Instructors can use these references to expand upon specific points, and students can use them to research papers and projects.

New Learning Aids

"**Solving a Problem**" sections present a step-by-step sample computation that leads to a genetic analysis and conclusion. This approach applies to the obvious—Mendel's laws, X-linked inheritance, and the Hardy-Weinberg equation—but also the not-so-obvious—such as comparing the "indels" (insertions and deletions) that distinguish the human from the chimp genome.

Case studies found after each chapter apply and sometimes extend concepts. These case studies supplement those in the *Case Workbook in Human Genetics* by Ricki Lewis. Relevant cases from the workbook are also listed for each chapter. New case studies include:

- a form of long-QT syndrome that causes excited children to collapse and die (chapter 5, "Extensions and Exceptions to Mendel's Laws")
- the Jukes family and inherited criminality (chapter 16, "Human Origins and Evolution")
- a woman who's ex-partner refuses to let her implant their frozen embryos (chapter 21, "Reproductive Technologies")
- a researcher who patented the use of what others once termed "junk" DNA to diagnose disease and is now charging licensing fees (chapter 22, "The Age of Genomics").

Web activities have been added for each chapter to encourage students to dig deeper. They provide an opportunity to find the newest genetic information and to use some of the latest tools and databases in genetic analysis. An appendix lists the reference information for diseases mentioned in the text to the web resource **Online Mendelian Inheritance in Man.**

What's New in This Edition?

Like a genome, a textbook evolves. This sixth edition has undergone a few insertions, deletions, and rearrangements.

Emphasis on control of gene expression

- Chapter 10 has undergone binary fission: It now focuses on "Gene Action."
- Chapter 11 presents "Control of Gene Expression." This new chapter explores gene expression through time and tissue; chromatin remodeling via the histone code and RNA interference; and the enigma of a genome that devotes only 1.5 percent of its information to encoding proteins, and the fact that those proteins greatly outnumber the genes that specify them.
- The theme of gene expression continues in a practical sense in chapter 18, "The Genetics of Cancer." Figure 18.2 presents data that have saved lives—DNA microarrays that revealed why some people with a rare form of leukemia do not survive given standard treatments for the more common form; they have a different illness, apparent only at the level of gene expression.

Unparalleled coverage of stem cell biology

- To accompany chapter 2's ("Cells") clear descriptions, four illustrations progress from basic to applied views of stem cells. Unlike most textbook depictions, figures 2.22 and 2.23 show stem cells giving rise to other stem cells, as well as daughter cells that go on to yield differentiated cells. Figure 2.24 takes the reader through the steps of somatic cell nuclear transfer, and figure 2.25 looks at stem cells from adults to heal a young man's heart.
- The stem cell theme continues in figure 11.4, which depicts how differential gene expression guides development of the pancreas into a uniquely dual structure—from a single type of progenitor cell.

Classical genetic observations viewed from a genomic perspective

- Redundancy in gene function sheds new light on chapter 5's "Extensions and Exceptions to Mendel's Laws," a group of important topics ignored in some other books.
- In chapter 7, "Multifactorial Traits," eye color is no longer considered a simple blue or brown, but includes the specks and flecks, shading and intensity that arise from the landscape at the back of the eye, providing great variability. Figure 7.13 summarizes the gene-controlled hormonal interactions that regulate body weight, also a phenotype not as simple as we once thought.

Updated examples

- Chapter 15, "Changing Allele Frequencies," discusses the emerging infectious diseases SARS and West Nile virus illness. Discussion of the possible effect of long-ago cannibalism on resistance to prion diseases fleshes out the coverage of balancing selection.
- New topics in Chapter 16, "Human Origins and Evolution," include targeted comparative sequencing to track shared ancestries; the 160,000-year-old *H. sapiens idaltu*, who looked amazingly like us; and a consideration of the many clues pointing to a duplication of the entire human genome.
- Chapter 22, "The Age of Genomics," has translocated material to earlier chapters, and has deleted descriptions of techniques no longer used, yet it preserves the telling of the historic race to sequence the human genome. New topics include "$1000 genome" sequencing technologies; the National Human Genome Research Institute's three-tiered architectural metaphor for the future of genomics; studies that focus on the healthy, rather than people with rare disorders; and a better understanding of the roots of disease. New genetic knowledge is not only providing information for the development of new diagnostic tests and treatments, but is easing identification of non-genetic factors that compromise health.

New "Stories" Integrated into the Narrative

- **Callipyge sheep,** whose giant rears illustrate genomic imprinting (chapter 6, "Matters of Sex")

- **Christina Vena,** a college student with lipodystrophy, cured with leptin shots (chapter 7, "Multifactorial Traits")

- **Let sleeping dogs lie:** how dogs with narcolepsy led to discovery of the gene in humans (chapter 8, "The Genetics of Behavior")

- **Rosalind Franklin's famed "photo 51"** (chapter 9, "DNA Structure and Replication")

- **The "blue people of Troublesome Creek"** (chapter 12, "Gene Mutation").

New Boxes

- The cast of real characters who have shared their experiences in past editions in "In Their Own Words" boxes update their stories, and are joined by some new voices.

- In "The Y Wars" (chapter 6), researcher Jennifer Marshall-Graves laments "The Rise and Fall of the Human Y Chromosome," while David Page describes "Rethinking the Rotting Y Chromosome."

- On a more serious note, parents tell the sad but inspiring tales of their children who have familial dysautonomia (chapter 12) and Li-Fraumeni family cancer syndrome (chapter 18).

New Design, New Tables, and New Figures Throughout

- A bright, modern, bold design sets the stage for the fascinating topic of genetics.

- Tables present the main points to ease studying.

- New figures add historical depth, highlight genomic approaches to traditional ideas, introduce technology, present news, and even offer artists' renditions of genetics.

Teaching and Learning Supplements

McGraw-Hill offers various tools and teaching products to support the sixth edition of *Human Genetics: Concepts and Applications.* Students can order supplemental study materials by contacting their local bookstore. Instructors can obtain teaching aids by calling the Customer Service Department at 800-338-3987, visiting the text website at www.mhhe.com/lewisgenetics6, or contacting your local McGraw-Hill sales representative.

Digital Content Manager

This multimedia collection of visual resources allows instructors to utilize artwork from the text in multiple formats to create customized classroom presentations, visually based tests and quizzes, dynamic course website content, or attractive printed support materials. The digital assets on this cross-platform CD-ROM are grouped by chapter within the following easy-to-use folders:

- **Art Libraries**—All text art in a format compatible with presentation or word processing software.

- **PowerPoint Presentations**—Ready-made presentations cover each chapter of the text.

- **Active Art Library**—Key figures from the text are saved in manipulable layers that can be isolated and customized to meet the needs of the lecture environment. Build images from simple to complex to suit your lecture style.

- **Animations Library**—Numerous full-color animations of key processes are provided. Harness the visual impact of processes in motion by importing these files into classroom presentations or course websites.

Instructor Testing and Resource CD-ROM (ITRCD)

The ITRCD is a cross-platform CD-ROM providing a wealth of resources for the instructor. Supplements featured on this CD-ROM include a computerized test bank utilizing Brownstone Diploma testing software to quickly create customized exams.

This user-friendly program allows instructors to search for questions by topic or format, edit existing questions or add new ones, and scramble questions and answer keys for multiple versions of the same test.

Other assets on the ITRCD are grouped within easy-to-use folders. The Instructor's Manual is available on this CD. Word files of the test bank are included for those instructors who prefer to work outside of the test generator software.

Instructor's Manual

The Instructor's Manual, prepared by Cran Lucas of Louisiana State University, is available through the Instructor Resources of the Online Learning Center, (www.mhhe.com/lewisgenetics6). The manual includes chapter outlines and overviews, a chapter-by-chapter resource guide to use of visual supplements, answers to questions in the text, additional questions and answers for each chapter, and Internet resources and activities.

Overhead Transparencies

A set of 100 full-color transparencies showing key illustrations from the text is available for adopters.

For the Student
Genetics: From Genes to Genomes CD-ROM:

This easy-to-use CD covers the most challenging concepts in the course and makes them more understandable through presentation of full-color animations and interactive exercises.

Online Learning Center

Get online at www.mhhe.com/lewisgenetics6. The OLC offers an extensive array of learning and teaching tools. Explore this dynamic site designed to help you get ahead and stay ahead in your study of human genetics. Some of the activities you will find on the website include:

- Self-quizzes to help you master material in each chapter

- Flash cards to ease learning of new vocabulary

- Case studies to practice application of your knowledge of human genetics
- Links to resource articles, popular press coverage, and support groups

Case Workbook in Human Genetics, fourth edition, by Ricki Lewis

This workbook is specifically designed to support the concepts presented in *Human Genetics* through real cases adapted from recent scientific and medical journals, with citations included. The workbook provides practice for constructing and interpreting pedigrees; applying Mendel's laws; reviewing the relationships of DNA, RNA, and proteins; analyzing the effects of mutations; evaluating phenomena that distort Mendelian ratios; designing gene therapies; and applying new genomic approaches to understanding inherited disease. An answer key is available for the instructor.

Acknowledgements

Human Genetics: Concepts and Applications, sixth edition, would not have been possible without the editorial and production dream team: many thanks to Deborah Allen, an extraordinary editor; Toni Michaels, Carrie Burger and Chris Hammond, photo editors; Anne Cody, copyeditor; Rose Koos, project manager, and Michelle Whitaker, designer.

I also thank my wonderful family: Larry, daughters Heather, Sarah, and Carly, and our legions of felines.

Reviewers

Hessel Bouma III
Calvin College

Ruth Chesnut
Eastern Illinois University

Joseph Chinnici
Virginia Commonwealth University

William Cushwa
Clark College

David P. Fan
University of Minnesota

Gail Gasparich
Towson University

Meredith Hamilton
Oklahoma State University

Mary Kananen and her students
Pennsylvania State University at Altoona

Jennifer Knight
University of Colorado at Boulder

Kari Krieger
University of Wisconsin at Green Bay

Clint Magill
Texas A & M University

Mary Murnik
Ferris State University

Gail Palmer
Hudson Valley Community College

Regina Rector
William Rainey Harper College

Laura Rhoads
State University of New York at Potsdam

Stefan Surzycki
Indiana University

Visual Preview

Instructional Art Program

The art program puts molecular information into a familiar context.

- Spectacular in appearance
- Easy to follow
- Complex processes focus on essentials

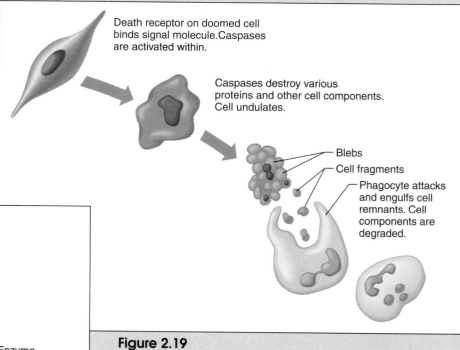

Death receptor on doomed cell binds signal molecule. Caspases are activated within.

Caspases destroy various proteins and other cell components. Cell undulates.

Blebs

Cell fragments

Phagocyte attacks and engulfs cell remnants. Cell components are degraded.

Figure 2.19

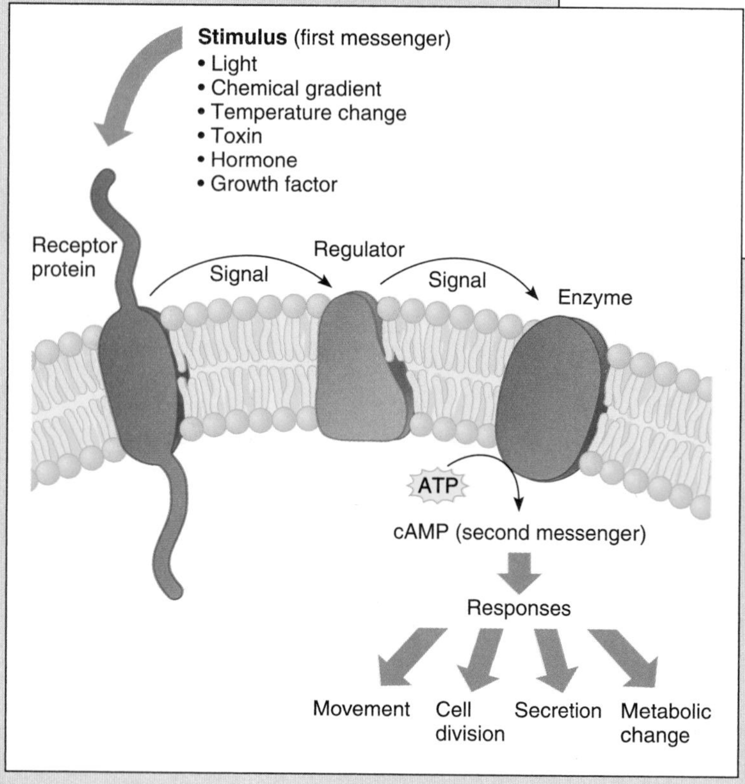

Stimulus (first messenger)
- Light
- Chemical gradient
- Temperature change
- Toxin
- Hormone
- Growth factor

Receptor protein

Signal   Regulator   Signal   Enzyme

ATP

cAMP (second messenger)

Responses

Movement   Cell division   Secretion   Metabolic change

Figure 2.20

Photographs bring illustrations to life

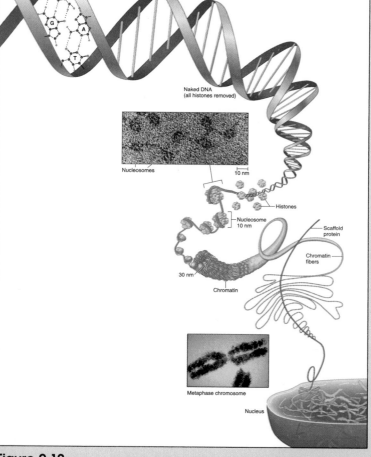

C   G   A   T

Naked DNA (all histones removed)

Nucleosomes   10 nm

Histones

Nucleosome 10 nm

Scaffold protein

Chromatin fibers

30 nm

Chromatin

Metaphase chromosome

Nucleus

Figure 9.12

Macro and micro views

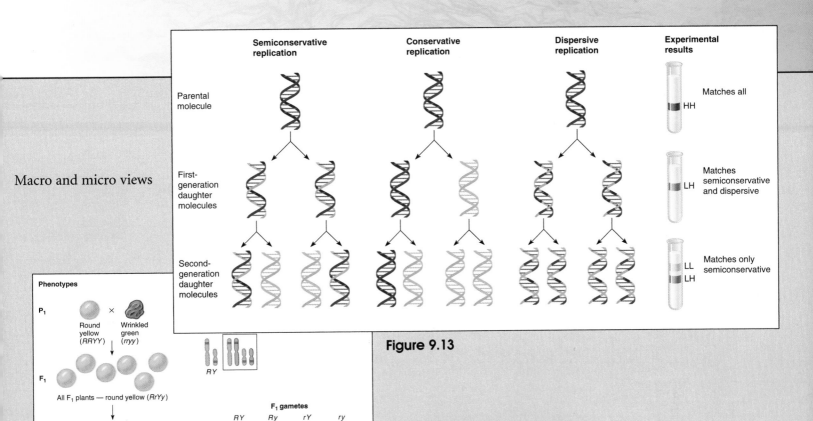

Figure 9.13

Molecular information appears in a familiar context

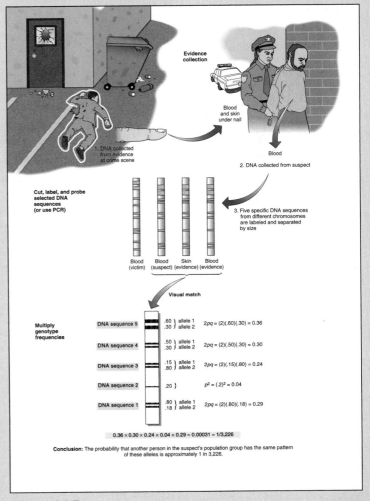

Figure 14.7

Figure 4.10

Extraordinary Learning Aids

Pedagogical aids ensure that students can identify the basic concepts presented and exemplified within each chapter.

- **Annotated outline** previews the chapter contents.
- **Key concepts** are summarized to reinforce important core material.
- **Chapter summaries** review the contents of the chapter, calling attention to important new vocabulary.
- **Review questions** measure content knowledge.
- **Applied questions** guide students in solving challenges that genetic information presents.
- **Answers** to all questions are at the end of the book.
- **Suggested readings** are useful in learning more about a particular topic.

CHAPTER

1

Overview of Genetics

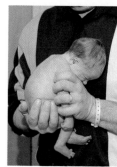

CHAPTER CONTENTS

1.1 Genetic Testing
Testing for inherited diseases and susceptibilities will become standard practice, making health care increasingly individualized. Tests that detect specific variations in genetic material will enable physicians to select treatments that a person can tolerate and that are most likely to be effective.

1.2 The Breadth of Genetics
DNA sequences that constitute genes carry information that tells cells how to manufacture specific proteins. A gene's effects are evident at the cell, tissue, organ, and organ system levels. Traits with large inherited components can be traced and predicted in families. Genetic change at the population level underlies evolution. Comparing genomes reveals that humans have much in common with other species.

1.3 Genes Do Not Usually Function Alone
In the twentieth century, genetics dealt almost entirely with single-gene traits and disorders. Today it is becoming clear that multiple genes and the environment mold most traits.

1.4 Geneticists Use Statistics to Represent Risks
Risk is an estimate of the likelihood that a particular individual will have a particular trait. It may be absolute for an individual, or relative based on comparison to other people.

1.5 Applications of Genetics
Genetics impacts our lives in diverse ways. Genetic tests can establish identities and diagnose disease. Genetic manipulations can provide new agricultural variants.

The genome tucked into each of this new-born's cells will influence much of the new individual's future—but the environment has a powerful effect too.

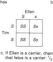

surrogate mothers and artificial insemination by donor (chapter 21). Moreover, many people cannot trace their families back more than three or four generations, so they lack sufficient evidence to reveal a mode of inheritance. Still, the pedigree is perhaps the most classic genetic tool, and it remains a powerful way to see, at a [glance, how a trait] passes from generation to [generation, just] as Gregor Mendel did wit[...]

Figure 4.18 Making predictions. Ellen's brother, Michael, has sickle cell disease, as depicted in this pedigree (a). Ellen wonders what the chance is that her fetus has inherited the sickle cell allele from her. First, she must calculate the chance that she is a carrier. The Punnett square in (b) shows that this risk is 2 in 3. (She must be genotype SS or Ss, but cannot be ss because she does not have the disease.) The risk that the fetus is a carrier, assuming that the father is not a carrier, is half Ellen's risk of being a carrier, or 1 in 3 (c).

Key Con[cepts]

Pedigrees are charts [that depict] family relationships a[nd] transmission of inherit[ed traits...] represent males, an[d...] horizontal lines link tw[o...] lines show generation[s...] horizontal lines depic[t...] for heterozygotes are [...] and symbols for indiv[iduals...] express the trait under[...] completely shaded. [Pedigrees] reveal mode of inher[itance...] with Punnett squares. [Geneticists] that apply Mendel's [laws...] predict the recurren[ce...] inherited disorders or [traits.]

Summary

4.1 Following the Inheritance of One Gene—Segregation

1. Gregor Mendel described the two basic laws of inheritance using pea plant crosses. The laws, which derive from the actions of chromosomes during meiosis, apply to all diploid organisms.

2. Mendel used a statistical approach to investigate why some traits seem to disappear in the hybrid generation. The **law of segregation** states that alleles of a gene are distributed into separate gametes during meiosis. Mendel demonstrated this using seven traits in pea plants.

3. A diploid individual with two identical alleles of a gene is **homozygous**. A **heterozygote** has two different alleles of a gene. A gene may have many alleles.

4. A **dominant** allele masks the expression of a **recessive** allele. An individual may be homozygous dominant, homozygous recessive, or heterozygous.

5. Mendel repeatedly found that when he crossed two true-breeding types, then bred the resulting hybrids to each other, the two variants of the trait appeared in a 3:1 phenotypic ratio. Crossing these progeny further revealed a genotypic ratio of 1:2:1.

6. A **Punnett square** is a chart used to follow the transmission of alleles. It is based on probability.

4.2 Single-Gene Inheritance in Humans

7. Traits or disorders caused by single genes are called Mendelian or unifactorial traits.

8. **Modes of inheritance** enable geneticists to predict phenotypes. In **autosomal dominant** inheritance, males and females may be affected, and the trait does not skip generations. Inheritance of an **autosomal recessive** trait may affect either males or females and may skip generations. Autosomal recessive conditions are more

likely to occur in famil[ies with] **consanguinity.** Recessi[ve...] be more severe and ca[...] earlier than dominant [...]

9. Genetic problems can [...] alleles as gametes form[...] in a new individual.

10. Dominance and reces[sivity...] alleles affect the abund[ance...] the gene's protein prod[uct.]

4.3 Following the Inh[eritance of] Two Genes—Ind[ependent] Assortment

11. Mendel's second law, [the law of] **independent assortm[ent...]** transmission of two or [more genes on] different chromosome[s...] random assortment of [maternally and] paternally derived chr[omosomes in] meiosis results in gam[etes with] different combination[s of genes.]

Chapter 4 Mendelian Inhe[ritance]

---

12. The chance that two independent genetic events will both occur is equal to the product of the probabilities that each event will occur on its own. This principle, called the product

rule, is useful in calculating the risk that certain individuals will inherit a particular genotype and in following the inheritance of two genes on different chromosomes.

4.4 Pedigree Analysis

13. A **pedigree** is a chart that depicts family relationships and patterns of inheritance for particular traits. A pedigree can be inconclusive.

Review Questions

1. How does meiosis explain Mendel's laws of segregation and independent assortment?

2. How was Mendel able to derive the two laws of inheritance without knowing about chromosomes?

3. Distinguish between
   a. autosomal recessive and autosomal dominant inheritance.
   b. Mendel's first and second laws.
   c. a homozygote and a heterozygote.
   d. a monohybrid and a dihybrid cross.
   e. a Punnett square and a pedigree.

4. Why would Mendel's results for the dihybrid cross have been different if the genes for the traits he followed were located near each other on the same chromosome?

5. Why are extremely rare autosomal recessive disorders more likely to appear in families in which blood relatives have children together?

6. How does the pedigree of the ancient Egyptian royal family in figure 4.14a differ from a pedigree a genetic counselor might use today?

7. People who have Huntington disease inherit one mutant and one normal allele. How would a person who is homozygous dominant for the condition arise?

8. What is the probability that two individuals with an autosomal recessive trait, such as albinism, will have a child with the same genotype and phenotype as they do?

Applied Questions

1. Achondroplasia is a common form of hereditary dwarfism that causes very short limbs, stubby hands, and an enlarged forehead. Below are four pedigrees depicting families with this specific type of dwarfism. What is the most likely mode of inheritance? Cite a reason for your answer.

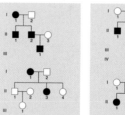

2. Draw a pedigree to depict the following family:
One couple has a son and a daughter with normal skin pigmentation. Another couple has one son and two daughters with normal skin pigmentation. The daughter from the first couple has three children with the son of the second couple. Their son and one daughter have albinism; their other daughter has normal skin pigmentation.

3. Chands syndrome is an autosomal recessive condition characterized by very curly hair, underdeveloped nails, and abnormally shaped eyelids. In the following pedigree, which individuals must be carriers?

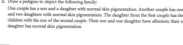

4. Caleb has a double row of eyelashes, which he inherited from his mother as a dominant trait. His maternal grandfather is the only other relative to have the trait. Veronica, a woman with normal eyelashes, falls madly in love with Caleb, and they marry. Their

PART TWO Transmission Genetics

New Learning Aids

"Solving a Problem" sections appear throughout the book where students are faced with learning how to perform a genetic analysis. Each new section presents a step-by-step sample computation.

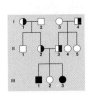
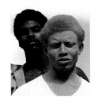

Figure 4.15   A pedigree for an autosomal recessive trait. Albinism affects males and females and can skip generations, as it does here in generations I and II. The homozygous recessive individual lacks an enzyme needed to produce melanin, which colors the eyes, skin, and hair.

carriers. One partner from each pair of grandparents must also be a carrier, which can sometimes be determined using a carrier test, inferred from family history, or deduced from a map of DNA sequence of the affected chromosome.

An autosomal dominant trait does not skip generations and can affect both sexes. A typical pedigree for an autosomal dominant trait has some squares and circles filled in to indicate affected individuals in each generation (**figure 4.16**).

A pedigree may be inconclusive, which means that either autosomal recessive or autosomal dominant inheritance can explain the pattern of filled-in symbols. **Figure 4.17** shows one such pedigree, for a type of hair loss called alopecia. According to the pedigree, this trait can be passed in an autosomal dominant mode because it affects both males and females and is present in every generation. However, the pedigree can also depict autosomal recessive inheritance if the individuals represented by unfilled symbols are carriers. Inconclusive pedigrees tend to arise when families are small and the trait is not severe enough to impair fertility.

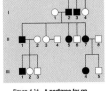

Figure 4.16   A pedigree for an autosomal dominant trait. Autosomal dominant traits do not skip generations. This trait is brachydactyly, or short fingers.

Figure 4.17   An inconclusive pedigree. This pedigree could account for an autosomal dominant trait or an autosomal recessive trait that does not prevent affected individuals from having children. (Unfilled symbols could represent carriers.)

Solving a Problem: Conditional Probability

Often genetic counselors are asked to predict the probability that a condition will occur in a particular individual, such as an offspring. Mendel's laws, pedigrees, and Punnett squares provide clues, as do logic and common sense. Consider the family depicted in **figure 4.18**.

Michael Stewart has sickle cell disease, which is inherited as an autosomal recessive condition. This means that his unaffected parents, Kate and Brad, must each be heterozygotes (carriers). Michael's sister, Ellen, also healthy, is expecting her first child. Ellen's husband, Tim, has no family history of sickle cell disease. Ellen wants to know the risk that her child will inherit the mutant allele from her and be a carrier.

Ellen's request really contains two questions. First, what is the risk that she herself is a carrier? Because Ellen is the product of a monohybrid cross, and we know that she is not homozygous recessive, she has a 2 in 3 chance of being a carrier, as the Punnett square indicates. If Ellen is a carrier, what is the chance that she will pass the mutant allele to an offspring? It is 1 in 2, because she has two copies of the gene, and according to Mendel's first law, only one goes into each gamete.

To calculate the overall risk to Ellen's child, we can apply the product rule and multiply the probability that Ellen is a carrier by the chance that, if she is, she will pass the mutant allele on. This result, following two events, is a conditional probability, because the likelihood of the second event—the child being a carrier—depends upon the first event—that Ellen is a carrier. If we assume Tim is not a carrier, Ellen's chance of giving birth to a child who carries the mutant allele is therefore 2/3 times 1/2, which equals 2/6, or 1/3. Ellen thus has a theoretical 1 in 3 chance of giving birth to a child who is a carrier for sickle cell disease.

Pedigrees can be difficult to construct and interpret for several reasons. People sometimes hesitate to supply information because they are embarrassed by symptoms affecting behavior or mental stability. Family relationships can be complicated by adoption, children born out of wedlock, serial relationships, blended families, and assisted reproductive technologies such as

Applied Questions

1. In Hunter syndrome, lack of the enzyme iduronate sulfatase leads to buildup of carbohydrates called mucopolysaccharides. In severe cases, this may swell the liver, spleen, and heart. In mild cases, deafness may be the only symptom. A child with this syndrome is deaf and has unusual facial features. Hunter syndrome is X-linked recessive. Intellect is usually unimpaired and life span can be normal. Suppose a man who has mild Hunter syndrome has a child with a carrier.

   a. What is the probability that a male child would inherit Hunter syndrome?
   b. What is the chance that a female child would inherit Hunter syndrome?
   c. What is the chance that a girl will be a carrier?
   d. How might a carrier of this condition experience symptoms?

2. Coffin-Lowry syndrome causes short, tapered fingers; abnormal finger and toe bones; puffy hands; soft, elastic skin; curved fingernails; facial anomalies; and sometimes hearing loss and heart problems. Evidence suggests that the syndrome is X-linked recessive, but girls are affected to a much lesser degree than boys. Suggest two explanations for why girls tend to have milder cases.

3. Amelogenesis imperfecta is an X-linked dominant condition that affects tooth enamel. Affected males have extremely thin enamel layers all over each tooth. Female carriers have grooved teeth from the uneven deposition of enamel. Explain the difference in phenotype between the sexes.

4. A prenatal test finds that cells of a fetus have two Barr bodies. What sex is the fetus?

5. Huntington disease (see Bioethics: Choices for the Future, Chapter 4) begins earlier and symptoms progress faster if the affected person inherits the disorder from his or her father. Explain this observation.

Web Activities

6. Identify an X-linked disorder at http://www.ncbi.nlm.nih.gov/disease/chr21-Y.html, then find it in OMIM and describe it.

7. From the Imprinted Gene Catalogue at http://cancer.otago.ac.nz/IGC/web/home.html, click on "search by species name" and then click on "complete list." Find two disorders that involve imprinting, one transmitted from the mother and one from the father, and use OMIM to describe them.

Case Studies

8. Reginald has mild hemophilia A that he can control by taking a clotting factor. He marries Lydia, whom he met at the hospital where he and Lydia's brother, Marvin, receive their treatment. Lydia and Marvin's mother and father, Emma and Clyde, do not have hemophilia. What is the probability that Reginald and Lydia's son will inherit hemophilia A?

9. Harold works in a fish market, but the odor does not bother him because he has anosmia, an X-linked recessive lack of sense of smell. Harold's wife, Shirley, has a normal sense of smell. Harold's sister, Maude, also has a normal sense of smell, as does her husband, Phil, and daughter, Marsha, but their identical twin boys, Alvin and Simon, cannot detect odors. Harold and Maude's parents, Edgar and Florence, can smell normally. Draw a pedigree for this family, indicating people who must be carriers of the anosmia gene.

10. Metacarpal 4-5 fusion is an X-linked recessive condition in which certain finger bones are fused. It occurs in many members of the Flabudgett family, depicted in the pedigree to the left:

    a. Why are three females affected, considering that this is an X-linked condition?
    b. What is the risk that individual III-1 will have an affected son?
    c. What is the risk that individual III-5 will have an affected son?

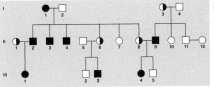

Case studies found after each chapter apply, and sometimes extend, concepts. These case studies supplement those in the *Case Workbook in Human Genetics* by Ricki Lewis.

Web activities encourage students to find information about human genetics that particularly interests them. They also provide an opportunity to find the latest genetic information and to use some of the latest tools and databases in genetic analysis. An appendix lists the reference information for diseases mentioned in the text to the web resource, **Online Mendelian Inheritance in Man.**

CHAPTER

Overview of Genetics

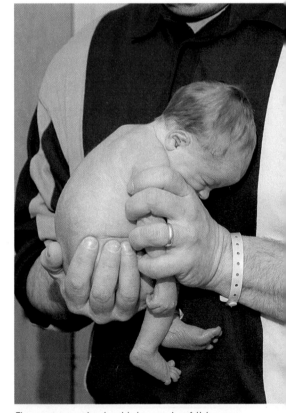

The genome tucked into each of this newborn's cells will influence much of the new individual's future—but the environment has a powerful effect too.

Genetics is the study of inherited traits and their variation. Sometimes people confuse genetics with genealogy, which considers relationships but not traits. With the advent of tests that can predict genetic illness, some people have even compared genetics to fortunetelling! But genetics is neither genealogy nor fortunetelling—it is a life science.

Genes are the units of heredity. They are biochemical instructions that tell **cells,** the basic units of life, how to manufacture certain proteins. These proteins ultimately underlie specific traits; they provide a great variety of characteristics that create much of our individuality, from our hair and eye color, to the shapes of our body parts, to our talents and personality traits (**figure 1.1**). For example, proteins called keratins comprise our hair and fill our skin cells. One consequence of impaired keratin production is the "scaly skin" disease ichthyosis, shown in figure 6.7.

A gene is composed of the molecule **deoxyribonucleic acid,** more familiarly known as **DNA.** Some traits are determined nearly entirely by genes; most traits, however, also have environmental components. The complete set of genetic information characteristic of an organism, including protein-encoding genes and other DNA sequences, constitutes a **genome.** Researchers at both a multinational public consortium and a private company deciphered the DNA building block sequence of the human genome in 2000 and will be analyzing those results for many years.

Genetics is unlike other life sciences in how directly and intimately it affects our lives, as well as those of our descendants. It obviously impacts our health, because we inherit certain diseases and disease susceptibilities. But principles of genetics also touch history, politics, economics, sociology, art, and psychology, and they force us to wrestle with concepts of benefit and risk, even tapping our deepest feelings about right and wrong. A field of study called **bioethics** was founded in the 1970s to address many of the personal issues that arise in applying medical technology. Bioethicists have more recently addressed concerns that new genetic knowledge raises, such as privacy, confidentiality, and discrimination.

An even newer field is **genomics,** which considers many genes at a time. The genomic approach is broader than the emphasis on single-gene traits that pervaded genetics during the twentieth century. Genomics addresses the more common illnesses influenced by many genes that interact with each other and the environment. Considering genomes also enables us to compare ourselves to other species—the similarities can be astonishing and quite humbling.

1.1 Genetic Testing

It may take much of the new century to understand our genetic selves. A few individuals have stepped forward to be among the first to probe their genomes. In late 2002, a journalist wrote in *Wired* magazine about undergoing a battery of genetic tests. And J. Craig Venter, who led the private effort to sequence the human genome, acknowledged that his was one of the genomes analyzed. He knows the results, and he has acted on some of them—for example, by taking cholesterol-lowering medication before his cholesterol actually rises to a dangerous level. Venter says that he volunteered his own genetic material to show the world that genome sequencing is not frightening, harmful, or magical and that it can instead be a powerful tool to improve health.

Past editions of this textbook began with a scenario of two college students undergoing genetic testing sometime in the near future. The future is now. Although a laser-based technology that can sequence a genome in minutes is in development, it is more cost-effective, for now, to tailor single, focused tests to detect health-related genetic variants most likely to be present in a particular individual, based on traditional clues such as personal health, family history, and ethnic background. Tests may look for gene variants known to cause illness or DNA sequences statistically associated with increased risk of developing a particular condition in a particular population. Researchers at several biotechnology companies predict that by 2006, genetic screening for many disorders and disease susceptibilities will be routine.

Young people might take genetic tests to prevent, delay, control, or treat symptoms that have a high probability of occurring, or to gain information, perhaps to make decisions about whether to have children or not. Consider two 19-year-old college roommates, Mackenzie and Laurel, who choose to undergo limited and tailored genetic testing. Each has her genome scanned for several hundred genes and DNA sequences. Some of the results illustrate the type of information that lies in our DNA.

Mackenzie requests three panels of tests, based on her family background. An older brother and

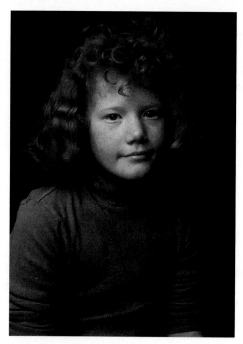

a.

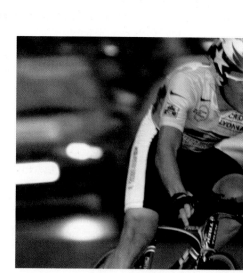

b.

Figure 1.1 Inherited traits. Genes control many familiar traits, from hair color **(a)** to athletic prowess **(b)**.

her father smoke cigarettes and are prone to alcoholism, and her father's mother, also a smoker, died of lung cancer. Two relatives on her mother's side had colon cancer. Mackenzie also has older relatives on both sides who have Alzheimer disease. She asks for tests to detect genes that predispose her to developing addictions, certain cancers, and inherited forms of Alzheimer disease.

Laurel requests different tests. She frequently has bronchitis and pneumonia, so she has a test for cystic fibrosis (CF), because CF's milder forms increase susceptibility to respiratory infections. These cases often go unrecognized as CF, as Laurel knows from her genetics class. Because her sister and mother also have bronchitis often, she suspects mild CF in the family.

Laurel also requests tests for type II (non-insulin-dependent) diabetes mellitus, because several of her relatives developed this condition as adults. Medication can control the abnormal blood glucose level, but dietary and exercise plans are essential, too. If Laurel knows she is at high risk, she'll adopt these habits now. However, Laurel refuses a test for inherited susceptibility to Alzheimer disease, even though a grandfather died of it. She does not want to know if this currently untreatable condition is likely to lie in her future. Finally, because past blood tests revealed elevated cholesterol, Laurel seeks information about her risk of developing heart and blood vessel (cardiovascular) disease.

Each student proceeds through the steps outlined in **figure 1.2.** The first step is to register a complete family history. Next, each young woman swishes a cotton swab on the inside of her cheek to obtain cells, which are then sent to a laboratory for analysis. There, DNA is extracted and cut into pieces, then tagged with molecules that

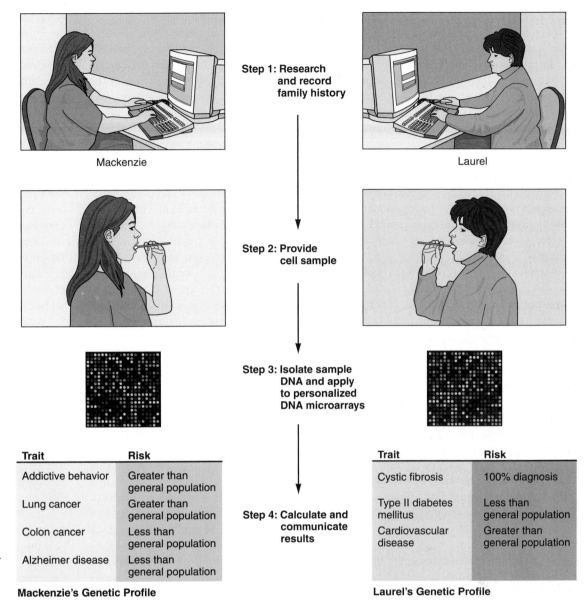

Figure 1.2 Genetic testing. Genetic tests are slowly becoming part of health care, revealing probabilities of developing certain conditions and refining medical diagnoses.

fluoresce under certain types of light. The students' genetic material is then applied to "DNA chips," postage-stamp-sized pieces of glass or nylon with particular sequences of DNA attached. Because the genes on the chip are aligned in fixed positions, this device is technically called a **DNA microarray.**

A typical DNA microarray bears hundreds or even thousands of DNA pieces. (Several companies offer the entire human genome on a chip.) One of Mackenzie's DNA chips bears genes that regulate her circadian (daily) rhythms and encode the receptor proteins on nerve cells that bind neurotransmitters. If Mackenzie indulges in addictive substances

or activities, certain variants of these genes may increase her risk of developing addictive behaviors. Another DNA chip screens for gene variants that greatly increase the risk for lung cancer, and a third DNA chip detects genes associated with colon cancer. Her fourth DNA chip is smaller, bearing genes that cause Alzheimer disease and several DNA sequences that are associated with increased risk of developing other types of dementia.

Laurel's chips suit her background and requests. The microarray panel for CF holds 600 DNA sequences from variants of the CF gene associated with milder symptoms. The DNA microarray for diabetes bears gene variants that reflect how Laurel's circulation transports glucose and how efficiently her cells take it up. The DNA microarray for cardiovascular disease is the largest and most diverse. It includes thousands of genes whose protein products influence blood pressure, blood clotting, and the synthesis, transport, and metabolism of cholesterol and other lipids.

The next day, a **genetic counselor** explains the findings. Mackenzie learns that she is indeed predisposed to develop addictive behaviors and lung cancer—a dangerous combination. But she does not face increased risk for inherited forms of colon cancer or Alzheimer disease.

Laurel does have mild CF, which explains her frequent respiratory infections. The DNA microarray indicates which types of infections she is most susceptible to, and which antibiotics will most effectively treat them—very useful information. She might even be a candidate for gene therapy—periodically inhaling a preparation containing the normal version of the CF-causing gene delivered in a "disabled" virus that would otherwise cause a respiratory infection. The diabetes test panel reveals her risk is lower than that for the general population. Laurel also has several gene variants that raise her blood cholesterol level. The cardiovascular disease DNA microarray panel indicates which cholesterol-lowering drug she will respond to best, should diet and exercise habits be insufficient to counter her inherited tendency to accumulate lipids in the bloodstream.

The DNA tests that Mackenzie and Laurel undergo will become part of their medical records, with tests added as their interests and health status change. For example, shortly before each young woman tries to become pregnant, she and her partner will take tests to detect whether they are carriers for any of several hundred illnesses, because two carriers of the same condition can pass it to offspring even when they are not themselves affected. If Laurel or Mackenzie are in this situation, DNA microarray tests on DNA from a fetus can determine whether it has inherited the illness. Such an alert can ensure that treatment begins soon enough to prevent or minimize symptoms in infants.

Illness may also prompt Laurel or Mackenzie to seek further genetic testing. If either young woman suspects she may have cancer, for example, a type of DNA micro-

array called an expression panel can determine which genes are turned on or off in affected cells compared to nonaffected cells of the same type. **"Gene expression"** refers to the cell's use of the information in the DNA sequence to synthesize a particular protein. In contrast, the DNA from cheek lining cells that Mackenzie and Laurel have tested reveals specific gene variants and DNA sequences that are present in *all* their cells. An expression panel displays the genes that actively produce specific proteins in the cell types that are affected in an illness.

DNA expression microarrays are very useful in diagnosing and treating cancer. They can identify cancer cells very early, when treatment is more likely to work. These devices also identify a set of 128 key gene variants that indicate cancer, as well as others that reveal if and how quickly the disease will progress. DNA microarrays can also show how tumor cells and the individual's immune system are likely to respond to particular drugs, and which drugs will produce intolerable side effects.

The first DNA microarray to analyze cancer, the "lymphochip," identifies cancer-causing and associated genes in white blood cells (see figure 18.2). A different DNA microarray test, for breast cancer, is used on samples of breast tissue to track the course of the disease and assess treatment. In one study, DNA tests were performed on tumor cells of 20 women with advanced breast cancer before and after a 3-month regimen of chemotherapy. The gene expression pattern returned to normal only in the three women who ultimately responded to the treatment. Therefore, the chip can predict which women are likely to respond to which drugs. A prostate cancer DNA microarray predicts the likelihood that a tumor will spread, information that is important in planning initial treatment.

Though Laurel and Mackenzie will gain much useful information from the genetic tests, their health records will be kept confidential. Laws prevent employers and insurers from discriminating against anyone based on genetic information. This is a practical matter—everyone has some gene variants associated with disease. In general, insurance companies decide whom to insure and at what rates based on symptoms present before or at the time of request for coverage. The results of genetic tests are not clinical diagnoses, but proba-

bility statements about how likely certain symptoms are to arise in an individual. The section on health care later in the chapter returns to the issue of insurer or employer discrimination based on genetic test results.

New health care professionals are being trained in genetics and the new field of genomics; older health care workers are also learning how to integrate new genetic knowledge and technology into medical practice. Another change has occurred in the breadth of genetics. In the past, physicians typically encountered genetics only as rare disorders caused by single genes or as chromosome disorders such as trisomy 21 Down syndrome. Today, medical science is beginning to recognize the role that genes play in many common types of conditions.

Key Concepts

Genetics investigates inherited traits and their variations. Genes, composed of DNA, are the units of inheritance, and they specify particular proteins, though not all DNA encodes protein. A genome is the complete set of genetic instructions for an organism. Human genome information will personalize medicine and predict future illness.

1.2 The Breadth of Genetics

Genetics considers the transmission of information at several levels, from the molecular level to populations and even to the evolution of species (**figure 1.3**).

DNA

Genes consist of sequences of four types of DNA building blocks—adenine, guanine, cytosine, and thymine, abbreviated A, G, C, and T. Each base bonds to a sugar and a phosphate group to form a unit called a nucleotide. DNA bases are nitrogen-containing, or nitrogenous, bases. In genes, DNA bases provide an alphabet of sorts. Each consecutive three DNA bases specifies the code for a particular amino acid, and amino acids are the building blocks of proteins.

An intermediate language, also encoded in nitrogenous base sequences, is contained in **ribonucleic acid (RNA)**. One type of RNA carries a copy of a DNA sequence and presents

Figure 1.3 From molecule to population. Genetics can be considered at several levels, from DNA, to chromosome, to individual, families, and populations.

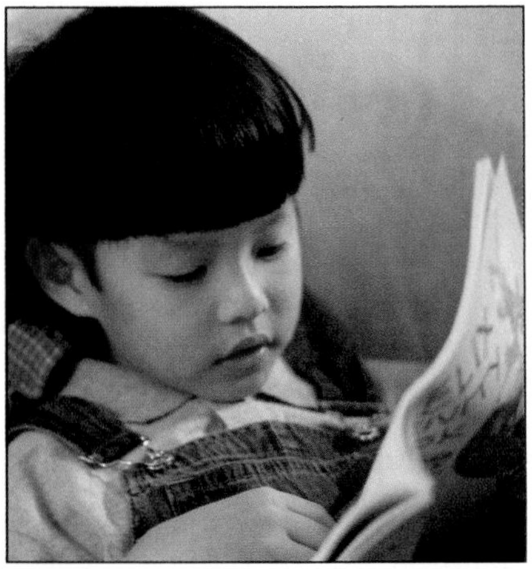

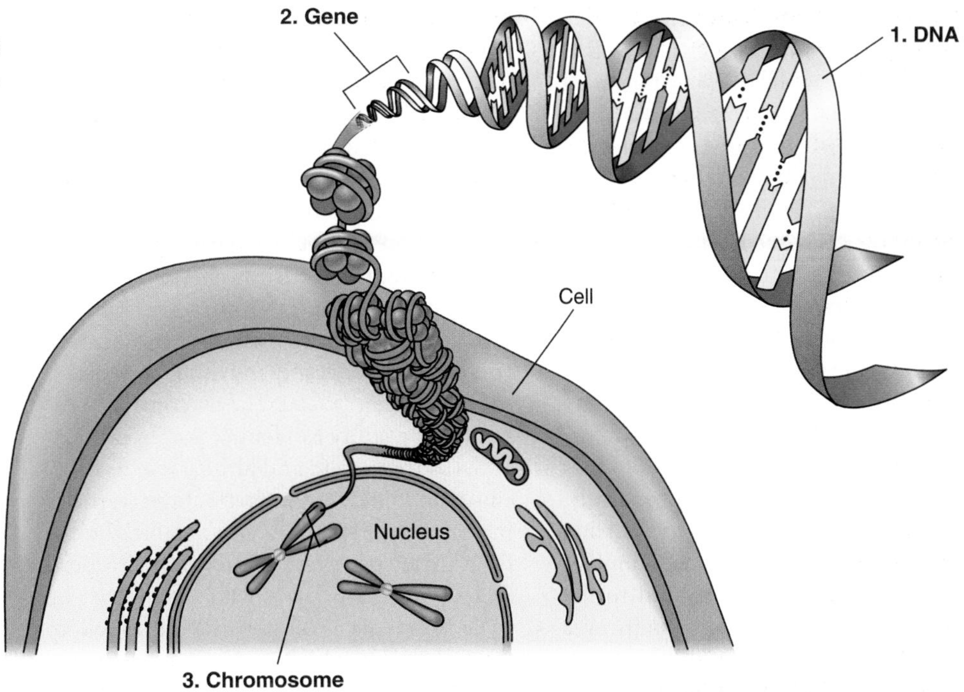
2. Gene
1. DNA
Cell
Nucleus
3. Chromosome

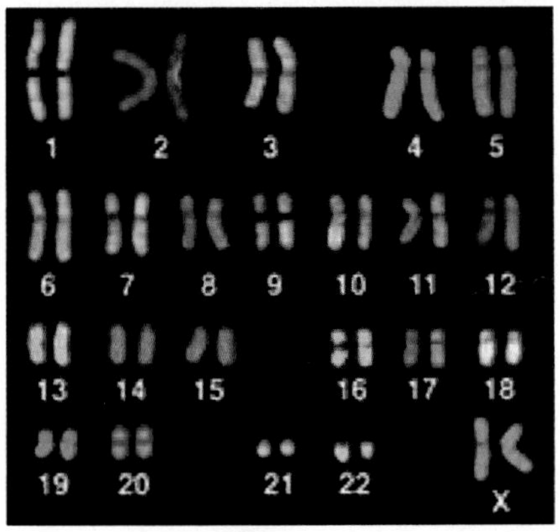
4. Human genome (23 chromosome pairs)
1 2 3 4 5
6 7 8 9 10 11 12
13 14 15 16 17 18
19 20 21 22 X

5. Individual

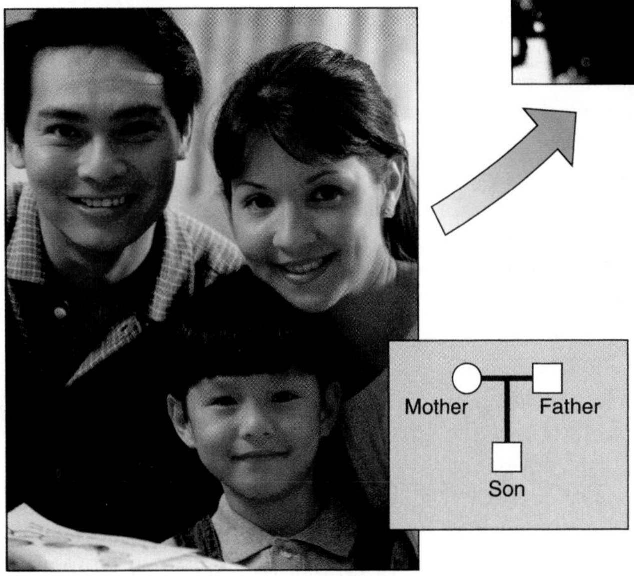
6. Family (pedigree)
Mother
Father
Son

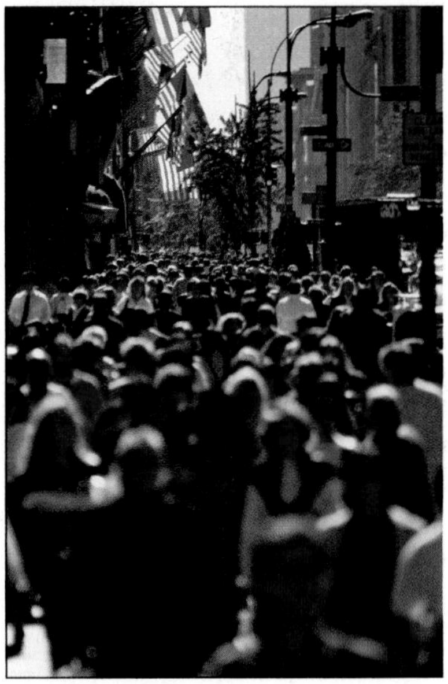

7. Population

it to other parts of the cell. In this way, the information encoded in DNA can be used to produce RNA molecules, which are then used to manufacture proteins. **Proteomics** is a new field that considers the proteins made in a particular cell type. DNA remains in the nucleus to be passed on when a cell divides.

Only about 1.5 percent of the DNA in the human genome encodes protein. The rest of the DNA includes many highly repeated sequences with unknown functions; sequences that activate or suppress protein-encoding genes; viral nucleic acid sequences that have inserted into the human genome; and other sequences whose origin and function are yet to be discovered. Only recently, for example, have researchers discovered that RNA actually controls itself. Small, double-stranded RNA molecules can bind to the single-stranded, protein-encoding messenger type of RNA, squelching a gene's activity. This process is called **RNA interference,** or RNAi, discussed in chapter 11. Its discovery not only helps to explain how genes are controlled, but illustrates how we are constantly learning about new aspects of gene function.

Genes, Chromosomes, and Genomes

Individual protein-encoding genes may differ from each other by small changes in the DNA base sequence. The variants of a gene are called **alleles,** and these changes in DNA sequence arise by a process called **mutation.** Some mutations cause disease; others provide variation, such as freckled skin; and some mutations may help. For example, one mutation makes a person's cells unable to manufacture a surface protein that binds HIV. These people are resistant to HIV infection. This genetic variant might have remained unknown had AIDS not arisen. Many mutations have no visible effect at all because they do not change the encoded protein in a way that affects its function, just as a minor spelling error does not obscure the meaning of a sentence.

Parts of the DNA sequence can vary among individuals, yet not change external appearance or health. A variant in sequence that is present in at least 1 percent of a population is called a **polymorphism.** A polymorphism can occur in a part of the DNA that encodes protein, or in a part that does not.

Polymorphism is also a general term that means "many forms." A polymorphism can be helpful, harmful, or, in most instances, have no obvious effect.

Researchers have identified millions of **single nucleotide polymorphisms** (SNPs, pronounced "snips"), which are single base sites that differ among individuals. The human genome may include up to 20 million SNPs, or 1 in every 1,250 or so DNA nucleotides, although they are not evenly distributed. DNA microarrays can include both disease-causing mutations and SNPs that merely mark places where people differ. Researchers conduct an association study to identify combinations of SNPs that are found almost exclusively among people with a particular disorder. In this way, SNP patterns detected with DNA microarrays are associated with disease risks.

Genes are part of larger structures called **chromosomes,** which also include proteins that the DNA wraps around. A human cell has 23 pairs of chromosomes. Twenty-two pairs are **autosomes,** or chromosomes that do not differ between the sexes. The autosomes are numbered from 1 to 22, with 1 the largest. The other two chromosomes, the X and the Y, are **sex chromosomes.** The Y chromosome bears genes that determine maleness. In humans, a female has two X chromosomes and a male has one X and one Y.

Charts called **karyotypes** order the chromosome pairs from largest to smallest. The chromosomes are stained with dyes or fluorescent chemicals bound to specific DNA sequences to create different patterns, which can reveal abnormalities.

The 23 chromosome pairs in a human cell hold two complete sets of genetic information. The human genome contains 24,000 or more protein-encoding genes, scattered among 3 billion DNA bases among each set of 23 chromosomes. Two entire genomes are tucked into each of a person's many cells. Geneticist Hermann J. Muller wrote in 1947, "In a sense we contain ourselves, wrapped up within ourselves, trillions of times repeated."

Cells, Tissues, and Organs

A human body consists of trillions of cells. All cells except red blood cells (which are actually fragments) contain all of the genetic instructions, but cells differ in appearance and function because they use only some of their genes, a process called **differentiation.** Specialized cells aggregate and interact to form tissues, which in turn form the organs and organ systems.

Organs include rare, less specialized cells, called **stem cells,** that can divide to yield another stem cell and a cell that goes on to differentiate. Thanks to stem cells, organs can grow and repair damage. When researchers better understand how stem cells function, these cells may be used to heal injuries or replace cells destroyed in degenerative disorders such as Parkinson disease and Alzheimer disease.

Individual

Two terms distinguish the alleles that are *present* in an individual from the alleles that are *expressed.* The **genotype** refers to the underlying instructions (alleles present), while the **phenotype** is the visible trait, biochemical change, or effect on health (alleles expressed). Alleles are further distinguished by how many copies it takes to affect the phenotype. A **dominant** allele produces an effect when present in just one copy (on one chromosome), whereas a **recessive** allele must be present on both chromosomes to be expressed. (Alleles on the Y chromosome are an exception; recessive alleles on the X chromosome in males are expressed because there is no second X chromosome to block expression.)

Family

Individuals are genetically connected into families. A person has half his or her genes in common with each parent and each sibling, and one-quarter with each grandparent. First cousins share one-eighth of their genes.

Traditionally, the study of traits in families has been called transmission genetics or Mendelian genetics, for Gregor Mendel, who pioneered the study of single genes using pea plants. Molecular genetics, which considers DNA, RNA, and proteins, often begins with transmission genetics, when an interesting trait or illness in a family comes to a researcher's attention. Charts called pedigrees represent the members of a family and indicate which individuals have particular inherited traits. Figure 1.3 includes a pedigree for a mother, father, and son.

Population

Above the family level of genetic organization is the population. In a strict biological sense, a population is a group of interbreeding individuals. In a genetic sense, a population is a large collection of alleles, distinguished by their frequencies. People from a Swedish population, for example, would have a greater frequency of alleles that specify light hair and skin than people from a population in Ethiopia who tend to have dark hair and skin. The fact that groups of people look different and may suffer from different health problems reflects the frequencies of their distinctive sets of alleles. All the alleles in a population constitute the **gene pool.** (An individual does not have a gene pool.)

Population genetics is very important in applications such as health care and forensics. It is also the very basis of evolution. In fact, evolution is technically defined as changing allele frequencies in populations. These small-scale genetic changes foster the more obvious species distinctions we most often associate with evolution.

Evolution

Comparing DNA sequences for individual genes, or the amino acid sequences of the proteins that the genes encode, can reveal how closely related different types of organisms are (**figure 1.4**). The underlying assumption is that the more similar the sequences are, the more recently two species diverged from a shared ancestor.

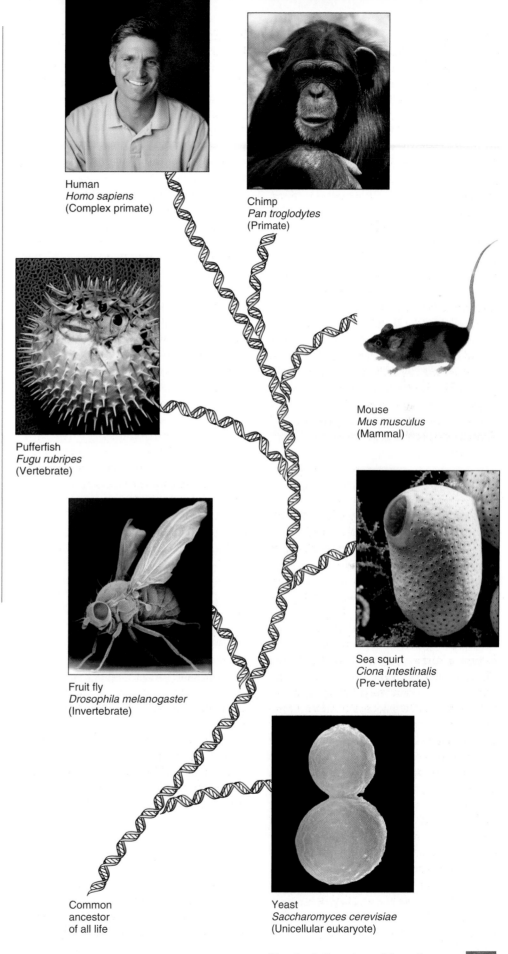

Figure 1.4 Genes and genomes reveal our place in the world. All life is related, and different species share a basic set of genes that makes life possible. The more closely related we are to another species, the more genes we have in common. This illustration depicts how humans are related to certain contemporaries who are also having their genomes sequenced—a process that will reveal just how closely related we are.

During evolution, species diverged from shared ancestors. For example, humans diverged more recently from chimps, our closest relative, than from mice, pufferfish, sea squirts, flies, or yeast. Said one researcher who works with the sea squirt, "These little sardinelike guys illuminate where we came from. They are our relatives, as icky as they might look." We even share genes with yeast, a single-celled fungus that nonetheless uses the same biochemical pathways that we do to acquire energy and carry out metabolism.

Human
Homo sapiens
(Complex primate)

Chimp
Pan troglodytes
(Primate)

Mouse
Mus musculus
(Mammal)

Pufferfish
Fugu rubripes
(Vertebrate)

Sea squirt
Ciona intestinalis
(Pre-vertebrate)

Fruit fly
Drosophila melanogaster
(Invertebrate)

Common
ancestor
of all life

Yeast
Saccharomyces cerevisiae
(Unicellular eukaryote)

Genome sequence comparisons reveal more about evolutionary relationships than comparing single genes. Humans, for example, share more than 98 percent of the DNA sequence with chimpanzees. Our genomes differ from theirs more in gene organization and in the number of copies of genes than in the overall sequence. Still, learning the functions of the human-specific genes may explain the differences between us and them. Genome comparisons can clarify our kinship with other species, too. Consider the aardvark, a mammal with a distinctive long snout, also known as the "earth pig." A study that compared specific genes on the chromosomes of various placental mammals found that humans differ the most from the aardvark. This suggests that the aardvark is the most primitive placental mammal (a mammal that nurtures its unborn young through a maternal organ called a placenta).

Humans also share many DNA sequences with mice, pufferfish, and fruit flies. At the level of genetic instructions for building a body, we are not very different from other organisms. We even share some genes necessary for life with single-celled organisms such as yeast.

Comparisons of person to person at the genome level reveal that we are incredibly like one another. Studies of polymorphisms among different modern ethnic groups reveal that modern humans arose in Africa and haven't changed very much since. The gene pools of all groups are subsets of the modern African gene pool. One study compared 377 highly variable genome regions among people in 52 populations from Africa, Eurasia, East Asia, Oceania, and the Americas. The study found 99.9 percent of the DNA examined identical in sequence.

Genome analyses also confirm that race, as defined by skin color, is a social concept, not a biological one. "Race" is actually defined by fewer than 0.01 percent of our genes. Put another way, two members of different races may have more alleles in common than two members of the same race. Very few, if any, gene variants are unique to any one racial or ethnic group. Imagine if we defined race by a different small set of genes, such as the ability to taste bitter substances!

Table 1.1 defines some of the terms used in this section, and is a summary of most of this book.

Key Concepts

Genetics can be considered at different levels: DNA, genes, chromosomes, genomes, individuals, families, and populations. • A gene can exist in more than one form, or allele. • Comparing genomes among species reveals evolutionary relatedness.

Table 1.1

A Mini-Glossary of Genetic Terms

Term	Definition
Allele	An alternate form of a gene; a gene variant.
Autosome	A chromosome not involved in determining sex.
Chromosome	A structure, consisting of DNA and protein, that carries the genes.
DNA	Deoxyribonucleic acid; the molecule whose building block sequence encodes the information that a cell uses to construct a particular protein.
Dominant	An allele that exerts a noticeable effect when present in just one copy.
Gene	A sequence of DNA that has a known function, such as encoding protein or controlling gene expression.
Gene expression	A cell's use of DNA information to manufacture specific proteins.
Gene pool	All of the genes in a population.
Genome	A complete set of genetic instructions in a cell, including DNA that encodes protein as well as other DNA.
Genomics	The new field of investigating how genes interact and comparing genomes.
Genotype	The allele combination in an individual.
Karyotype	A size-order display of chromosomes.
Mendelian trait	A trait that is completely determined by a single gene.
Multifactorial trait	A trait that is determined by one or more genes and by the environment. Also called a complex trait.
Mutation	A change in a gene that affects the individual's health, appearance, or biochemistry.
Pedigree	A diagram used to follow inheritance of a trait in a family.
Phenotype	The observable expression of an allele combination.
Polymorphism	A site in a genome that varies in 1 percent or more of a population.
Recessive	An allele that exerts a noticeable effect only when present in two copies.
RNA	Ribonucleic acid; the molecule that enables a cell to synthesize proteins using the information in DNA sequences.
Sex chromosome	A chromosome that carries genes whose presence or absence determines sex.

1.3 Genes Do Not Usually Function Alone

For much of its short history, the field of genetics dealt almost exclusively with the few thousand traits and illnesses that are clearly determined by single genes, also called **Mendelian traits.** A database called "Online Mendelian Inheritance in Man (OMIM)" lists and describes all known single-gene traits and disorders in humans. OMIM numbers are noted in the appendix for disorders that are mentioned in the text.

Genetics is much more complicated, however, than a one-gene-one-disease paradigm. Most genes do not function alone, but are influenced by the actions of other genes, and sometimes by factors in the environment as well. Traits that are determined by one or more genes and the environment are called **multifactorial,** or complex, traits (**figure 1.5**). (The term *complex traits* has different meanings in a scientific and a popular sense, so this book uses the more precise term *multifactorial*.)

Confusing matters further is the fact that some illnesses occur in different forms—some inherited, some not, some Mendelian, some multifactorial. Usually the inherited forms are rarer, as is the case for Alzheimer disease, breast cancer, and Parkinson disease.

Researchers can develop treatments based on the easier-to-study inherited form of an illness that physicians can then use to treat more common, multifactorial forms. For example, the drugs called statins that millions of people take to lower cholesterol were developed from work on the one-in-a-million children with familial hypercholesterolemia (see figure 5.2).

Knowing whether a trait or illness is Mendelian or multifactorial is important for predicting the risk of recurrence. The probability that a Mendelian trait will occur in another family member is simple to calculate using the laws that Mendel derived, discussed in chapter 4. In contrast, predicting the recurrence of a multifactorial trait is difficult because several contributing factors are in play. Inherited breast cancer illustrates how the fact that genes rarely act alone can complicate calculation of risk.

Mutations in a gene called *BRCA1* cause fewer than 5 percent of all cases of breast cancer. But studies of the disease incidence in different populations have yielded confusing results. In Jewish families of eastern European descent (Ashkenazim) with many members affected at a young age, inheriting the most common *BRCA1* mutation confers an 86 percent chance of developing the disease over a lifetime. But women from other ethnic groups who inherit this allele may have only a 45 percent chance of developing breast cancer. A possible explanation is that the second group has different alleles of other genes that interact with *BRCA1* than do the eastern European Jewish families.

Environmental factors may also affect the gene's expression. For example, exposure to pesticides that mimic the effects of estrogen may be an environmental contributor to breast cancer. It can be difficult to tease apart genetic and environmental contributions to disease. BRCA1 breast cancer, for example, is especially prevalent in Long Island, New York. This population includes both many Ashkenazim and many people exposed to pesticides.

Increasingly, predictions of inherited disease are considered in terms of "modified genetic risk," which takes into account single genes as well as environmental and family background information. A modified genetic risk is necessary to predict BRCA1 breast cancer occurrence in a family.

The fact that the environment modifies gene actions counters the concept of **genetic determinism,** or the idea that an inherited trait is unchangeable and its appearance inevitable. The idea that "we are our genes" can be very dangerous. In predictive testing for inherited disease, the potential for environmental effects requires that results be presented as risks rather than foregone conclusions. That is, a person might be told that she has a 45 percent chance of developing BRCA1 breast cancer, not, "You will get breast cancer." Conversely, a person can inherit the normal form of the *BRCA1* gene and still develop breast cancer from a different cause. One danger of do-it-yourself at-home testing for genetic disease is that a person may conclude that the detection of a mutation means unavoidable disease. Such test results only predict risk, and they must be considered with other factors.

Genetic determinism as part of social policy can be particularly harmful. In the past, for example, the assumption that one ethnic group is genetically less intelligent than another led to lowered expectations and fewer educational opportunities for those perceived as biologically inferior. Environment, in fact, has a huge impact on intellectual development. The bioethics essay in chapter 8 considers genetic determinism further.

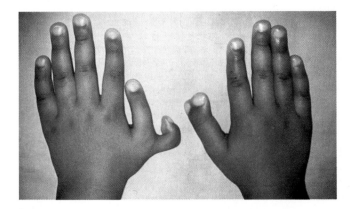

a.

Figure 1.5 Mendelian versus multifactorial traits.
(a) Polydactyly—extra fingers and/or toes—is a Mendelian trait, determined by a single gene. **(b)** Hair color is multifactorial, controlled by at least three genes plus environmental factors such as the bleaching effects of sun exposure.

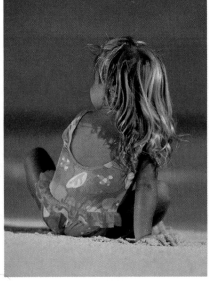

b.

Key Concepts

Inherited traits are determined by one gene (Mendelian) or by one or more genes and the environment (multifactorial). Even the expression of single genes is affected to some extent by the actions of other genes. Genetic determinism is the idea that an inherited trait cannot be modified.

1.4 Geneticists Use Statistics to Represent Risks

Predicting the inheritance of traits in individuals is not a precise science, largely because of the many influences on gene function and the uncertainties of analyzing multiple factors. Genetic counselors calculate risks for clients who want to know the chance that a new family member will inherit a particular disease—or has inherited it, but does not yet exhibit the symptoms.

In general, risk assessment estimates the degree to which a particular event or situation represents a danger to a population. In genetics, that event is the likelihood of inheriting a particular gene or gene combination. The genetic counselor can infer that information from a detailed family history, or from the results of tests that identify a gene variant or an absent or abnormal protein.

Risks can be expressed as absolute or relative figures. **Absolute risk** is the probability that an individual will develop a particular condition. **Relative risk** is the likelihood that an individual from a particular population will develop a condition in comparison to individuals from another group, usually the general population. Relative risk is expressed as a ratio of the probability in one group compared to another. In genetics, relative risks might be calculated by evaluating any situation that might elevate the risk of developing a particular condition, such as one's ethnic group, age, or exposure to a certain danger. The threatening situation is called a **risk factor.** For example, chromosome abnormalities are more common in the offspring of older mothers. Pregnant women who undergo testing for Down syndrome caused by an extra chromosome 21 are compared by age to the general population of pregnant women to derive the relative risk that they are carrying a fetus that has the syndrome. The risk factor is age.

Determining a relative risk may seem unnecessary, because an absolute risk applies to an individual. However, relative risks help health care providers identify patients most likely to have the conditions for which absolute risks can be calculated, and patients most likely to benefit from particular medical tests. A problem that genetic counselors face in assessing risk, however, is that statistics tend to lose their meaning in a one-on-one situation. To a couple learning that their fetus has Down syndrome, it is immaterial that the relative risk was low based on population statistics pertaining to their age group.

Mathematically, absolute and relative risk are represented in different ways. Odds and percentages are used to depict absolute risk. For example, Mackenzie's absolute risk of developing inherited Alzheimer disease over her lifetime is 4 in 100 (the odds), or 4 percent. Determining her relative risk requires knowing the risk to the general population. If that risk is 10 in 100, then Mackenzie's relative risk is 4 percent divided by 10 percent, or 0.4. A relative risk of less than 1 indicates the chance of developing a particular illness is less than that for the general population; a value greater than 1 indicates risk greater than that for the general population. Mackenzie's 0.4 relative risk means she has 40 percent as much risk of inheriting Alzheimer disease as the average person in the general population; a relative risk of 8.4, by contrast, would indicate a greater-than-8-fold risk compared to an individual in the general population.

Determining the risks for Alzheimer disease is actually more complicated than depicted in this hypothetical case. Several genes are involved, the percentage of inherited cases isn't known, and prevalence is highly associated with age. Elevated risk is linked to having more than one affected relative and to an early age of onset. But Alzheimer disease is a very common illness—about 40 percent of people over age 85 have the condition.

Risk estimates can change depending upon how groups being compared are defined. For a couple who has a child with an extra chromosome, such as a child with Down syndrome, the risk of recurrence is 1 in 100, a figure derived from looking at many families who have at least one such child. Therefore, the next time the couple has a child, two risk estimates are possible for Down syndrome—1 in 100, based on the fact that they already have an affected child, and the risk associated with the woman's age. The genetic counselor presents the highest risk, to describe a worst-case scenario. Consider a 23-year-old and a 42-year-old woman who have each had one child with the extra chromosome of Down syndrome. Each faces a recurrence risk of 1 in 100 based on medical history, but the two women have different age-associated risks—the 23-year-old's is 1 in 500, but the 42-year-old's is 1 in 63. The counselor provides the 1 in 100 figure to the younger woman, but the age-associated 1 in 63 figure to the older woman.

Geneticists derive risk figures in several ways. **Empiric risk** comes from population-level observations, such as the 1 in 100 risk of having a second child with an extra chromosome. Another type of risk estimate derives from Mendel's laws. A child whose parents are both carriers of sickle cell disease, for example, faces a 1 in 4, or 25 percent, chance of inheriting the disease. This child also has a 1 in 2, or 50 percent, chance of being a carrier, like the parents. The risk is the same for each offspring. It is a common error to conclude that if two carrier parents have a child with an inherited disorder, the next three children are guaranteed to be healthy. This isn't so, because each conception is an independent event.

Key Concepts

Risk is an estimate of the likelihood that a particular individual will develop a particular condition. Absolute risk is the probability that an individual will develop a certain condition. Relative risk is based on the person's population group compared to another population group.

1.5 Applications of Genetics

Barely a day goes by without some mention of genetics in the news. Genetics is impacting many areas of our lives, from health care choices, to what we eat and wear, to unraveling our pasts and controlling our futures.

Thinking about genetics evokes fear, hope, anger, and wonder, depending on context and circumstance. **Figure 1.6** shows an artistic view of genetics. Following are glimpses of applications of genetics that we will explore more fully in subsequent chapters.

Establishing Identity and Origins

Comparing DNA sequences to establish or rule out identity, relationships, or ancestry is becoming routine. This approach, called **DNA profiling,** has many applications.

Forensics

Before September 11, 2001, the media reported on DNA profiling only sporadically, usually in the wake of plane crashes where victims needed to be identified or in spectacular criminal cases. The terrorist attacks on the World Trade Center and the Pentagon made DNA profiling a daily task for many months, as investigators meticulously compared DNA sequences in bone and teeth collected from the scenes to hair and skin samples from hairbrushes, toothbrushes, and clothing of missing people, as well as to DNA samples from relatives.

A more conventional forensic application matches a rare DNA sequence in tissue left at a crime scene to that of a sample from a suspect. This is statistically strong evidence that the accused person was at the crime scene, or that someone cleverly planted evidence of his or her presence. Although DNA evidence is usually considered along with eyewitness testimony and other evidence, states that maintain DNA databases of convicted felons often get "cold hits"—when DNA at a crime scene matches a criminal's DNA in the database.

The United Kingdom, where DNA profiling was pioneered in the middle 1980s, has for years collected DNA from all convicts. In the United States, Virginia was the first state to establish such a database. Since 1989, law enforcement officials in Virginia have scored cold hits in hundreds of robberies, rapes, homicides, carjackings, woundings, and various other crimes. The database currently includes the DNA of more than 187,000 felons.

DNA profiling has been equally successful in overturning convictions. Illinois has led the way; there, in 1996, DNA tests exonerated the Ford Heights Four, men convicted of a gang rape and double murder who had spent eighteen years in prison, two of them on death row. In 1999, the men received compensation of $36 million for their wrongful conviction. A journalism class at Northwestern University initiated the investigation that gained the men their freedom. The case led to new state laws granting death row inmates new DNA tests if their convictions could have arisen from mistaken identity, or if DNA tests were performed when they were far less accurate. In 2003, Governor George Ryan was so disturbed by the number of overturned convictions based on DNA evidence that shortly before he left office, he commuted the sentences of everyone on death row to life imprisonment, much to the dismay of the families of murder victims.

Maintaining DNA databases on convicted felons is generally accepted because criminals give up certain civil rights. Establishing such databases on the general public is another story. Bioethics: Choices for the Future discusses some of the first general population databases.

Rewriting History

DNA can help to flesh out details of history, and sometimes springs surprises. Consider the offspring of Thomas Jefferson's slave, Sally Hemings (**figure 1.7**). Rumor at the

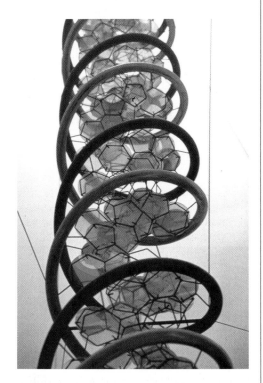

Figure 1.6 Genetic science inspires art. This sleek, symmetrical depiction of the double helix of DNA adorns the four-story spiral staircase in the Life Sciences building at the University of California in Davis.

Bread lists for 1815. 148

Monticello	farm	Tufton	Lego.
Betty Brown	Abram	Bagwell	Charles
Edwin	Doll	Minerva	Aggy
Robert	Shepherd	Willis	Polly
Mary.	Barnaby	Archy	James B.
Sally	Stannard	Jordan.	Rachael
Beverly	Bartlet.	Mary	Joe
Harriet	Davy senr.	Washington	Lania.
Madison	Isabel	John B.	Gloster
Eston.	Indridge	Virginia.	Washington
Billy B.	Thrimston	Robert	Edmund
Burwell	Lovilo.	Esther.	Eve.

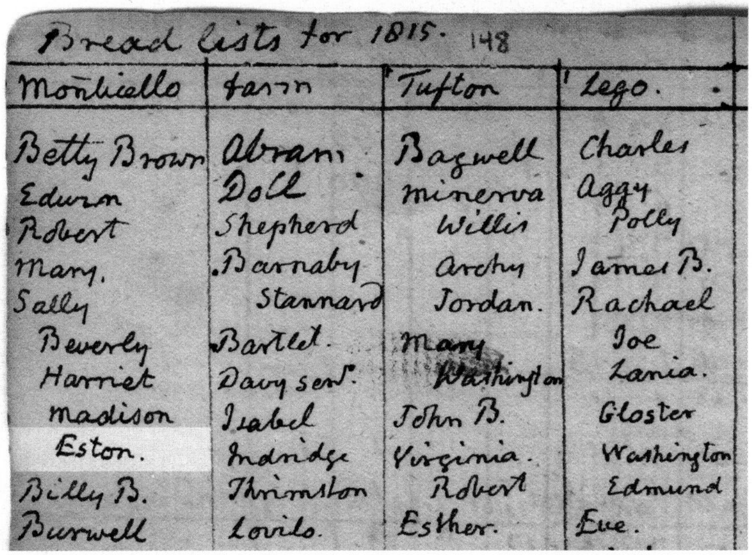

Figure 1.7 DNA clarifies history. Analysis of DNA sequences on the Y chromosomes of some of Thomas Jefferson's descendants indicate that either the president, his brother, or one of his nephews fathered Eston Hemings, a son of slave Sally Hemings.

Population Genetic Databases—Beyond Iceland

More than a dozen nations are recording genetic, genealogical, lifestyle, and health information on citizens to discover the inherited and environmental influences on common disorders. The plans vary in how people participate, but they raise similar concerns: Who will have access to the information? How can people benefit from providing it? How might it be abused?

The first country to make headlines for collecting genetic information on a population level was Iceland. In 1998, a company called deCODE Genetics received government permission to collect existing health and genealogy records and to add DNA sequence data. Many Icelandic families can trace their families back more than a thousand years and have family tree diagrams etched in blood on old leather. Participation in the database is presumed—citizens must file a special form to opt out of the project. DeCODE has used the information to identify genes that contribute to several common disorders (**table 1**). Their strategy groups people by clinical condition and identifies parts of the genome that they uniquely share, then finds genes in these regions whose functions could explain the symptoms.

The Estonian Genome Project uses registries for patients with cancers, Parkinson disease, diabetes mellitus, and osteoporosis. When patients show up for appointments, they learn about the project and are asked for details of their health histories and to donate DNA. Researchers then match variations in the DNA sequence to particular medical conditions.

Researchers in the United Kingdom are recruiting half a million individuals between the ages of 45 and 69, the age range when many common illnesses begin, to donate DNA to a "biobank." Investigators will search for connections among DNA sequence variants, health, and lifestyle characteristics as the population ages over the next three decades. Another effort, called GenomeEUtwin, has amassed data on more than 600,000 pairs of twins from eight European nations for decades. The Estonian, UK Biobank, GenomeEUtwin, and a Canadian project, called Cartagene, have joined to form the Public Population Project in Genomics. All are public. Like deCODE, the other population genetic databases share the goal of using genetic information to develop diagnostic tests and treatments. Bioethicists have suggested

Table 1

Disease-Related Genes Identified in Iceland

Alzheimer disease

Anxiety disorder

Hypertension

Myocardial infarction

Osteoarthritis

Osteoporosis

Schizophrenia

Stroke

Type II diabetes mellitus

strategies to ensure that individuals benefit from such projects, such as:

- Preserving choice in seeking genetic tests.

- Protecting privacy by legally restricting access to genome information.

- Tailoring genetic tests to genes that are most relevant to an individual.

- Refusing to screen for trivial traits in embryos or fetuses.

---

time placed Jefferson near Hemings nine months before each of her seven children was born, and the children themselves claimed to be presidential offspring. A Y chromosome analysis revealed that Thomas Jefferson could have fathered Heming's youngest son, Eston—but so could any of several other Jefferson family members. The Y chromosome, because it is present only in males, is faithfully passed from father to son. Researchers identified very unusual DNA sequences on the Y chromosomes of descendants of Thomas Jefferson's paternal uncle, Field Jefferson. These men were checked because the president's only son with wife Martha had died in infancy, making it impossible to check his direct descendants. The Jefferson family's unusual Y chromosome matched that

of descendants of Eston Hemings, supporting the talk of the time.

Tracing Origins

DNA profiling can provide details of times past. For example, bone cells from a child buried in a Roman cemetery in the year 450 A.D. had DNA sequences from the parasite that causes malaria. This genetic evidence is consistent with other signs of malaria, such as very porous bones and historical accounts of an epidemic contributing to the fall of the Roman Empire.

Reaching farther back, DNA profiling can clarify relationships from Biblical times. Consider a small group of Jewish people, the cohanim, who share distinctive Y chromosome DNA sequences. The

cohanim have a special status as priests in the religion. By considering the number of DNA differences between cohanim and other Jewish people, how long it takes DNA to mutate, and the average human generation time of 25 years, researchers extrapolated that the cohanim Y chromosome pattern originated 2,100 to 3,250 years ago—which includes the time when Moses lived. According to religious documents, Moses' brother Aaron was the first priest.

The Jewish priest DNA signature also appears today among the Lemba, a population of South Africans with black skin. Researchers thought to look at them for the telltale gene variants because their customs suggest a Jewish origin—they do not eat pork (or hippopotamus), they circumcise their newborn sons, and they celebrate a weekly day of rest. Today, the Lemba clearly practice Judaism (**figure 1.8**).

DNA profiling can also trace origins for organisms other than humans. For example, researchers analyzed DNA from the leaves of 300 varieties of wine grapes, in search of the two parental strains that gave rise to the sixteen major types of wine grapes existing today (**figure 1.9**). One parent was already known—the bluish-purple Pinot grape. But the second parent, revealed in the DNA, was a surprise—a variety of white grape called Gouais blanc that was so unpopular it hadn't been cultivated for years and was actually banned during the Middle Ages. Thanks to DNA analysis, vintners now know to maintain both parental stocks, to preserve the gene pool from which all wines descend.

Peeks at Evolution—Dog Origins

DNA evidence has refined our ideas of where and how domestic dogs originated. Instead of evolving from the gray wolf in North America some 15,000 years ago, as had been thought, dogs more likely descended from

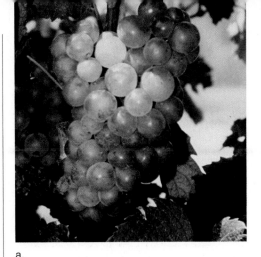
a.

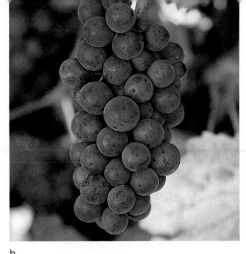
b.

Figure 1.9 Surprising wine origins. (a) Gouais blanc and (b) Pinot (noir) grapes gave rise to nineteen modern popular wines, including Chardonnay.

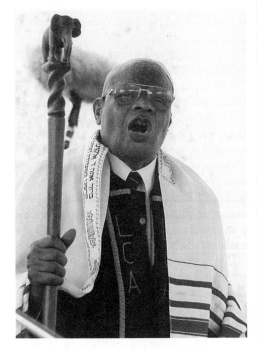

Figure 1.8 Y chromosome DNA sequences reveal origins.
The Lemba, a modern people with dark skin, have the same Y chromosome DNA sequences as the cohanim, a group of Jewish priests. The Lemba practiced Judaism long before DNA analysis became available.

wolves in China 25,000 or more years ago. Comparisons of DNA sequences among dogs from all over the globe and among their nearest relatives—wolves, jackals, and coyotes—point to one origin, followed by several separations into populations that led to the very diverse hundreds of modern breeds. The dogs of Eurasia have the most variable genomes—that is, the genomes of other dogs are subsets of the Eurasian canines—suggesting that the ancestral dogs were Eurasian, most likely from China. Archaeological evidence indicates that five basic types of dogs accompanied humans across the Bering Strait 15,000 to 10,000 years ago (see figure 15.14), and later, Europeans brought others—yet all ultimately came from China. Such breed names as the Mexican hairless, Alaskan husky, Chesapeake Bay retriever, and Newfoundland are not true to their genetic heritage (**figure 1.10**)!

Determining how dogs became our best friends requires some speculation and imagination, but genetics is involved here, too. A widely accepted scenario is that dogs gradually descended from wolves as they learned to live with people. One view envisions people befriending the more docile wolves, perhaps keeping them as pets or hunters. When these wolf-dogs bred, they passed on the genes that impart their gentleness, and over time, a new breed was selected. An alternate view is that the founding wolves separated themselves from their herds by being bold enough to forage around human settlements to find food. Experiments on dogs today indicate that they may possess certain

skills that enable them to uncannily interpret human communication cues. For example, monkeys are unable to identify under which of two objects a person has hidden food; dogs do it with ease, presumably watching the person for clues. The fact that dogs raised with people as well as those raised only with other dogs are equally good at following and remembering where the person put the food suggests that this skill is inborn—that is, inherited.

However and whenever the modern dog separated itself from its wolf brethren, humans then controlled their breeding to create such divergent-looking animals as the chihuahua and the St. Bernard. The dog genome sequence, published in draft form in 2003, will provide guidelines to identify the gene variant combinations that distinguish a poodle from a pug, a beagle from a boxer. Reading 14.2 explores the genetics of dogs and cats further.

Health Care

Inherited illness caused by a variant in a single gene differs from other types of illnesses in several ways (**table 1.2**). First, the recurrence risk of single-gene disorders can be predicted using the laws of inheritance chapter 4 describes. In contrast, an infectious disease requires that a pathogen be passed from one person to another—a much less predictable circumstance.

A second key distinction of inherited illness is that the risk of developing symptoms can be predicted. This is because all genes are present in all cells, even if they are not

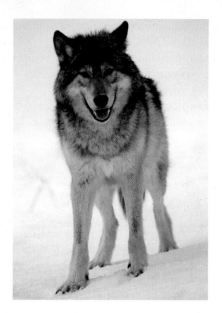

a.

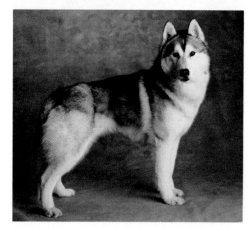

b.

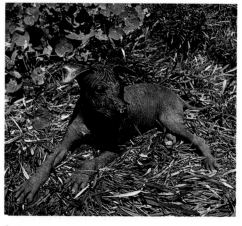

c.

Figure 1.10 Dog origins. It's easy to see that dogs descended from gray wolves **(a)** when we look at a Siberian husky **(b)**, but the relationship isn't as clear for many of the other 576 breeds, such as the Mexican hairless **(c)**. Despite their names, the Alaskan husky and the Mexican hairless trace their roots to Asia, not North America.

Table 1.2
How Genetic Diseases Differ from Other Diseases
1. One can predict recurrence risk in other family members.
2. Predictive testing is possible.
3. Different populations may have different characteristic frequencies.
4. Correction of the underlying genetic abnormality may be possible.

expressed in every cell. The use of genetic testing to foretell disease is termed predictive medicine. For example, some women who have lost several relatives at young ages to BRCA1 breast cancer and who know they have inherited the gene variant that causes the illness call themselves "previvors," in contrast to survivors. Some BRCA1 "previvors" have their breasts removed to prevent the cancer. A medical diagnosis, however, is still made based on existing symptoms. This is because some people who inherit gene variants associated with particular symptoms never develop them, because of interactions with other genes or environmental factors.

A third feature of genetic disease is that an inherited disorder may be much more common in some populations than others. Certain genes do not "like" or "dislike" certain types of people, but we tend to pick partners in nonrandom ways that can cause particular gene variants to cluster in certain groups. This phenomenon has economic consequences. While it might not be "politically correct" to offer a "Jewish genetic disease screen," as several companies do, it makes biological sense—a dozen disorders are much more common among Ashkenazim.

So far, tests are available to identify about 1,000 single-gene disorders, but each year, only about 250,000 people in the United States take these tests. Many people fear that employers or insurers will discriminate based on the results of genetic tests—or even on the simple action of taking the tests. Yet millions regularly have their cholesterol checked! However, studies from Canada on more than a decade of offering predictive genetic testing for Huntington disease indicate that fear of health insurance discrimination might not be a major factor in not taking a test—Canada has national health care. More older people took the test, to guide financial decisions and future plans, than did younger people to help make decisions about having children. Investigations in London showed that testing for cystic fibrosis did not significantly affect reproductive decisions either.

Despite the slow start to predictive genetic testing in some nations, in the U.S. legislation to prevent the misuse of genetic information in the insurance industry has been in development since 1993. The 1996 Health Insurance Portability and Accountability Act passed by the U.S. Congress stated that genetic information, without symptoms, does not constitute a preexisting condition, and individuals could not be excluded from group coverage on the basis of a detected genetic predisposition. But the law did not cover individual insurance polices, nor did it stop insurers from asking people to have genetic tests. In February 2000, U.S. President Bill Clinton issued an executive order prohibiting the federal government from obtaining genetic information for employees or job applicants and from using such information in promotion decisions. Since then, more than a dozen bills have been introduced in Congress to prevent genetic discrimination, and most states have enacted antidiscrimination legislation. Yet because the legislation is still in flux, and because the media reports anecdotal cases of health insurance denial or higher premiums following a genetic test, many people continue to fear the misuse of genetic information. For example, in Germany a young healthy woman was refused employment as a teacher because a relative has Huntington disease.

Balancing the perceived risks to privacy that genetic tests present are the possibilities that such tests can lower health care costs. If people know their inherited risks, they can take measures to forestall or ease symptoms that environmental factors might trigger—for example, by eating healthy foods, not smoking, exercising regularly, avoiding risky behaviors, having frequent medical exams, and beginning treatments earlier. Genetic tests can also enable people to make more informed reproductive decisions. People who know that they can transmit an inherited illness may elect not to have children, or to use one of the assisted reproductive technologies chapter 21 discusses.

A few genetic diseases can be treated. Supplying a missing protein can prevent some symptoms, such as providing a clotting factor to a person who has the bleeding disorder hemophilia. **Gene therapy,** in contrast, theoretically provides a more lasting cure by replacing the instructions for producing the protein. In Their Own Words on page 17 describes gene therapy to treat hemophilia. Unfortunately, the word *theoretically* in the last sentence is important, because gene therapy has been less successful than researchers hoped when the first experiments went well in 1990. In recent years, an 18-year-old died in a gene therapy experiment, and young children developed leukemia when the healing gene healed, but also inserted into a cancer-causing gene, as discussed in chapter 20. These and other gene therapies currently being developed alter cells that are affected in the particular illness. The changes cannot be passed to offspring, unless the healing gene enters sperm or eggs (which has happened). Gene therapy that intentionally alters sperm or eggs is more controversial and unlikely to be pursued.

Agriculture

The field of genetics arose from agriculture. Traditional agriculture is the controlled breeding of plants and animals to select individuals with certain combinations of useful inherited traits, such as seedless fruits or lean meat. **Biotechnology** is the use of organisms to produce goods (including foods and drugs) or services, and it is an ancient art as well as a modern science. One ancient example of biotechnology is using microorganisms to ferment fruits to manufacture alcoholic beverages, a technique the Babylonians used by 6000 B.C.

Traditional agriculture is imprecise, because it shuffles many genes—and, therefore, many traits—at a time. The application of DNA-based techniques, part of modern biotechnology, enables researchers to manipulate one gene at a time, adding control and precision to agriculture. Biotechnology that creates organisms that harbor new genes or that over- or underexpress their own genes is often popularly called "genetic engineering," but the resulting organisms are technically termed genetically modified (GM). More specifically, an organism with genes from another species is termed transgenic. Golden rice, for example, manufactures beta carotene (a vitamin A precursor) using "transgenes" from petunia and bacteria. It also stores twice as much iron as unaltered rice because one of its own genes is over-expressed (**figure 1.11**). These nutritional boosts bred into edible rice strains may help prevent vitamin A and iron deficiencies in people who eat them. Another genetically modified crop is *bt* corn, which contains a gene from the bacterium *Bacillus thuringiensis* that enables the plant to produce a protein that kills certain leaf-devouring insect larvae pests. Organic farmers have used the protein as a pesticide for decades, but *bt* corn can make its own. Growing the GM crop has greater yield using less synthetic pesticide than growing non-GM corn.

GM animals secrete into their milk "foreign" proteins, such as clotting factors, that serve as human pharmaceuticals. This provides a much purer and safer preparation than the pooled blood extracts that once transmitted infections. Plants can also be genetically modified to produce proteins that serve as drugs, called "pharm crops."

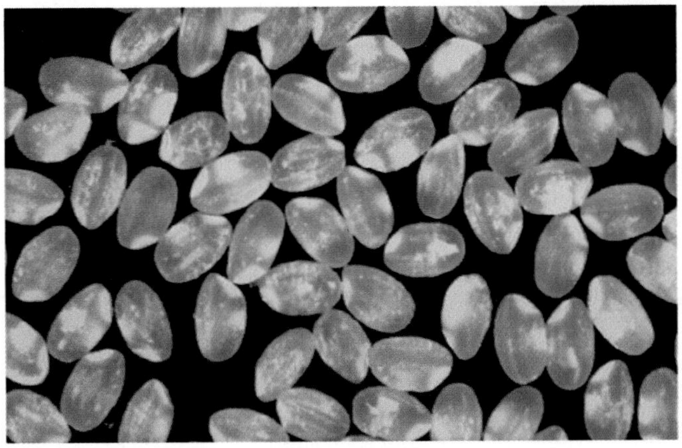

Figure 1.11 **Nutrient-boosted crops, courtesy of biotechnology.** Golden rice, a transgenic plant, will be made available to farmers everywhere. Its extra nutrients can help combat vitamin A and iron deficiencies.

An organism's own gene expression can be boosted too. GM cows given extra copies of their genes that encode the milk protein casein produce protein-rich milk that eases cheese manufacture.

People in the United States have been safely eating GM foods for a decade. But in Europe, many people object to GM foods, seemingly on ethical grounds or based on fear. Officials in France and Austria have called such crops "not natural," "corrupt," and "heretical." **Figure 1.12** shows an artist's rendition of some of these fears. Food labels in Europe indicate whether a product is "GM-free." Europe has a moratorium on approving GM foods, and if it is ever lifted, stricter labeling requirements will be imposed. Some objections to GM foods arise from lack of knowledge. A public opinion poll in the United Kingdom discovered, for example, that a major reason citizens avoid eating GM foods is that they do not want to eat DNA! One British geneticist wryly observed that the average meal provides about 150,000 kilometers (about 93,000 miles) of DNA. Ironically, British people ate GM foods for years before concern arose. For example, tomatoes with a gene added to delay ripening vastly outsold regular tomatoes in England, because they were cheaper.

Other concerns about GM organisms may be better founded. For example, labeling can prevent a person from having an allergic reaction to an ingredient in a food that wouldn't naturally be there, such as a peanut protein in corn. An ecological concern is that field tests may not adequately predict the effects of GM plants on ecosystems. GM crops have been found to grow in places beyond where they were planted, thanks to wind pollination. Corn genetically modified to produce a pig vaccine, for example, was found growing in a soybean field near the test plot in Nebraska. Some GM organisms, such as fish that grow to twice normal size or become able to survive at temperature extremes, may be so unusual that they disrupt ecosystems.

The success of genetically modified crops also depends upon where they are cultivated. Consider *bt* cotton, which, like *bt* corn, produces its own insecticide. In field tests on small farms in India, where pests are common and chemical pesticides are usually not used, GM cotton yields were nearly double those of unaltered cotton. The same GM cotton was less successful in China, the United States, and Europe, where most pests are killed with chemical pesticides. The GM cotton did not fare better in these regions because pests were already well-controlled. The experiment therefore suggests that this GM cotton might be valuable in southeast Asian and sub-Saharan Africa, where insect pests are prevalent. In other nations, using the GM cotton may lessen reliance on chemical pesticides.

Genetics from a Global Perspective

Because genetics so intimately affects us, it cannot be considered solely as a branch of life science. Equal access to testing, misuse of information, and abuse of genetics to intentionally cause harm are compelling issues that parallel scientific progress.

Genetics and genomics are rapidly spawning technologies that promise to vastly improve quality of life. But at least for the next few years, tests and treatments will be costly and not widely available to most people. While those in economically and politically stable nations may look forward to genome-based individualized health care, what some have called "Cadillac medicine," those in other nations just try to survive, often lacking basic vaccines and medicines. In an African nation where two out of five children suffer from AIDS and many die from other infectious diseases, newborn screening for rare single-gene defects hardly seems important. However, genetic disorders weaken people so that they become more susceptible to infectious diseases, which they can pass to others.

Human genome information can ultimately benefit everyone. Consider drug development. Today, there are fewer than 500 types of drugs. Genome information from humans and our pathogens and parasites is revealing new drug targets. **Table 1.3**

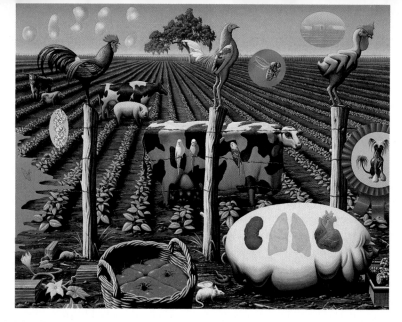

Figure 1.12　Biotechnology and art.　Artist Alexis Rockman vividly captures some fears of biotechnology, including a pig used to incubate spare parts for sick humans, a muscle-boosted, boxy cow, a featherless chicken with extra wings, a mini-warthog, and a mouse with a human ear growing out of its back.

Table 1.3

Pathogens with Sequenced Genomes

Pathogen	Human Disease
Bacterial	
Borrelia burgdorferi	Lyme disease
Brucella suis	Fever (infertility in other animals)
Campylobacter jejuni	Food poisoning
Clostridium perfringens	Food poisoning
Enterococcus faecalis	Urinary tract, wound, intestinal, and heart infections
Listeria monocytogenes	Lethal infection in newborns
Mycobacterium tuberculosis	Tuberculosis
Neisseria meningitides	Meningitis and septicemia (brain membrane inflammation and blood poisoning)
Streptococcus pyogenes	Puerperal fever, scarlet fever, pharyngitis, impetigo, cellulitis, "flesh-eating bacteria"
Treponema pallidum	Syphilis
Vibrio cholerae	Cholera
Yersinia pestis	Plague
Nonbacterial	
Brugia malayi (a worm)	Elephantiasis (grossly enlarged lymph nodes)
Entamoeba histolytica	Intestinal infection
Plasmodium falciparum	Malaria
Schistosoma mansoni	Schistosomiasis
Toxoplasma gondii	Birth defects, opportunistic infection in AIDS
Trypanosoma brucei	African sleeping sickness
Trypanosoma cruzi	Chagas disease

Living with Hemophilia

Don Miller was born in 1949 and is semi-retired from running the math library at the University of Pittsburgh. Today he has a sheep farm. On June 1, 1999, he was the first hemophilia patient to receive a disabled virus that delivered a functional gene for clotting factor VIII to his bloodstream. Within weeks he began to experience results. Miller is one of the first of a new breed of patient—people helped by gene therapy. Here he describes his life with hemophilia and his treatment. It worked—today his disease is under control.

The hemophilia was discovered when I was circumcised, and I almost bled to death, but the doctors weren't really sure until I was about 18 months old. No one where I was born was familiar with it.

When I was three, I fell out of my crib and I was black and blue from my waist to the top of my head. The only treatment then was whole blood replacement. So I learned not to play sports. A minor sprain would take a week or two to heal. One time I fell at my grandmother's house and had a 1-inch-long cut on the back of my leg. It took five weeks to stop bleeding, just leaking real slowly. I didn't need whole blood replacement, but if I moved a little the wrong way, it would open and bleed again.

I had transfusions as seldom as I could. The doctors always tried not to infuse me until it was necessary. Of course there was no AIDS then, but there were problems with transmitting hepatitis through blood transfusions, and other blood-borne diseases. All that whole blood can kill you from kidney failure. When I was nine or ten I went to the hospital for intestinal polyps. I was operated on and they told me I'd have a 10 percent chance of pulling through. I met other kids there with hemophilia who died from kidney failure due to the amount of fluid from all the transfusions. Once a year I went to the hospital for blood tests. Some years I went more often than that. Most of the time I would just lay there and bleed. My joints don't work from all the bleeding.

By the time I got married at age 20, treatment had progressed to gamma globulin from plasma. By then I was receiving gamma globulin from donated plasma and small volumes of cryoprecipitate, which is the factor VIII clotting protein that my body cannot produce pooled from many donors. We decided not to have children because that would end the hemophilia in the family.

I'm one of the oldest patients at the Pittsburgh Hemophilia Center. I was HIV negative, and over age 25, which is what they want. By that age a lot of people with hemophilia are HIV positive, because they lived through the time period when we had no choice but to use pooled cryoprecipitate. I took so little cryoprecipitate that I wasn't exposed to very much. And, I had the time. The gene therapy protocol involves showing up three times a week.

The treatment is three infusions, one a day for three days, on an outpatient basis. So far there have been no side effects. Once the gene therapy is perfected, it will be a three-day treatment. A dosage study will follow this one, which is just for safety. Animal studies showed it's best given over three days. I go in once a week to be sure there is no adverse reaction. They hope it will be a one-time treatment. The virus will lodge in the liver and keep replicating.

In the eight weeks before the infusion, I used eight doses of factor. In the fourteen weeks since then, I've used three. Incidents that used to require treatment no longer do. As long as I don't let myself feel stressed, I don't have spontaneous bleeding. I've had two nosebleeds that stopped within minutes without treatment, with only a trace of blood on the handkerchief, as opposed to hours of dripping.

I'm somewhat more active, but fifty years of wear and tear won't be healed by this gene therapy. Two of the treatments I required started from overdoing activity, so now I'm trying to find the middle ground.

Don Miller

lists some of the pathogens whose genomes have been sequenced and the illnesses they cause. Global organizations, including the United Nations, World Health Organization, and the World Bank, are discussing how nations can share new diagnostic tests and therapeutics that arise from genome information.

Key Concepts

Genetics has applications in diverse areas. Matching DNA sequences can clarify relationships, which is useful in forensics, establishing identity, and understanding certain historical events. • Inherited disease differs from other disorders in its predictability; the possibility of predictive testing; characteristic frequencies in different populations; and the potential of gene therapy to correct underlying abnormalities.
- Agriculture, both traditional and biotechnological, applies genetic principles.
- Human genome information has tremendous potential but must be carefully managed.

Summary

1.1 Genetic Testing

1. Genes are the instructions to manufacture proteins, which determine inherited traits.

2. A **genome** is a complete set of genetic information. A cell contains two genomes of DNA.

3. People can choose specific gene tests, based on family and health history, to detect or even predict risk of developing certain conditions. **DNA microarrays** detect many genes at once. Expression arrays indicate which proteins a cell makes.

1.2 The Breadth of Genetics

4. **Genes** are sequences of **DNA** that encode both the amino acid sequences of proteins and the RNA molecules that carry out protein synthesis. **RNA** carries the gene sequence information so that it can be utilized, while the DNA is transmitted when the cell divides. Much of the genome does not encode protein.

5. Variants of a gene arise by **mutation.** Variants of the same gene are **alleles.** They may differ slightly from one another, but they encode the same product. A **polymorphism** is a general term for a particular site or sequence of DNA that varies in one percent or more of a population. The **phenotype** is the gene's expression. An allele combination constitutes the **genotype.** Alleles may be **dominant** (exerting an effect in a single copy) or **recessive** (requiring two copies for expression).

6. **Chromosomes** consist of DNA and protein. The 22 types of **autosomes** do not include genes that specify sex. The X and Y **sex chromosomes** bear genes that determine sex.

7. The human genome contains about 3 billion DNA bases. Cells **differentiate** by expressing subsets of genes. **Stem cells** divide to yield other stem cells and cells that differentiate.

8. Pedigrees are diagrams used to study traits in families.

9. Genetic populations are defined by their collections of alleles, termed the **gene pool.**

10. Genome comparisons among species reveal evolutionary relationships.

1.3 Genes Do Not Usually Function Alone

11. Single genes determine **Mendelian traits.**

12. **Multifactorial traits** reflect the influence of one or more genes and the environment. Recurrence of a Mendelian trait is predicted based on Mendel's laws; predicting recurrence of a multifactorial trait is more difficult.

13. **Genetic determinism** is the idea that expression of an inherited trait cannot be changed.

1.4 Geneticists Use Statistics to Represent Risks

14. Risk assessment estimates the probability of inheriting a particular gene. **Absolute risk,** expressed as odds or a percentage, is the probability that an individual will develop a particular trait or illness over his or her lifetime.

15. **Relative risk** is a ratio that estimates how likely a person is to develop a particular phenotype compared to another group, usually the general population.

16. Risk estimates are **empiric,** based on Mendel's laws, or modified to account for environmental influences.

1.5 Applications of Genetics

17. **DNA profiling** can establish identity, relationships, and origins.

18. In inherited diseases, recurrence risks are predictable and a causative mutation may be detected before symptoms arise. Some inherited disorders are more common among certain population groups. **Gene therapy** attempts to correct certain genetic disorders.

19. Genetic information can be misused, especially by employers and insurers.

20. Agriculture is selective breeding. **Biotechnology** is the use of organisms or their parts for human purposes. A **transgenic** organism harbors a gene or genes from a different species.

Review Questions

1. Place the following terms in size order, from largest to smallest, based on the structures or concepts they represent:
   a. chromosome
   b. gene pool
   c. gene
   d. DNA
   e. genome

2. Distinguish between:
   a. an autosome and a sex chromosome
   b. genotype and phenotype
   c. DNA and RNA
   d. recessive and dominant traits
   e. absolute and relative risks
   f. pedigrees and karyotypes
   g. gene and genome

3. List four ways that inherited disease differs from other types of illnesses.

4. Cystic fibrosis is a Mendelian trait; height is a multifactorial trait. How do the causes of these characteristics differ?

5. Mutants are often depicted in the media as being abnormal, ugly, or evil. Why is this not necessarily true?

6. Health insurance forms typically ask for applicants to list existing or preexisting symptoms. How do the results of a genetic test differ from this?

Applied Questions

1. Breast cancer caused by the *BRCA1* gene affects 1 in 800 women in the general U.S. population. Among Jewish people of eastern European descent, it affects 2 in 100. What is the relative risk for this form of breast cancer among eastern European Jewish women in the United States?

2. In a search for a bone marrow transplant donor, why would a patient's siblings be considered before first cousins?

3. Keeping DNA databases of convicted felons has led to the solution of many crimes, and the exonerations of many innocent people. What might be the benefits and dangers of establishing databases on everyone? How should such a program be instituted?

4. How is *genetic engineering* a vague term, while *transgenic organism* is more precise?

5. Researchers have always published genome sequences, including those of organisms and viruses that cause disease (pathogens). Such freely available data are essential to scientific research, as they provide researchers with information that could be used to develop treatments. Since the terrorist attacks of September 11, 2001, however, some editors of scientific journals have considered restricting the publication of the genome sequences of pathogens for fear that terrorists would use the information to create "weaponized" versions—bacteria or viruses that spread more easily or cause more severe symptoms, for example. Do you think publication of genome sequences should be restricted? Cite a reason for your answer.

Web Activities

6. Many artists have been inspired by aspects of genetics, from the elegance of nucleic acid molecules to common fears of genetic technologies. Look at the following websites, select a work of art, and describe what it represents.

   http://www.dna50.org/main.htm

   http://gnn.tigr.org/articles/art_gallery.shtml

7. Genetics inspires cartoonists, too. Look at http://cartoonbank.com, and search under "DNA." Select a cartoon that misrepresents genetics, and explain how it is inaccurate, misleading, or sensationalized.

8. The website from GeneLink Inc. (http://www.bankdna.com/dnabanking.asp) announces "the world's first family-centered DNA bank and hereditary genetic information services." A client sends a sample of his or her DNA, obtained with a cheekbrush, to the company, which then examines certain genes. Explore the website, and discuss the pros and cons of using this type of service to learn about your DNA.

Case Studies

9. Morris has a DNA microarray test for several genes that predispose to developing prostate cancer. He learns that his overall relative risk is 1.5, compared to the risk in the general population. Overjoyed, he tells his wife that his risk of developing prostate cancer is only 1.5 percent. She says no, his risk is 50 percent greater than that of the average individual in the general population. Who is correct?

10. Benjamin undergoes a genetic screening test and receives the following relative risks:

– addictive behaviors	0.6
– coronary artery disease	2.3
– kidney cancer	1.4
– lung cancer	5.8
– diabetes	0.3
– depression	1.2

    Which conditions is he more likely to develop than someone in the general population, and which conditions is he less likely to develop?

11. The Larsons have a child who has inherited cystic fibrosis. Their physician tells them that if they have other children, each faces a 1 in 4 chance of also inheriting the illness. The Larsons tell their friends, the Espositos, of their visit with the doctor. Mr. and Mrs. Esposito are expecting a child, so they ask their physician to predict whether he or she will one day develop multiple sclerosis—Mr. Esposito is just beginning to show symptoms. They are surprised to learn that, unlike the situation for cystic fibrosis, recurrence risk for multiple sclerosis cannot be easily predicted. Why not?

12. Burlington Northern Santa Fe Railroad asked its workers for a blood sample, and then supposedly tested for a gene variant that predisposes a person for carpal tunnel syndrome, a disorder of the wrists caused by repetitive motions. The company threatened to fire a worker who refused to be tested; the worker sued the company. The Equal Employment Opportunity Commission ruled in the worker's favor, agreeing that the company's action violated the Americans with Disabilities Act.

    a. Do you agree with the company or the worker? What additional information would be helpful in taking sides?

    b. How is the company's genetic testing not based on sound science?

    c. How can tests such as those described for the two students at the beginning of this chapter be instituted in a way that does not violate a person's right to privacy, as the worker in the railroad case contended?

Learn to apply the skills of a genetic counselor with additional cases found in the *Case Workbook in Human Genetics.*

Genetics in the news

Suggested Readings

Burgermeister, Jane. October 11, 2003. Teacher was refused job because relatives have Huntington's disease. *The British Medical Journal* 327:827. Genetic discrimination is more likely in some nations than others.

Duncan, David Ewing. November 2002. 100% genetically analyzed. *Wired.* A journalist learns his possible genetic future—a bit melodramatic, but a fairly accurate look at where health care is headed.

Gavaghans, Helen. November 11, 2002. UK Biobank to go on the political agenda. *The Scientist* 16(22):24–25. As the British population ages, disease-causing genes will be identified.

Kirkness, Ewen, et al. September 26, 2003. The dog genome: Survey sequencing and comparative analysis. *Science* 301:1898–1903. Dogs have counterparts to 360 human diseases.

Kristof, Nicholas D. February 11, 2003. Staying alive, staying human. *The New York Times,* p. F1. Another reporter has his genome scanned.

Lee, Henry C. and Frank Tirnady. 2003. *Blood Evidence.* Cambridge, Mass.: Perseus Publishing. How DNA is revolutionizing forensics.

Lewis, Ricki. October 20, 2003. A genetic check-up: Lessons from Huntington disease and cystic fibrosis. *The Scientist* 17(20):24–26. Testing for common disorders is more complex than testing for single gene disorders.

Lewis, Ricki. February 12, 2002. Race and the clinic: Good science or political correctness? *The Scientist* 16(4):14. Race may not be a biological concept, but differences in gene frequencies among people of different skin colors may be clinically significant.

Lewis, Ricki. September 3, 2001. Where the bugs are: Forensic entomology. *The Scientist* 15(17):10. DNA profiling of insects provides helpful clues to solving crimes.

Lewis, Ricki. July 24, 2000. Keeping up: Genetics to genomics in four editions. *The Scientist* 14:46. A look at the evolution of this textbook.

Paabo, Svante. February 16, 2001. The human genome and our view of ourselves. *Science* 291:1219. Knowing the sequence of the human genome provides new ways of looking at ourselves.

Savolainen, Peter et al. November 22, 2002. Genetic evidence for an East Asian origin of domestic dogs. *Science* 298:1610–13. All dogs may descend from Chinese wolves.

Singer, Peter A. and Abdallah S. Daar. October 5, 2001. Harnessing genomics and biotechnology to improve global health equity. *Science* 294:87–89. The New African Initiative is an effort to ensure that all cultures have access to biotechnology.

Vastag, Brian. January 8, 2003. Gene chips inch toward the clinic. *The Journal of the American Medical Association* 289(2):155–56. Applications of DNA microarray technology are now regular reading in medical journals.

Ye, Xudong, et al. January 14, 2000. Engineering the provitamin A (beta carotene) biosynthetic pathway into (carotenoid-free) rice endosperm. *Science* 287:303–5. "Golden rice" may prevent human malnutrition.

Cells

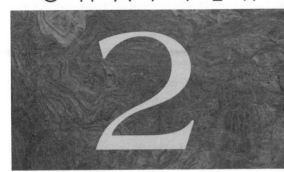

CHAPTER CONTENTS

2.1 The Components of Cells

Inherited characteristics can ultimately be explained at the cellular level. DNA in the genetic headquarters, the nucleus, coordinates the functions of organelles, the plasma membrane, and the cytoskeleton.

2.2 Cell Division and Death

As a human grows, develops, and heals, cells form and die. Both cell division and cell death are highly regulated, stepwise events under genetic control.

2.3 Cell-Cell Interactions

Cells must communicate with each other. They do so by receiving and responding to signals, and by physical contact. Signal transduction and cellular adhesion are genetically controlled processes.

2.4 Stem Cells and Cell Specialization

Stem cells and progenitor cells enable organs to grow and heal. Stem cell biology suggests many medical applications.

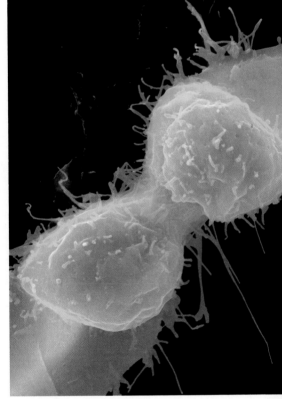

Cell division: one becomes two.

The activities and abnormalities of cells underlie inherited traits, quirks, and illnesses. The muscles of a boy with muscular dystrophy weaken because they lack a protein that normally supports the cells' shape during forceful contractions. A child with cystic fibrosis chokes on sticky mucus because the cells lining her respiratory tract produce a misshaped protein that in its normal form would prevent too much water from leaving the secretions. The red blood cells of a person with sickle cell disease contain an abnormal form of hemoglobin that aggregates into a gel-like mass when the oxygen level is low. The mass bends the red cells into sickle shapes, and they wedge within the tiniest vessels, painfully cutting off the blood supply to vital organs (**figure 2.1**).

Understanding what goes wrong in certain cells when a disease occurs suggests ways to treat the condition—we learn what must be repaired or replaced. Understanding cell function also reveals how a healthy body works, and how it develops from one cell to trillions. Our bodies include many variations on the cellular theme, with such specialized cell types as bone and blood, nerve and muscle, and even variations of those. Equally important are unspecialized cells that are nestled into organs. These **stem cells,** able to replicate themselves as well as to generate specialized cells, enable a body to develop, grow, and repair damage.

Cells interact. They send, receive, and respond to information. Some aggregate with others of like function, forming tissues, which in turn interact to form organs and organ systems. Other cells move about the body. Cell numbers are important, too—they are critical to development, growth, and healing. These processes reflect a precise balance between cell division and cell death.

2.1 The Components of Cells

All cells share certain features that enable them to perform the basic life functions of reproduction, growth, response to stimuli, and energy use. Body cells also have specialized features, such as the contractile proteins in a muscle cell, and the hemoglobin that fills red blood cells. The more than 260 specialized or differentiated cell types in a human body arise because the cells express different subsets of genes.

Figure 2.1 illustrates three cell types in humans, and figure 2.23 shows some others. The human body's cells fall into four broad categories: epithelium (lining cells), muscle, nerve, and connective tissues (including blood, bone, cartilage, and adipose cells).

Other multicellular organisms, including other animals, fungi, and plants, also have differentiated cells. Some single-celled

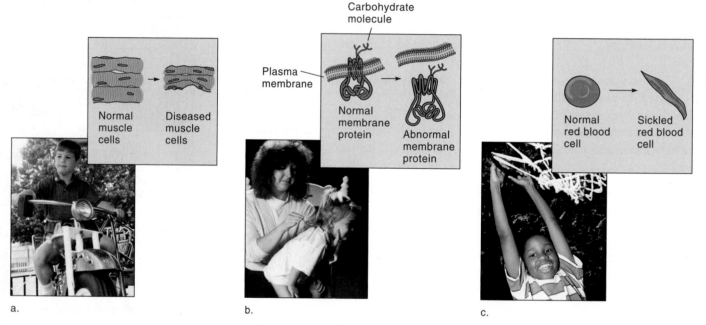

a. b. c.

Figure 2.1 Genetic disease at the whole-person and cellular levels. **(a)** This young man has Duchenne muscular dystrophy. The condition has not yet severely limited his activities, but he shows an early sign of the illness—overdeveloped calf muscles that result from his inability to rise from a sitting position the usual way. Lack of the protein dystrophin causes his skeletal muscle cells to collapse when they contract. **(b)** A parent gives this child "postural drainage" therapy twice a day to shake free the sticky mucus that clogs her lungs due to cystic fibrosis. The cells lining her respiratory passages lack a plasma membrane protein that controls the entry and exit of salts and water. **(c)** Seye Arise was born with sickle cell disease, enduring the pain of blocked circulation and even several strokes. At age four, he received a bone marrow transplant from his brother Moyo. Today he is fine! The new bone marrow produced red blood cells with a healthy doughnut shape—not the sickle shape his genes dictated.

organisms, such as the familiar paramecium and ameba, have very distinctive cells as complex as our own. Most of the planet, however, is populated by simpler single-celled organisms that are nonetheless successful life forms, because they occupied earth long before we did and are still abundant today.

Biologists recognize three broad varieties of cells that define three major "domains" of life: the Archaea, the Bacteria, and the Eukarya. A domain is a broader classification than the familiar kingdom.

The archaea and bacteria are both single-celled, but they differ in the sequences of many of their genetic molecules and in the types of molecules in their membranes. Archaea and bacteria are both **prokaryotes,** because they lack a **nucleus,** the structure that contains the genetic material in the cells of other types of organisms.

The third domain of life, the Eukarya or **eukaryotes,** includes single-celled organisms that have nuclei, as well as all multicellular organisms such as ourselves. Eukaryotic cells are also distinguished from prokaryotic cells by structures called **organelles,** which perform specific functions. The cells of all three domains contain globular structures of RNA and protein called **ribosomes.** Ribosomes provide structural support for protein synthesis.

Chemical Constituents of Cells

Cells are composed of molecules. Some of the chemicals of life (biochemicals) are so large that they are called macromolecules.

The major macromolecules that make up and fuel cells are **carbohydrates** (sugars and starches), **lipids** (fats and oils), **proteins,** and **nucleic acids.** Cells require vitamins and minerals in much smaller amounts, but they are also essential to health.

Carbohydrates provide energy and contribute to cell structure. Lipids form the basis of several types of hormones, provide insulation, and store energy. Proteins have many diverse functions in the human body. They participate in blood clotting, nerve transmission, and muscle contraction and form the bulk of the body's connective tissue. **Enzymes** are proteins that are especially important because they facilitate, or catalyze, biochemical reactions so that they occur swiftly enough to sustain life.

Most important to the study of genetics are the nucleic acids deoxyribonucleic acid (DNA) and ribonucleic acid (RNA). DNA and RNA form a living language that translates information from past generations into specific collections of proteins that give a cell its individual characteristics. Recall that the set of proteins that a cell can manufacture is called its proteome.

Macromolecules often combine to form larger structures within cells. For example, the membranes that surround cells and compartmentalize their interiors consist of double layers (bilayers) of lipids embedded with carbohydrates, proteins, and other lipids.

Life is based on the chemical principles that govern all matter; genetics is based on a highly organized subset of the chemical reactions of life. Reading 2.1 describes some drastic effects that result from major biochemical abnormalities.

Organelles

A eukaryotic cell holds a thousand times the volume of a bacterial or archaeal cell (**figure 2.2**). In order to carry out the activities of life in such a large cell, organelles divide the labor, partitioning off certain areas or serving a specific function. Saclike organelles sequester biochemicals that might harm other cellular constituents. Some organelles consist of membranes studded with enzymes arranged in the order in which they participate in the chemical reactions that produce a particular molecule. In general, organelles keep related biochemicals and structures close enough to one another to interact efficiently. This eliminates the need to maintain a high concentration of a particular biochemical throughout the cell.

Organelles enable a cell to retain as well as use its genetic instructions; acquire energy; secrete substances; and dismantle debris. The coordinated functioning of the organelles in a eukaryotic cell is much like the organization of departments in a department store (**figure 2.3**).

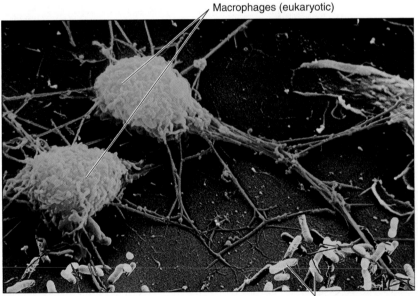

Macrophages (eukaryotic)

Bacteria (prokaryotic)

Figure 2.2 Eukaryotic and prokaryotic cells. A human cell is eukaryotic and much more complex than a bacterial cell, while an archaean cell looks much like a bacterial cell. Here, human macrophages (blue) capture bacteria (yellow). Note how much larger the human cells are.

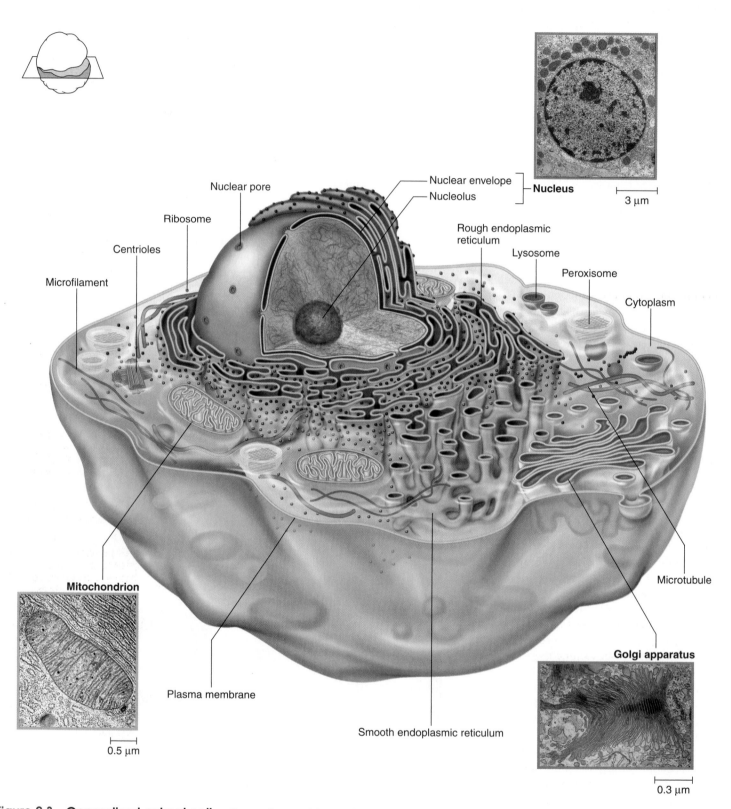

Nuclear pore

Ribosome

Centrioles

Microfilament

Nuclear envelope

Nucleolus

Nucleus

3 µm

Rough endoplasmic
reticulum

Lysosome

Peroxisome

Cytoplasm

Microtubule

Mitochondrion

0.5 µm

Plasma membrane

Smooth endoplasmic reticulum

Golgi apparatus

0.3 µm

Figure 2.3   Generalized animal cell.   Organelles provide specialized functions for the cell. Most of these structures are transparent; colors are used to distinguish them.

The most prominent organelle, the nucleus, is enclosed in a layer called the nuclear envelope. Nuclear pores are rings of proteins that allow certain biochemicals to exit or enter the nucleus (**figure 2.4**). Within the nucleus, an area that appears darkened under a microscope, the nucleolus ("little nucleus"), is the site of ribosome production. The nucleus is filled with DNA complexed with many proteins to form chromosomes. Other proteins form fibers that give the nucleus a roughly spherical shape. RNA is abundant too, as are enzymes and protein factors required to synthesize RNA from DNA. The material in the nucleus, minus these contents, is called nucleoplasm.

The remainder of the cell—that is, everything but the nucleus, organelles, and the outer boundary, or **plasma membrane**—is the **cytoplasm.** Other cellular components include stored proteins, carbohydrates, and lipids; pigment molecules; and various other small chemicals.

Secretion—The Eukaryotic Production Line

Organelles interact to coordinate basic life functions and sculpt the characteristics of specialized cell types. The activities of several types of organelles may be coordinated to perform a complex function such as secretion.

Secretion begins when the body sends a biochemical message to a cell to begin producing a particular substance. For example, an infant suckling a mother's breast causes her brain to release hormones that signal cells in her breast to begin producing the complex mixture that makes up milk (**figure 2.5**). In response, information in certain genes is copied into molecules of **messenger RNA** (mRNA), which then exit the nucleus (see step 2 in figure 2.5). In the cytoplasm, the messenger RNAs, with the help of ribosomes and another type of RNA called **transfer RNA,** direct the manufacture of milk proteins.

Most protein synthesis occurs on a maze of interconnected membranous tubules and sacs called the **endoplasmic reticulum** (ER). The ER winds from the nuclear envelope outwards to the plasma membrane. The portion of the ER nearest the nucleus, which is flattened and studded with ribosomes, is called the rough ER

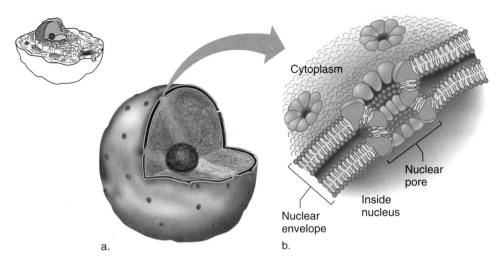

Cytoplasm

Nuclear pore

Inside nucleus

Nuclear envelope

a.   b.

Figure 2.4   The nucleus.   (a) The largest structure within a typical human cell, the nucleus lies within two membrane layers that make up the nuclear envelope **(b).** Pores through the envelope allow specific molecules to move in and out of the nucleus.

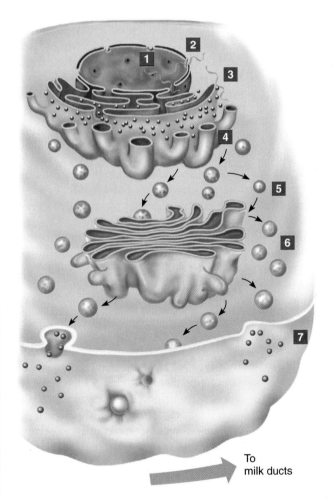

To milk ducts

1 Milk protein genes are transcribed into mRNA.

2 mRNA exits through nuclear pores.

3 mRNA forms complex with ribosomes and moves to surface of rough ER, where proteins are made.

4 Enzymes in smooth ER manufacture lipids.

5 Milk proteins and lipids are packaged into vesicles from both rough and smooth ER for transport to Golgi.

6 Final processing of proteins, addition of sugars, and packaging for export out of cell occurs in Golgi.

7 Proteins and lipids are released from cell by fusion of vesicles with plasma membrane.

**Figure 2.5   Secretion.   Milk production and secretion illustrate organelle functions and interactions in a cell from a mammary gland: (1) through (7) indicate the order in which organelles participate in this process. Lipids are secreted in separate droplets from proteins and their attached sugars.

Inborn Errors of Metabolism Affect the Major Biomolecules

Enzymes are proteins that catalyze (speed or facilitate) specific chemical reactions. Therefore, enzymes control a cell's production of all types of macromolecules. When the gene that encodes an enzyme mutates so that the enzyme is not made or cannot function, the result can be too much or too little of the product of the specific biochemical reaction that the enzyme catalyzes. Genetic disorders that result from deficient or absent enzymes are called inborn errors of metabolism. Figures 20.1, 20.2, and 20.3 show how three inborn errors result from a buildup of the biochemical whose synthesis is controlled by a particular enzyme. The In Their Own Words essay in chapter 5 shows another example, alkaptonuria. Following are descriptions of inherited conditions that reflect an imbalance or abnormality in particular molecules.

Carbohydrates

The newborn yelled and pulled up her chubby legs in pain a few hours after each feeding. She developed a watery diarrhea, even though she was breastfed, and breast milk is supposed to be the "perfect" food. Finally, a doctor identified *lactase deficiency*—the baby lacked the enzyme lactase, which enables the digestive system to break down milk sugar, which is the carbohydrate lactose. Bacteria multiplied in the undigested lactose in the child's intestines, producing gas, cramps, and bloating. Switching to a soybean-based, lactose-free infant formula helped. A different disorder with similar (although milder) symptoms is lactose intolerance, common in adults.

Lipids

A sudden sharp pain began in the man's arm and spread to his chest—the first sign of a heart attack. At age 36, he was younger than most people who suffer heart attacks, but he had inherited a gene that halved the number of protein receptors for cholesterol on his liver cells. Because cholesterol could not enter the liver cells efficiently, it built up in his arteries, constricting blood flow in his heart and eventually causing a mild heart attack. A fatty diet had accelerated his *familial hypercholesterolemia,* an inherited form of heart disease.

Proteins

The first sign that the infant was ill was also the most innocuous—his urine smelled like maple syrup. Tim slept most of the time, and he vomited so often that he hardly grew. A blood test revealed that Tim had inherited *maple syrup urine disease.* He could not digest three types of amino acids (protein building blocks), so these amino acids accumulated in his bloodstream. A diet very low in these amino acids has helped Tim, but this treatment is new and his future uncertain.

Nucleic Acids

From birth, Michael's wet diapers contained orange, sandlike particles, but otherwise he seemed healthy. By six months of age, though, he was obviously in pain when urinating. A physician also noted that Michael's writhing movements were involuntary rather than normal attempts to crawl.

The orange particles in Michael's diaper indicated *Lesch-Nyhan syndrome,* caused by deficiency of an enzyme called HGPRT. The near absence of the enzyme blocked Michael's body from recycling two of the four types of DNA building blocks, instead converting them into uric acid, which crystallizes in urine. Other symptoms that would appear later were not as easy to explain—severe mental retardation, seizures, and aggressive and self-destructive behavior. By age three or so, Michael would respond to stress by uncontrollably biting his fingers, lips, and shoulders. He would probably die before the age of 30 of kidney failure or infection.

Vitamins

Vitamins enable the body to use the carbohydrates, lipids, and proteins we eat. Julie inherited *biotinidase deficiency,* which greatly slows the rate at which her body can use the vitamin biotin. If Julie hadn't been diagnosed as a newborn and quickly started on biotin supplements, by early childhood she would have shown biotin deficiency symptoms: mental retardation, seizures, skin rash, and loss of hearing, vision, and hair. Her slow growth, caused by her body's inability to extract energy from nutrients, would have eventually proved lethal.

Minerals

Ingrid is in her thirties, but she lives in the geriatric ward of a state mental hospital, unable to talk or walk. Although her grin and drooling make her appear mentally deficient, Ingrid is alert and communicates using a computer. When she was a healthy high-school senior, symptoms of *Wilson disease* began to appear, as her weakened liver could no longer control the excess copper her digestive tract absorbed from food. The initial symptoms were stomachaches, headaches, and an inflamed liver (hepatitis). Then very odd changes began—slurred speech; loss of balance; a gravelly, low-pitched voice; and altered handwriting. Ingrid received many incorrect diagnoses before a psychiatrist noted the telltale greenish rings around her irises, caused by copper buildup, and diagnosed Wilson disease. Only then did Ingrid receive penicillamine, which enabled her to excrete the excess copper in her urine, which turned the color of bright new pennies. Although Ingrid's symptoms did not improve, the treatment halted the course of the illness, saving her life.

because it appears fuzzy when viewed under an electron microscope due to the ribosomes. Messenger RNA attaches to the ribosomes on the rough ER. Amino acids from the cytoplasm are then linked, following the instructions in the mRNA's sequence, to form particular proteins that will either exit the cell or become part of membranes (step 3, figure 2.5). Proteins are also synthesized on ribosomes not associated with the ER. These proteins remain in the cytoplasm.

The ER acts as a quality control center for the cell. Its chemical environment enables the protein that the cell is manufacturing to start folding into the three-dimensional shape necessary for its specific function. Misfolded proteins are pulled out of the ER and degraded, much as an obviously defective toy might be pulled from an assembly line at a toy factory and discarded. Misfolded proteins that are not destroyed can cause disease, as discussed further in chapter 10.

As the rough ER winds out toward the plasma membrane, the ribosomes become fewer, and the diameters of the tubules widen, forming a section called the smooth ER. Here, lipids are made and added to the proteins arriving from the rough ER (step 4, figure 2.5). The lipids and proteins travel until the tubules of the smooth ER eventually narrow and end. Then the proteins exit in membrane-bounded, saclike organelles called **vesicles** that pinch off from the tubular endings of the membrane (step 5, figure 2.5). Lipids—a major component of human milk—exit the plasma membrane directly, taking bits of it with them.

A loaded vesicle takes its contents to the next stop in the secretory production line, the **Golgi apparatus.** This processing center is a stack of flat, membrane-enclosed sacs. Here, sugars are synthesized and linked to form starches, or they attach to proteins to form **glycoproteins** or to lipids to form **glycolipids.** Proteins finish folding in the Golgi apparatus (step 6, figure 2.5). The components of complex secretions, such as milk, are temporarily stored here. Droplets then bud off the Golgi apparatus in vesicles that move outward to the plasma membrane, fleetingly becoming part of the membrane until they are secreted to the cell's exterior (step 7, figure 2.5).

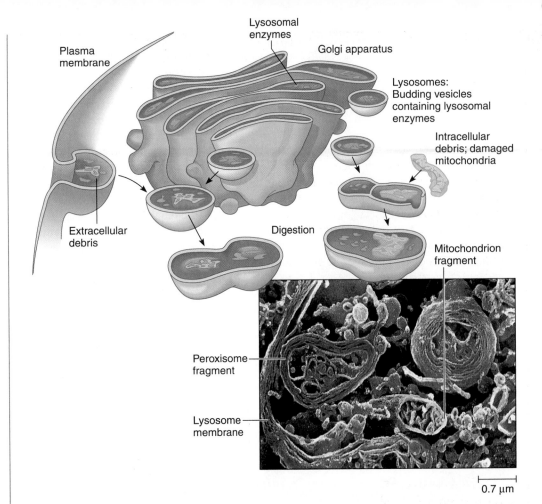

Figure 2.6 Lysosomes. Lysosomes fuse with vesicles or damaged organelles, activating the enzymes within to recycle the molecules for the cell's use. Lysosomal enzymes also dismantle bacterial remnants. These enzymes require a very acidic environment to function.

Intracellular Digestion— Lysosomes and Peroxisomes

Eukaryotic cells break down molecules and other structures as well as produce them. Organelles called **lysosomes** are membrane-bounded sacs that contain enzymes that dismantle captured bacterial remnants, worn-out organelles, and other debris (**figure 2.6**). Lysosomal enzymes also break down some digested nutrients into forms that the cell can use. Lysosomes fuse with vesicles carrying debris from outside or within the cell, and the lysosomal enzymes then degrade the contents. A lysosome loaded with such "garbage" moves toward the plasma membrane and fuses with it, dumping its contents to the outside. The word *lysosome* means "body that lyses;" *lyse* means "to cut." Lysosomes maintain the very acidic environment that their enzymes require to function, without harming other cellular constituents.

Cells differ in the number of lysosomes they contain. Certain white blood cells and macrophages (see figure 2.2) are the body's scavengers, moving about and engulfing bacteria. They are loaded with lysosomes. Liver cells require many lysosomes to break down cholesterol and toxins.

All lysosomes contain more than 40 types of digestive enzymes, which must maintain a correct balance. Absence or malfunction of an enzyme causes a lysosomal storage disease. In these inherited disorders, the molecule that the missing or abnormal enzyme normally degrades accumulates. The lysosome swells, crowding organelles and interfering with the cell's functions. In Tay-Sachs disease, for example, an enzyme that normally breaks down lipid in the cells that surround nerve cells is deficient, burying the nervous system in lipid. An affected infant begins to lose skills at about six months of age, then gradually loses sight, hearing, and

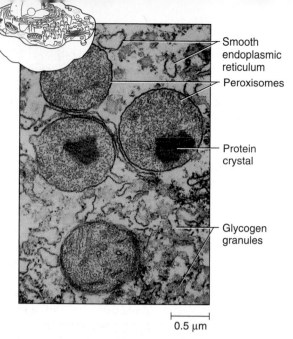

Smooth
endoplasmic
reticulum

Peroxisomes

Protein
crystal

Glycogen
granules

|— 0.5 µm —|

Figure 2.7 Peroxisomes. The high concentration of enzymes within a peroxisome results in the crystallization of the proteins, giving peroxisomes a characteristic appearance. Peroxisomes are abundant in liver cells, where they assist in detoxification.

Cristae

Outer
membrane

Inner
membrane

|— 0.5 µm —|

Figure 2.8 A mitochondrion. Cristae, infoldings of the inner membrane, increase the available surface area containing enzymes for energy reactions in a mitochondrion.

the ability to move, typically dying within three years. Even before birth, the lysosomes of affected cells swell.

Peroxisomes are sacs with outer membranes that are studded with several types of enzymes. These enzymes perform a variety of functions, including breaking down certain lipids and rare biochemicals, synthesizing bile acids used in fat digestion, and detoxifying compounds that result from exposure to damaging oxygen free radicals. Peroxisomes are large and abundant in liver and kidney cells (**figure 2.7**).

The 1992 film *Lorenzo's Oil* recounted the true story of a child with an inborn error of metabolism caused by an absent peroxisomal enzyme. Six-year-old Lorenzo Odone had adrenoleukodystrophy (ALD). His peroxisomes lacked a normally abundant protein that transports an enzyme into peroxisomes, where the enzyme catalyzes a reaction that helps break down a certain type of lipid called a very-long-chain fatty acid. Without the enzyme transporter protein, the cells of the brain and spinal cord accumulate the fatty acid. Early symptoms include low blood sugar, skin darkening, muscle weakness, and heartbeat irregularities. The patient eventually loses control over the limbs and usually dies within a few years. Ingesting a type of lipid in rapeseed (canola) oil—the oil in the film's title—slows buildup of the very-long-chain fatty acids in blood plasma and the liver. But the rapeseed lipid cannot enter the brain, where it is required to combat the symptoms.

Energy Production—Mitochondria

The activities of secretion, as well as the many chemical reactions taking place in the cytoplasm, require enormous and continual energy. Organelles called **mitochondria** provide energy by breaking down the products of digestion (nutrients).

A mitochondrion has an outer membrane similar to those in the ER and Golgi apparatus and an inner membrane that is folded into structures called cristae (**figure 2.8**). These folds hold enzymes that catalyze the

biochemical reactions that release energy from the chemical bonds of nutrient molecules. The bonds that hold together a molecule called adenosine triphosphate (ATP) store this energy. ATP, therefore, serves as a cellular energy currency.

The number of mitochondria in a cell varies from a few hundred to tens of thousands, depending upon the cell's activity level. A typical liver cell, for example, has about 1,700 mitochondria, but a muscle cell, with its very high energy requirements, has many more.

Mitochondria are especially interesting because, like the nucleus, they contain DNA, although a very small amount. Another unusual characteristic of mitochondria is that they are almost always inherited from the mother only, because mitochondria are in the middle regions of sperm cells but usually not in the head regions that enter eggs. Moreover, mitochondria that do enter with a sperm are usually destroyed in the very early embryo. A class of inherited diseases whose symptoms result from abnormal mitochondria are always passed from mother to offspring. These illnesses usually produce extreme muscle weakness, because muscle activity requires so many mitochondria. Chapter 5 discusses mitochondrial inheritance. Evolutionary biologists study mitochondrial genes to trace the beginnings of humankind, as discussed in chapter 15.

Table 2.1 summarizes the structures and functions of organelles.

The Plasma Membrane

Just as the character of a community is molded by the people who enter and leave it, the special characteristics of different cell types are shaped in part by the substances that enter and leave. The plasma membrane controls this process. It forms a selective barrier that completely surrounds the cell and monitors the movements of molecules in and out of the cell. How the chemicals that comprise the plasma membrane associate with each other determines which substances can enter or leave the cell. Similar membranes form the outer boundaries of several organelles, and some organelles consist entirely of membranes. A cell's membranes are more than mere coverings. Some of their constituent or associated molecules carry out specific functions.

Table 2.1

Structures and Functions of Organelles

Organelle	Structure	Function
Endoplasmic reticulum	Membrane network; rough ER has ribosomes, smooth ER does not	Site of protein synthesis and folding; lipid synthesis
Golgi apparatus	Stacks of membrane-enclosed sacs	Site where sugars are made and linked into starches or joined to lipids or proteins; proteins finish folding; secretions stored
Lysosome	Sac containing digestive enzymes	Degrades debris, recycles cell contents
Mitochondrion	Two membranes; inner membrane enzyme-studded	Releases energy from nutrients, participates in cell death
Nucleus	Porous sac containing DNA	Separates DNA from rest of cell
Peroxisome	Sac containing enzymes	Catalyzes several reactions
Ribosome	Two associated globular subunits of RNA and protein	Scaffold and catalyst for protein synthesis
Vesicle	Membrane-bounded sac	Temporarily stores or transports substances

A biological membrane is built of a double layer (bilayer) of molecules called **phospholipids (figure 2.9).** A phospholipid is a fat molecule with attached phosphate groups. A phosphate group (PO_4) is a phosphorus atom bonded to four oxygen atoms. The ability of phospholipid molecules to organize themselves into sheetlike structures makes membrane formation possible. Phospholipids do this because their ends have opposite reactions to water. The phosphate end of a phospholipid is attracted to water, and thus is hydrophilic (water-loving); the other end, which consists of two chains of fatty acids, moves away from water, and is therefore hydrophobic (water-fearing). Because of these water preferences, phospholipid molecules in water spontaneously arrange into bilayers, with the hydrophilic surfaces exposed to the watery exterior and interior of the cell, and the hydrophobic surfaces facing each other on the inside of the bilayer, away from the water.

The phospholipid bilayer forms the structural backbone of a biological membrane. Embedded in the bilayer are proteins, some traversing the entire bilayer, others poking out from either or both faces. Other molecules can attach to these membrane proteins, forming **glycoproteins** and **glycolipids.** (Other types of lipids include cholesterol and triglycerides.) The proteins, glycoproteins, and glycolipids that jut from a plasma membrane create the surface topographies that are so important in a cell's interactions with other cells. The surfaces of your unique cells indicate that they are part of your body, and also that they have differentiated in a particular way.

Many molecules that extend from the plasma membrane function as **receptors,** structures that have indentations or other shapes that fit and hold molecules outside the cell. The molecule that binds to the receptor, called the **ligand,** sets into motion a cascade of chemical reactions that carries out a particular cellular activity. This process of communication from outside to inside the cell is termed **signal transduction.** Other membrane proteins enable a cell to stick to other cells in a process called **cellular adhesion.** Signal transduction and cellular adhesion are discussed in greater detail in section 2.3.

The phospholipid bilayer is oily, and many of the proteins move within it like ships on a sea. Some proteins with related functions cluster on "lipid rafts" that float on the phospholipid bilayer. The rafts are rich in cholesterol and other types of lipids. This clustering of proteins eases their interaction. The proteins aboard the lipid rafts contribute to the cell's identity; act as transport shuttles into the cell; serve as gatekeepers; and can let in certain toxins and pathogens. HIV, for example, enters a cell by breaking a lipid raft. The inner hydrophobic region of the phospholipid bilayer blocks entry and exit to most substances that dissolve in water. However, certain molecules can cross the membrane through proteins that form passageways, or when they are escorted by a "carrier" protein. Some membrane proteins form channels for ions, which are atoms or molecules that bear an electrical charge. Reading 2.2 describes how faulty ion channels can cause disease.

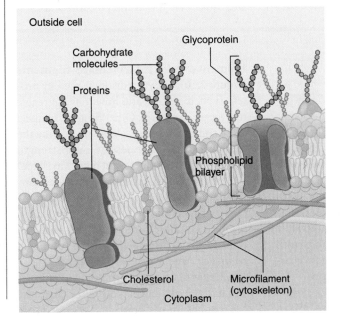

Outside cell

Carbohydrate molecules

Glycoprotein

Proteins

Phospholipid bilayer

Cholesterol

Microfilament (cytoskeleton)

Cytoplasm

Figure 2.9 Anatomy of a plasma membrane.
In a plasma membrane, mobile proteins are embedded throughout a phospholipid bilayer, producing a somewhat fluid structure. Other types of lipids aggregate to form "rafts," and an underlying mesh of protein fibers supports the plasma membrane. Jutting from the membrane's outer face are carbohydrate molecules linked to proteins (glycoproteins) and lipids (glycolipids).

Inherited Diseases Caused by Faulty Ion Channels

What do collapsing horses, irregular heartbeats in teenagers, and cystic fibrosis have in common? All result from abnormal ion channels in plasma membranes.

Ion channels are protein-lined tunnels in the phospholipid bilayer of a biological membrane. These passageways permit electrical signals in the form of ions (charged particles) to pass through membranes.

Ion channels are specific for calcium (Ca^{+2}), sodium (Na^+), potassium (K^+), or chloride (Cl^-). A plasma membrane may have a few thousand ion channels specific for each of these ions. Ten million ions can pass through an ion channel in one second! The following disorders result from abnormal ion channels.

Hyperkalemic Periodic Paralysis and Sodium Channels

The quarterhorse was originally bred in the 1600s to run the quarter mile, but one of the four very fast stallions used to establish much of today's population of 3 million animals inherited *hyperkalemic periodic paralysis* (HPP). The horse, otherwise a champion, collapsed from sudden attacks of weakness and paralysis.

HPP results from abnormal sodium channels in the plasma membranes of muscle cells. But the trigger for the temporary paralysis is another ion: potassium. A rising blood potassium level, which may follow intense exercise, slightly alters the electrical charge in the plasma membranes of muscle cells. Normally, this slight change would have no effect, but in horses with HPP, sodium channels open too widely, allowing too much sodium into muscle cells. The cells cannot respond to nervous stimulation for awhile, and the racehorse falls.

People can inherit HPP, too. In one family, several members collapsed suddenly after eating bananas! These fruits are very high in potassium, which caused the symptoms.

Long-QT Syndrome and Potassium Channels

Four children in a Norwegian family were born deaf, and three of them died at ages four, five, and nine. All of the children had inherited from unaffected carrier parents *long-QT syndrome associated with deafness.* ("QT" refers to part of a normal heart rhythm.) These children had abnormal potassium channels in the cells of the heart muscle and in the inner ear. In the heart cells, the malfunctioning ion channels disrupted electrical activity, causing a fatal disturbance to the heart rhythm. In the cells of the inner ear, the abnormal ion channels increased the extracellular concentration of potassium ions, impairing hearing. Some cases of long-QT syndrome are caused not by faulty ion channels, but by the proteins, called ankyrins, that hold the channels in place within the plasma membrane.

Cystic Fibrosis and Chloride Channels

A seventeenth century English saying, "A child that is salty to taste will die shortly after birth," described the consequence of abnormal chloride channels in CF. The chloride channel is called CFTR, for cystic fibrosis transductance regulator. In most cases of CF, CFTR protein remains in the cytoplasm, unable to reach the plasma membrane, where it would normally function (see figure 2.1*b*). CF is inherited from carrier parents. The major symptoms of difficulty breathing, frequent severe respiratory infections, and a clogged pancreas that disrupts digestion all result from buildup of extremely thick mucous secretions.

Abnormal chloride channels in cells lining the lung passageways and ducts of the pancreas cause the symptoms of CF. The primary defect in the chloride channels also causes sodium channels to malfunction. The result: salt trapped inside cells draws moisture in and thickens surrounding mucus.

The Cytoskeleton

The **cytoskeleton** is a meshwork of tiny protein rods and tubules that molds the distinctive structures of a cell, positioning organelles and providing three-dimensional shape. The proteins of the cytoskeleton are broken down and built up as a cell performs specific activities. Some cytoskeletal elements function as rails, forming conduits that transport cellular contents; other parts of the cytoskeleton, called motor molecules, power the movement of organelles along these rails by converting chemical energy to mechanical energy.

The cytoskeleton includes three major types of elements—**microtubules, micro**filaments, and **intermediate filaments** (**figure 2.10**). They are distinguished by protein type, diameter, and how they aggregate into larger structures. Other proteins connect these components to each other, creating the meshwork that provides the cell's strength and ability to resist force and maintain shape.

Long, hollow microtubules provide many cellular movements. A microtubule is composed of pairs (dimers) of a protein, called tubulin, assembled into a hollow tube. The cell can change the length of the tubule by adding or removing tubulin molecules.

Cells contain both formed microtubules and individual tubulin molecules. When the cell requires microtubules to carry out a specific function—in cell division, for example—the free tubulin dimers self-assemble into more tubules. After the cell divides, some of the microtubules fall apart into individual tubulin dimers. This replenishes the cell's supply of building blocks. Cells are in a perpetual state of flux, building up and breaking down microtubules. Some drugs used to treat cancer affect the microtubules that pull a cell's duplicated chromosomes apart, either by preventing tubulin from assembling into microtubules, or by preventing microtubules from breaking down into free tubulin dimers. In each case, cell division stops.

Microtubules also form moving structures called cilia, which sometimes enable cells to move. Cilia are hairlike structures that move in a coordinated fashion, producing a wavelike motion. An individual cilium is constructed of nine microtubule pairs that surround a central, separated pair. A type of motor protein called dynein connects the outer microtubule pairs and also links them to the central pair. Dynein supplies the energy to slide adjacent microtubules against each other, bending the cilium. Coordinated movement of cilia generates a wave that moves the cell or propels substances along its surface. Cilia beat particles up and out of respiratory tubules, and move egg cells in the female reproductive tract. Reading 2.3 describes a condition caused by abnormal dynein that alters the positions of certain organs in the body.

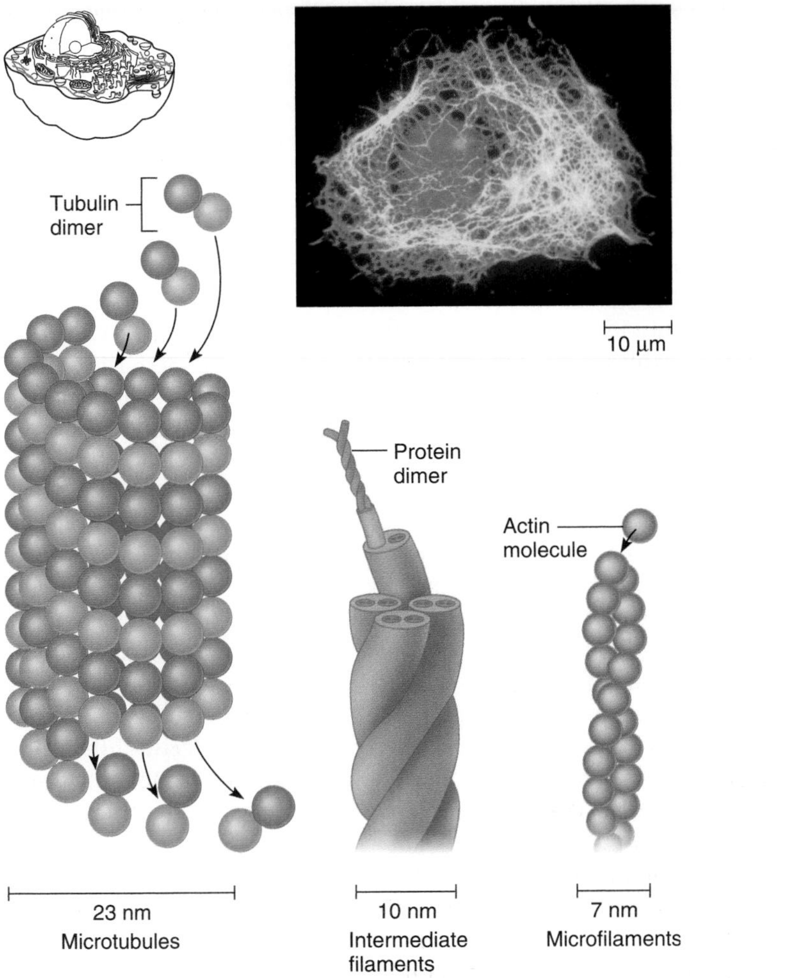

Another component of the cytoskeleton, the microfilament, is a long, thin rod composed of the protein actin. In contrast to microtubules, microfilaments are solid, not hollow, and are narrower. Microfilaments provide strength for cells to survive stretching and compressive forces. They also help to anchor one cell to another and provide many other functions within the cell through proteins that interact with actin. When any of these proteins is absent or abnormal, a genetic disease results.

Intermediate filaments are so named because their diameters are intermediate between those of the other cytoskeletal elements. Unlike microtubules and microfilaments, which consist of a single protein type, intermediate filaments are made of different proteins in different specialized cell types. However, all intermediate filaments share a common overall organization of dimers entwined into nested coiled rods. Intermediate filaments are scarce in many cell types, but are very abundant in cells of the skin.

The intermediate filaments in actively dividing skin cells in the bottommost layer of the epidermis (the upper skin layer) form a strong inner framework that firmly attaches the cells to each other and to the underlying tissue. These cellular attachments are crucial to the skin's barrier function. In a group of inherited conditions called epidermolysis bullosa, intermediate filaments are abnormal. The skin blisters easily as tissue layers separate (**figure 2.11**).

Tubulin dimer

10 µm

Protein dimer

Actin molecule

23 nm
Microtubules

10 nm
Intermediate filaments

7 nm
Microfilaments

Figure 2.10 **The cytoskeleton is made of protein rods and tubules.** The three major components of the cytoskeleton are microtubules, intermediate filaments, and microfilaments. Through special staining, the cytoskeleton in this cell glows yellow under the microscope. (The abbreviation nm stands for nanometer, which is a billionth of a meter.)

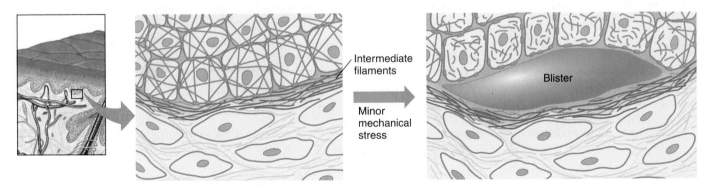

Intermediate filaments

Minor mechanical stress

Blister

Figure 2.11 **Intermediate filaments in skin.** Keratin intermediate filaments internally support cells in the basal (bottom) layer of the epidermis. Abnormal intermediate filaments in the skin cause epidermolysis bullosa, a disease characterized by skin that easily blisters.

A Heart in the Wrong Place

In the original *Star Trek* television series, Dr. McCoy often complained when examining Mr. Spock that Vulcan organs weren't where they were supposed to be, based on human anatomy. The good doctor would have had a hard time examining humans with a condition called *situs inversus,* in which certain normally asymmetrically located organs develop on the wrong side of the body.

In a normal human body, certain organs lie either on the right or the left of the body's midline. The heart, stomach, and spleen are on the left, and the liver is on the right. The right lung has three sections, or lobes; the left lung has two. Other organs twist and turn in either a right or left direction. All these organs originate in the center of an initially symmetrical embryo, and then the embryo turns, and the organs migrate to their final locations.

Misplaced body parts are a symptom of *Kartagener syndrome,* in which the heart, spleen, or stomach may be on the right, both lungs may have the same number of lobes, the small intestine may twist the wrong way, or the liver may span the center of the body (**figure 1**). Many people with this syndrome die in childhood from heart abnormalities. Kartagener syndrome was first described in 1936 by a Swiss internist caring for a family with several members who had strange symptoms—chronic cough, sinus pain, poor sense of smell, male infertility, and misplaced organs—usually a heart on the right.

Many years later, researchers identified another anomaly in patients with Kartagener syndrome, which explained how the heart winds up on the wrong side of the chest. All affected individuals lack dynein, the protein that enables microtubules to slide past one another and generate motion. Without dynein, cilia cannot wave. In the respiratory tract, immobile cilia allow debris and mucus to accumulate, causing the cough, clogged sinuses, and poor sense of smell. Lack of dynein also paralyzes sperm tails, producing male infertility. But how could dynein deficiency explain a heart that develops on the right instead of the left?

One hypothesis is based on the fact that dynein helps establish the spindle, the structure that determines the orientation of dividing cells in the embryo with respect to each other. The dynein defect may, early on, set cells on a developmental pathway that diverts normal migration of the heart from the embryo's midline to the left.

Another explanation for how organs end up in the wrong locations comes from mice genetically altered to lack a gene whose protein product is required for assembling cilia. About 50 percent of the mice have reversed organs. All of the animals either lack cilia that are normally present on cells of the early embryo, called node cells, or their cilia cannot move. Node cells are the sites where the first differences between right and left arise, and they set the pattern for organ placement. Normally, the cilia rotate counterclockwise, which moves fluids to the left. This movement creates a gradient (changing concentration across an area) of molecules, called morphogens, that control development. The differing concentrations of specific morphogens in different parts of the body may send signals that guide the development of organs. Without cilia that can move, organs wind up on the left or the right at random. This is why only 50 percent of the genetically altered mice, and presumably not all people who inherit Kartagener syndrome, have organs in the wrong place. Just by chance, some of them develop normally.

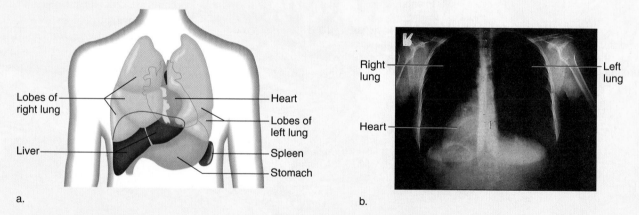

Lobes of right lung
Liver
Heart
Lobes of left lung
Spleen
Stomach
a.

Right lung
Left lung
Heart
b.

Figure 1   Situs inversus.   The drawing on the left **(a)** shows the normal position of the heart, lungs, liver, spleen, and stomach. In situs inversus, certain organs form on the wrong side of the body **(b).** Note the location of the heart.

Disruption in the structures of cytoskeletal proteins, or in how they interact, can be devastating. Consider hereditary spherocytosis, which disturbs the interface between the plasma membrane and the cytoskeleton in red blood cells.

The doughnut shape of normal red blood cells enables them to squeeze through the narrowest blood vessels. Rods of a protein called spectrin form a meshwork beneath the plasma membrane, strengthening the cell, and proteins called ankyrins attach the spectrin rods to the plasma membrane (**figure 2.12**). Spectrin also attaches to the microfilaments and microtubules of the cytoskeleton. Spectrin molecules are like steel girders, and ankyrins are like nuts and bolts. If either molecule is absent, the cell collapses.

In hereditary spherocytosis, the ankyrins are abnormal, and parts of the red blood cell plasma membrane disintegrate, causing the cell to balloon out. The bloated cells obstruct narrow blood vessels—especially in the spleen, the organ that normally disposes of aged red blood cells. Anemia develops as the spleen destroys red blood cells more rapidly than the bone marrow can replace them, producing great fatigue and weakness. Removing the spleen can treat the condition.

Key Concepts

Cells are the units of life. They consist mostly of carbohydrates, lipids, proteins, and nucleic acids. • Organelles subdivide specific cell functions. They include the nucleus, the endoplasmic reticulum (ER), Golgi apparatus, mitochondria, lysosomes, and peroxisomes. • The plasma membrane is a flexible, selective phospholipid bilayer with embedded proteins and lipid rafts. • The cytoskeleton is an inner structural framework made of protein rods and tubules, connectors and motor molecules.

2.2 Cell Division and Death

The cell numbers in a human body must be in balance to promote normal growth and development. The process of mitotic cell division, or **mitosis,** provides new cells by forming two cells from one. Mitosis occurs in **somatic cells** (all cells but the sperm and eggs). Although it seems counterintuitive, some cells must die as a body forms, just as a sculptor must take away some clay to shape the desired object. A foot, for example, might start out as a webbed triangle of tissue, with digits carved from it as certain cells die. This type of cell death, a normal part of development, is termed **apoptosis,** from the Greek for leaves falling from a tree. Apoptosis is a precise, genetically programmed sequence of events, as is mitosis (**figure 2.13**).

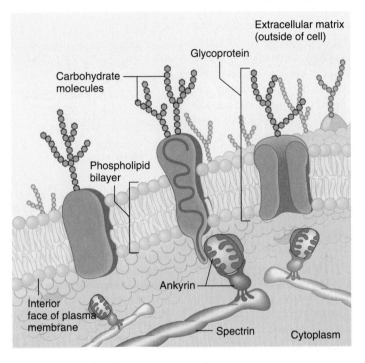

Figure 2.12 The red blood cell plasma membrane. The cytoskeleton that supports the plasma membrane of a red blood cell is specialized to withstand the great turbulent force of circulation. In the plasma membrane, proteins called ankyrins bind molecules of spectrin from the cytoskeleton to the inner membrane surface. On its other end, ankyrin binds proteins that help ferry molecules across the plasma membrane. In hereditary spherocytosis, abnormal ankyrin causes the plasma membrane to collapse, and the cell then balloons out—a problem for a cell whose function depends upon its shape.

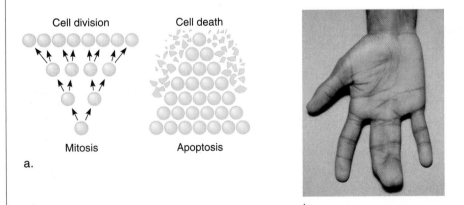

Figure 2.13 Mitosis and apoptosis mold a body. Biological structures in animal bodies enlarge, allowing organisms to grow, as opposing processes regulate cell number. **(a)** Cell numbers increase from mitosis and decrease from apoptosis. **(b)** Fingers and toes are carved from webbed structures. In syndactyly, normal apoptosis fails to carve digits, and webbing persists.

The Cell Cycle

Many cell divisions transform a single fertilized egg into a many-trillion-celled person. A series of events called the **cell cycle** describes the sequence of events as a cell prepares for division and then divides.

Cell cycle rate varies in different tissues at different times. A cell lining the small intestine's inner wall may divide throughout life; a cell in the brain may never divide; a cell in the deepest skin layer of a 90-year-old may divide more if the person lives long enough. Frequent mitosis enables the embryo and fetus to grow rapidly. By birth, the mitotic rate slows dramatically. Later, mitosis must maintain the numbers and positions of specialized cells in tissues and organs.

The cell cycle is a continual process, but we divide it into stages based on what we see. The two major stages are **interphase** (not dividing) and mitosis (dividing) (**figure 2.14**). In mitosis, a cell duplicates its chromosomes, then apportions one set into each of two daughter cells. This maintains the set of 23 chromosome pairs characteristic of a human somatic cell. Another form of cell division, meiosis, produces sperm or eggs, which have half the usual amount of genetic material, or 23 single chromosomes. Chapter 3 discusses meiosis.

Interphase—A Time of Great Activity

Interphase is a very active time. The cell continues the basic biochemical functions of life and also replicates its DNA and other subcellular structures for distribution to daughter cells.

Interphase is divided into two **gap (G) phases** and one **synthesis (S) phase.** A cell can exit the cell cycle at G_1 to enter a quiescent phase called G_0. A cell in G_0 can maintain its specialized characteristics, but not replicate its DNA or divide. It may also proceed to mitosis and divide, or die. Apoptosis may ensue if the cell's DNA is so damaged that the cell might become cancerous. G_0 then, is when a cell's fate is either decided, or put on hold.

During the first gap phase (G_1), the cell resumes synthesis of proteins, lipids, and carbohydrates following mitosis. These molecules will surround the two new cells that form from the original one. G_1 is the period of the cell cycle that varies the most in duration among different cell types.

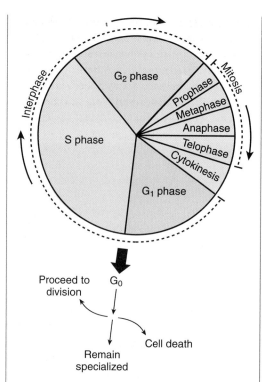

Figure 2.14   **The cell cycle.** The cell cycle is divided into interphase, when cellular components are replicated to prepare for division, and mitosis, when the cell splits in two, distributing its contents into two daughter cells. Interphase is divided into two gap phases (G_1 and G_2), when the cell duplicates specific molecules and structures, and a synthesis phase (S), when it replicates the genetic material. Mitosis is divided into four stages plus cytokinesis, which is when the cells physically separate. Another stage, G_0, is a "time-out" phase when a cell "decides" which course of action to follow.

Slowly dividing cells, such as those in the liver, may exit at G_1 and enter G_0, where they remain for years. In contrast, the rapidly dividing cells in bone marrow speed through G_1 in 16 to 24 hours. Cells of the early embryo may skip G_1 entirely.

During the next period of interphase, S phase, the cell replicates its entire genome, so that each chromosome consists of two copies joined at an area called the **centromere.** In most human cells, S phase takes 8 to 10 hours. Many proteins are also synthesized during this phase, including those that form the mitotic **spindle** that will pull the chromosomes apart. Microtubules form structures called **centrioles** near the nucleus. Centriole microtubules are oriented at right angles to each other, forming paired oblong structures that organize other microtubules into the spindle.

The second gap phase, G_2, occurs after the DNA has been replicated but before

mitosis begins. More proteins are synthesized during this phase. Membranes are assembled from molecules made during G_1 and stored as small, empty vesicles beneath the plasma membrane. These vesicles will merge with the plasma membrane to enclose the two daughter cells.

Mitosis—The Cell Divides

As mitosis begins, the replicated chromosomes are condensed enough to be visible, when stained, under a microscope. The two long strands of identical chromosomal material in a replicated chromosome are called **chromatids** (**figure 2.15**). At a certain point during mitosis, a replicated chromosome's centromere splits, allowing its chromatid pair to separate into two individual chromosomes. (Although the centromere of a replicated chromosome appears as a constriction, its DNA is replicated.)

During **prophase,** the first stage of mitosis, DNA coils tightly, shortening and thickening the chromosomes and enabling them to more easily separate (**figure 2.16**). Micro-

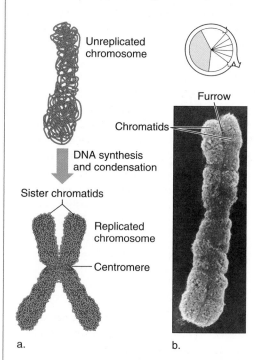

Figure 2.15   **Replicated and unreplicated chromosomes.** Chromosomes are replicated during S phase, before mitosis begins. Two genetically identical chromatids of a replicated chromosome join at the centromere **(a).** In the photograph **(b),** a human chromosome is in the midst of forming two chromatids. A longitudinal furrow extends from the chromosome tips inward.

tubules assemble from tubulin building blocks in the cytoplasm to form the spindles. Toward the end of prophase, the nuclear membrane breaks down. The nucleolus is no longer visible.

Metaphase follows prophase. Chromosomes attach to the spindle at their centromeres and align along the center of the cell, which is called the equator. Metaphase chromosomes are under great tension, but they appear motionless because they are pulled with equal force on both sides, like a tug-of-war rope pulled taut.

Next, during **anaphase,** the plasma membrane indents at the center, where the metaphase chromosomes line up. A band of microfilaments forms on the inside face of the plasma membrane, constricting the cell down the middle. Then the centromeres part, which relieves the tension and releases one chromatid from each pair to move to opposite ends of the cell—like a tug-of-war rope breaking in the middle and the participants falling into two groups. Microtubule movements stretch the dividing cell. During the very brief anaphase stage, a cell temporarily contains twice the normal number of chromosomes because each chromatid becomes an independently moving chromosome, but the cell has not yet physically divided.

In **telophase,** the final stage of mitosis, the cell looks like a dumbbell with a set of chromosomes at each end. The spindle falls apart, and nucleoli and the membranes around the nuclei re-form at each end of the elongated cell. Division of the genetic material is now complete. Next, during a process called **cytokinesis,** organelles and macromolecules are distributed between the two daughter cells. Finally, the microfilament band contracts like a drawstring, separating the newly formed cells.

Control of the Cell Cycle

When and where a somatic cell divides is crucial to health, and regulation of mitosis is a daunting task. Quadrillions of mitoses occur in a lifetime, and these cell divisions do not occur at random. Too little mitosis, and an injury may go unrepaired; too much, and an abnormal growth forms.

Groups of interacting proteins function at times in the cell cycle called **checkpoints** to ensure that chromosomes are faithfully replicated and apportioned into daughter cells (**figure 2.17**). A "DNA damage checkpoint,"

for example, temporarily pauses the cell cycle while special proteins repair damaged DNA. An "apoptosis checkpoint" turns on as mitosis begins. During this checkpoint, proteins called survivins override signals telling the cell to die, ensuring mitosis rather than apoptosis. Later during mitosis, the "spindle assembly checkpoint" oversees construction of the spindle and the binding of chromosomes to it.

Cells obey an internal "clock" that tells them approximately how many times to divide. Mammalian cells grown (cultured) in a dish divide about 40 to 60 times. A connective tissue cell from a fetus, for example, divides on average about 50 times. But a similar cell from an adult divides only 14 to 29 times. The number of divisions left declines with age.

How can a cell "know" how many divisions it has undergone and how many remain? The answer lies in the chromosome tips, called **telomeres (figure 2.18).** Telomeres function like a cellular fuse that burns down as pieces are lost from the very ends. Telomeres have hundreds to thousands of repeats of a specific six-nucleotide DNA sequence. At each mitosis, the telomeres lose 50 to 200 individual nucleotides, gradually shortening the chromosome. After about 50 divisions, a critical amount of telomere DNA is lost, which signals mitosis to stop. The cell may remain alive but not divide again, or it may die. An enzyme called telomerase keeps chromosome tips long in eggs and sperm, in cancer cells, and in a few types of normal cells (such as bone marrow cells) that must continually supply many new cells (see figure 18.3). However, most cells do not produce telomerase, and their chromosomes gradually shrink.

Outside factors also affect a cell's mitotic clock. Crowding can slow or halt mitosis. Normal cells growing in culture stop dividing when they form a one-cell-thick layer lining the container. If the layer tears, the cells that border the tear grow and divide to fill in the gap, but stop dividing once it is filled. Perhaps a similar mechanism in the body limits mitosis.

Chemical signals control the cell cycle from outside as well as from inside the cell. Hormones and growth factors are biochemicals from outside the cell that influence mitotic rate. A hormone is a substance synthesized in a gland and transported in the bloodstream to another part of the body, where it exerts a specific effect. Hormones secreted in the brain, for example, signal the

cells lining a woman's uterus to build up each month by mitosis in preparation for possible pregnancy. Growth factors act more locally. Epidermal growth factor, for example, stimulates cell division beneath a scab.

Two types of proteins, cyclins and kinases, interact inside cells to activate the genes whose products carry out mitosis. The two types of proteins form pairs. Cyclin levels fluctuate regularly throughout the cell cycle, while kinase levels stay the same. A certain number of cyclin-kinase pairs turn on the genes that trigger mitosis. Then, as mitosis begins, enzymes degrade the cyclin. The cycle starts again as cyclin begins to build up during the next interphase.

Apoptosis

Apoptosis rapidly and neatly dismantles a cell into neat, membrane-enclosed pieces that a phagocyte (a cell that engulfs and destroys another) can mop up. It is a little like taking the contents of a messy room and packaging them into garbage bags—then disposing of it all. In contrast is necrosis, a form of cell death associated with inflammation, rather than a neat, contained destruction.

Like mitosis, apoptosis is a continuous process that occurs in a series of steps. It begins when a "death receptor" on the doomed cell's plasma membrane receives a signal to die. Within seconds, enzymes called caspases are activated inside the cell, stimulating each other and snipping apart various cell components. These killer enzymes take several actions at once. They

- destroy the cytoskeletal threads that support the nucleus so that it collapses, causing the genetic material within to condense.

- demolish the enzymes that replicate and repair DNA.

- activate enzymes that chew DNA up into similarly sized small pieces.

- tear apart the rest of the cytoskeleton.

- cause mitochondria to release molecules that trigger further caspase activity, end the cell's energy supply, and destroy these organelles.

- destroy the cell's ability to adhere to other cells.

- send a certain phospholipid from the plasma membrane's inner face to its outer surface, where it attracts phagocytes.

A dying cell has a characteristic appearance (**figure 2.19**). It rounds up as contacts with other cells are cut off, and the plasma membrane undulates and forms bulges called blebs. The nucleus bursts, releasing DNA pieces that align in a way that resemble ladders when the pieces are dyed and displayed in an electrical field. The mitochondria decompose. Then the cell shatters. Almost instantly, pieces of membrane encapsulate the cell fragments, which prevents inflammation. Within an hour, the cell is gone.

From the embryo onward through development, mitosis and apoptosis are synchronized, so that tissue neither overgrows nor shrinks. In this way, a child's liver retains much the same shape as she grows into adulthood. During early development, mitosis and apoptosis orchestrate the ebb and flow of cell number as new structures form. Later, these processes protect. Mitosis produces new skin to heal a scraped knee; apoptosis peels away sunburnt skin cells that might otherwise become cancerous. Cancer is a profound derangement of the balance between cell division and death, with mitosis occurring too frequently or too many times, or apoptosis too infrequently. Chapter 18 discusses cancer in detail.

Key Concepts

Mitosis and apoptosis regulate cell numbers during development, growth, and repair. • The cell cycle includes interphase and mitosis. During G_0, the cell "decides" to divide, die, or stay differentiated. Interphase includes two gap (G) phases and a synthesis (S) phase that prepares the cell for mitosis. During S phase, DNA is replicated. Proteins, carbohydrates, and lipids are synthesized during G_1 and more proteins are synthesized in G_2. During prophase, metaphase, anaphase, and telophase, replicated chromosomes condense, align, split, and distribute into daughter cells. The cell cycle is controlled by checkpoints, telomeres, hormones, growth factors from outside the cell, and cyclins and kinases from within. • During apoptosis, cells receive a death signal, activate caspases, and break apart in an orderly fashion.

Figure 2.16 Mitosis in a human cell. In a separate process, cytokinesis, the cytoplasm and other cellular structures distribute and pinch off into two daughter cells. (For simplicity, not all 23 chromosome pairs are depicted.)

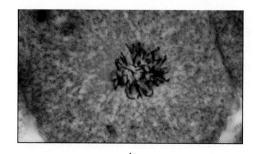

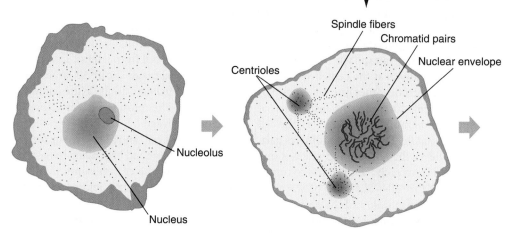

Interphase
Chromosomes are uncondensed.

Prophase
Condensed chromosomes take up stain. The spindle assembles, centrioles appear, and the nuclear envelope breaks down.

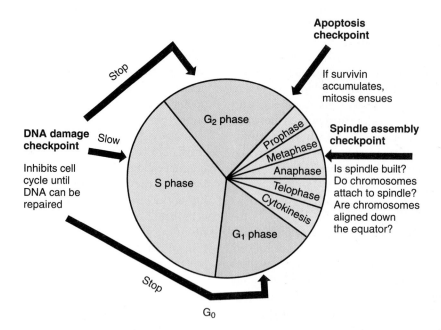

Figure 2.17 Cell cycle checkpoints. Checkpoints ensure that mitotic events occur in the correct sequence. Many types of cancer result from faulty checkpoints.

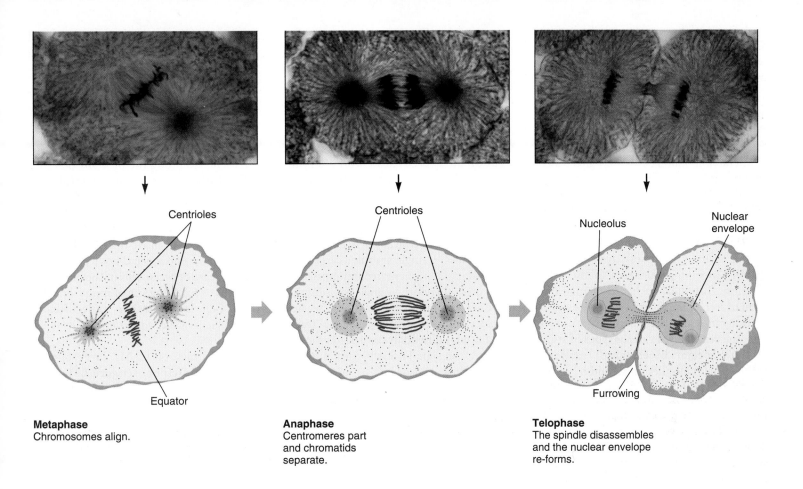

Metaphase
Chromosomes align.

Anaphase
Centromeres part and chromatids separate.

Telophase
The spindle disassembles and the nuclear envelope re-forms.

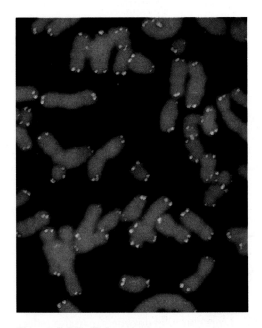

Figure 2.18 Telomeres. Fluorescent tags mark the telomeres in this human cell.

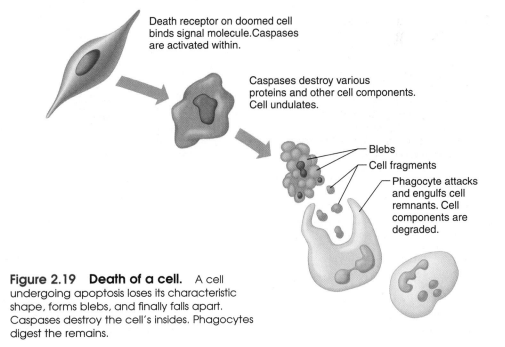

Death receptor on doomed cell binds signal molecule. Caspases are activated within.

Caspases destroy various proteins and other cell components. Cell undulates.

Blebs

Cell fragments

Phagocyte attacks and engulfs cell remnants. Cell components are degraded.

Figure 2.19 Death of a cell. A cell undergoing apoptosis loses its characteristic shape, forms blebs, and finally falls apart. Caspases destroy the cell's insides. Phagocytes digest the remains.

2.3 Cell-Cell Interactions

Precisely coordinated biochemical steps orchestrate the cell-cell interactions that make multicellular life possible. Defects in cell communication and interaction cause certain inherited illnesses. Two broad types of interactions among cells are signal transduction and cellular adhesion.

Signal Transduction

In signal transduction, molecules on the plasma membrane assess, transmit, and amplify incoming messages to the cell's interior. *Transduce* means to change one form of something (such as energy or information) into another. In signal transduction, the cell changes various types of stimuli into specific biochemical reactions. Some signal molecules must bind receptors for the cell to function normally; others, such as a signal to divide when cell division is not warranted, must be ignored.

Signal transduction is carried out by the interaction between cytoplasmic proteins and proteins embedded in the plasma membrane that extend from one or both faces. The transduction process is a complex series of chemical interactions that begins at the cell surface. In the first step, a receptor directly binds an incoming stimulus called the first messenger (**figure 2.20**). The responding receptor contorts in a way that touches a nearby protein called a regulator. Next, the regulator protein activates a nearby enzyme, which catalyzes (speeds) a specific chemical reaction. The product of this reaction is called the second messenger. The second messenger lies at the crux of the entire process; it elicits the cell's response, typically by activating certain enzymes. A single stimulus can trigger the production of many second messenger molecules; therefore, signal transduction amplifies incoming information. Because cascades of proteins carry out signal transduction, it is a genetically controlled process.

Defects in signal transduction underlie many inherited disorders. In neurofibromatosis type 1 (NF1), for example, tumors (usually benign) grow in nervous tissue under the skin and in parts of the nervous system. At the cellular level, NF1 occurs when cells fail to block transmission of a growth factor signal that triggers cell division. Affected cells misinterpret the signal and divide when it is inappropriate. Several new cancer drugs work by plugging receptors for growth factors on cancer cells.

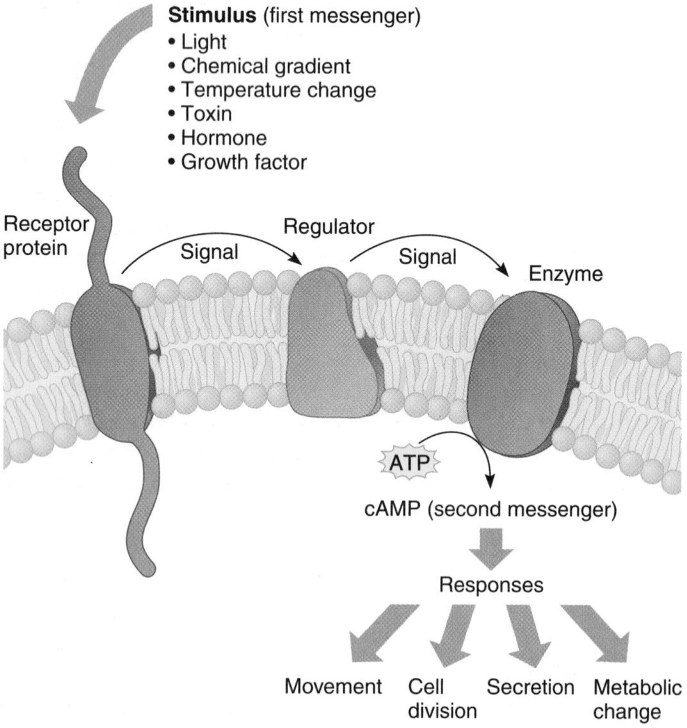

Cellular Adhesion

Cellular adhesion is a precise sequence of interactions among the proteins that join cells. Inflammation—the painful, red swelling at a site of injury or infection—illustrates one type of cellular adhesion. Inflammation occurs when white blood cells (leukocytes) move through the blood vessels to the endangered body part, where they squeeze between cells of the blood vessel walls to reach the site of injury or infection. **Cellular adhesion molecules,** or CAMs, help guide white blood cells to the injured area.

Three types of CAMs carry out the inflammatory response (**figure 2.21**). First, selectins attach to the white blood cells, and slow them to a roll by also binding to carbohydrates on the capillary wall. (This is a little like putting out your arms to slow your ride down a slide.) Next, clotting blood, bacteria, or decaying tissues release chemical attractants that signal white blood cells to stop. The chemical attractants activate CAMs called integrins, which latch onto the white blood cells, and CAMs called adhesion receptor proteins, which extend from the capillary wall at the injury site. The integrins and adhesion receptor proteins then guide the white blood cells between the tilelike lining cells to the other side—the injury site.

What happens if the signals that direct white blood cells to injury sites fail? A young woman named Brooke Blanton knows the answer all too well. Her first symptom was teething sores that did not heal. These and other small wounds never accumulated the pus (bacteria, cellular debris, and white blood cells) that indicates the body is fighting infection. Brooke has leukocyte-adhesion deficiency. Her body lacks the CAMs that enable white blood cells to stick to blood vessel walls, and so her blood cells zip right past wounds. Brooke must avoid injury and infection, and she receives anti-infective treatments for even the slightest wound.

More common disorders may also reflect abnormal cellular adhesion. Without cellular adhesion, cancer cells journey easily from one part of the body to another. Arthritis may occur when the wrong adhe-

Stimulus (first messenger)
- Light
- Chemical gradient
- Temperature change
- Toxin
- Hormone
- Growth factor

Receptor protein

Signal   Regulator   Signal   Enzyme

ATP

cAMP (second messenger)

Responses

Movement   Cell division   Secretion   Metabolic change

Figure 2.20 **Signal transduction.** A receptor binds a first messenger, triggering a cascade of biochemical activity at the cell's surface. An enzyme catalyzes a reaction inside the cell that circularizes ATP to cyclic AMP, the second messenger. cAMP then stimulates various responses, such as cell division, metabolic changes, and muscle contraction. Splitting ATP also releases energy.

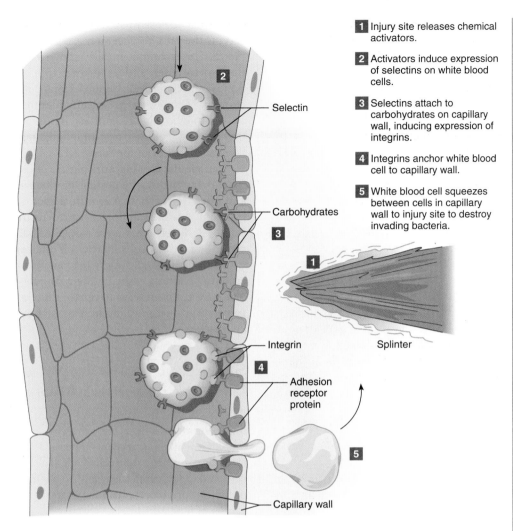

1 Injury site releases chemical activators.

2 Activators induce expression of selectins on white blood cells.

3 Selectins attach to carbohydrates on capillary wall, inducing expression of integrins.

4 Integrins anchor white blood cell to capillary wall.

5 White blood cell squeezes between cells in capillary wall to injury site to destroy invading bacteria.

Figure 2.21 **Cellular adhesion.** Cellular adhesion molecules (CAMs), including selectins, integrins, and adhesion receptor proteins, direct white blood cells to injury sites.

sion molecules rein in white blood cells, inflaming a joint where no injury exists.

Cellular adhesion is critical to many other functions. CAMs guide cells surrounding an embryo to grow toward maternal cells and form the placenta, the supportive organ linking a pregnant woman to the fetus. Sequences of CAMs also help establish connections among the nerve cells that underlie learning and memory.

Key Concepts

In signal transduction, cell surface receptors receive information from first messengers (stimuli) and pass them to second messengers, which then trigger a cellular response. • Cellular adhesion molecules (CAMs) guide white blood cells to injury sites using a sequence of cell-protein interactions.

2.4 Stem Cells and Cell Specialization

Bodies grow and heal thanks to cells that retain the ability to divide, generating both new cells like themselves and cells that go on to specialize. Stem cells and **progenitor cells** renew tissues so that as the body grows, or loses cells to apoptosis, injury, and disease, others arise to take their place.

Cell Lineages

A stem cell divides by mitosis to yield either two daughter cells like itself, or one that is a stem cell and one that is a partially specialized progenitor cell (**figure 2.22**). A progenitor cell's daughters usually specialize as any of a restricted number of cell types. A fully differentiated cell, such as a mature blood cell, descends from a sequence of increas-

ingly specialized progenitor cell intermediates, each one less like a stem cell and more like a blood cell. Our 260 or so differentiated cell types develop from lineages of stem and progenitor cells. **Figure 2.23** shows parts of a few lineages.

Stem cells and progenitor cells are described in terms of potential—that is, according to the number of possible fates of their daughter cells. A fertilized ovum and the cells of the very early embryo, when it is just a small ball of identical-appearing cells, are **totipotent,** which means that they can give rise to every cell type. In contrast, stem cells that persist until later in development and progenitor cells are **pluripotent:** Their daughter cells have fewer possible fates. This is a little like a freshman's consideration of many majors, compared to a junior's more narrowed focus in selecting courses.

As cells specialize, they express some genes and ignore others. An immature bone cell forms from a progenitor cell by manufacturing mineral-binding proteins and enzymes. In contrast, an immature muscle cell forms from a muscle progenitor cell that accumulates contractile proteins. The bone cell does not produce muscle proteins, nor does the muscle cell produce bone proteins. All cells, however, synthesize proteins for basic "housekeeping" functions, such as energy acquisition and protein synthesis.

Many, if not all, of the organs in an adult human body harbor stem or progenitor cells that are activated when injury or illness occurs. Stem cells in the adult may be set aside in the embryo or fetus in particular organs as repositories of future healing. Alternatively, or perhaps also, stem cells or progenitor cells may travel from the bone marrow to replace damaged or dead cells in response to signals that are released when injury or disease occurs. Some stem and progenitor cells are actually more "plastic" than researchers had first thought—for example, hematopoietic stem cells in bone marrow can form not only blood cells, but also nerve, muscle, liver, and blood vessel lining cells. Because every cell contains all of an individual's genetic material, it is theoretically possible that, given appropriate signals, any cell type can become any other. But this may not occur naturally, or may only happen under certain unusual conditions, such as catastrophic injury.

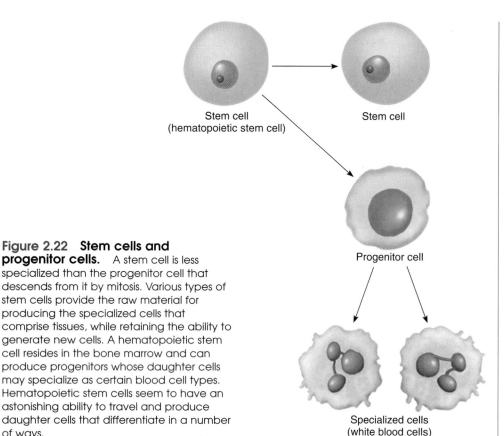

Stem cell
(hematopoietic stem cell)

Stem cell

Progenitor cell

Specialized cells
(white blood cells)

Figure 2.22 Stem cells and progenitor cells. A stem cell is less specialized than the progenitor cell that descends from it by mitosis. Various types of stem cells provide the raw material for producing the specialized cells that comprise tissues, while retaining the ability to generate new cells. A hematopoietic stem cell resides in the bone marrow and can produce progenitors whose daughter cells may specialize as certain blood cell types. Hematopoietic stem cells seem to have an astonishing ability to travel and produce daughter cells that differentiate in a number of ways.

Stem Cell Technology Using Embryos

Physicians are beginning to use stem cells to treat particular disorders or injuries. Using stem cell biology to heal is one type of "regenerative medicine," a field in its infancy.

Stem cells that may be used in regenerative medicine have several sources, some controversial, most not. Although rare, stem cells probably exist everywhere in the body. They can be derived from the earliest embryos through old age, and even from deceased adults and medical waste, such as the fatty material discarded after liposuction and surgically removed organs. According to many biologists, the most promising cells for therapy are embryonic stem (ES) cells. These are obtained and cultured from a 5-day embryo, called a blastocyst, which is a hollow ball of cells with a few cells comprising the inner cell mass on the inside. These inner cell mass cells, given appropriate biochemical signals, become totipotent ES cells (they can generate any cell type), in contrast to the more limited repertoire of possibilities for stem or progenitor cells in adult tissues. ES cells are

also less likely to provoke rejection by the recipient's immune system. From an ethical standpoint, however, ES cells are controversial because they must come from embryos.

There are two sources for obtaining ES cells. One is to use embryos from fertility clinics where couples undergoing *in vitro* fertilization (IVF) freeze the extras. This approach could create banks of stored cell types, though they would not precisely match the cell surfaces of a particular individual. "Typing" would have to be done, as it is for blood transfusions and organ transplants. If not used, these embryos would be discarded.

The second source of ES cells is to create an embryo using the nucleus from a somatic cell from a patient, such as a person who has suffered a spinal cord injury **(figure 2.24)**. The nucleus is injected into or fused with a donated egg cell whose nucleus has been removed. The resulting cell—not really a fertilized egg—develops for 5 days. Inner cell mass cells are removed and cultured to become ES cells, then given "cocktails" of growth factors to differentiate as needed—into nerve cells (neurons) to patch a spinal

cord injury, for example. The person's body accepts the cells because they are a genetic match. This technique is called **somatic cell nuclear transfer,** and its medical application is nonscientifically termed therapeutic cloning. (Clones are genetically identical cells or individuals.) In contrast, reproductive cloning creates a new individual (see Bioethics: Choices for the Future 3.1.)

Therapeutic cloning works in cattle and rodents, but may not be possible for humans and other primates that require a sperm's contribution. Ethical objections focus on intent: IVF leftovers were conceived to produce a child, and somatic cell nuclear transfer creates and destroys an early embryo. Nations vary in their policies: some permit both ways to obtain ES cells, some allow one only, and others ban both approaches.

Stem Cell Technology Using Cells from Adults

Using stem cells from adults may eventually make the debate over ES cell technology moot. Bone marrow transplants have delivered hematopoietic stem cells for half a century, and today, using such cells from stored umbilical cord blood is routine in treating a variety of blood disorders.

Continuing basic research on stem cells from the adult may lead to other clinical applications. For example, new drugs to treat breast cancer seek the rare stem cells tucked between the lining and muscular layers of the milk ducts, where cancer begins. The fact that progenitor cells in bone marrow can travel to an injured liver, then produce new liver cells, suggests a less invasive way of treating liver disease—via the bloodstream.

Hearts were once thought to be unrepairable, but recent stem cell discoveries have changed that view **(figure 2.25)**. When several men who had received heart transplants from women died, autopsies showed that their hearts had differentiated cells with Y chromosomes, which indicated that the cells came from the recipient. The new "heart patches" also included progenitor cells marked with the telltale Y. The mens' bodies had apparently recruited progenitor cells to become part of the new heart—either from the bone marrow, or from stem cells in the bit of their own tissue to which the new heart

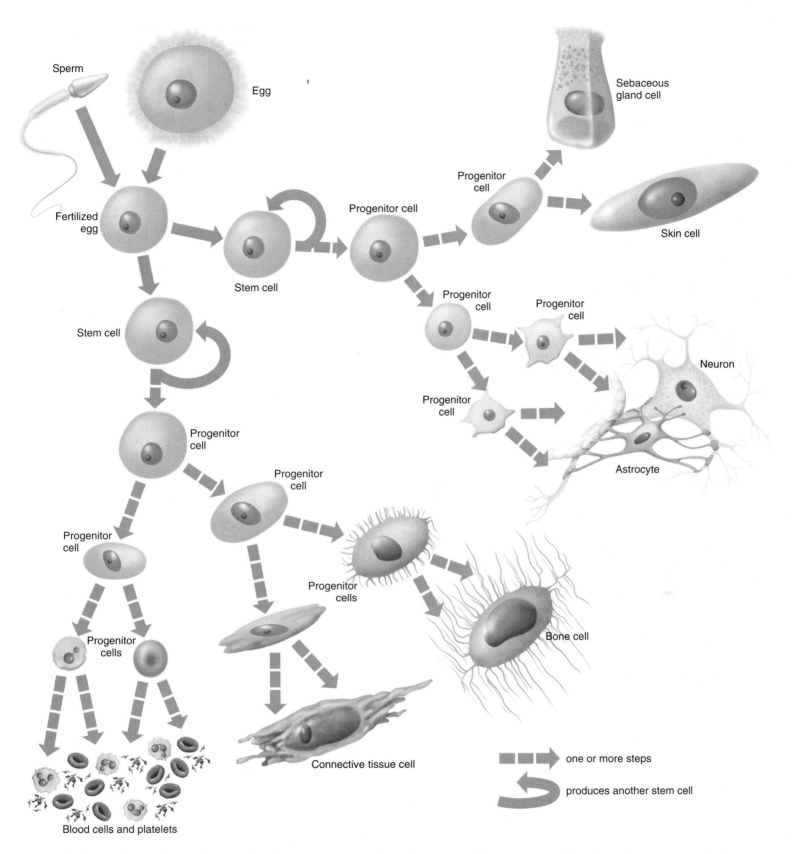

Figure 2.23 Pathways to cell specialization. All cells in the human body descend from stem cells, through the processes of mitosis and differentiation. The differentiated cells on the left are all connective tissues (blood, connective tissue, and bone), but the blood cells are more closely related to each other than they are to the other two cell types. On the right, the skin and sebaceous gland cells share a recent progenitor, and both share a more distant progenitor with neurons and supportive astrocytes. Imagine how complex the illustration would be if it embraced all 260-plus types of cells in a human body!

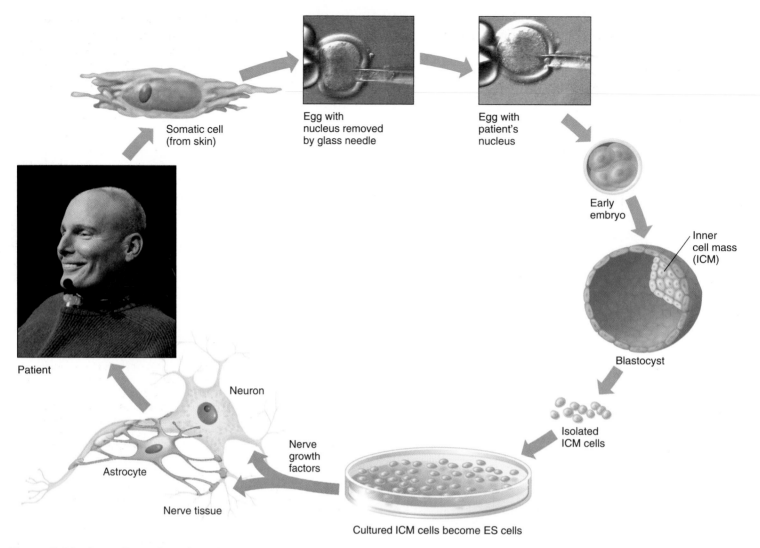

Figure 2.24 **Somatic cell nuclear transfer yields embryonic stem cells genetically matched to a patient.** A new way to possibly treat degenerative diseases and injuries is to culture cells whose nuclei come from a patient's own cells, and use the new cells to replace diseased or damaged cells. The immune system would not reject these cells, because they contain the patient's genome. An alternative approach to treat nervous system problems is to use neural stem cells taken from cadavers, but these would not match cells from the patient. The prospective patient in this illustration is the actor Christopher Reeve, who has a spinal cord injury.

was stitched. Perhaps a smaller female heart, stressed in a sick man's chest cavity, released growth factors and other signals that activated the recipient's stem and progenitor cells.

The heart transplant study inspired experimental treatment for 16-year-old Dmitri Bonnville, who was shot in the chest with a nail gun while working at a construction site. With no other option except to do a heart transplant, physicians gave Dmitri a drug to coax his bone marrow to produce stem cells that could travel to the heart. The young man improved and did not require the transplant. Early evidence suggests that the stem cells induced

blood vessel growth in and around the heart, rather than replacing heart muscle.

Brain neurons, too, were once thought unable to divide. Then researchers discovered that new neurons arise in the brains of birds when they learn songs. Looking at animals more closely related to humans, researchers used a stain called BrdU to reveal small clusters of neural stem cells in the brains of tree shrews and marmosets. These stem cells can differentiate into neurons or the cells that support them. Demonstrating stem cells in human brains proved difficult, since no one was willing to provide a sample of what one researcher

calls "brain marrow." Then, in the late 1990s, researchers found volunteers—people with cancer of the tongue or larynx being treated with BrdU. After death, their brains revealed pockets of neural stem cells stained with BrdU. Researchers may one day be able to treat spinal cord injuries and neurodegenerative conditions such as Parkinson disease or multiple sclerosis by coaxing a person's own neural stem cells to heal the damage.

Stem cell technology may be used to treat less serious conditions, too. For example, a single stem cell in the skin can give rise to skin cells, hair follicle cells, and sebaceous (oil) gland cells. Manipulating these

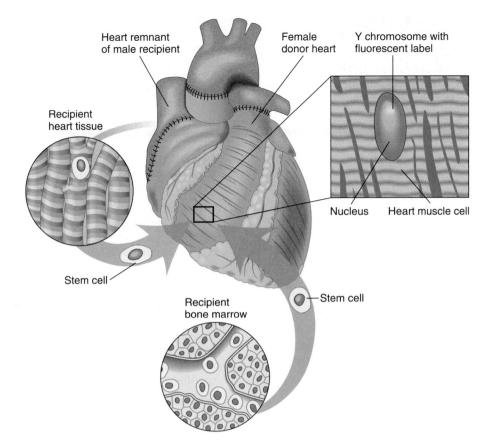

Figure 2.25 Can stem cells heal hearts? A study of the hearts of eight men who had received transplants from women revealed that stem cells from the recipients' bodies helped to accept the new organs. The stem cells came from the bone marrow or from remnants of the mens' hearts—or both. The new organs contained progenitor cells and specialized cells that had Y chromosomes—meaning that they must have come from male recipients.

stem cells might lead to treatments for baldness, acne, and hair removal!

We still have much to learn about stem cells. For example, what makes a stem cell a stem cell? Researchers have identified 216 genes that must be expressed to impart a state of "stemness" to a cell. Many of these genes are involved in signal transduction. All but four of the 216 genes are also expressed in non-stem cells. As analysis of the human genome continues, researchers will be able to more precisely define the genetic functions that enable a cell to retain developmental potential—essential to building and maintaining bodies, the subject of the next chapter.

Key Concepts

All cells descend from progenitor and stem cells, most of which are pluripotent. The fertilized egg and cells of the early embryo are totipotent. Differential gene expression underlies cell specialization. • Stem cells are found at all stages of development and throughout the body. Embryonic stem cells are the most promising for regenerative medicine. They derive from fertilized ova stored at fertility clinics and from somatic cell nuclear transfer from a patient's own cell nucleus to an enucleated donor egg. Stem cells from adults may have a variety of medical applications.

Summary

2.1 The Components of Cells

1. Cells are the fundamental units of life and comprise the human body. Inherited traits and illnesses can be understood at the cellular and molecular levels.

2. All cells share certain features, but they are also specialized because they express different subsets of genes. Cells consist primarily of water and several types of macromolecules: **carbohydrates, lipids, proteins,** and **nucleic acids.**

3. The three domains of life—Archaea, Bacteria, and Eukarya—have characteristic cells. The archaea and bacteria are simple, small, and lack **nuclei** and other **organelles. Eukaryotic** cells have

organelles, and their genetic material is contained in a nucleus.

4. Organelles sequester related biochemical reactions, improving efficiency of life functions and protecting the cell. Along with organelles, the cell consists of **cytoplasm** and other chemicals.

5. The nucleus contains DNA and a nucleolus, which is a site of ribosome synthesis. **Ribosomes** provide scaffolds for protein synthesis; they exist free in the cytoplasm or complexed with the **rough ER.**

6. In secretion, the rough ER is the site of protein synthesis and folding, the **smooth ER** is the site of lipid synthesis, transport, and packaging, and the **Golgi apparatus**

packages secretions into vesicles, which exit through the **plasma membrane.** Enzymes in **mitochondria** extract energy from nutrients. **Lysosomes** contain enzymes that dismantle debris, and **peroxisomes** house enzymes that perform a variety of functions.

7. The plasma membrane is a protein-studded **phospholipid bilayer.** It controls which substances exit and enter the cell, and how the cell interacts with other cells.

8. The **cytoskeleton** is a protein framework of hollow **microtubules,** made of tubulin, and solid **microfilaments,** which consist of actin. **Intermediate filaments** are made of more than one protein type and are

abundant in skin. The cytoskeleton and the plasma membrane distinguish different types of cells.

2.2 Cell Division and Death

9. Coordination of cell division (**mitosis**) and cell death (**apoptosis**) maintains cell numbers, enabling structures to enlarge during growth and development but preventing abnormal growth.

10. The **cell cycle** describes whether a cell is dividing (mitosis) or not (**interphase**). Interphase consists of two gap phases, when proteins and lipids are produced, and a synthesis phase, when DNA is replicated.

11. Mitosis proceeds in four stages. In **prophase**, replicated chromosomes consisting of two **chromatids** condense, the **spindle** assembles, the nuclear membrane breaks down, and the nucleolus is no longer visible. In **metaphase**, replicated chromosomes align along the center of the cell. In **anaphase**, the **centromeres** part, equally dividing the now unreplicated chromosomes into two daughter cells. In **telophase**, the new cells separate. **Cytokinesis** apportions other components into daughter cells.

12. Internal and external factors control the cell cycle. **Checkpoints** are times when proteins regulate the cell cycle. **Telomere** size determines how many more mitoses will occur. Crowding, hormones, and growth factors signal cells from the outside; the interactions of cyclins and kinases trigger mitosis from inside.

13. In apoptosis, a receptor on the plasma membrane receives a death signal, then activates caspases that tear apart the cell in an orderly fashion. Membrane surrounds the pieces, preventing inflammation.

2.3 Cell-Cell Interactions

14. In **signal transduction**, a stimulus (first messenger) activates a cascade of action among membrane proteins, culminating in production of a second messenger that turns on enzymes that provide the response.

15. **Cellular adhesion molecules** enable cells to interact. Selectins slow the movement of white blood cells, or leukocytes, and integrins and adhesion receptor proteins guide the blood cell through a capillary wall to an injury site.

2.4 Stem Cells and Cell Specialization

16. Stem cells produce daughter cells that retain the ability to divide and that specialize in particular ways.

17. **Totipotent** stem cells can become anything. **Pluripotent** stem cells can differentiate as any of a variety of cell types. **Progenitor cells** can specialize as any of a restricted number of cell types.

18. Embryonic stem (ES) cells have more medical applications and are less likely to be rejected than stem cells from adults.

19. ES cells can be obtained from existing embryos (IVF "leftovers") or be tailor-made (through **somatic cell nuclear transfer**).

20. Researchers are developing ways to use the body's stem and progenitor cells to heal.

Review Questions

1. List the steps of each of the following processes:
   a. signal transduction
   b. cellular adhesion
   c. the cell cycle
   d. apoptosis
   e. mitosis
   f. secretion

2. Explain the functions of the following proteins:
   a. tubulin and actin
   b. caspases
   c. cyclins and kinases
   d. checkpoint proteins
   e. cellular adhesion molecules

3. List four types of controls on cell cycle rate.

4. How can all of a person's cells contain exactly the same genetic material, yet specialize as bone cells, nerve cells, muscle cells, and connective tissue cells?

5. Distinguish between
   a. a bacterial cell and a eukaryotic cell.
   b. interphase and mitosis.
   c. mitosis and apoptosis.
   d. rough ER and smooth ER.
   e. microtubules and microfilaments.
   f. a stem cell and a progenitor cell.
   g. totipotent and pluripotent.

6. What functions do each of the following organelles perform?
   a. mitochondria
   b. lysosomes
   c. peroxisomes
   d. smooth ER
   e. rough ER
   f. Golgi apparatus
   g. nucleus

7. What advantage does compartmentalization provide to a large and complex cell?

8. What role does the plasma membrane play in signal transduction?

9. Explain how stem cells obtained from IVF leftovers and somatic cell nuclear transfer differ in terms of their genomes.

Applied Questions

1. How might abnormalities in each of the following contribute to cancer?

   a. cellular adhesion

   b. signal transduction

   c. balance between mitosis and apoptosis

   d. cell cycle control

   e. telomerase activity

2. Why do many inherited conditions result from defective enzymes?

3. In neuronal ceroid lipofuscinosis, the nervous system degenerates after birth. The child experiences seizures, loss of vision, and lack of coordination, dying in early childhood. At the molecular level, the child lacks an enzyme that normally breaks down certain proteins, causing them to accumulate and destroying the nervous system. Name two organelles that are involved in this illness.

4. How do stem cells maintain their populations within tissues that consist of mostly differentiated cells?

5. Explain why mitosis that is too frequent or too infrequent, or apoptosis that is too frequent or too infrequent, can endanger health.

6. Why wouldn't a cell in an embryo likely be in phase G_0?

7. A defect in which organelle would cause fatigue?

8. Describe three ways that drugs can be used to treat cancer, based on disrupting microtubule function, telomere length, and signal transduction.

9. How can signal transduction, the plasma membrane, and the cytoskeleton function together?

10. What abnormality at the cellular or molecular level lies behind each of the following disorders?

    a. cystic fibrosis

    b. adrenoleukodystrophy

    c. neurofibromatosis type 1

    d. leukocyte adhesion deficiency

    e. syndactyly

11. A child with sickle cell disease endures periods of crisis, when circulation becomes painfully poor, starving parts of the body of oxygen. The blood of a child in crisis contains many more stem cells, sent from the bone marrow, than does the blood of a child not in crisis. What does this observation suggest about stem cell function?

12. The thymus gland in the chest manufactures white blood cells that protect against infection. It begins to shrink in adolescence. Researchers have discovered that a single variety of stem cell can, in a dish, be stimulated to regrow a thymus. List the steps to use somatic cell nuclear transfer to create a thymus gland to help a person suffering from AIDS.

Web Activities

13. The Coalition for the Advancement of Medical Research (www.camradvocacy.org) includes scientists, foundations, and patients advocating stem cell research for regenerative medicine. Consult the website to learn the latest news on legislative efforts to either ban or spare stem cell research, and explain which types of research the bills would and would not allow.

14. Select ten nations and using a web search engine, research whether they allow use of IVF leftovers to obtain human ES cells, somatic cell nuclear transfer to obtain the cells, neither, or both.

Case Study

15. Anthony Wright and Julia Green are 32-year-old participants in a clinical trial to evaluate stem cell therapy for multiple myeloma, a cancer of certain bone marrow cells. They are assigned to different treatment groups. Both receive standard therapy, which is alpha interferon. Anthony's group also receives conventional doses of four chemotherapeutic drugs, which kill any rapidly dividing cells. Julia's group's treatment is more drastic. She receives extremely high doses of the four drugs, enough to kill her bone marrow cells, then she has an umbilical cord stem cell transplant, which is an infusion of the material in a vein in her arm. Julia survives a year longer (5 years total) than Anthony, and the other people in the study had similar outcomes—those receiving stem cells lived longer. The conclusion: stem cell therapy is more effective for treating multiple myeloma than combination chemotherapy alone.

    a. It takes several weeks for Julia and Anthony to recover from the effects of the treatments. Which would have been more likely to have suffered serious side effects? Cite a reason for your answer.

    b. Julia's father reads about the experimental treatment in the newspaper and is outraged. "It is unethical to use embryos as spare parts," he tells her. How has he misunderstood the procedure?

    c. Why might Julia have eventually relapsed?

Learn to apply the skills of a genetic counselor with these additional cases found in the *Case Workbook for Human Genetics:*

   Carnitine-acylcarnitine translocase deficiency

   Combined factors V and VIII deficiency

Suggested Readings

Duncan, Rory R., et al. March 13, 2003. Functional and spatial segregation of secretory vesicle pools according to vesicle age. *Nature* 422:176. Researchers track the interaction of organelles in secretion.

Inwald, D., et al. January 2001. Adhesion molecule deficiencies. *Journal of Clinical Pathology* 54:1. The discovery of cellular adhesion molecules explained disorders in which wounds do not heal.

Lewis, Ricki. January 13, 2003. A state of stemness: What if ...? *The Scientist* 17(1):9. Stem cells may be more plastic than anyone imagined.

Lewis, Ricki. June 30, 2003. The neurobiology of rehabilitation. *The Scientist* 17(13):22–25. The human brain may be able to heal itself.

Lewis, Ricki. March 24, 2003. Deciphering death's circuitry. *The Scientist* 17(6):32. Complex signaling orchestrates apoptosis.

Lewis, Ricki. September 16, 2002. Mike West: Cloning for human therapeutics. *The Scientist* 16(8):60. An interview with the first person to clone a human embryo.

Mazzarello, Paolo, and Marina Bentivoglio. April 9, 1998. The centenarian Golgi apparatus. *Nature* vol. 392. The Golgi apparatus was discovered a century ago.

Renehan, Andrew G., et al. June 21, 2001. What is apoptosis and why is it important? *The British Medical Journal* 322:1536.

Weekly updates of current news related to human genetics are available through Power Web on your Online Learning Center.

Development

CHAPTER CONTENTS

3.1 The Reproductive System
Males and females have paired gonads that house reproductive cells, and networks of tubes and associated glands that nurture the development of sperm and oocytes, the gametes.

3.2 Meiosis
Meiosis is a form of cell division that halves the two genomes of a somatic cell to produce haploid gametes. It ensures that the chromosome number remains constant from generation to generation, and it also recombines the genetic contributions of each parent, creating great genetic variability.

3.3 Gamete Maturation
A sperm and an oocyte look nothing alike, yet each houses a haploid package of genetic material. A sperm is specialized to deliver its package; an oocyte accumulates reserves to support early development.

3.4 Prenatal Development
Nearly all human prenatal development occurs during the first eight weeks, the period of the embryo. During the remaining months of gestation, structures grow and specialize.

3.5 Birth Defects
Malfunctioning genes or environmental insults can derail development, with devastating results. The nature of a birth defect depends upon which structures were forming at the time of the abnormal gene action or environmental exposure.

3.6 Maturation and Aging
Development hardly ceases with birth—decades of growth and elaboration of structures continue. Single-gene and multifactorial conditions may be expressed at different times, or speed aging-associated changes. Genomewide comparisons between people who live very long and those who die of certain disorders may reveal genes that control longevity.

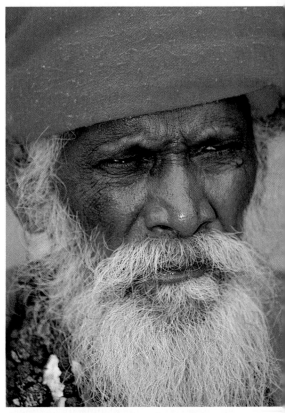

Aging of a person is obvious, but cells begin to die of "old age" even in the fetus.

Genes orchestrate our physiology from shortly after conception through adulthood. As a result, disorders caused by the malfunction of single genes, or genetic predispositions, affect people of all ages. Certain single gene mutations act before birth, causing broken bones, dwarfism, or even cancer. Many other mutant genes exert their effects during childhood, and it may take parents months or even years to realize their child has a health problem. Duchenne muscular dystrophy (figure 2.1*a*), for example, usually begins as clumsiness in early childhood. Inherited forms of heart disease and breast cancer can appear in early or middle adulthood, earlier than multifactorial forms of these conditions typically begin. Pattern baldness is an inherited trait that may not become obvious until well into adulthood.

This chapter explores the stages of the human life cycle, the developmental backdrop against which genes function.

3.1 The Reproductive System

The formation of a new individual begins with a **sperm** from a male and an ovum (more precisely, an **oocyte**) from a female. Sperm and oocytes are **gametes,** or sex cells. They provide a mechanism for forming a new individual and mix genetic contributions from past generations. As a result, each person (except for identical multiples) has a unique combination of inherited traits.

Sperm and oocytes are produced in the reproductive system, which is organized similarly in the male and female. Each system has paired structures, called **gonads,** where the sperm and oocytes are manufactured; tubules to transport these cells; and hormones and secretions that control the process.

The Male

Sperm cells develop within a 125-meter-long network of **seminiferous tubules,** which are packed into paired, oval organs called **testes** (sometimes called testicles) (**figure 3.1**). The testes are the male gonads. They lie outside the abdomen within a sac

called the scrotum. Lying outside the abdominal cavity exposes the testes to a lower temperature than the rest of the body, which is necessary for sperm to develop. Leading from each testis is a tightly coiled tube, the **epididymis,** in which sperm cells mature and are stored; each epididymis continues into another tube, the **vas deferens.** Each vas deferens bends behind the bladder to join the **urethra,** the tube that carries both sperm and urine out through the penis.

Along the sperm's path, three glands produce secretions. The vasa deferentia pass through the **prostate gland,** which produces a thin, milky, alkaline fluid that activates the sperm to swim. Opening into the vas deferens is a duct from the **seminal vesicles,** which secrete fructose (a sugar that supplies sperm with energy), plus hormonelike prostaglandins, which may stimulate contractions in the female that help sperm and oocyte meet. Each about the size of a pea, the **bulbourethral glands** join the urethra where it passes through the body wall. They secrete an alkaline mucus that coats the urethra before sperm are released. All of these secretions combine to form the **seminal fluid** that carries sperm.

During sexual arousal, the penis becomes erect so that it can penetrate and deposit sperm in the female reproductive tract. At the peak of sexual stimulation, a pleasurable sensation called **orgasm** occurs, accompanied by rhythmic muscular contractions that eject the sperm from each vas deferens through the urethra and out the penis. The discharge of sperm from the penis, called ejaculation, delivers about 200 to 600 million sperm cells.

The Female

The female sex cells develop within paired organs in the abdomen called **ovaries** (**figure 3.2**), which are the female gonads. Within each ovary of a newborn female are about a million immature oocytes. Each individual oocyte is surrounded by nourishing **follicle cells,** and each ovary houses oocytes in different stages of development. After puberty, about once a month, one ovary releases the most mature oocyte. Beating cilia sweep the

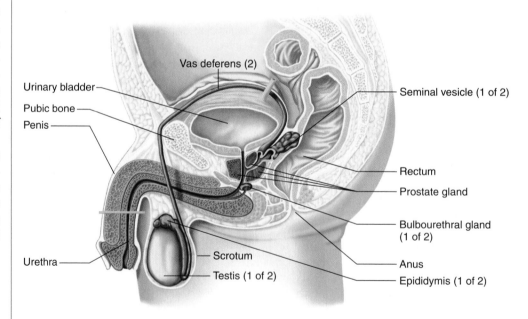

Figure 3.1 The human male reproductive system. Sperm cells are manufactured within the seminiferous tubules, tightly wound within the testes, which descend into the scrotum. The prostate gland, seminal vesicles, and bulbourethral glands add secretions to the sperm cells to form seminal fluid. Sperm mature and are stored in the epididymis and exit through the vas deferens. The paired vasa deferentia join in the urethra, through which seminal fluid exits the body.

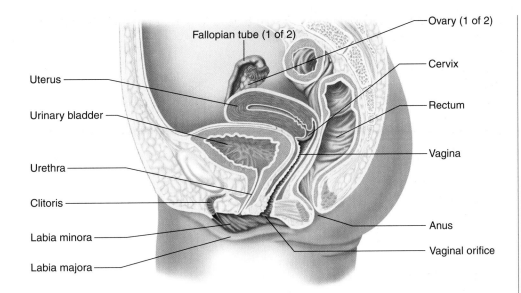

Fallopian tube (1 of 2)

Ovary (1 of 2)

Cervix

Uterus

Rectum

Urinary bladder

Vagina

Urethra

Clitoris

Anus

Labia minora

Vaginal orifice

Labia majora

Figure 3.2 The human female reproductive system. Oocytes are packed into the paired ovaries. Once a month after puberty, an ovary releases one oocyte, which is drawn into a nearby fallopian tube. If a sperm fertilizes the oocyte in the fallopian tube, the fertilized ovum continues into the uterus, where for nine months it develops into a new individual. If the oocyte is not fertilized, the body expels it, along with the built-up uterine lining.

mature oocyte into the fingerlike projections of one of two **fallopian tubes.** The tube carries the oocyte into a muscular, saclike organ called the **uterus,** or womb.

The released oocyte may encounter a sperm, usually in a fallopian tube. If the sperm enters the oocyte so that the genetic material of the two cells merges into a new nucleus, the result is a **fertilized ovum.** This cell undergoes a series of rapid cell divisions while moving through the tube and within days nestles into the lining of the uterus. Here, if all goes well, it will continue to develop. If fertilization does not occur, the oocyte, along with much of the uterine lining, is shed as the menstrual flow. Hormones coordinate the monthly menstrual cycle.

The lower end of the uterus narrows and leads to the **cervix,** which opens into the tubelike vagina that exits from the body. The vaginal opening is protected on the outside by two pairs of fleshy folds. At the upper juncture of both pairs is a 2-centimeter-long structure called the clitoris, which is anatomically similar to the penis. Rubbing the clitoris triggers female orgasm. Hormones control the cycle of oocyte maturation and the preparation of the uterus to nurture a fertilized ovum.

Key Concepts

Sperm develop in the seminiferous tubules, mature and collect in each epididymis, enter the vasa deferentia, and move through the urethra in the penis. The prostate gland adds an alkaline fluid, seminal vesicles add fructose and prostaglandins, and bulbourethral glands secrete mucus to form seminal fluid. • In the female, ovaries contain oocytes. Each month, an ovary releases an oocyte, which enters a fallopian tube leading to the uterus. If the oocyte is fertilized, it begins a series of rapid cell divisions and nestles into the uterine lining to develop. Otherwise, the oocyte exits the body with the menstrual flow. Hormones control the monthly cycle of oocyte development.

3.2 Meiosis

Gametes form from special cells, called germline cells, in a type of cell division called **meiosis** that halves the chromosome number. A further process, maturation, sculpts the distinctive characteristics of sperm and oocyte. The organelle-packed oocyte has 90,000 times the volume of the sperm. Unlike other cells in the

human body, gametes contain 23 different chromosomes—half the usual amount of genetic material, but still a complete genome. **Somatic** (nonsex) **cells** contain 23 pairs, or 46 chromosomes. The chromosome pairs are called **homologous pairs,** or *homologs* for short. Homologs have the same genes in the same order but may carry different alleles, or forms of the same gene. Gametes are **haploid** ($1n$), which means that they have only one of each type of chromosome and therefore one copy of the human genome. Somatic cells are **diploid** ($2n$), signifying that they have two copies of the genome.

Halving the number of chromosomes during gamete formation makes sense. If the sperm and oocyte each contained 46 chromosomes, the fertilized ovum would contain twice the normal number of chromosomes, or 92. Such a genetically overloaded cell, called a polyploid, usually does not develop. About one in a million newborns is polyploid, but these infants have abnormalities in all organ systems and usually only live a few days. However, studies on spontaneously aborted embryos indicate that about 1 percent of conceptions have three chromosome sets instead of the normal two, so that these embryos do not survive to be born.

Meiosis mixes up trait combinations. For example, a person might produce one gamete containing alleles encoding green eyes and freckles, yet another encoding brown eyes and no freckles. Meiosis explains why siblings genetically differ from each other and from their parents.

In a much broader sense, meiosis, as the mechanism of sexual reproduction, provides genetic diversity, which can help a population to survive a challenging environment. A population of sexually reproducing organisms is made up of individuals with different genotypes and phenotypes. In contrast, a population of asexually reproducing organisms consists of identical individuals. Should a new threat arise, such as an infectious disease that kills only individuals with a certain genotype, then the entire asexual population could be wiped out. In a sexually reproducing population, by contrast, individuals that inherited a certain combination of genes might survive. This differential survival of certain genotypes is

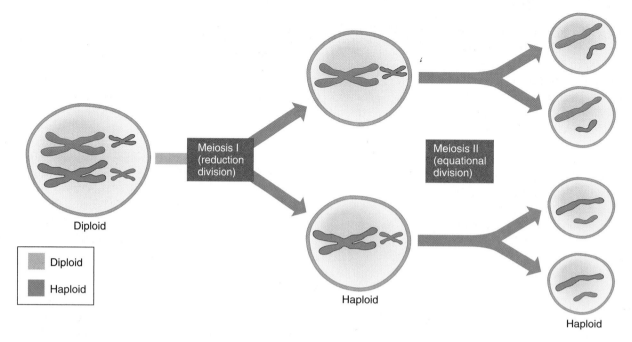

Diploid

Meiosis I (reduction division)

Meiosis II (equational division)

Diploid

Haploid

Haploid

Haploid

Haploid

Figure 3.3 Overview of meiosis. Meiosis is a form of cell division in which certain cells are set aside, and give rise to haploid gametes. The first meiotic division reduces the number of chromosomes to 23, all in the replicated form. In the second meiotic division, the cells essentially undergo mitosis. The result of the two meiotic divisions is four haploid cells. In this illustration, homologous pairs of chromosomes are indicated by size, and parental origin of chromosomes by color.

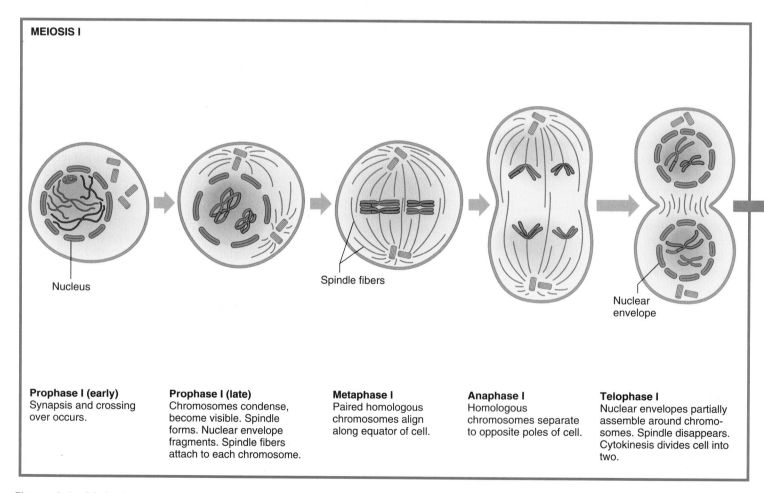

MEIOSIS I

Nucleus

Spindle fibers

Nuclear envelope

Prophase I (early)
Synapsis and crossing over occurs.

Prophase I (late)
Chromosomes condense, become visible. Spindle forms. Nuclear envelope fragments. Spindle fibers attach to each chromosome.

Metaphase I
Paired homologous chromosomes align along equator of cell.

Anaphase I
Homologous chromosomes separate to opposite poles of cell.

Telophase I
Nuclear envelopes partially assemble around chromosomes. Spindle disappears. Cytokinesis divides cell into two.

Figure 3.4 Meiosis.

the basis of evolution, discussed in chapter 16. Some microorganisms that can reproduce asexually or sexually revert to the sexual route when the environment changes.

Meiosis entails two divisions of the genetic material. The first division is called **reduction division** (or meiosis I) because it reduces the number of replicated chromosomes from 46 to 23. The second division, called the **equational division** (or meiosis II), produces four cells from the two cells formed in the first division by splitting the replicated chromosomes. **Figure 3.3** shows an overview of the process, and **figure 3.4** depicts the major events of each stage.

As in mitosis, meiosis occurs after an interphase period when DNA is replicated (doubled) **(table 3.1)**. For each chromosome pair in the cell undergoing meiosis, one homolog comes from the person's mother, and one from the father. In figures 3.3 and 3.4, the colors represent the contributions

Table 3.1

Comparison of Mitosis and Meiosis

Mitosis	Meiosis
One division	Two divisions
Two daughter cells per cycle	Four daughter cells per cycle
Daughter cells genetically identical	Daughter cells genetically different
Chromosome number of daughter cells same as that of parent cell (2n)	Chromosome number of daughter cells half that of parent cell (1n)
Occurs in somatic cells	Occurs in germline cells
Occurs throughout life cycle	In humans, completes after sexual maturity
Used for growth, repair, and asexual reproduction	Used for sexual reproduction, producing new gene combinations

of the two parents, whereas size indicates different chromosomes.

After interphase, prophase I (so called because it is the prophase of meiosis I) begins as the replicated chromosomes con-

dense and become visible when stained. A spindle forms. Toward the middle of prophase I, the homologs line up next to one another, gene by gene, in an event called **synapsis.** A mixture of RNA and protein

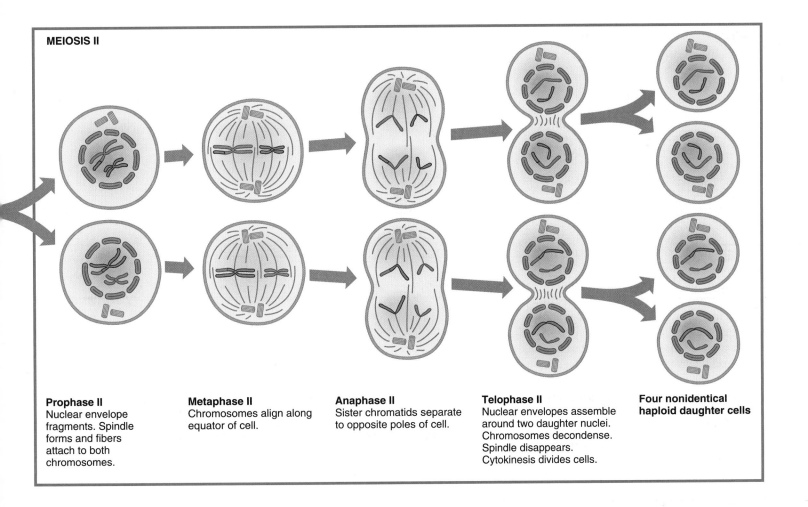

Prophase II
Nuclear envelope fragments. Spindle forms and fibers attach to both chromosomes.

Metaphase II
Chromosomes align along equator of cell.

Anaphase II
Sister chromatids separate to opposite poles of cell.

Telophase II
Nuclear envelopes assemble around two daughter nuclei. Chromosomes decondense. Spindle disappears. Cytokinesis divides cells.

Four nonidentical haploid daughter cells

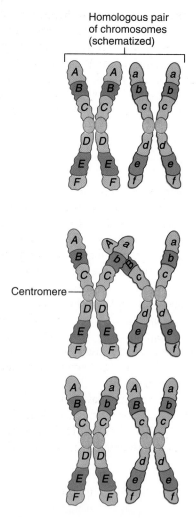

Figure 3.5 **Crossing over recombines genes.** Crossing over helps to generate genetic diversity by mixing parental traits. The capital and lowercase forms of the same letter represent different forms (alleles) of the same gene.

holds the chromosome pairs together. At this time, the homologs exchange parts in a process called **crossing over (figure 3.5).** All four chromatids that comprise each homologous chromosome pair are pressed together as exchanges occur. The four-chromatid arrangement is called a tetrad. After crossing over, each homolog contains genes from each parent. (Prior to this, all of the genes on a homolog were derived from one parent.) New gene combinations arise from crossing over when the parents carry different alleles. Toward the end of prophase I, the synapsed chromosomes separate but remain attached at a few points along their lengths.

To understand how crossing over mixes trait combinations, consider a simplified example. Suppose that homologs carry genes for hair color, eye color, and finger length. One of the chromosomes carries alleles for blond hair, blue eyes, and short fingers. Its homolog carries alleles for black hair, brown eyes, and long fingers. After crossing over, one of the chromosomes might bear alleles for blond hair, brown eyes, and long fingers, and the other might bear alleles for black hair, blue eyes, and short fingers. The daughter cells that result from meiosis carry a mix of the parent cell traits.

Meiosis continues in metaphase I, when the homologs align down the center of the cell. Each member of a homolog pair attaches to a spindle fiber at opposite poles. The pattern in which the chromosomes align during metaphase I is important in generating genetic diversity. For each homolog pair, the pole the maternally or paternally derived member goes to is random. The situation is analogous to the number of different ways that 23 boys and 23 girls could line up in boy-girl pairs. The greater the number of chromosomes, the greater the genetic diversity generated at this stage.

For two pairs of homologs, four (2^2) different metaphase configurations are possible. For three pairs of homologs, eight (2^3) different combinations can occur. Our 23 chromosome pairs can line up in 8,388,608 (2^{23}) different ways. This random arrangement of the members of homolog pairs in metaphase is called **independent assortment (figure 3.6).** It accounts for a basic law of inheritance discussed in the next chapter.

Homologs separate in anaphase I and finish moving to opposite poles by telophase I, establishing a haploid set of still-replicated chromosomes at each end of the stretched-out cell. Unlike in mitosis, the centromeres of each homolog in meiosis I remain together. During a second interphase, chromosomes unfold into very thin threads. Proteins are manufactured, but the genetic material is not repli-

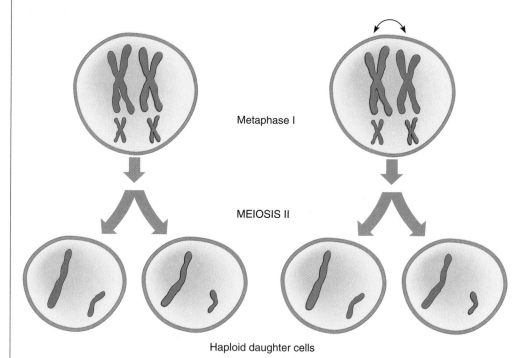

Metaphase I

MEIOSIS II

Haploid daughter cells

Figure 3.6 **Independent assortment.** The pattern in which homologs align during metaphase I determines the combination of maternally and paternally derived chromosomes in the daughter cells. Two pairs of chromosomes can align in two different ways to produce four different possibilities in the daughter cells. The potential variability that meiosis generates skyrockets when one considers all 23 chromosome pairs and the effects of crossing over.

cated a second time. The single DNA replication, followed by the double division of meiosis, halves the chromosome number.

Prophase II marks the start of the second meiotic division. The chromosomes are again condensed and visible. In metaphase II, the replicated chromosomes align down the center of the cell. In anaphase II, the centromeres part, and the newly formed chromosomes, each now in the unreplicated form, move to opposite poles. In telophase II, nuclear envelopes form around the four nuclei, which then separate into individual cells. The net result of meiosis is four haploid cells, each carrying a new assortment of genes and chromosomes that represent a single copy of the genome.

Meiosis generates astounding genetic variety. Any one of a person's more than 8 million possible combinations of chromosomes can meet with any one of the more than 8 million combinations of a partner, raising potential variability to more than 70 trillion $(8,388,608^2)$ genetically unique individuals! Crossing over contributes even more genetic variability.

Key Concepts

The haploid sperm and oocyte are derived from diploid germline cells by meiosis and maturation. Meiosis maintains the chromosome number over generations and mixes gene combinations. In the first meiotic (or reduction) division, the number of replicated chromosomes is halved. In the second meiotic (or equational) division, each of two cells from the first division divides again, yielding four cells from the original one. Chromosome number is halved because the DNA replicates once, but the cell divides twice. Crossing over and independent assortment generate further genotypic diversity by creating new combinations of alleles.

3.3 Gamete Maturation

Meiosis occurs in both sexes, but the sperm and oocyte look very different. Although each type of gamete is haploid, different distributions of other cell components create their distinctions. The cells of the maturing male and female proceed through similar stages, but with sex-specific terminology and different timetables. A male begins manufacturing sperm at puberty and continues throughout life, whereas a female begins meiosis when she is a fetus. Meiosis in the female is completed only if a sperm fertilizes the oocyte.

Sperm Development

Spermatogenesis, the formation of sperm cells, begins in a diploid cell called a **spermatogonium (figure 3.7).** This cell divides mitotically, yielding two daughter cells: one daughter cell continues to specialize into a mature sperm, and the other remains an unspecialized stem cell.

Bridges of cytoplasm join several spermatogonia, and their daughter cells enter meiosis together. As they mature, these spermatogonia accumulate cytoplasm and replicate their DNA, becoming **primary spermatocytes.**

During reduction division (meiosis I), each primary spermatocyte divides, forming two equal-sized haploid cells called **secondary spermatocytes.** In meiosis II,

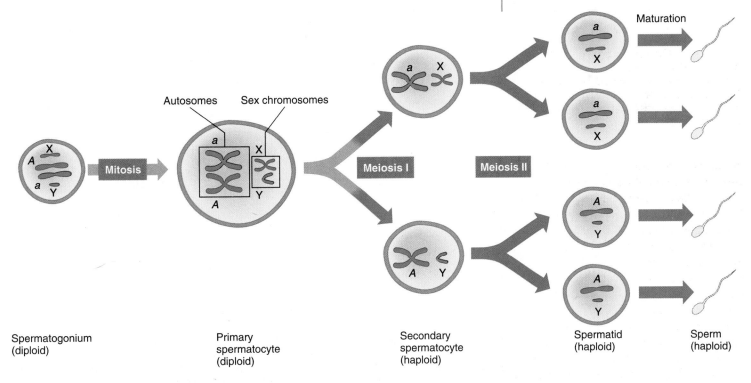

Autosomes   Sex chromosomes

Mitosis   Meiosis I   Meiosis II   Maturation

Spermatogonium (diploid)   Primary spermatocyte (diploid)   Secondary spermatocyte (haploid)   Spermatid (haploid)   Sperm (haploid)

Figure 3.7   Sperm formation (spermatogenesis).   Primary spermatocytes have the normal diploid number of 23 chromosome pairs. The large pair of chromosomes represents autosomes (non-sex chromosomes). The X and Y chromosomes are sex chromosomes.

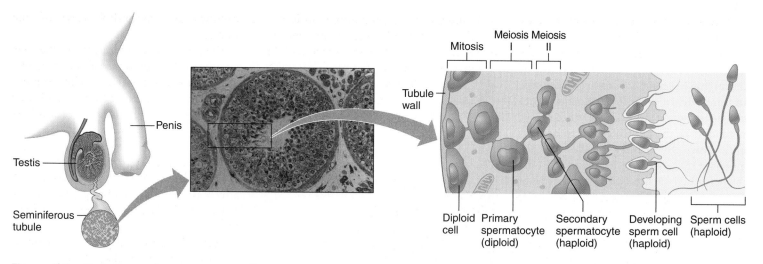

Figure 3.8 Meiosis produces sperm cells.   Diploid cells divide through mitosis in the linings of the seminiferous tubules. Some of the daughter cells then undergo meiosis, producing haploid spermatocytes, which differentiate into mature sperm cells.

each secondary spermatocyte divides to yield two equal-sized **spermatids.** Each spermatid then develops the characteristic sperm tail, or flagellum. The base of the tail has many mitochondria, which produce ATP molecules that propel the sperm inside the female reproductive tract. After spermatid differentiation, some of the cytoplasm connecting the cells falls away, leaving mature, tadpole-shaped **spermatozoa,** or sperm. **Figure 3.8** presents an anatomical view showing the stages of spermatogenesis within the seminiferous tubules.

A sperm, which is a mere 0.006 centimeters (0.0023 inch) long, must travel about 18 centimeters (7 inches) to reach an oocyte. Each sperm cell consists of a tail, body or midpiece, and a head region (**figure 3.9**). A membrane-covered area on the front end, the **acrosome,** contains enzymes that help the cell penetrate the protective layers around the oocyte. Within the bulbous sperm head, DNA is wrapped around proteins. The sperm's DNA at this time is genetically inactive. A male manufactures trillions of sperm in his lifetime. Although many of these will come close to an oocyte, very few will actually touch one.

Meiosis in the male has built-in protections that help prevent sperm from causing birth defects. Spermatogonia that are exposed to toxins tend to be so damaged that they never mature into sperm. More mature sperm cells exposed to toxins are often so damaged that they cannot swim.

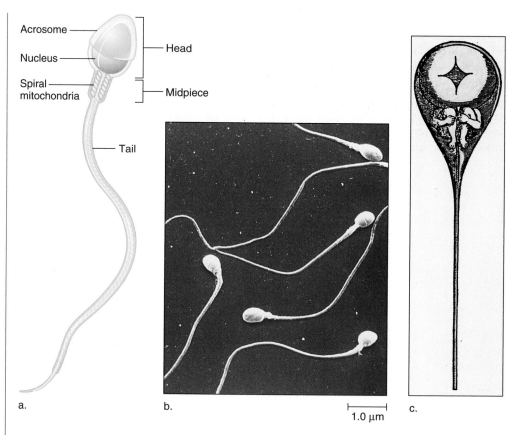

Figure 3.9 Sperm.   **(a)** A sperm contains distinct regions that assist in delivering DNA to an oocyte. **(b)** Scanning electron micrograph of human sperm cells. **(c)** This 1694 illustration by Dutch histologist Niklass Hartsoeker presents a once-popular hypothesis that a sperm carries a preformed human called a homunculus.

Oocyte Development

Meiosis in the female, called **oogenesis** (egg making), begins, as does spermatogenesis, with a diploid cell. This cell is an **oogonium.** Unlike the male cells, oogonia are not attached, but follicle cells surround each one. Each oogonium grows, accumulates cytoplasm, and replicates its DNA, becoming a **primary oocyte.** The ensuing meiotic division in oogenesis, unlike that in spermatogenesis, produces cells of different sizes.

In meiosis I, the primary oocyte divides into two cells: a small cell with very little cytoplasm, called a first **polar body,** and a much larger cell called a **secondary oocyte** (**figure 3.10**). Each cell is haploid, with the chromosomes in replicated form. In meiosis II, the tiny first polar body may divide to yield two polar bodies of equal size, with unreplicated chromosomes; or it may simply decompose. The secondary oocyte, however, divides unequally in meiosis II to produce another small polar body, with unreplicated chromosomes, and the mature egg cell, or ovum, which contains a large volume of cytoplasm. **Figure 3.11** summarizes meiosis in the female, and **figure 3.12** provides an anatomical view of the process.

Most of the cytoplasm among the four meiotic products in the female concentrates in only one cell, the ovum. The woman's body absorbs the polar bodies, and they normally play no further role in development. Rarely, a sperm fertilizes a polar body. The woman's hormones respond as if she is pregnant, but a clump of cells that is not an embryo grows for a few weeks, and then leaves the woman's body. This event is a type of miscarriage called a "blighted ovum."

Before birth, a female's million or so oocytes arrest in prophase I. By puberty, around 400,000 oocytes remain. After puberty, meiosis I continues in one or several oocytes each month, but halts again at metaphase II. In response to specific hormonal cues each month, one ovary releases a secondary oocyte; this event is **ovulation.** If a sperm penetrates the oocyte membrane, then female meiosis completes, and a fertilized ovum forms. If the secondary oocyte is not fertilized, it degenerates and leaves the body in the menstrual flow, meiosis never completed.

Figure 3.10 Meiosis in a female produces a secondary oocyte and a polar body. Unequal division enables the cell destined to become a fertilized ovum to accumulate the bulk of the cytoplasm and organelles from the primary oocyte, but with only one genome's worth of DNA. (×700)

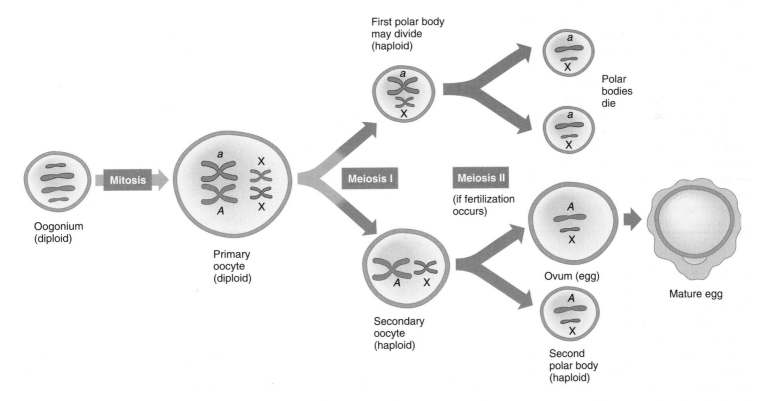

Figure 3.11 Ovum formation (oogenesis). Primary oocytes have the diploid number of 23 chromosome pairs. Meiosis in females is uneven, concentrating most of the cytoplasm into one large cell called an oocyte (or egg). The other products of meiosis, called polar bodies, contain the other three sets of chromosomes and are normally discarded.

Figure 3.12 The making of oocytes. Oocytes develop within the ovary in protective follicles. An ovary contains many oocytes in various stages of maturation. After puberty, the most mature oocyte in one ovary bursts out each month, an event called ovulation.

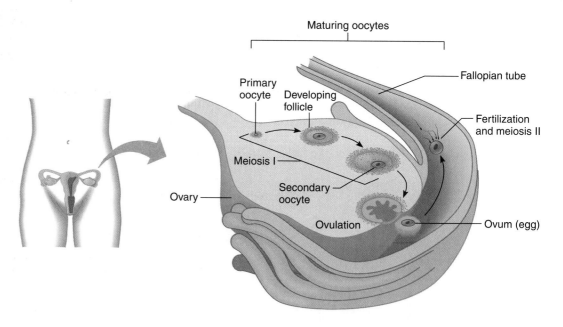

A female ovulates about 400 oocytes between puberty and menopause. Sperm cells are likely to enter only a few of these oocytes. Only one in three of the oocytes that do meet and merge with a sperm cell will continue to grow, divide, and specialize to eventually form a new individual.

Key Concepts

Spermatogonia divide mitotically, yielding one stem cell and one cell that accumulates cytoplasm and becomes a primary spermatocyte. In meiosis I, each primary spermatocyte halves its genetic material to form two secondary spermatocytes. In meiosis II, each secondary spermatocyte divides, yielding two equal-sized spermatids attached by bridges of cytoplasm. Maturing spermatids separate and shed some cytoplasm. A mature sperm has a tail, body, and head, with an enzyme-containing acrosome covering the head. • An oogonium accumulates cytoplasm and replicates its chromosomes, becoming a primary oocyte. In meiosis I, the primary oocyte divides, forming a small polar body and a large, haploid secondary oocyte. In meiosis II, the secondary oocyte divides, yielding another small polar body and a mature haploid ovum. Oocytes arrest at prophase I until puberty, after which one or several oocytes complete the first meiotic division during ovulation each month. The second meiotic division completes at fertilization.

3.4 Prenatal Development

A prenatal human is considered an **embryo** for the first eight weeks. During this time, rudiments of all body parts form. The embryo in the first week is considered to be in a "preimplantation" stage because it has not yet settled into the uterine lining. Prenatal development after the eighth week is the fetal period, when structures grow and specialize. The human organism between the start of the ninth week and birth is a **fetus.**

Fertilization

Hundreds of millions of sperm cells are deposited in the vagina during sexual intercourse. A sperm cell can survive in the woman's body for up to six days, but the oocyte can only be fertilized in the 12 to 24 hours after ovulation.

The woman's body helps sperm reach an oocyte. A process in the female called **capacitation** chemically activates sperm, and the oocyte secretes a chemical that attracts sperm. Sperm are also assisted by contractions of the female's muscles, by their moving tails, and by upwardly moving mucus propelled by cilia on cells of the female reproductive tract. Still, only 200 or so sperm come near the oocyte.

A sperm first contacts a covering of follicle cells, called the corona radiata, that guards a secondary oocyte. The sperm's acrosome then bursts, releasing enzymes that bore through a protective layer of glyco-protein, called the zona pellucida, beneath the corona radiata. Fertilization, or conception, begins when the outer membranes of the sperm and secondary oocyte meet (**figure 3.13**). The encounter is dramatic. A wave of electricity spreads physical and chemical changes across the entire oocyte surface—changes that keep other sperm out. More than one sperm can enter an oocyte, but the resulting cell has too much genetic material for development to follow.

Usually only the sperm's head enters the oocyte. Within 12 hours of the sperm's penetration, the ovum's nuclear membrane disappears, and the two sets of chromosomes, called **pronuclei,** approach one another. Within each pronucleus, DNA replicates. Fertilization completes when the two genetic packages meet and merge, forming the genetic instructions for a new individual. The fertilized ovum is called a zygote. The Bioethics: Choices for the Future reading on cloning and stem cell technology describes cloning, another way for an organism to begin development.

Early Events—Cleavage and Implantation

About a day after fertilization, the zygote divides by mitosis, beginning a period of frequent cell division called **cleavage** (**figure 3.14**). The resulting early cells are called **blastomeres.** When the blastomeres form a solid ball of sixteen or more cells, the embryo is called a **morula** (Latin for "mulberry," which it resembles).

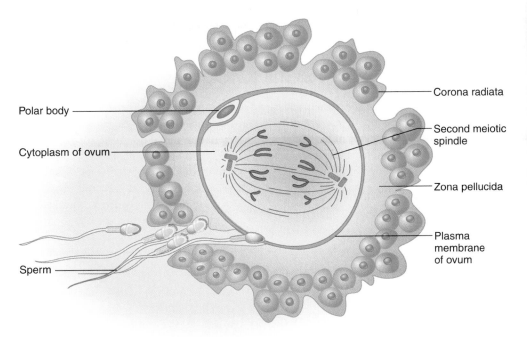

Polar body

Cytoplasm of ovum

Sperm

Corona radiata

Second meiotic spindle

Zona pellucida

Plasma membrane of ovum

a.

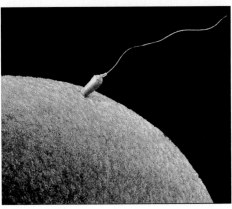

b.

Figure 3.13 Fertilization.
(a) Fertilization by a sperm cell induces the oocyte (arrested in metaphase II) to complete meiosis. Before fertilization occurs, the sperm's acrosome bursts, spilling enzymes that help the sperm's nucleus enter the oocyte. **(b)** A series of chemical reactions ensues that helps to ensure that only one sperm nucleus enters an oocyte.

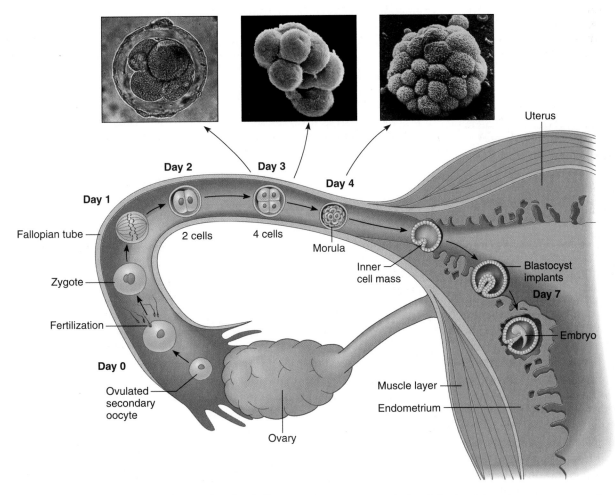

Figure 3.14 Cleavage: From ovulation to implantation. The zygote forms in the fallopian tube when a sperm nucleus fuses with the nucleus of an oocyte. The first divisions ensue while the zygote moves toward the uterus. By day 7, the zygote, now called a blastocyst, begins to implant in the uterine lining.

Considering Cloning and Stem Cell Technology

Fictional scientists have cloned Nazis, politicians, and dinosaurs. In actuality, the closest that cloning has come to humans is a sheep named Dolly, a mouse named Cumulina, a few farm animals, a cat named Cc, and a six-celled human embryo at a Massachusetts biotechnology company. Others have claimed to have cloned humans, but without evidence.

Cloning is the creation of a genetic replica of an individual. The technique transfers a nucleus from a somatic cell into an oocyte whose nucleus has been removed, and then develops new cells or a new individual from the manipulated cell. Figure 2.24 illustrates cloning taken to the 5-day stage of the embryo, to supply stem cells tailored to the individual, to treat disease or injury. In contrast, reproductive cloning seeks to create a baby using the nucleus from the cell of a particular individual who will then, supposedly, be duplicated. Creating a "copy" of a child killed in an accident by transferring a nucleus from one of her cells into an enucleated oocyte is reproductive cloning. Many people object to reproductive cloning of humans on ethical and practical grounds—it isn't necessary, and may not even work in humans.

The premises behind the technology may be biologically flawed, for a clone is not an exact replica of an individual. Many of the distinctions between an individual and a clone arise from epigenetic phenomena—effects that do not change genes themselves, but alter their expression. There are other distinctions, too (parentheses indicate chapters that discuss these subjects further):

- Telomeres of chromosomes in the donor nucleus are shorter than those in the recipient cell (chapter 2).

- Premature aging, as evidenced in shortened telomeres, may be why the first cloned mammal, Dolly, contracted a severe respiratory infection at six years. She was euthanized. Her immune system function may have been more like that of the other sheep living with her who also became ill, but were twice her age (**figure 1**).

- In normal development, for some genes, one copy is turned off, depending upon which parent transmits it. That is, some genes must be inherited from either the father or the mother to be active, a phenomenon called genomic imprinting. Genes in a donor nucleus do not pass through a germline before they go back to the beginning of development, and thus are not imprinted. Effects of lack of imprinting in clones aren't known, but it's clear that a first cell of an embryo derived from a somatic cell nucleus is not equivalent to a fertilized ovum (chapter 5).

- DNA from a donor cell has had years to accumulate mutations. Such a somatic mutation might not be noticeable if it occurs in one of millions of somatic cells, but it could be devastating if that somatic cell nucleus is used to program the development of an entire new individual. Donor DNA introducing mutations from the previous life may contribute to the very low success rates of animal cloning experiments (chapter 11).

- At a certain time in early prenatal development in all female mammals, one X chromosome is inactivated. Whether the inactivated X chromosome is from the mother or the father occurs at random in each cell, creating an

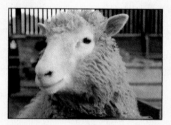

Figure 1 Dolly, the first cloned mammal. She was put to sleep when she contracted a respiratory illness in 2003. Dolly lived six years and had several healthy lambs.

During cleavage, organelles and molecules from the secondary oocyte's cytoplasm still control cellular activities, but some of the embryo's genes begin to function. The ball of cells hollows out, and its center fills with fluid, creating a **blastocyst**—the "cyst" referring to the fluid-filled center. Some of the cells form a clump. This is the **inner cell mass** that is used to derive embryonic stem cells (see figure 2.24). Formation of the inner cell mass is the first event that distinguishes cells from each other in terms of their relative positions, other than the inside and outside of the morula. The cells of the inner cell mass will continue developing to form the embryo.

A week after conception, the blastocyst begins to nestle into the rich lining of the woman's uterus. This event, called implantation, takes about a week. As it starts, the outermost cells of the embryo, called the **trophoblast,** secrete the "pregnancy hormone," **human chorionic gonadotropin** (hCG), which prevents menstruation. hCG detected in a woman's urine or blood is one sign of pregnancy.

The Embryo Forms

During the second week of prenatal development, a space called the **amniotic cavity** forms between the inner cell mass and the outer cells anchored to the uterine lining. Then the inner cell mass flattens into a two-layered disc. The layer nearest the amniotic cavity is the **ectoderm** (Greek for "outside skin"). The inner layer, closer to the blastocyst cavity, is the **endoderm** (Greek for "inside skin"). Shortly after, a third layer, the **mesoderm** ("middle skin"), forms in the middle. This three-layered structure is called the primordial embryo, or the **gastrula.**

Once these three layers, called **primary germ layers,** form, the fates of many cells are determined, which means that they are destined to develop as a specific cell type. Each layer gives rise to certain structures (**figure 3.15**). Cells in the ectoderm become

overall mosaic pattern of expression for genes on the X chromosome. The pattern of X inactivation of a female clone would most likely not match that of her nucleus donor (chapter 6).

- Mitochondria contain DNA. A clone's mitochondria descend from the recipient oocyte, not the donor cell.

The environment is another powerful factor in why a clone isn't really an identical copy. **Figure 2** shows one effect of the environment on gene expression. Although the calves in the figure were cloned from identical nuclei, they have slightly different coat color patterns. When the calves were embryos, cells destined to produce pigment moved about in a unique way in each calf, producing different color patterns. In humans, experience, nutrition, stress, exposure to infectious diseases, and other environmental influences join our genes in molding who we are. Identical twins, although they have the same DNA sequence (except for somatic mutations), are not exact replicas of each other. Similarly, cloning a deceased child would probably disappoint parents seeking to recapture their lost loved one.

A compelling argument against reproductive cloning that embraces both ethics and biology is that it would be cruel to create a child who would most likely suffer. Cloning rarely works in other types of animals. In the 1980s, a company called

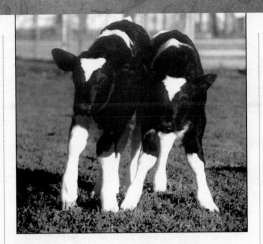

Figure 2 Cloned calves, George and Charlie.   Clones are not identical in phenotype. The color patterns on these cloned calves differ because of cell movements when they were embryos.

Granada Genetics cloned cattle from fetal cell nuclei, but the newborns were huge and required a great deal of care, a problem repeatedly seen in other cloned animals since then. There is no reason to assume that a newborn human clone will fare any better than other species.

Why does cloning so often fail? The reasons may lie in the fact that, as one researcher puts it, "The whole natural order [meaning meiosis] is broken." Recall that meiosis in the female completes at fertilization. In cloning, a diploid nucleus is plunked into oocyte cytoplasm, where signals direct it to

do what a female secondary oocyte tends to do—shed half of itself as a polar body. If the out-of-place donor nucleus does this, the new cell is haploid and will not develop. In humans and some other primates, the absence of an organelle, called a centrosome, from the sperm prevents chromosomes from aligning in metaphase so that division cannot occur. Another possible problem is that the donor nucleus may replicate its DNA. A genetic overload results, stopping development.

If human cloning ever becomes reality, we will probably learn that we are not merely the products of our genes. Consider cat Rainbow and her clone, Carbon Copy, or "Cc." Rainbow is hefty, Cc trim; Rainbow is shy, Cc aggressive and playful. The cats differ so greatly in personality and temperament that the company that created Cc, Genetic Savings and Clone, abandoned its original business plan to bring back dead pets, telling would-be clients that a clone is not a duplicate after all. Similarly, pig clones are no more alike than pig sibs. Cloned pigs differ in number of bristles and teeth, temperament, food favorites, and whether or not they like to cuddle with humans!

On a more serious note, the essence of the ethical objection to cloning is that we are dissecting and defining our very individuality, reducing it to a biochemistry so supposedly simple that we can duplicate it. We probably can't.

skin, nervous tissue, or parts of certain glands. Endoderm cells form parts of the liver and pancreas and the linings of many organs. The middle layer of the embryo, the mesoderm, forms many structures, including muscle, connective tissues, the reproductive organs, and the kidneys.

The idea that cell fates are set in the gastrula, however, is changing. Certain progenitor cells can **transdifferentiate,** which means that they can divide to yield cells specialized in a different way. For example, hematopoietic stem cells in the bone marrow can give rise to neurons, and vice versa. This was at first very surprising to researchers, because they had thought for many years that once a

cell was in a particular primary germ layer, it didn't stray. Yet in this example, bone marrow stem cells arise from mesoderm, while neurons normally derive from ectoderm. The word *normally* may be important here—transdifferentiation may occur naturally only in response to a certain type of injury. Perhaps no one noticed it in the past because nobody thought to look for it!

Table 3.2 summarizes the stages of early prenatal development.

Supportive Structures

As the embryo develops, structures form that support and protect it. These include chori-

onic villi, the placenta, the yolk sac, the allantois, the umbilical cord, and the amniotic sac.

By the third week after conception, fingerlike projections called **chorionic villi** extend from the area of the embryonic disc close to the uterine wall, projecting into pools of the woman's blood. Her blood system and the embryo's are separate, but nutrients and oxygen diffuse across the chorionic villi from her circulation to the embryo, and wastes leave the embryo's circulation and enter the woman's circulation to be excreted.

By 10 weeks, the placenta is fully formed. It links woman and fetus for the rest of the pregnancy. The placenta secretes hormones that maintain pregnancy and alter the

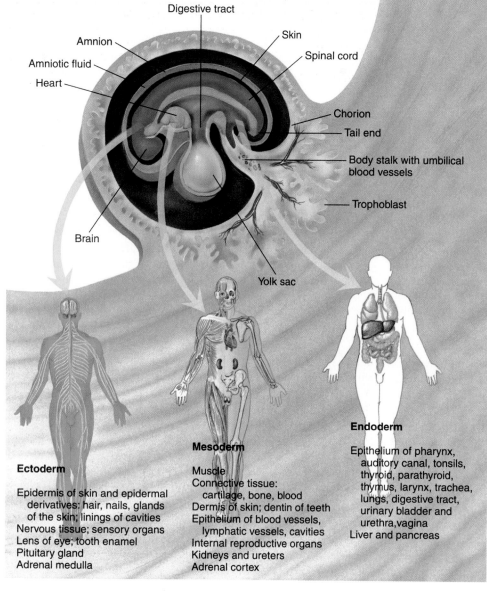

Figure 3.15 The primordial embryo. When the three basic layers of the embryo form, many cells become "determined" to follow a specific developmental pathway. However, each layer retains stem cells as the organism develops, and these cells may be capable of producing daughter cells that can specialize as any of many cell types, including some not associated with the layer of origin.

Labels in figure:
Digestive tract
Amnion
Amniotic fluid
Heart
Skin
Spinal cord
Chorion
Tail end
Body stalk with umbilical blood vessels
Trophoblast
Brain
Yolk sac

Ectoderm

Epidermis of skin and epidermal derivatives; hair, nails, glands of the skin; linings of cavities
Nervous tissue; sensory organs
Lens of eye; tooth enamel
Pituitary gland
Adrenal medulla

Mesoderm

Muscle
Connective tissue: cartilage, bone, blood
Dermis of skin; dentin of teeth
Epithelium of blood vessels, lymphatic vessels, cavities
Internal reproductive organs
Kidneys and ureters
Adrenal cortex

Endoderm

Epithelium of pharynx, auditory canal, tonsils, thyroid, parathyroid, thymus, larynx, trachea, lungs, digestive tract, urinary bladder and urethra, vagina
Liver and pancreas

woman's metabolism to send nutrients to the fetus.

Other structures nurture the developing embryo. The **yolk sac** manufactures blood cells, as does the **allantois,** a membrane surrounding the embryo that gives rise to the umbilical blood vessels. The umbilical cord forms around these vessels and attaches to the center of the placenta. Toward the end of the embryonic period, the yolk sac shrinks, and the amniotic sac swells with fluid that cushions the embryo and maintains a con-

stant temperature and pressure. The amniotic fluid contains fetal urine and cells.

Two of the supportive structures that develop during pregnancy provide the material for prenatal tests (see figure 13.6), discussed in chapter 13. Chorionic villus sampling examines chromosomes from cells snipped off the chorionic villi at 10 weeks. Because the villi cells and the embryo's cells come from the same fertilized ovum, an abnormal chromosome detected in villi cells should also be in the

embryo. In amniocentesis, a sample of amniotic fluid is taken after the fourteenth week of pregnancy, and fetal cells in the fluid are examined for biochemical, genetic, and chromosomal anomalies.

Multiples

Twins and other multiples arise early in development.

Twins are either fraternal or identical. Fraternal, or **dizygotic** (DZ), twins result when two sperm fertilize two oocytes. This can happen if ovulation occurs in two ovaries in the same month, or if two oocytes leave the same ovary and are both fertilized. DZ twins are no more alike than any two siblings, although they share a very early environment in the uterus. The tendency to have DZ twins may run in families if certain women tend to ovulate two oocytes a month.

Identical, or **monozygotic** (MZ), twins descend from a single fertilized ovum and therefore are genetically identical. They are natural clones. Three types of MZ twins form, depending upon when the fertilized ovum or very early embryo splits (**figure 3.16**). This difference in timing determines which supportive structures the twins share. About a third of all MZ twins have completely separate chorions and amnions, and about two-thirds share a chorion but have separate amnions. Slightly fewer than 1 percent of MZ twins share both amnion and chorion. (The amnion is the sac that contains fluid that surrounds the fetus. The chorion develops into the placenta.) The significance of these differences, if any, is that they determine whether MZ twins develop in slightly different uterine environments. For example, if one chorion develops more attachment sites to the maternal circulation, one twin may receive more nutrients and gain more weight.

In 1 in 50,000 to 100,000 pregnancies, an embryo divides into twins after the point at which the two groups of cells can develop as two individuals, between days 13 and 15. The result is conjoined or "Siamese" twins. The latter name comes from Chang and Eng, who were born in Thailand, then called Siam, in 1811. They were joined by a band of tissue from the navel to the breastbone, and could easily have been separated today. Chang and Eng lived for 63 years, attached. They fathered 22 children and divided each week between their wives.

In the case of Abigail and Brittany Hensel, shown in **figure 3.17,** the separation occurred after day 9 of development, but before day 14. Biologists determined this because the girls' shared organs contain representatives of ectoderm, mesoderm, and endoderm; that is, when the lump of cells divided incompletely, the three primary germ layers had not yet completely sorted themselves out. The Hensel girls are extremely rare "incomplete twins." Each girl has her own neck, head, heart, stomach, and gallbladder. Each has one leg and one arm, and a third arm between their heads was surgically removed. Each girl also has her own

Table 3.2

Stages and Events of Early Human Prenatal Development

Stage	Time Period	Principal Events
Fertilized ovum	12–24 hours following ovulation	Oocyte fertilized; zygote has 23 pairs of chromosomes and is genetically distinct
Cleavage	30 hours to third day	Mitosis increases cell number
Morula	Third to fourth day	Solid ball of cells
Blastocyst	Fifth day through second week	Hollowed ball forms trophoblast (outside) and inner cell mass, which implants and flattens to form embryonic disc
Gastrula	End of second week	Primary germ layers form

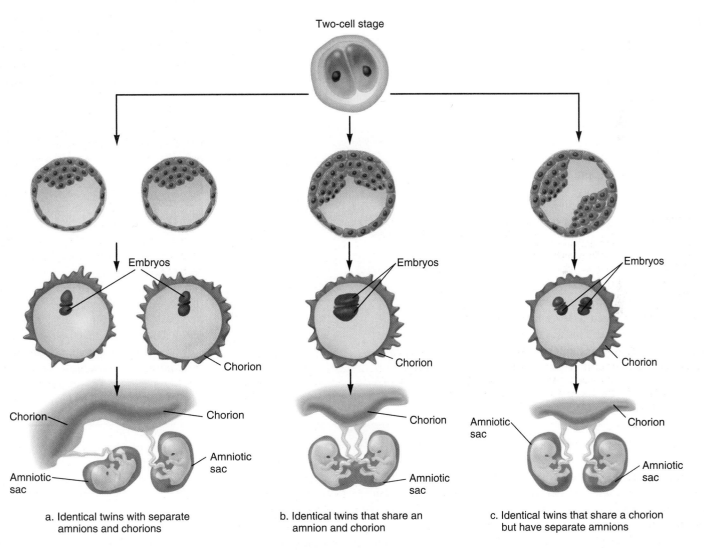

a. Identical twins with separate amnions and chorions

b. Identical twins that share an amnion and chorion

c. Identical twins that share a chorion but have separate amnions

Figure 3.16 Facts about twins. Identical twins originate at three points in development. **(a)** In about one-third of identical twins, separation of cells into two groups occurs before the trophoblast forms on day 5. These twins have separate chorions and amnions. **(b)** About 1 percent of identical twins share a single amnion and chorion, because the tissue splits into two groups after these structures have already formed. **(c)** In about two-thirds of identical twins, the split occurs after day 5 but before day 9. These twins share a chorion but have separate amnions. Fraternal twins result from two sperm fertilizing two secondary oocytes. These twins develop their own amniotic sacs, yolk sacs, allantois, placentae, and umbilical cords.

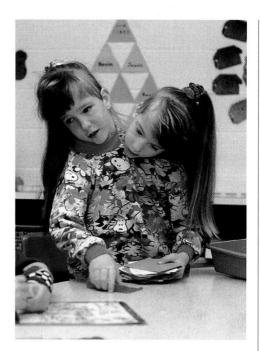

Figure 3.17 Conjoined twins.
Abby and Britty Hensel are the result of incomplete twinning during the first two weeks of prenatal development.

nervous system! The twins share a large liver, a single bloodstream, and all organs below the navel. They have three lungs and three kidneys. Because Abby and Britty were strong and healthy, doctors suggested surgery to separate them. But their parents, aware from other cases that only one child would likely survive a separation, chose to let their daughters be.

Surgical separation of conjoined twins is more likely to succeed if fewer body parts are shared or attached. This was the case for Maria de Jesus and Maria Teresa, born in Guatemala in 2001 and separated before they celebrated their first birthday. They were joined at the head, but facing opposite directions, so they could not do much more than roll around. The surgery took 23 hours! Today they are well. The outcome wasn't good for Landan and Laleh Bijani, 29-year-old Iranian conjoined twins who could no longer stand being joined along their heads, with their brains fused. They died shortly after 50 hours of surgery in 2003.

MZ twins occur in 3 to 4 pregnancies per 1,000 births worldwide. In North America, twins occur in about 1 in 81 pregnancies, which means that 1 in 40 of us is a twin. However, not all twins survive to be born. One study of twins detected early in pregnancy showed that up to 70 percent of the eventual births are of a single child. This is called the "vanishing twin" phenomenon.

The Embryo Develops

As the days and weeks proceed, different rates of cell division in different parts of the embryo fold the forming tissues into intricate patterns. In a process called embryonic induction, the specialization of one group of cells causes adjacent groups of cells to specialize. Gradually, these changes mold the three primary germ layers into organs and organ systems. **Organogenesis** is the transformation of the simple three layers of the embryo into distinct organs. During the weeks of organogenesis, the developing embryo is particularly sensitive to environmental influences such as chemicals and viruses.

During the third week of prenatal development, a band called the **primitive streak** appears along the back of the embryo. The primitive streak gradually elongates to form an axis that other structures organize around as they develop. The primitive streak eventually gives rise to connective tissue precursor cells and the **notochord,** a structure that forms the basic framework of the skeleton. The notochord induces overlying ectoderm to specialize into a hollow **neural tube,** which develops into the brain and spinal cord (central nervous system). Some nations designate day 14 of prenatal development and primitive streak formation as the point beyond which they ban research on the human embryo. The reason is that the primitive streak is the first sign of a nervous system, and day 14 is also the time at which implantation is complete.

Appearance of the neural tube marks the beginning of organ development. Shortly after, a reddish bulge containing the heart appears. The heart begins to beat around day 18, and this is easily detectable by day 22. Soon the central nervous system starts to form.

The fourth week of embryonic existence is one of spectacularly rapid growth and

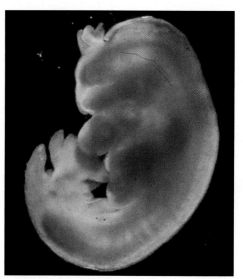

a. 28 days   4–6 mm

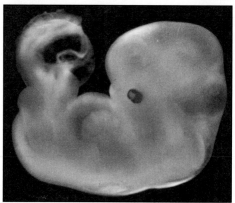

b. 42 days   12–15 mm

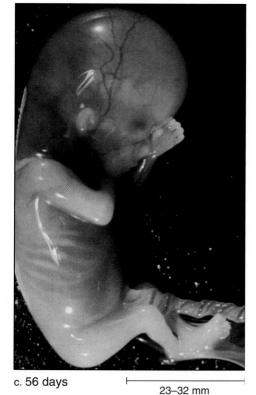

c. 56 days   23–32 mm

Figure 3.18 Human embryos.
Embryos at **(a)** 28 days, **(b)** 42 days, and **(c)** 56 days.

differentiation (**figure 3.18**). Arms and legs begin to extend from small buds on the torso. Blood cells form and fill primitive blood vessels. Immature lungs and kidneys appear.

If the neural tube does not close normally by about day 28, a neural tube defect results, leaving an area of the spine open and allowing parts of the brain or spinal cord to protrude (see Reading 16.1). If this happens, a substance from the fetus's liver called alpha fetoprotein (AFP) leaks at an abnormally rapid rate into the pregnant woman's circulation. A maternal blood test at the fifteenth week of pregnancy measures AFP levels. If they are elevated, further tests measure AFP in the amniotic fluid, and ultrasound is used to visualize a defect. (Ultrasound scanning bounces sound waves off the fetus, creating an image; see figure 13.7.)

By the fifth and sixth weeks, the embryo's head appears to be too large for the rest of its body. Limbs end in platelike structures with tiny ridges, and gradually apoptosis sculpts the fingers and toes. The eyes are open, but they do not yet have lids or irises. By the seventh and eighth weeks, a skeleton composed of cartilage forms. The embryo is now about the length and weight of a paper clip. At eight weeks of gestation, the prenatal human has rudiments of all of the structures that will be present at birth. It is now a fetus.

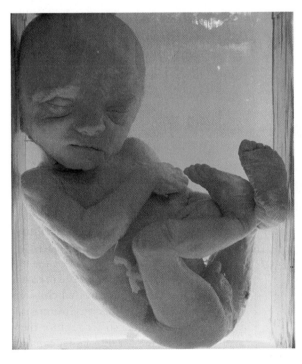

Figure 3.19   A fetus at 24 weeks.
At this stage and beyond, a fetus can survive outside of the uterus—but many do not.

The Fetus

During the fetal period, body proportions approach those of a newborn (**figure 3.19**). Initially, the ears lie low, and the eyes are widely spaced. Bone begins to replace the softer cartilage. As nerve and muscle functions become coordinated, the fetus moves.

Sex is determined at conception, when a sperm bearing an X or Y chromosome meets an oocyte, which always carries an X chromosome. An individual with two X chromosomes is a female, and one with an X and a Y is a male. A gene on the Y chromosome, called SRY (for "sex-determining region of the Y"), determines maleness. Differences between the sexes do not appear until week 6, after the SRY gene is activated in males. Male hormones then stimulate male reproductive organs and glands to differentiate from existing, indifferent structures. In a female, the indifferent structures of the early embryo develop as female organs and glands. Differences may begin to be noticeable on ultrasound scans by 12 to 15 weeks. Sexuality is discussed further in chapter 6.

By week 12, the fetus sucks its thumb, kicks, makes fists and faces, and has the beginnings of teeth. It breathes amniotic fluid in and out, and urinates and defecates into it. The first trimester (three months) of pregnancy ends.

By the fourth month, the fetus has hair, eyebrows, lashes, nipples, and nails. By 18 weeks, the vocal cords have formed, but the fetus makes no sounds because it doesn't breathe air. By the end of the fifth month, the fetus curls into a head-to-knees position. It weighs about 454 grams (1 pound). During the sixth month, the skin appears wrinkled because there isn't much fat beneath it (figure 3.19). The skin turns pink as capillaries fill with blood. By the end of the second trimester, the woman feels distinct kicks and jabs and may even detect a fetal hiccup. The fetus is now about 23 centimeters (9 inches) long.

In the final trimester, fetal brain cells rapidly form networks as organs elaborate and grow. A layer of fat forms beneath the skin. The digestive and respiratory systems mature last, which is why infants born prematurely often have difficulty digesting milk and breathing. Approximately 266 days after a single sperm burrowed its way into an oocyte, a baby is ready to be born.

The birth of a live, healthy baby is against the odds. Of every 100 secondary oocytes exposed to sperm, 84 are fertilized. Of these 84, 69 implant in the uterus, 42 survive one week or longer, 37 survive six weeks or longer, and only 31 are born alive. Of the fertilized ova that do not survive, about half have chromosomal abnormalities that cause problems too severe for development to proceed.

Key Concepts

Following sexual intercourse, sperm are capacitated and drawn to the secondary oocyte. Acrosomal enzymes assist the sperm's penetration of the oocyte, and chemical and electrical changes in the oocyte's surface block additional sperm from entering. The two sets of chromosomes meet, forming a zygote. • Cleavage cell divisions form a morula and then a blastocyst. The outer layer of cells invades and implants in the uterine lining. The inner cell mass develops into the embryo. Certain blastocyst cells secrete hCG. • Germ layers form in the second week. Cells in a specific germ layer later become parts of particular organ systems as a result of differential gene expression. • During week 3, chorionic villi extend toward the maternal circulation, and the placenta begins to form. Nutrients and oxygen enter the embryo, and wastes pass from the embryo into the maternal circulation. The yolk sac and allantois manufacture blood cells, the umbilical cord forms, and the amniotic sac expands with fluid. • Monozygotic twins arise from a single fertilized ovum and may share supportive structures. Dizygotic twins arise from two fertilized ova. • During week 3, the primitive streak appears, followed rapidly by the notochord, neural tube, heart, central nervous system, limbs, digits, facial features, and other organ rudiments. By week 8, all of the organs that will be present in the newborn have begun to develop. • During the fetal period, structures grow, specialize, and begin to interact. Bone replaces cartilage in the skeleton, body growth catches up with the head, and sex organs become more distinct. In the final trimester, the fetus moves and grows rapidly, and fat fills out the skin.

3.5 Birth Defects

When genetic abnormalities or toxic exposures affect an embryo or fetus, developmental problems occur, resulting in birth defects. Only a genetically caused birth defect can be passed to future generations. Although development can be derailed in many ways, about 97 percent of newborns appear healthy at birth.

The Critical Period

The specific nature of a birth defect usually depends on which structures are developing when the damage occurs. The time when genetic abnormalities, toxic substances, or viruses can alter a specific structure is its **critical period (figure 3.20)**. Some body parts, such as fingers and toes, are sensitive for short periods of time. In contrast, the brain is sensitive throughout prenatal development, and connections between nerve cells continue to change throughout life. Because of the brain's continuous critical period, many birth defect syndromes include mental retardation.

About two-thirds of all birth defects arise from a disruption during the embryonic period. More subtle defects, such as learning disabilities, that become noticeable only after infancy are often caused by interventions during the fetal period. A disruption in the first trimester might cause mental retardation; in the seventh month of pregnancy, it might cause difficulty in learning to read.

Some birth defects can be attributed to an abnormal gene that acts at a specific point in prenatal development. In a rare inherited condition called phocomelia, for example, an abnormal gene halts limb development from the third to the fifth week of the embryonic period, causing the infant to be born with "flippers" in place of arms and legs. The risk that a genetically caused birth defect will affect a particular family member can be calculated.

Many birth defects are caused not by genes but by toxic substances the pregnant woman encounters. These environmentally caused problems will not affect another family member unless the exposure occurs again. Chemicals or other agents that cause birth defects are called **teratogens** (Greek for "monster-causing"). While it is best to avoid teratogens while pregnant, some women may need to remain on a potentially teratogenic drug to maintain their own health.

Teratogens

Most drugs are not teratogens. **Table 3.3** lists some that are.

Thalidomide

The idea that the placenta protects the embryo and fetus from harmful substances was tragically disproven between 1957 and 1961, when 10,000 children were born in Europe with what seemed, at first, to be phocomelia. Because doctors realized that this genetic disorder is very rare, they began to look for another cause. They soon discovered that the mothers had all taken a mild tranquilizer, thalidomide, early in pregnancy, during the time an embryo's limbs form, to alleviate the nausea of morning sickness. "Thalidomide babies" were often born with incomplete or missing legs and arms.

The United States was spared from the thalidomide disaster because an astute government physician noted the drug's adverse effects on laboratory monkeys. Still, several "thalidomide babies" were born in South America in 1994, where pregnant women were given the drug. In spite of its teratogenic effects, thalidomide is still a valuable drug—it is used to treat leprosy and certain blood and bone marrow cancers.

Cocaine

Cocaine is very dangerous to the unborn. It can cause spontaneous abortion by inducing a stroke in the fetus. Cocaine-exposed infants who do survive are more distracted and unable to concentrate on their surroundings than unexposed infants. Other health and behavioral problems arise as these children grow.

One problem in evaluating the prenatal effects of cocaine is that affected children are often exposed to other environmental influences that could also account for their symptoms. Cocaine use by a father can also affect an embryo because the cocaine binds to sperm.

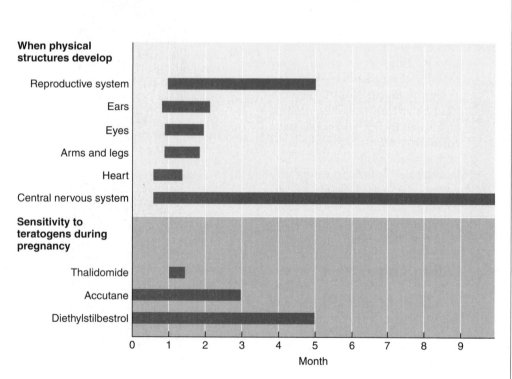

Figure 3.20 Critical periods of development. The nature of a birth defect resulting from drug exposure depends upon which structures were developing at the time of exposure. The time when a particular structure is vulnerable is called its critical period. Accutane is an acne medication. Diethylstilbestrol (DES) was used in the 1950s to prevent miscarriage. Thalidomide was used to prevent morning sickness.

Table 3.3

Teratogenic Drugs

Drug	Medical Use	Risk to Fetus
Alkylating agents	Cancer chemotherapy	Growth retardation
Aminopterin, methotrexate	Cancer chemotherapy	Skeletal and brain malformations
Coumadin derivatives	Seizure disorders	Tiny nose Hearing loss Bone defects Blindness
Diethylstilbestrol (DES)	Repeat miscarriage	Vaginal cancer, vaginal adenosis Small penis
Diphenylhydantoin (Dilantin)	Seizures	Cleft lip, palate Heart defects Small head
Isotretinoin (Accutane)	Severe acne	Cleft palate Heart defects Abnormal thymus Eye defects Brain malformation
Lithium	Bipolar disorder	Heart and blood vessel defects
Penicillamine	Rheumatoid arthritis	Connective tissue abnormalities
Progesterone in birth control pills	Contraception	Heart and blood vessel defects Masculinization of female structures
Tetracycline	Antibiotic	Stained teeth
Thalidomide	Morning sickness	Limb defects

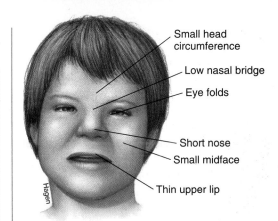

Small head circumference
Low nasal bridge
Eye folds
Short nose
Small midface
Thin upper lip

Hagen

a.

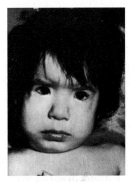

b.

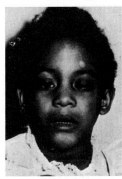

c.

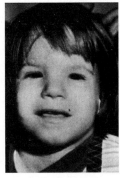

d.

Figure 3.21   Fetal alcohol syndrome. Some children whose mothers drank alcohol during pregnancy have characteristic flat faces **(a)** that are strikingly similar in children of different races **(b, c,** and **d).**

Cigarettes

Chemicals in cigarette smoke stress a fetus. Carbon monoxide crosses the placenta and prevents the fetus's hemoglobin molecules from adequately binding oxygen. Other chemicals in smoke prevent nutrients from reaching the fetus. Smoke-exposed placentas lack important growth factors, causing poor growth before and after birth. Cigarette smoking during pregnancy increases the risk of spontaneous abortion, stillbirth, prematurity, and low birth weight.

Alcohol

A pregnant woman who has just one or two alcoholic drinks a day, or perhaps a large amount at a single crucial time in prenatal development, risks fetal alcohol syndrome (FAS) in her unborn child. In the future, tests for gene variants that encode proteins that regulate alcohol metabolism will be able to predict which women and fetuses are at elevated risk for developing fetal alcohol syndrome.

A child with FAS has a characteristic small head, and a flat face and nose (**figure 3.21**). Growth is slow before and after birth. Intellectual impairment ranges from minor learning disabilities to mental retardation. Teens and young adults who have FAS are short and have small heads. More than 80 percent of them retain the facial characteristics of a young child with FAS.

The long-term mental effects of prenatal alcohol exposure are more severe than the physical vestiges. Many adults with FAS function at early grade-school level. They often lack social and communication skills and find it difficult to understand the consequences of actions, form friendships, take initiative, and interpret social cues.

Aristotle noticed problems in children of alcoholic mothers more than 23 centuries ago. In the United States today, 1 to 3 of every 1,000 infants has the syndrome, meaning 2,000 to 6,000 affected children are born each year. Many more children have milder "alcohol-related effects." A fetus of a woman with active alcoholism has a 30 to 45 percent chance of harm from prenatal alcohol exposure.

Nutrients

Certain nutrients ingested in large amounts, particularly vitamins, act as drugs. The acne medicine isotretinoin (Accutane) is a vitamin A derivative that causes spontaneous abortion and defects of the heart, nervous system, and face in exposed embryos. Physicians first noted the tragic effects of this drug nine months after dermatologists began prescribing it to young women in the early 1980s. Another vitamin A-based drug used to treat psoriasis, as well as excesses of vitamin A itself, also cause birth defects. Some forms of vitamin A are stored in body fat for up to three years.

Excessive exposure to vitamin C can also harm a fetus. The fetus becomes accustomed to the large amounts the woman takes; after birth, when the vitamin supply suddenly plummets, the baby may develop symptoms of vitamin C deficiency (scurvy). Such a baby bruises easily and is prone to infection.

Malnutrition threatens the fetus as well. A woman must consume extra calories while she is pregnant or breastfeeding. Obstetrical records of pregnant women before, during, and after World War II link inadequate nutrition in early pregnancy to an increase in the incidence of spontaneous abortion. The aborted fetuses had very little brain tissue. Poor nutrition later in pregnancy affects the development of the placenta and can cause low birth weight, short stature, tooth decay, delayed sexual development, and learning disabilities. Some effects of prenatal malnutrition may not become apparent for years, as is discussed in the next section.

Occupational Hazards

Some people encounter teratogens in the workplace. Researchers note increased rates of spontaneous abortion and children born with birth defects among women who work with textile dyes, lead, certain photographic chemicals, semiconductor materials, mercury, and cadmium. Men whose jobs expose them to sustained heat, such as smelter workers, glass manufacturers, and bakers, may produce sperm that can fertilize an oocyte and then cause spontaneous abortion or a birth defect. A virus or a toxic chemical carried in semen may also cause a birth defect.

Viral Infection

Viruses are small enough to cross the placenta and reach a fetus. Some viruses that cause mild symptoms in an adult, such as the virus that causes chickenpox, may devastate a fetus. Men can transmit infections to an embryo or fetus during sexual intercourse.

HIV can reach a fetus through the placenta or infect a newborn via blood contact during birth. Fifteen to 30 percent of infants born to HIV-positive women are HIV positive themselves. The risk of transmission is significantly reduced if the woman takes anti-HIV drugs while pregnant. All fetuses of HIV-infected women are at higher risk for low birth weight, prematurity, and stillbirth if the woman's health is failing.

German measles (rubella) is a well-known viral teratogen. Australian physicians first noted its effects in 1941. In the United States, rubella did not gain public attention until the early 1960s, when an epidemic of the usually mild illness caused 20,000 birth defects and 30,000 stillbirths. Women who contract the virus during the first trimester of pregnancy run a high risk of bearing children with cataracts, deafness, and heart defects. In fetuses exposed during the second or third trimesters of pregnancy, rubella may cause, much later, learning disabilities, speech and hearing problems, and type I diabetes mellitus.

The incidence of these problems, called congenital rubella syndrome, has dropped markedly thanks to widespread vaccination. However, the syndrome resurfaces in unvaccinated populations. A resurgence in 1991 was attributed to a cluster of unvaccinated Amish women in rural Pennsylvania. In that isolated group, 14 of every 1,000 newborns had congenital rubella syndrome, compared to an incidence of 0.006 per 1,000 in the general U.S. population.

Herpes simplex virus can harm a fetus or newborn whose immune system is not yet completely functional. Forty percent of babies exposed to active vaginal herpes lesions become infected, and half of these infants die. Of those infants who are infected but survive, 25 percent sustain severe nervous system damage, and another 25 percent have widespread skin sores. A woman who has sores at the time of delivery can have a surgical delivery to protect the child.

Pregnant women are routinely checked for hepatitis B infection, which in adults causes liver inflammation, great fatigue, and other symptoms. Each year in the United States, 22,000 infants are infected with this virus during birth. These babies are healthy, but they are at high risk for developing serious liver problems as adults. When infected women are identified, a vaccine can be given to their newborns to help prevent complications.

Key Concepts

The critical period is the time during prenatal development when a structure is sensitive to damage from a faulty gene or environmental insult. Most birth defects develop during the embryonic period and are more severe than problems that arise during fetal development. • Teratogens are agents that cause birth defects.

3.6 Maturation and Aging

Aging begins at conception. Later on, as we age, the limited life spans of cells are reflected in the waxing and waning of biological structures and functions. Although some aspects of our anatomy and physiology peak very early—such as the number of brain cells or hearing acuity, which do so in childhood—age 30 seems to be a turning point for decline. Some researchers estimate that, after this age, the human body becomes functionally less efficient by about 0.8 percent each year.

Many diseases that begin in adulthood, or are associated with aging, have genetic components. Often these disorders are multifactorial, because it takes many years for environmental exposures to alter gene expression in ways that noticeably affect health. Following is a closer look at how genes may affect health throughout life.

Adult-Onset Inherited Disorders

Human prenatal development is a highly regulated program of genetic switches that are turned on at specific places and times. Environmental factors can affect how certain genes are expressed before birth, creating risks that appear much later. Specifically, adaptations that enable a fetus to grow despite near-starvation become risk factors for certain common illnesses of adulthood, such as coronary artery disease, stroke, hypertension, and type II diabetes mellitus. A fetus that does not receive adequate nutrition has intrauterine growth retardation (IUGR). Such an individual is born on time, but is very small. Premature infants, in contrast, are small but are born early, and are not predisposed to conditions resulting from IUGR.

More than one hundred studies clearly correlate low birth weight due to IUGR with increased incidence of cardiovascular disease. Much of the data come from war records—enough time has elapsed to study the effects of prenatal malnutrition as people age. A study of nearly 15,000 people born in Sweden from 1915 to 1929 correlates IUGR to heightened cardiovascular disease risk after age 65. Similarly, an analysis of individuals who were fetuses during a seven-month famine in the Netherlands in 1943 indicates a high rate of diabetes today. Experiments on intentionally starved sheep and rat fetuses support these historical findings.

How can poor nutrition before birth reverberate as disease many decades later? Perhaps to survive, the starving fetus redirects its circulation to protect vital organs such as the brain, as muscle mass and hormone production change to conserve energy. Growth-retarded babies have too little muscle tissue, and since muscle is the primary site of insulin action, glucose metabolism is altered. Thinness at birth, and the accelerated weight gain in childhood that often occurs to compensate, sets the stage for coronary heart disease and type II diabetes.

Symptoms of a genetic disease may begin at any time. In general, conditions that affect children are recessive. A fetus who has inherited osteogenesis imperfecta ("brittle bone disease"), for example, may already have broken bones. Dominantly inherited conditions more often start to affect health in early to middle adulthood. This is the case for polycystic kidney disease. Cysts that may have been present in the kidneys during one's twenties begin causing bloody urine, high blood pressure, and abdominal pain as one enters the thirties. Similarly, hundreds of benign polyps, symptomatic of familial polyposis of the colon (discussed in chapter 18), may coat the inside of the large intestine of a 20-year-old, but they do not cause bloody stools until the fourth decade, when some of them may become cancerous. The joint destruction of osteoarthritis may begin in one's thirties, but not become painful for another ten or twenty years. The personality changes, unsteady gait, and diminishing mental faculties of Huntington disease typically begin near age 40.

Five to 10 percent of Alzheimer disease cases are inherited and first produce symptoms in the forties and fifties. (Chapter 12 discusses mutations that cause Alzheimer disease.) German neurologist Alois Alzheimer first identified the condition in 1907 as affecting people in mid-adulthood. It strikes four million people in the United States annually, although most cases are not inherited. The noninherited cases usually begin later in life.

Alzheimer disease starts gradually. Mental function declines steadily for three to ten years after the first symptoms appear. Confused and forgetful, Alzheimer patients often wander away from family and friends. Finally, the patient cannot perform basic functions such as speaking or eating and usually must be cared for in a hospital or nursing home.

On autopsy, the brains of Alzheimer disease patients are found to contain deposits of a protein called beta amyloid in learning and memory centers. Alzheimer brains also contain structures called neurofibrillary tangles, which consist of a protein called tau. Tau binds to and disrupts microtubules in nerve cell branches, destroying the shape of the cell.

Accelerated Aging Disorders

Genes control aging both passively (as structures break down) and actively (by initiating new activities). A class of inherited diseases that accelerate the aging timetable vividly illustrates the role genes play in aging.

The most severe rapid aging disorders are the segmental progeroid syndromes. They were once called progerias, but the newer terminology reflects the fact that they do not hasten all aspects of aging. Most of these disorders, and possibly all of them, are caused by cells' inability to adequately repair DNA. This enables mutations that would ordinarily be corrected to persist. Over time, the accumulation of mutations destabilizes the entire genome, and even more mutations occur in somatic cells. The various changes that we associate with aging occur.

Table 3.4 lists the more common segmental progeroid syndromes. Those with more symptoms end life sooner. People

Table 3.4

Rapid Aging Syndromes

Disorder	Incidence	Average Life Span	OMIM Number
Ataxia telangiectasia	1/60,000	20	208900
Cockayne syndrome	1/100,000	20	216400
Hutchinson-Gilford syndrome	<1/1,000,000	13	176670
Rothmund-Thomson syndrome	<1/100,000	normal	268400
Trichothiodystrophy	<1/100,000	10	601675
Werner syndrome	<1/100,000	50	277700

The Centenarian Genome

The human genome is like a vast library that holds the clues to good health. One way to identify those clues is to probe the genomes of those who have lived the longest, past 100 years. These fortunate people are called centenarians. Usually they enjoy excellent health, remaining active and interested in community affairs, then succumb rapidly to a disease that usually claims people decades earlier.

Centenarians fall into three broad groups—about 20 percent of them never get the diseases that kill most people; 40 percent get these diseases, but at a much older age than average; and the other 40 percent live with and survive the more common disorders of aging. Researchers hope that learning which gene variants offer this protection will lead to better understanding of the disorders that strike most of us in later adulthood—including heart disease,

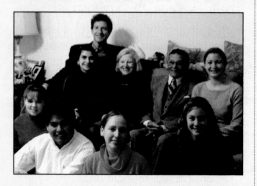

This centenarian (seated second from the right in the back row) was born in 1901. Centenarians are 1 in 10,000.

stroke, cancers, type II diabetes mellitus, and Alzheimer disease and other dementias.

While the environment seems to play an important role in the deaths of people ages 60 to 85, past that age, genes seem to predominate. That is, someone who dies at age 68 of lung cancer can probably blame a lifetime of cigarette smoking. But a smoker who dies at age 101 of the same disease probably had gene variants that protected against lung cancer. Centenarians have higher levels of large lipoproteins that carry cholesterol (HDL) than other people, which researchers estimate adds 20 years of life.

Evidence that longevity is largely inherited includes commonsense observations, such as the fact that the children and siblings of centenarians tend to be long-lived as well. Specifically, brothers of centenarians are 17 times as likely to live past age 100 than the average man, and sisters are 8.5 times as likely. The fact that some people more than 100 years of age have less-than-healthful habits suggests that genes are protecting them. One researcher suggests that the saying, "The older you get, the sicker you get" be replaced with "The older you get, the healthier you've been."

Centenarians have luckily inherited two types of gene variants—those that directly protect them, and variants of genes that, when mutant, cause disease. Research focuses on individual genes as well as genomewide scans to identify variants that make it more

likely one will live past age 100. **Table 1** lists some "candidate" gene types that may control longevity. To find other gene variants that promote long life, researchers are comparing the genomes of centenarians with those of people with particular conditions associated with aging. For example, a group of these very old people all have certain gene variants that differ from those in people with type II diabetes mellitus, suggesting that these DNA sequences may somehow protect against deranged glucose metabolism.

The New England Centenarian Study, headed at Boston University, began in 1988 to amass information on families of the oldest citizens in the United States. By studying those who have lived past the century mark, and have lived well, researchers will be able to identify a "healthy standard genome." Perhaps it will provide information that will help the majority of us who do not live as long.

Table 1
Single genes important in aging affect:
• control of insulin secretion and glucose metabolism.
• immune system functioning.
• control of the cell cycle.
• lipid (cholesterol) metabolism.
• response to stress.
• production of antioxidant enzymes.

with Rothmund-Thomson syndrome, for example, may lead a normal life span, but develop gray hair or baldness, cataracts, cancers, and osteoporosis at young ages. The brothers in **figure 3.22,** in contrast, show the extremely rapid aging of Hutchinson-Gilford syndrome. An affected child appears normal at birth but slows in growth by the first birthday. Within just a few years, the child ages with shocking rapidity, acquiring wrinkles, baldness, and the facial features characteristic of advanced

age. The body ages on the inside as well, as arteries clog with fatty deposits. The child usually dies of a heart attack or a stroke by age 13, although some patients live into their twenties. Only a few dozen cases of this syndrome have ever been reported.

An adult form of segmental progeroid syndrome called Werner syndrome becomes apparent before age 20, causing death before age 50 from diseases associated with aging. Young adults with Werner syndrome develop atherosclerosis, diabetes

mellitus, hair graying and loss, osteoporosis, cataracts, and wrinkled skin.

Not surprisingly, the cells of segmental progeroid syndrome patients show aging-related changes. Recall that normal cells growing in culture divide about 50 times before dying. Cells from progeroid syndrome patients die in culture after only 10 to 30 divisions. Understanding how and why these cells race through the aging process may help us to understand genetic control of normal aging.

Is Longevity Inherited?

Aging reflects genetic activity plus a life-time of environmental influences. Families with many very aged members have a fortuitous collection of genes plus shared environmental influences such as good nutrition, excellent health care, devoted

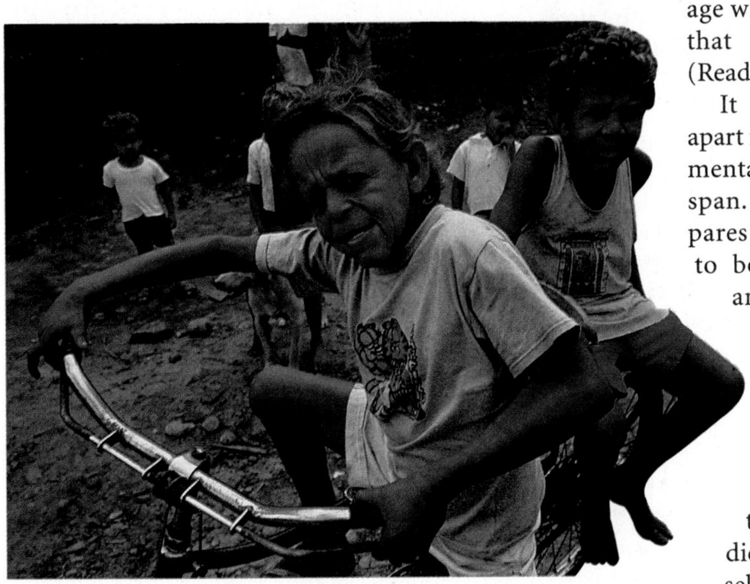

Figure 3.22 Segmental progeroid syndromes.
The Luciano brothers inherited Rothmund-Thomson syndrome and appear much older than their years.

relatives, and other advantages. A genome-level approach to identifying causes of longevity has identified a region of chromosome 4 that houses gene variants associated with long life. Ongoing genomewide comparisons between people who've passed their 100th birthdays and those who have died of the common illnesses of older age will reveal other genes that influence longevity (Reading 3.1).

It is difficult to tease apart inborn from environmental influences on life span. One approach compares adopted individuals to both their biological and adoptive parents. In one study, Danish adoptees with one biological parent who died of natural causes before age 50 were more than twice as likely to die before age 50 themselves as were adoptees whose biological parents lived beyond this age. This suggests an inherit-

ed component to longevity. Interestingly, adoptees whose natural parents died early due to infection were more than five times as likely to also die early of infection, perhaps because of inherited immune system deficiencies. The adoptive parents' ages at death had no influence on that of their adopted children. Chapter 7 explores the "nature versus nurture" phenomenon more closely.

Summary

3.1 The Reproductive System

1. The male and female reproductive systems include paired **gonads** and networks of tubes in which **sperm** and **oocytes** are manufactured.

2. Male **gametes** originate in **seminiferous tubules** within the paired **testes.** They then pass through the **epididymis** and **vasa deferentia,** where they mature before exiting the body through the **urethra** during sexual intercourse. The **prostate gland,** the **seminal vesicles,** and the **bulbourethral glands** add secretions.

3. Female gametes originate in the **ovaries.** Each month after puberty, one ovary releases an oocyte into a **fallopian tube.** The oocyte then moves to the **uterus** for implantation (if fertilized) or expulsion.

3.2 Meiosis

4. **Meiosis** reduces the chromosome number in gametes to one genome. This maintains the chromosome number from generation to generation. Meiosis ensures genetic variability by partitioning different combinations of genes into gametes as a result of **crossing over** and **independent assortment** of chromosomes.

5. Meiosis I, **reduction division,** halves the number of chromosomes. Meiosis II, **equational division,** produces four cells from the two that result from meiosis I, without another DNA replication.

6. Crossing over occurs during prophase I. It mixes up paternally and maternally derived genes on homologous chromosome pairs.

7. Chromosomes segregate and independently assort in metaphase I, which determines the distribution of genes from each parent in the gamete.

3.3 Gamete Maturation

8. **Spermatogenesis** begins with **spermatogonia,** which accumulate cytoplasm and replicate their DNA to become **primary spermatocytes.** After meiosis I, the cells become haploid **secondary spermatocytes.** In meiosis II, the secondary spermatocytes divide to each yield two **spermatids,** which then differentiate into **spermatozoa.**

9. In **oogenesis,** some oogonia grow and replicate their DNA, becoming **primary oocytes.** In meiosis I, the primary oocyte divides to yield one large **secondary oocyte**

and a much smaller **polar body.** In meiosis II, the secondary oocyte divides to yield the large ovum and another small polar body. Female meiosis is completed at fertilization.

3.4 Prenatal Development

10. In the female, sperm are **capacitated** and drawn chemically and physically toward a secondary oocyte. One sperm burrows through the oocyte's protective layers with **acrosomal** enzymes. Fertilization occurs when the sperm and oocyte fuse and their genetic material combines in one nucleus, forming the **zygote.** Electrochemical changes in the egg surface block additional sperm from entering. Cleavage begins and a 16-celled **morula** forms. Between days 3 and 6, the morula arrives at the uterus and hollows, forming a **blastocyst** made up of **blastomeres.** The **trophoblast** and **inner cell mass** form. Around day 6 or 7, the blastocyst implants, and trophoblast cells secrete **hCG,** which prevents menstruation.

11. During the second week, the **amniotic cavity** forms as the inner cell mass flattens. **Ectoderm** and **endoderm** form, and then **mesoderm** appears, establishing the **primary germ layers.** Cells in each germ layer begin to develop into specific organs. During the third week, the **placenta, yolk sac, allantois,** and umbilical cord begin to form as the amniotic cavity swells with fluid. **Monozygotic** twins result when one fertilized ovum splits. **Dizygotic** twins result from two fertilized ova. Organs form throughout the embryonic period. Structures including the **primitive streak,** the **notochord** and **neural tube,** arm and leg buds, the heart, facial features, and the skeleton gradually appear.

12. The **fetal** period begins after the eighth week. Organ rudiments laid down in the embryo grow and specialize. The developing organism moves and reacts, and gradually, its body proportions resemble those of a newborn baby. In the last trimester, the brain develops rapidly, and fat is deposited beneath the skin. The digestive and respiratory systems mature last.

3.5 Birth Defects

13. Birth defects can result from a malfunctioning gene or an environmental intervention.

14. A substance that causes birth defects is a **teratogen.** Environmentally caused birth defects are not transmitted to future generations.

15. The time when a structure is sensitive to damage from an abnormal gene or environmental intervention is its critical period.

3.6 Maturation and Aging

16. Genes cause or predispose us to illness throughout life. Single-gene disorders that strike early tend to be recessive, whereas adult-onset single-gene conditions are often dominant.

17. Malnutrition before birth can alter gene expression to increase the risk of type II diabetes mellitus and cardiovascular disease much later in life.

18. The **segmental progeroid syndromes** are single-gene disorders that increase the rate of aging-associated changes.

19. Long life is due to genetics and environmental influences.

Review Questions

1. How many sets of human chromosomes are present in each of the following cell types?
   a. an oogonium
   b. a primary spermatocyte
   c. a spermatid
   d. a cell from either sex during anaphase of meiosis I
   e. a cell from either sex during anaphase of meiosis II
   f. a secondary oocyte
   g. a polar body derived from a primary oocyte

2. List the structures and functions of the male and female reproductive systems.

3. A dog has 39 pairs of chromosomes. Considering only the independent assortment of chromosomes, how many genetically different puppies are possible when two dogs mate? Is this number an underestimate or overestimate of the actual total? Why?

4. How does meiosis differ from mitosis?

5. What do oogenesis and spermatogenesis have in common, and how do they differ?

6. How does gamete maturation differ in the male and female?

7. Describe the events of fertilization.

8. Exposure to teratogens tends to produce more severe health effects in an embryo than in a fetus. Why?

9. List four teratogens, and explain how they disrupt prenatal development.

10. Cite two pieces of evidence that genes control aging.

Applied Questions

1. Based on your knowledge of human prenatal development, at what stage do you think it is ethical to ban experimentation? Cite reasons for your answer. (The options of banning the research altogether, or of allowing research at any stage, are as valid an option as pinpointing a particular stage.)

2. Under a microscope, a first and second polar body look alike. What would a researcher have to look at to distinguish them?

3. Armadillos always give birth to identical quadruplets. Are the offspring clones?

4. Some Vietnam War veterans who were exposed to the herbicide Agent Orange claim that their children—born years after the exposure—have birth defects caused by dioxin, a contaminant in the herbicide. What types of cells would the chemical have to affect in these men to cause birth defects years later?

5. In about 1 in 200 pregnancies, a sperm fertilizes a polar body instead of an oocyte. A mass of tissue that is not an embryo develops. Why can't a polar body support development of an entire embryo?

6. Should a woman be held legally responsible if she drinks alcohol, smokes, or abuses drugs during pregnancy and it harms her child? Should liability apply to all substances that can harm a fetus, or only to those that are illegal?

7. Would you want to one day have your genome scanned to estimate how long you are likely to live? Why or why not?

8. What types of evidence have led researchers to hypothesize that a poor prenatal environment can raise the risk for certain adult illnesses? How are genes part of this picture?

Web Activities

9. Look over the "Living to 100 life expectancy calculator" at http://www.livingto100.com/quiz.htm and list ten ways that you can change your behavior to possibly live longer. What does this quiz suggest about the relative role of genes and the environment in determining longevity?

10. Go to http://www.advancedcell.com/pg_page1.html and look at the photographs of Lily, Daffodil, Crocus, Forsythia, and Rose. What is the evidence that these calf clones are not identical?

Case Study

11. Miguel and Maria know that they are each carriers of cystic fibrosis, and that the condition is quite severe in their families. So, they elect to have a procedure called preimplantation genetic diagnosis (see fig. 21.6) to ensure that their child does not inherit the condition. Maria's oocyte is fertilized with Miguel's sperm in a laboratory dish, a technique called *in vitro* fertilization, and allowed to develop to the 8 cell stage. One cell is removed, and a DNA probe is used to test for the mutant CF allele that is on both sides of the family. Only the wild type allele is detected.

Anna and Peter are also carriers of a genetic disorder that can affect either sex. They cannot get into a preimplantation genetic diagnosis clinical trial, which would be free, their insurance will not cover the procedure, and they cannot afford it. So, they choose chorionic villus sampling, in which a cell from the developing placenta is tested for the presence of a mutant allele at the tenth week of gestation. Their fetus is found to be a carrier, like them.

A third couple, Vivian and Max, are not willing to take the higher risk of miscarriage that chorionic villus sampling poses, so they wait until the sixteenth week, and Vivian has amniocentesis. Vivian knows from her family history that she may be a carrier for hemophilia A. If she is, a son would face a 50 percent chance of inheriting the disorder. The amniocentesis indicates a daughter.

a. How can a gene test performed on one cell of an 8-celled embryo, the developing placenta, or shed from a fetus into the fluid surrounding it, predict the future health of the individual?

b. At the time of preimplantation genetic diagnosis, is the embryo a cleavage embryo, an inner cell mass, or a gastrula?

c. What structures are present in Vivian and Max's fetus that have not yet developed in Anna and Peter's at the time of their prenatal tests?

Learn to apply the skills of a genetic counselor with this additional case found in the *Case Workbook in Human Genetics:*

Embryos and fetuses in research

Suggested Readings

Barzilai, Nir, et. al. October 15, 2003. Unique lipoprotein phenotype and genotype associated with exceptional longevity. *The Journal of the American Medical Association* 290:2030–40. The right cholesterol-carrier profile can add 20 years to life.

Cibelli, Jose B., et al. January 2002. The first human cloned embryo. *Scientific American* 286(1):44–51. It was only a few cells, but it caused a flutter of headlines.

Friedrich, M. J. November 13, 2002. Biological secrets of exceptional old age. *The Journal of the American Medical Association* 288(18):2247–53. Researchers are discovering the parts of the genome that control life span in people past the age of 100 and their families.

Hayflick, Leonard. January 27, 2000. New approaches to old age. *Nature* 403:365. We live longer than our genes dictate.

Lewis, Ricki. March 24, 2003. Porcine parts on the horizon? *The Scientist* 17(6):7. Cloned pigs whose cells lack molecules that stimulate the human immune system may one day provide organs.

Lewis, R. October 30, 2000. New light on fetal origins of adult disease. *The Scientist* 14(21):1. Starvation during prenatal development can alter gene expression in ways that raise the risks of developing certain multifactorial disorders in adulthood.

O'Connor, Anahad. March 25, 2003. Images of preserved embryos to become a learning tool. *The New York Times*, p. F1. The Virtual Human Embryo has images of miscarried embryos.

Perls, Thomas T., et al. June 11, 2002. Life-long sustained mortality advantage of siblings of centenarians. *Proceedings of the National Academy of Sciences* 99(12):8442–47. Siblings of people past the age of 100 also lead longer lives, indicating that genes contribute to longevity.

Puca, Annibale, et al. August 28, 2001. A genomewide scan for linkage to human exceptional longevity identifies a locus on chromosome 4. *Proceedings of the National Academy of Sciences* 98:10505–08. Comparing long-lived siblings revealed that part of chromosome 4 includes genes involved in life span.

Shermer, Michael. April 2003. I, clone. *Scientific American*. 288(4):38. Why a clone is not an exact duplicate.

Spitz, Lewis, and Edward M. Kiely. March 12, 2003. Conjoined twins. *The Journal of the American Medical Association* 289(10):1307–10. There are different types of conjoined twins.

The December 18, 2001 issue of *The New York Times*, section F, has several articles and spectacular illustrations and photos of human prenatal development.

Weekly updates of current news related to human genetics are available through Power Web on your Online Learning Center.

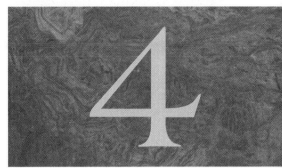

Mendelian Inheritance

CHAPTER CONTENTS

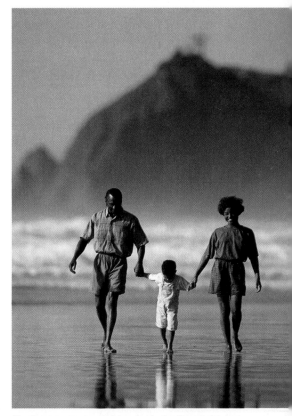

Pedigrees are used to study traits and relationships in families of humans as well as in families of some of our favorite mammals, such as purebred horses and dogs.

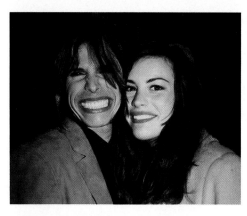

Figure 4.1 Inherited similarities.
Facial similarities are not always as obvious as those between rocker Steven Tyler of Aerosmith and his actress daughter, Liv.

Inherited similarities can be startling. When Aerosmith singer Steve Tyler first met his daughter, Liv, nine years old at the time, he knew with one glance that she was his child. He promptly burst into tears, so compelling was the resemblance. Even today, father and daughter have strikingly similar facial features (**figure 4.1**).

4.1 Following the Inheritance of One Gene—Segregation

Awareness of heredity appears in an ancient Jewish law that excuses a boy from circumcision if his male cousins bled to death from the ritual. Nineteenth-century biologists thought that body parts controlled trait transmission, and they gave the units of inheritance such colorful names as pangens, idioblasts, bioblasts, gemules, or just characters. An investigator who used the term *elementen* made the most lasting impression on what would become the science of genetics. His name was Gregor Mendel.

Mendel the Man

Mendel spent his early childhood in a small village in what is now the Czech Republic, near the Polish border. His father was a farmer, and his mother was the daughter of a gardener, so Mendel learned early how to tend fruit trees. At age 10 he left home to attend a special school for bright students,

supporting himself by tutoring. After a few years at a preparatory school, Mendel became a priest at the Augustinian monastery of St. Thomas in Brnö. At this atypical monastery, the priests were also teachers, and they did research in natural science. From them, Mendel learned how to artificially pollinate crop plants to control their breeding.

Mendel wanted to teach natural history, but had difficulty passing the necessary exams, a victim of test anxiety. At age 29, he was such an effective substitute teacher that he was sent to earn a college degree. At the University of Vienna, courses in the sciences and statistics fueled his enduring interest in plant breeding and got him thinking about experiments to address a question that had confounded other plant breeders—why did certain traits disappear in one generation, yet reappear in the next? To solve this puzzle, Mendel bred hybrids and applied the statistics he had learned in college.

From 1857 to 1863, Mendel crossed and cataloged some 24,034 plants, through several generations. He deduced that consistent ratios of traits in the offspring indicated that the plants transmitted distinct units, or "elementen." He derived two hypotheses to explain how inherited traits are transmitted. Mendel described his work to the Brnö Medical Society in 1865 and published it in the organization's journal the next year. The remarkably clear paper discusses plant hybridization, the reappearance of traits in the third generation, and the joys of working with peas, plus Mendel's data.

Mendel's hypotheses eventually became laws because they apply as much to all diploid species, including humans, as they do to pea plants. But it took years for his findings to be recognized. His treatise was published in English in 1901. Then three botanists (Hugo DeVries, Karl Franz Joseph Erich Correns, and Seysenegg Tschermak) independently rediscovered the laws of inheritance and then found Mendel's paper. All credited Mendel, who came to be regarded as the "father of genetics." As is the way of science, many others repeated and confirmed Mendel's work. However, researchers in this new field of genetics also identified situations that seem to disrupt Mendelian ratios, the subject of chapter 5.

Mendel deduced how chromosomes transmit genes to the next generation without knowing what either of these structures

are! In the twentieth century, researchers discovered the molecular basis of the pea plant traits that Mendel studied. The "short" and "tall" plants reflected the expression of a gene that enables a plant to produce the hormone gibberellin, which elongates the stem. One tiny change to the DNA, and a short plant results. Likewise, "round" and "wrinkled" peas arise from the *R* gene, whose encoded protein connects sugars into branching polysaccharides. Seeds with a mutant gene cannot attach the sugars; water exits the cells, and the peas wrinkle.

Mendel's Experiments

Peas were an ideal choice for probing trait transmission because they are easy to grow, develop quickly, and have many traits that take one of two easily distinguishable forms. It was this last quality of "differentiating characters" that particularly interested Mendel. **Figure 4.2** illustrates the seven traits that he followed.

Mendel's first experiments dealt with single traits with two expressions, such as "short" and "tall." He set up all combinations of possible artificial pollinations, manipulating fertilizations to cross tall with tall, short with short, and tall with short, which produces hybrids. Mendel noted that short plants crossed to other short plants were "true-breeding," always producing short plants.

The crosses of tall plants to each other were more confusing. Some tall plants were true-breeding, but others crossed with each other yielded short plants in about one-quarter of the next generation. It appeared as if in some tall plants, tallness could mask shortness (**figure 4.3**). One trait that masks another is said to be **dominant;** the masked trait is **recessive.** Wrote Mendel,

> **In the case of each of the seven crosses the hybrid character resembles that of one of the parental forms so closely that the other either escapes observation completely or cannot be detected with certainty. . . . The expression "recessive" has been chosen because the characters thereby designated withdraw or entirely disappear in the hybrids, but nevertheless reappear unchanged in their progeny.**

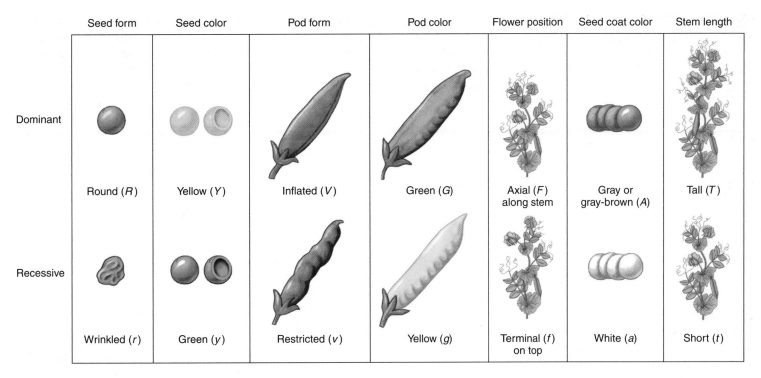

Figure 4.2 **Traits Mendel studied.** Gregor Mendel studied the transmission of seven traits in the pea plant. Each trait has two easily distinguished expressions, or phenotypes.

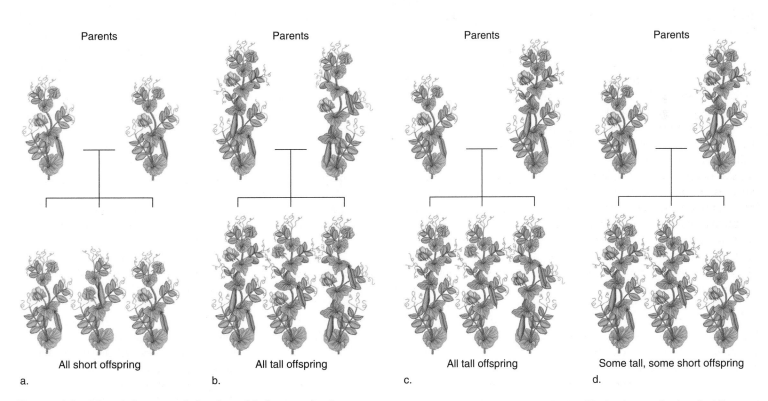

Figure 4.3 **Mendel crossed short and tall pea plants.** **(a)** When Mendel crossed short pea plants with short pea plants, all of the progeny were short. **(b)** Some tall plants crossed to tall plants yielded only tall plants. **(c)** Certain tall plants crossed with short plants produced all tall plants. **(d)** Other tall plants crossed with short plants produced some tall plants and some short plants.

Mendel conducted up to 70 hybrid crosses for each of the seven traits. (See figure 4.2). Because one trait is followed and the parents are hybrids, this is called a **monohybrid cross.**

To further investigate the non-true-breeding tall plants, Mendel set aside the short plants that had arisen from crossing the hybrid tall plants, and allowed the remaining tall offspring to undergo self-fertilization. He saw the ratio of one-quarter short to three-quarters tall plants. In further crosses, he found that two-thirds of the tall plants from the monohybrid cross were non-true-breeding, and the remaining third were true-breeding (**figure 4.4**).

In these experiments, Mendel confirmed that hybrids hide one expression of a trait, which reappears when hybrids are selfed. But Mendel went farther, trying to explain how this happened. He suggested that gametes distribute "elementen"—what we call genes—because these cells physically link generations. Paired sets of elementen would separate from each other as gametes form. When gametes join at fertilization, the elementen would group into new combinations. Mendel reasoned that each element was packaged in a separate gamete, and if opposite-sex gametes combine at random, then he could mathematically explain the different ratios of traits produced from his pea plant crossings. Mendel's idea that elementen separate in the gametes would later be called the **law of segregation.** Mendel eventually turned his energies to monastery administration when other scientists did not recognize the importance of his work.

When Mendel's ratios were demonstrated again and again in several species in the early 1900s, at the same time that chromosomes were being described for the first time, it became apparent that elementen and chromosomes had much in common. Both paired elementen and pairs of chromosomes separate at each generation and are transmitted—one from each parent—to offspring. Both elementen and chromosomes are inherited in random combinations. Chromosomes provided a physical mechanism for Mendel's hypotheses. In 1909, English embryologist William Bateson renamed Mendel's elementen *genes* (Greek for "give birth to"). It wasn't until the 1940s, however, that scientists began investigating the gene's chemical basis. We pick up the historical trail at this point in chapter 9.

Terms and Tools to Follow Segregating Genes

Figures 4.3 and 4.4 depict the law of segregation in pea plants. We can also describe it in terms of the behavior of chromosomes and genes during meiosis.

Because a gene is a long sequence of DNA, it can vary in many ways. An individual with two identical alleles for a gene is **homozygous** for that gene. An individual with two different alleles is **heterozygous.** Mendel's "non-true-breeding" plants were heterozygous, also called "hybrid."

When a gene has two alleles, it is common to symbolize the dominant allele with a capital letter and the recessive with the corresponding small letter. If both

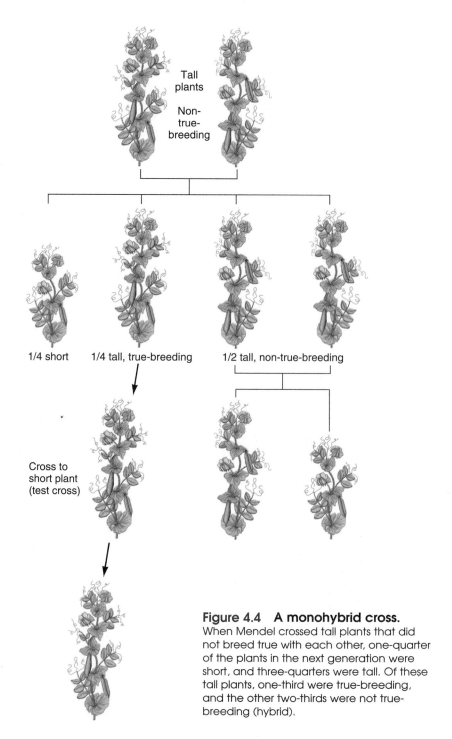

Tall plants

Non-true-breeding

1/4 short   1/4 tall, true-breeding   1/2 tall, non-true-breeding

Cross to short plant (test cross)

Figure 4.4   A monohybrid cross.
When Mendel crossed tall plants that did not breed true with each other, one-quarter of the plants in the next generation were short, and three-quarters were tall. Of these tall plants, one-third were true-breeding, and the other two-thirds were not true-breeding (hybrid).

alleles are recessive, the individual is homozygous recessive. Two small letters, such as *tt* for short plants, symbolize this. An individual with two dominant alleles is homozygous dominant. Two capital letters, such as *TT* for tall pea plants, represent this. Another possible allele combination is one dominant and one recessive allele—*Tt* for non-true-breeding tall pea plants, or heterozygotes.

An organism's appearance does not always reveal its alleles. Both a *TT* and a *Tt* pea plant are tall, but *TT* is a homozygote and *Tt* a heterozygote. The **genotype** describes the organism's alleles, and the **phenotype** describes the outward expression of an allele combination. A **wild type** phenotype is the most common expression of a particular allele combination in a population. A **mutant** phenotype is a variant of a gene's expression that arises when the gene undergoes a change, or **mutation.**

When analyzing genetic crosses, the first generation is the parental generation, or P₁; the second generation is the first filial generation, or F₁; the next generation is the second filial generation, or F₂, and so on. If you considered your grandparents the P₁

generation, your parents would be the F₁ generation, and you and your siblings are the F₂ generation.

Mendel's observations on the inheritance of single genes reflect the events of meiosis. When a gamete is produced, the two copies of a particular gene separate along with the homologs that carry them. In a plant of genotype *Tt*, for example, gametes carrying either *T* or *t* form in equal numbers during anaphase I. When gametes meet to start the next generation, they combine at random. That is, a *t*-bearing oocyte is neither more or less attractive to a sperm than is a *T*-bearing oocyte. These two factors—equal allele distribution into gametes and random combinations of gametes—underlie Mendel's law of segregation (**figure 4.5**).

Meiosis explains what Mendel saw when he crossed short and tall plants. When he crossed short plants (*tt*) with true-breeding tall plants (*TT*), the seeds grew into F₁ plants that were all tall (genotype *Tt*). Next, he self-crossed the F₁ plants. The three possible genotypic outcomes were *TT, tt,* and *Tt*. A *TT* individual resulted when a *T* sperm fertilized a *T* oocyte; a *tt* plant resulted when a *t* oocyte met a *t* sperm; and a *Tt*

individual resulted when either a *t* sperm fertilized a *T* oocyte, or a *T* sperm fertilized a *t* oocyte.

Because two of the four possible gamete combinations produce a heterozygote, and each of the others produces a homozygote, the genotypic ratio expected of a monohybrid cross is 1 *TT:* 2 *Tt:* 1 *tt.* The corresponding phenotypic ratio is three tall plants to one short plant, a 3:1 ratio. Mendel saw these results for all seven traits that he studied, although, as **table 4.1** shows, the ratios were not exact. Today we use a diagram called a **Punnett square** to derive these ratios (**figure 4.6**). A Punnett square represents particular genes in gametes and how they come together, assuming that they are carried on different chromosomes. Experiments yield numbers of offspring that approximate these ratios.

Mendel distinguished the two genotypes resulting in tall progeny—*TT* from *Tt*—with additional crosses. He bred tall plants of unknown genotype with short (*tt*) plants. If a tall plant crossed with a *tt* plant produced both tall and short progeny, Mendel knew it was genotype *Tt*; if it produced only tall plants, he knew it must be *TT*. Crossing an individual of unknown

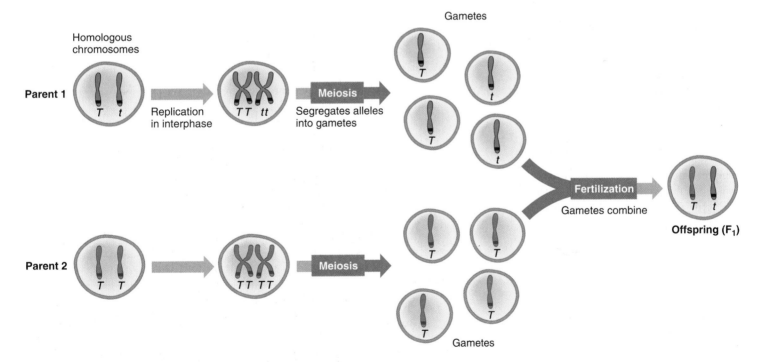

Figure 4.5   Mendel's first law—gene segregation.   During meiosis, homologous pairs of chromosomes (and the genes that compose them) separate from one another and are packaged into separate gametes. At fertilization, gametes combine at random to form the individuals of a new generation. Green and blue denote different parental origins of the chromosomes. In this example, offspring of genotype *TT* are also generated, along with genotype *Tt* .

genotype with a homozygous recessive individual is called a test cross. The homozygous recessive is the only genotype that can be identified by its phenotype—that is, a short plant is always *tt*. The homozygous recessive is therefore a "known" that can reveal the unknown genotype of another individual when the two are crossed.

Key Concepts

From observing crosses in which two tall pea plants produced short offspring, along with other crosses, Mendel deduced that "elementen" for height segregate during meiosis, then combine at random with those from the opposite gamete at fertilization. • A homozygote has two identical alleles, and a heterozygote has two different alleles. The allele expressed in a heterozygote is dominant; the allele not expressed is recessive. • A monohybrid cross yields a genotypic ratio of 1:2:1 and a phenotypic ratio of 3:1. Punnett squares help calculate expected genotypic and phenotypic ratios among progeny. A test cross uses a homozygous recessive individual to reveal an unknown genotype.

4.2 Single-Gene Inheritance in Humans

Mendel's first law addresses traits determined by single genes, as demonstrated in pea plants. Transmission of single genes in humans is called Mendelian, unifactorial, or single-gene inheritance.

Even the most familiar Mendelian disorders, such as sickle cell disease and Duchenne muscular dystrophy, are rare compared to infectious diseases, cancer, and multifactorial disorders. Most Mendelian conditions affect 1 in 10,000 or fewer individuals. **Table 4.2** lists some Mendelian disorders, and Reading 4.1 considers some interesting traits described in *Online Mendelian Inheritance in Man*.

Modes of Inheritance

Modes of inheritance are rules that explain the common patterns that inherited characteristics follow as they are passed through families. Knowing the mode of inheritance makes it possible to calculate the probability that a particular couple will have a child who inherits a particular condition.

Mendel derived his laws by studying traits carried on autosomes (non-sex chromosomes). The way those laws affect the modes of inheritance depend on whether a trait is transmitted on an autosome or a sex chromosome, and whether an allele is recessive or dominant. **Autosomal dominant** and **autosomal recessive** are the two modes of inheritance directly derived from Mendel's laws.

Autosomal Dominant Inheritance

In autosomal dominant inheritance, a trait can appear in either sex because an autosome carries the gene. If a child has the trait, at least one parent must also have it. Autosomal dominant traits do not skip generations. If no offspring inherit the trait in one generation, its transmission stops because the offspring can pass on only the recessive form of the gene. **Figure 4.7** uses a

Table 4.1
Mendel's Law of Segregation

Experiment	Total	Dominant	Recessive	F_2 Phenotypic Ratios
1. Seed form	7,324	5,474	1,850	2.96:1
2. Seed color	8,023	6,022	2,001	3.01:1
3. Seed coat color	929	705	224	3.15:1
4. Pod form	1,181	882	299	2.95:1
5. Pod color	580	428	152	2.82:1
6. Flower position	858	651	207	3.14:1
7. Stem length	1,064	787	277	2.84:1

Average = 2.98:1

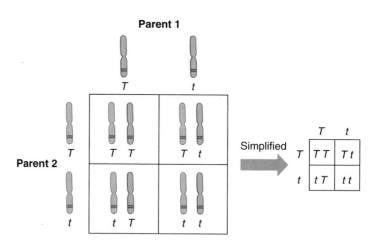

Figure 4.6 A Punnett square. A Punnett square is a diagram of how two alleles of a gene combine in a cross between two individuals. The different types of gametes of one parent are listed along the top of the square, with those of the other parent listed on the left-hand side. Each compartment within the square contains the genotype that results when gametes that correspond to that compartment join. The Punnett square here describes a monohybrid cross of two tall pea plants. Among the progeny, tall plants outnumber short plants 3:1. Can you determine the genotypic ratio? Punnett squares usually indicate only the alleles, as shown at the right.

Table 4.2

Some Mendelian Disorders in Humans

Disorder	Symptoms
Autosomal Recessive	
Ataxia telangiectasis	Facial rash, poor muscular coordination, involuntary eye movements, high risk for cancer, sinus and lung infections
Cystic fibrosis	Lung infections and congestion, poor fat digestion, male infertility, poor weight gain, salty sweat
Familial hypertrophic cardiomyopathy	Overgrowth of heart muscle, causing sudden death in young adults
Gaucher disease	Swollen liver and spleen, anemia, internal bleeding, poor balance
Hemochromatosis	Body retains iron; high risk of infection, liver damage, excess skin pigmentation, heart and pancreas damage
Maple syrup urine disease	Lethargy, vomiting, irritability, mental retardation, coma, and death in infancy
Phenylketonuria	Mental retardation, fair skin
Sickle cell disease	Joint pain, spleen damage, high risk of infection
Tay-Sachs disease	Nervous system degeneration
Autosomal Dominant	
Achondroplasia	Dwarfism with short limbs, normal size head and trunk
Familial hypercholesterolemia	Very high serum cholesterol, heart disease
Huntington disease	Progressive uncontrollable movements and personality changes, beginning in middle age
Lactose intolerance	Inability to digest lactose, causing cramps after ingestion
Marfan syndrome	Long limbs, sunken chest, lens dislocation, spindly fingers, weakened aorta
Myotonic dystrophy	Progressive muscle wasting
Neurofibromatosis (I)	Brown skin marks, benign tumors beneath skin
Polycystic kidney disease	Cysts in kidneys, bloody urine, high blood pressure, abdominal pain
Polydactyly	Extra fingers and/or toes
Porphyria variegata	Red urine, fever, abdominal pain, headache, coma, death

Punnett square to predict the genotypes and phenotypes of offspring of a mother who has an autosomal dominant trait and a father who does not.

A young man, James Poush, discovered an autosomal dominant trait in his family while in high school and published the first full report on distal symphalangism. James and certain relatives had stiff fingers and toes with tiny nails. When he studied genetics, he realized this might be a Mendelian trait. James identified 27 affected individuals among 156 relatives, and concluded that the trait is autosomal dominant. Of 63 relatives with an affected parent, 27 (43 percent) were affected—close to the 50 percent expected for autosomal dominant inheritance (**table 4.3**). Bioethics: Choices for the Future (page 82) considers the complexities of detecting autosomal dominant mutant genes before symptoms arise.

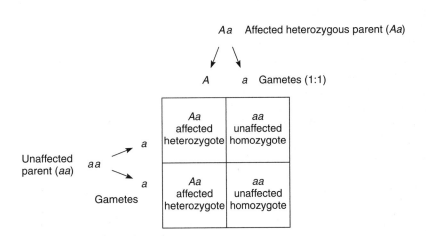

Figure 4.7 Autosomal dominant inheritance. When one parent has an autosomal dominant condition and the other does not, each offspring has a 50 percent probability of inheriting the mutant allele and the condition. The affected parent is *Aa* here, and not *AA*, because for many dominant disorders, the homozygous dominant (*AA*) phenotype is either lethal or very rare because both parents of the person with the *AA* genotype would have to have the disorder.

It's All in the Genes

Do you have uncombable hair, misshapen toes or teeth, or a pigmented tongue tip? Are you unable to smell a squashed skunk, or do you sneeze repeatedly in bright sunlight? Do you lack teeth, eyebrows, eyelashes, nasal bones, thumbnails, or fingerprints? If so, your unusual trait may be one of thousands described in *Online Mendelian Inheritance in Man* (OMIM, at www.ncbi.nlm.nih.gov/entrez/query.fcgi?db=OMIM). A team at Johns Hopkins University, led by renowned geneticist Victor McKusick, updates OMIM daily. Entering a disease name allows one to retrieve family histories, clinical descriptions, mode of inheritance, and molecular information on the causative gene and protein products. Woven amidst the medical terminology and genetic jargon are the stories behind some fascinating inherited traits.

Genes control whether hair is blond, brown, or black, has red highlights, and is straight, curly, or kinky. Widow's peaks, cowlicks, a whorl in the eyebrow, and white forelocks run in families; so do hairs with triangular cross-sections. Some people have multicolored hairs, like cats; others have hair in odd places, such as on the elbows, nose tip, knuckles, palms, or soles. Teeth can be missing or extra, protuberant or fused, present at birth, shovel-shaped, or "snow-capped." A person can have a grooved tongue, duckbill lips, flared ears, egg-shaped pupils, three rows of eyelashes, spotted nails, or "broad thumbs and great toes." Extra breasts are known in humans and guinea pigs, and one family's claim to genetic fame is a double nail on the littlest toe.

Unusual genetic variants can affect metabolism, producing either disease or harmless, yet noticeable, effects. Members of some families experience "urinary excretion of odoriferous component of asparagus" or "urinary excretion of beet pigment," producing a strange odor or dark pink urine stream after consuming the offending vegetable. In blue diaper syndrome, an infant's urine turns blue on contact with air, thanks to an inherited inability to break down an amino acid.

One bizarre inherited illness is the Jumping Frenchmen of Maine syndrome. This exaggerated startle reflex was first noted among French-Canadian lumberjacks from the Moosehead Lake area of Maine, whose ancestors were from the Beauce region of Quebec. Physicians first reported the condition at a medical conference in 1878. Geneticists videotaped the startle response in 1980, and the condition continues to appear in genetics journals. OMIM offers a most vivid description:

If given a short, sudden, quick command, the affected person would respond with the appropriate action, often echoing the words of command. . . . For example, if one of them was abruptly asked to strike another, he would do so without hesitation, even if it was his mother and he had an ax in his hand.

The Jumping Frenchmen of Maine syndrome may be an extreme variant of the more common Tourette syndrome, which causes tics and other uncontrollable movements. **Figure 1** illustrates some other genetic variants.

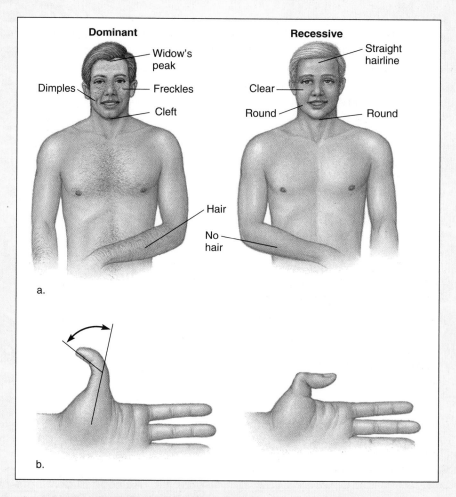

Figure 1 Inheritance of some common traits. (a) Freckles, dimples, hairy arms, widow's peak, and a cleft chin are examples of dominant traits. **(b)** The ability to bend the thumb backward or forward is inherited.

Table 4.3

Criteria for an Autosomal Dominant Trait

1. Males and females can be affected. Male-to-male transmission can occur.

2. Males and females transmit the trait with equal frequency.

3. Successive generations are affected.

4. Transmission stops if a generation arises in which no one is affected.

Autosomal Recessive Inheritance

An autosomal recessive trait can appear in either sex. Affected individuals have a homozygous recessive genotype, whereas in heterozygotes—also called carriers—the wild type allele masks expression of the mutant allele. Consider the Deford family. Sportswriter Frank Deford and his wife, Carol, had their daughter Alex in 1972. She died at age 8 of cystic fibrosis. Frank Deford wrote about his feelings at the time of diagnosis in a book, *Alex, the Life of a Child:*

I went to the encyclopedia and read about this cystic fibrosis. To me, at that point, it was one of those vague diseases you hear about now and then. . . . One out of every 20 whites carries the defective gene, as I do, as Carol does, as perhaps 10 million other Americans do—a population about the size of Illinois or Ohio. . . . If Carol and I had been lucky, if our second-born had not been cursed with cystic fibrosis, then we probably never would have had another child, and our bad genes would merely have been passed on, blissfully unknown to us.

Frank Deford described the very essence of recessive inheritance: skipped generations in the expression of a trait. Because the human generation time is so long—about 25 to 30 years—we can usually trace a trait or illness for only two or three generations. For this reason, the Defords did not know of any other affected relatives.

Alex had inherited a mutant allele on chromosome 7 from each of her parents. The adult Defords were unaffected by the illness because they each also had a dominant allele that encodes enough of a functional protein for health. They are carriers. **Figure 4.8** shows another monohybrid cross in humans.

Mendel's first law can be used to calculate the probability that an individual will have either of two phenotypes. The probabilities of each possible genotype are added. For example, the chance that a child whose parents are both carriers of cystic fibrosis will *not* have the condition is the sum of the probability that she has inherited two normal alleles (1/4) plus the chance that she herself is a heterozygote (1/2), or 3/4. Note that this also equals 1 minus the probability that she is a homozygous recessive who has the condition.

The ratios that Mendel's first law predicts for autosomal recessive inheritance apply to each offspring anew, just as a tossed coin has a 50 percent chance of coming up heads with each throw, no matter how many heads have already been thrown. Misunderstanding this concept leads to a common problem in genetic counseling. Many people conclude that if they have already had a child affected by an autosomal recessive illness, then their next three children are guaranteed to escape it. This isn't true. Each child faces the same 25 percent risk of inheriting the condition.

Most autosomal recessive conditions occur unexpectedly in families. However, blood relatives who have children together have a much higher risk of having a child with an autosomal recessive condition. Marriage between relatives produces **consanguinity,** which means "shared blood"—a figurative description, since genes are not passed in blood. Relatives can trace their families back to a common ancestor. An unrelated man and woman have eight different grandparents, but first cousins have only six, because they share one pair through their parents, who are siblings (see figure 4.14*c*). Consanguinity increases the likelihood of disease because the parents may have inherited the same mutant recessive allele from a shared grandparent. That is, the probability of two relatives inheriting the same disease-causing recessive allele is greater than that of two unrelated people having the same allele by chance.

The nature of the phenotype is important when evaluating transmission of Mendelian traits. For example, each adult sibling of a person who is a known carrier of Tay-Sachs disease has a two-thirds chance of being a carrier. The probability is two-thirds, and not one-half, because there are only three genotypic sources for an adult—homozygous for the normal allele, or a carrier who inherits the mutant allele from either mother or father. A homozygote would not have survived childhood.

Geneticists who study human traits and illnesses can hardly set up crosses as Mendel did, but they can pool information from families whose members have the same trait or illness based on symptoms, biochemical tests, or genetic tests. Consider a simplified example of 50 couples in which both partners are carriers of sickle cell disease. If 100 children are born, about 25 of them would be expected to have sickle cell disease. Of the remaining 75, theoretically 50 would be carriers like their parents, and the remaining 25 would have two wild type alleles. **Table 4.4** lists criteria for an autosomal recessive trait.

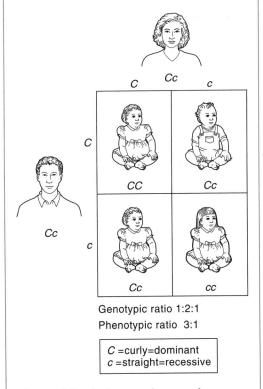

Genotypic ratio 1:2:1
Phenotypic ratio 3:1

C = curly = dominant
c = straight = recessive

Figure 4.8 Autosomal recessive inheritance. A 1:2:1 genotypic ratio results from a monohybrid cross, whether in peas or people. Curly hair (*C*) is dominant to straight hair (*c*). This pedigree depicts a monohybrid cross for hair curliness.

When Diagnosing a Fetus Also Diagnoses a Parent: Huntington Disease

Mendel's laws apply to all diploid organisms. They can have profound effects on families in which some members inherit a disease caused by a mutation in a single gene. The case of Huntington disease (HD) is particularly complex, because symptoms usually do not appear until about 38 to 40 years of age—often after people have had children and made career and other choices (see Tables 12.4 and 12.8). Initial symptoms of clumsiness and slurred speech progress to a near-constant writhing and repetitive, dancelike movements—ceasing, oddly, only during sleep. People typically live with the worsening disease for fifteen to twenty years, usually dying of infection. Some become demented; others remain aware. Drugs can dampen symptoms, but there is no cure.

HD is autosomal dominant. This means that each offspring of an affected individual has a 50 percent (1 in 2) chance of inheriting the condition. The child of an affected parent, or the sibling of an affected individual, is said to be at-risk. (They aren't really carriers because this is not a recessive disorder. *HH* and *Hh* genotypes cause the same symptoms.) In the United States, about 150,000 people are at-risk. Unlike the case in many other disorders with a genetic component, inheriting the mutant HD gene means that the disease will develop with close to 100 percent certainty. A genetic marker test, requiring that several family members be tested to establish a pattern, became available to some families in 1983, offering a prediction accuracy of 96 to 99 percent. In 1993, direct testing for the mutation became possible with the discovery of the HD gene on one tip of chromosome 4. It encodes a protein called huntingtin that, when mutant, contains a stretch of extra amino acids that causes it to misfold and form clumps in certain brain cells. This causes the symptoms.

The ability to predict HD posed psychological difficulties for at-risk individuals, who have usually seen what having the disease is like. Who should be tested? One study found that from 10 to 20 percent of at-risk individuals offered the gene test actually take it, generally after months of genetic counseling. Clinicians feared that receiving bad news would cause some people to commit suicide, but studies have indicated that this is not so. A study of at-risk individuals offered HD testing in Canada, where there is no fear of health insurance discrimination because there is national health care, found that older people were most likely to be tested. They used the information primarily to make financial decisions, rather than reproductive ones.

HD testing brought other surprises. Often individuals given a genetic reprieve are curious about their depression afterwards— "survivor guilt," rather than the expected euphoria, is a common reaction, particularly if one's siblings do not receive such good news. Some people who had made life decisions based on accepting a worst-case scenario—that they would one day have HD—found that they did not have the mutation after all, but had already made irreversible decisions, such as not having children. One young man, convinced he faced a future with HD, took up very risky behaviors—skydiving, bungee jumping, hang gliding, and gambling. He also had a vasectomy. What he didn't have was the mutation.

Yet predictive testing for HD is a relief for some people. Said one woman who did not have the mutation, "The devil you know is far better than the one you don't know." Her siblings refused to be tested. Researchers have found that those who psychologically could not handle the test results tend to refuse testing, which may explain why the suicide rate is lower than expected. A dilemma arises with testing, however, when a pregnancy is involved. Consider the following case:

> **Peter M. discovered at age 24 that his mother, age 45, has HD. She was adopted, so she did not know of a family history. Peter's wife Martha is pregnant, and she does not want to have a child who will have HD. She wants to have the fetus checked for the mutation. But Peter does not want to know his HD status. Should Martha have the test?**

The dilemma is that if the fetus is affected, Peter's fate will be revealed. A team of Australian doctors, lawyers, and ethicists pondered this family's situation. The clinicians decided it was right to offer testing to Peter first, and then test the fetus only if Peter had the mutation. This would be medically safer and would leave the choice with Peter. They discouraged Martha from having the test and keeping the results secret, because this would place great stress on all involved. The physicians acknowledged that Martha could insist and have the test, because it would be her body that would be tested, but they discouraged it because of the late-onset nature of the disorder—that is, even an affected child would have many good years. In contrast, the legal team concluded that only Martha's consent would be needed, but left the final recommendations to the doctors.

The ethicists advised support of the individual with the most compelling need. If Peter would become suicidal with a test result indicating HD, then his right to refuse to know should be paramount. However, if he could handle such information, then Martha should have the test, because not doing so would compromise her ability to make an informed choice about the pregnancy.

What would you do?

Table 4.4

Criteria for an Autosomal Recessive Trait

1. Males and females are affected.
2. Affected males and females can transmit the gene, unless it causes death before reproductive age.
3. The trait can skip generations.
4. Parents of an affected individual are heterozygous or have the trait.

Solving a Problem: Segregation

Using Mendel's laws to predict phenotypes and genotypes requires a careful reading of the problem to identify and organize relevant information. Sometimes common sense is useful, too. The following general steps can help to solve a problem that addresses Mendel's first law, the inheritance of a single-gene trait.

1. List all possible genotypes and phenotypes for the trait.
2. Determine the genotypes of the individuals in the first (P_1) generation. This may require deductive reasoning based on information about those people's parents.
3. After determining the genotypes, determine the possible alleles in gametes produced by each individual in the cross.
4. Unite these gametes in all combinations, using a Punnett square if necessary, to reveal all possible genotypes. Calculate ratios for the first generation of offspring (F_1).
5. To extend predictions to the second offspring (F_2) generation, use the genotypes of the specified F_1 individuals and repeat steps 3 and 4.

As an example, consider curly hair, depicted in figure 4.8. If C is the dominant allele, conferring curliness, and c is the recessive allele, then both CC and Cc genotypes result in curly hair. A person with cc genotype has straight hair.

Wendy has beautiful curls, and her husband Rick has straight hair. Wendy's father is bald, but once had curly hair, and her mother has stick-straight hair. What is the probability that Wendy and Rick's child will have straight hair? Steps 1 through 5 solve the problem:

1. State possible genotypes:
   CC, Cc = curly cc = straight
2. Determine genotypes: Rick must be cc, because his hair is straight. Wendy must be Cc, because her mother has straight hair and therefore gave her a c allele.
3. Determine gametes: Rick's sperm carry only c. Half of Wendy's oocytes carry C, and half carry c.
4. Unite the gametes:

		Wendy	
		C	c
Rick	c	Cc	cc

5. Conclusion: Each child of Wendy and Rick has a 50 percent chance of having curly hair (Cc) and a 50 percent chance of having straight hair (cc).

On the Meaning of Dominance and Recessiveness

Determining whether an allele is dominant or recessive is critical in medical genetics because it helps predict which individuals are at high risk of inheriting a particular condition. Dominance and recessiveness reflect the characteristics or abundance of a protein.

Mendel based his definitions of dominance and recessiveness on what he could see—one allele masked the other. Today we can often add a cellular or molecular explanation. Consider inborn errors of metabolism, which are caused by the absence of an enzyme. These disorders tend to be recessive; although cells of a carrier make half the normal amount of the enzyme, this is usually sufficient to maintain health. The one normal allele, therefore, compensates for the mutant one, to which it is dominant. The situation is similar in pea plants. Short stem length results from deficiency of an enzyme that activates a growth hormone, but the Tt plants produce enough hormone to attain the same height as TT plants.

A recessive trait is sometimes called a "loss of function" because the recessive allele usually causes the loss of normal protein production and function. In contrast, some dominantly inherited disorders result from the action of an abnormal protein that interferes with the function of the normal protein. Huntington disease is an example of such a "gain of function" disorder. The mutant allele, which is dominant, encodes an abnormally elongated protein that prevents the normal protein from functioning in the brain. Researchers determined that Huntington disease represents a gain of function because individuals who are missing one copy of the gene do not have the illness.

Recessive disorders tend to be more severe, and produce symptoms at much earlier ages, than dominant disorders. Disease-causing recessive alleles can remain, and even flourish, in populations because heterozygotes carry them without becoming ill and pass them to future generations. In contrast, if a dominant mutation arises that causes severe illness early in life, people who have the allele are either too ill or do not live long enough to reproduce, and the allele eventually becomes rare in the population unless it is replaced by mutation. Dominant disorders whose symptoms do not appear until adulthood, or that do not drastically disrupt health, tend to remain in a population because they do not affect health until after a person has reproduced. Therefore, the dominant conditions that persist tend to be those that first cause symptoms in middle adulthood.

Key Concepts

A Mendelian trait is caused by a single gene. Modes of inheritance reveal whether a Mendelian trait is dominant or recessive and whether the gene that controls it is carried on an autosome or a sex chromosome. Autosomal dominant traits do not skip generations and can affect both sexes; autosomal recessive traits can skip generations and can affect both sexes. Rare autosomal recessive disorders sometimes recur in families when blood relatives have children together. Mendel's first law, which can predict the probability that a child will inherit a Mendelian trait, applies anew to each child. • Genetic problems are solved with logic and by applying Mendel's laws to follow gametes. • At the biochemical level, dominance refers to the ability of a protein encoded by one allele to compensate for a missing or abnormal protein encoded by another allele.

4.3 Following the Inheritance of Two Genes—Independent Assortment

The law of segregation follows the inheritance of two alleles for a single gene. In a second set of experiments, Mendel examined the inheritance of two different traits, each attributable to a gene with two different alleles.

Mendel's Second Law

The second law states that for two genes on different chromosomes, the inheritance of one does not influence the chance of inheriting the other. The two genes thus "independently assort" because they are packaged into gametes at random, **figure 4.9.** Two genes that are far apart on the same chromosome also appear to independently assort, because so many crossovers occur between them that it is as if they are carried on separate chromosomes (see figure 3.5).

Mendel looked at seed shape, which was either round or wrinkled (determined by the *R* gene), and seed color, which was either yellow or green (determined by the *Y* gene). When he crossed true-breeding plants that had round, yellow seeds to true-breeding plants that had wrinkled, green seeds, all the progeny had round, yellow seeds. These offspring were double heterozygotes, or dihybrids, of genotype *RrYy*. From their appearance, Mendel deduced that round is dominant to wrinkled, and yellow to green.

Next, he self-crossed the dihybrid plants in a **dihybrid cross,** so named because two genes and traits are followed.

Mendel found four types of seeds in the next, third generation: 315 plants with round, yellow seeds; 108 plants with round, green seeds; 101 plants with wrinkled, yellow seeds; and 32 plants with wrinkled, green seeds. These classes occurred in a ratio of 9:3:3:1.

Mendel then took each plant from the third generation and crossed it to plants with wrinkled, green seeds (genotype *rryy*). These test crosses established whether each plant in the third generation was true-breeding for both genes (genotypes *RRYY* or *rryy*), true-breeding for one gene but heterozygous for the other (genotypes *RRYy, RrYY, rrYy,* or *Rryy*), or heterozygous for both genes (genotype *RrYy*). Mendel could explain the 9:3:3:1 proportion of progeny classes only if one gene does not influence transmission of the other. Each parent would produce equal numbers of four different types of gametes:

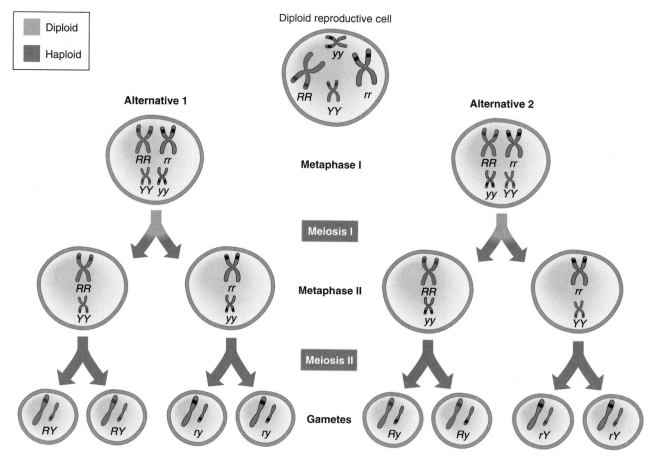

Figure 4.9 Mendel's second law—independent assortment. The independent assortment of genes carried on different chromosomes results from the random alignment of chromosome pairs during metaphase of meiosis I. An individual of genotype *RrYy*, for example, manufactures four types of gametes, containing the dominant alleles of both genes (*RY*), the recessive alleles of both genes (*ry*), and a dominant allele of one with a recessive allele of the other (*Ry* or *rY*). The allele combination depends upon which chromosomes are packaged together in a gamete—and this happens at random.

RY, Ry, rY, and *ry*. Note that each of these combinations has one gene for each trait. A Punnett square for this cross shows that the four types of seeds:

1. round, yellow (*RRYY, RrYY, RRYy,* and *RrYy*)

2. round, green (*RRyy* and *Rryy*)

3. wrinkled, yellow (*rrYY* and *rrYy*) and

4. wrinkled, green (*rryy*)

are present in the ratio 9:3:3:1, just as Mendel found (**figure 4.10**).

Solving a Problem: Following More Than One Segregating Gene

A Punnett square for three genes has 64 boxes; for four genes, 256 boxes. An easier way to predict genotypes and phenotypes in multi-gene crosses is to use the mathematical laws of probability on which Punnett squares are based. Probability predicts the likelihood of an event.

An application of probability theory called the product rule can predict the chance that parents with known genotypes can produce offspring of a particular genotype. The product rule states that the chance that two independent events will both occur equals the product of the chance that either event will occur alone. Consider the probability of obtaining a plant with wrinkled, green peas (genotype *rryy*) from dihybrid (*RrYy*) parents. Do the reasoning for one gene at a time, then multiply the results (**figure 4.11**).

A Punnett square for *Rr* crossed to *Rr* shows that the probability of *Rr* plants producing *rr* progeny is 25 percent, or 1/4. Similarly, the chance of two *Yy* plants producing a *yy* plant is 1/4. Therefore, the chance of dihybrid parents (*RrYy*) producing homozygous recessive (*rryy*) offspring is 1/4 multiplied by 1/4, or 1/16. Now consult the 16-box Punnett square for Mendel's dihybrid cross again (figure 4.10). Only one of the 16 boxes is *rryy*, just as the product rule predicts. **Figure 4.12** shows how probability and Punnett squares can be used to predict offspring genotypes and phenotypes for three human traits simultaneously.

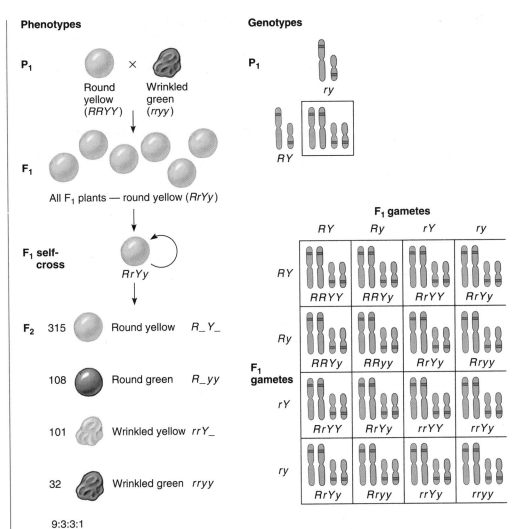

Figure 4.10 Plotting a dihybrid cross. A Punnett square can delineate the random combinations of gametes dihybrid individuals produce. An underline in a genotype (in the F$_2$ generation) indicates that either a dominant or recessive allele is possible. The numbers in the F$_2$ generation are Mendel's experimental data. The large Punnett square depicts random gamete combinations.

Until recently, Mendel's second law has not been nearly as useful in medical genetics as the first law, because not enough genes were known to follow the transmission of two or more traits at a time. But human genome information and DNA microarray technology are changing that practice. It is common now to screen for hundreds or thousands of gene variants or expressed genes at once. The increasingly computational nature of genetics in the twenty-first century has produced an entirely new field called bioinformatics. So, in this sense, genetics is continuing the theme of mathematical analysis that Gregor Mendel began more than a century ago.

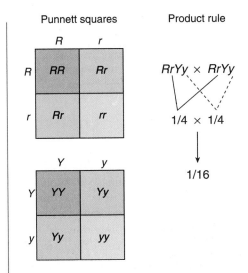

Figure 4.11 The product rule.

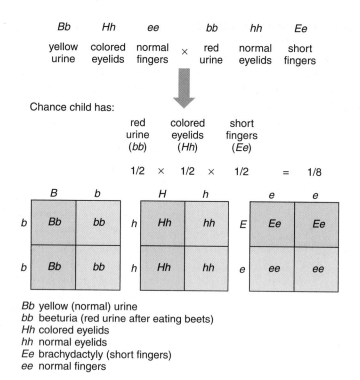

Bb *Hh* *ee*   *bb* *hh* *Ee*
yellow colored normal   red normal short
urine eyelids fingers × urine eyelids fingers

Chance child has:

red   colored   short
urine   eyelids   fingers
(*bb*)   (*Hh*)   (*Ee*)

1/2 × 1/2 × 1/2 = 1/8

Bb yellow (normal) urine
bb beeturia (red urine after eating beets)
Hh colored eyelids
hh normal eyelids
Ee brachydactyly (short fingers)
ee normal fingers

Figure 4.12   Using probability to track three traits.   A man with normal urine, colored eyelids, and normal fingers wants to have children with a woman who has red urine after she eats beets, normal eyelids, and short fingers. The chance that a child of theirs will have red urine after eating beets, colored eyelids, and short fingers is 1/8.

Key Concepts

Mendel's law of independent assortment considers genes transmitted on different chromosomes. In a dihybrid cross of heterozygotes for seed color and shape, Mendel saw a phenotypic ratio of 9:3:3:1. He concluded that transmission of one gene does not influence that of another. Meiotic events explain independent assortment. Punnett squares and probability can be used to follow independent assortment. Knowing the human genome sequence has made it possible to analyze more than one gene at a time.

4.4   Pedigree Analysis

In this era of genome sequencing, families are still often the starting point of genetic investigation—and families still represent the context in which most people think of genetics. For researchers, families are tools, and the bigger the family the better—the more children in a generation, the easier it is to discern modes of inheritance. Geneticists use charts called **pedigrees** to display family relationships and to depict which relatives have specific phenotypes and, sometimes, genotypes. A human pedigree serves the same purpose as one for purebred dogs or cats or thoroughbred horses—it helps keep track of relationships and traits.

A pedigree consists of shapes connected by lines. Vertical lines represent generations; horizontal lines that connect two shapes at their centers depict parents; shapes connected by vertical lines joined horizontally represent siblings. Squares indicate males; circles, females; and diamonds, individuals of unspecified sex. Roman numerals designate generations. Arabic numerals or names indicate individuals. **Figure 4.13** shows these and other commonly used pedigree symbols. Colored or shaded shapes indicate individuals who express the trait under study, and half-filled shapes represent known carriers. A genetic counselor will often sketch out a pedigree while interviewing a client, then use a computer program and add test results that might indicate genotypes to fill in the pedigree and finalize a report.

Pedigrees Then and Now

The earliest pedigrees were genealogical, indicating family relationships but not traits. **Figure 4.14** shows such a pedigree for

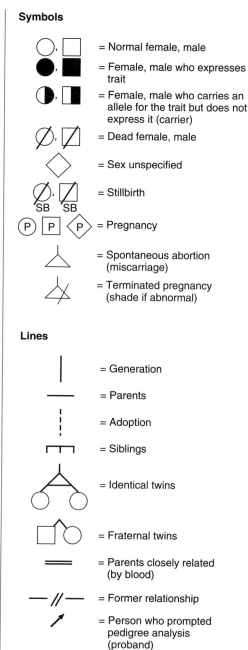

Symbols

○, □ = Normal female, male

● , ■ = Female, male who expresses trait

◐ , ◨ = Female, male who carries an allele for the trait but does not express it (carrier)

∅, ⊘ = Dead female, male

◇ = Sex unspecified

∅ SB, ⊘ SB = Stillbirth

Ⓟ, ☐P, ◇P = Pregnancy

△ = Spontaneous abortion (miscarriage)

△ = Terminated pregnancy (shade if abnormal)

Lines

| = Generation

— = Parents

┊ = Adoption

┌┴┐ = Siblings

= Identical twins

= Fraternal twins

= = Parents closely related (by blood)

—//— = Former relationship

↗ = Person who prompted pedigree analysis (proband)

Numbers

Roman numerals = generations

Arabic numerals = individuals in a generation

Figure 4.13   Pedigree components. Symbols representing individuals are connected to form pedigree charts, which display the inheritance patterns of particular traits.

a highly inbred part of the ancient Egyptian royal family. The term *pedigree* arose in the fifteenth century, from the French *pie de grue*, which means "crane's foot." Pedigrees at that time, typically depicting large families, showed parents linked by curved lines to their offspring. The overall diagram often resembled a bird's foot.

One of the first pedigrees to trace an inherited illness was an extensive family tree of several European royal families, indicating which members had the clotting disorder hemophilia (see figure 6.8). The mutant gene probably originated in Queen Victoria of England in the nineteenth century. In 1845, a genealogist named Pliny Earle constructed a pedigree of a family with colorblindness, using musical notation—half notes for unaffected females, quarter notes for colorblind females, and filled-in and squared-off notes to represent the many colorblind males. In the early twentieth century, pedigrees took on a negative note when eugenicists attempted to use the diagrams to show that traits such as criminality, feeblemindedness, and promiscuity were the consequence of faulty genes.

Today, pedigrees are important both for helping families identify the risk of transmitting an inherited illness and as starting points for identifying a gene from the human genome sequence. People who have kept meticulous family records are invaluable in helping researchers follow the inheritance of particular genes in groups such as the Mormons and the Amish. Very large pedigrees provide information on many individuals with a particular disorder. The researchers can then search these individuals' DNA to identify a particular sequence they have all inherited that is not found in healthy family members. Discovery of the gene that causes Huntington disease, for example, took researchers to a remote village in Venezuela to study an enormous family. The gene was eventually traced to a sailor who introduced the mutation in the nineteenth century.

Pedigrees Display Mendel's Laws

A person familiar with Mendel's laws can often tell a mode of inheritance just by looking carefully at a pedigree. Consider an autosomal recessive trait, albinism. Recall from Reading 2.2 that the homozygous recessive individual lacks an enzyme necessary to manufacture the pigment melanin and, as a result, has very pale hair and skin. Recall also that an autosomal recessive trait can affect both sexes and can (but doesn't necessarily) skip generations. **Figure 4.15** shows a pedigree for albinism. If a condition is known to be inherited as an autosomal recessive trait, carrier status can be inferred for individuals who have affected (homozygous recessive) children. In figure 4.15, because individuals III-1 and III-3 are affected, individuals II-2 and II-3 must be

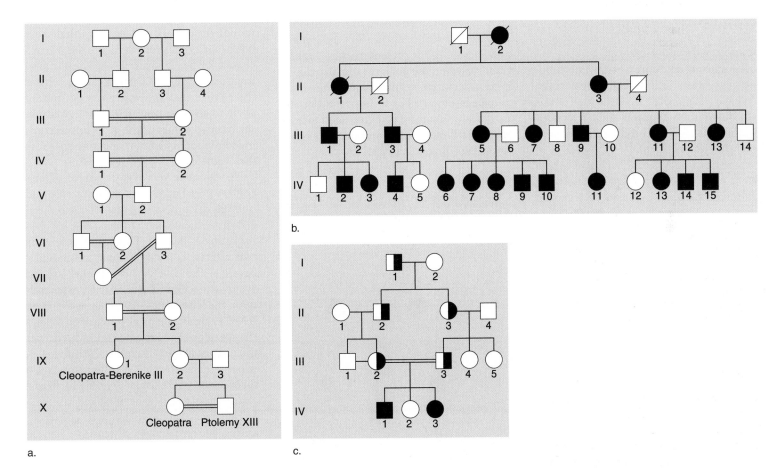

a.

b.

c.

Figure 4.14 Some unusual pedigrees. **(a)** A partial pedigree of Egypt's Ptolemy dynasty shows only genealogy, not traits. It appears almost ladderlike because of the extensive inbreeding. From 323 B.C. to Cleopatra's death in 30 B.C., the family experienced one cousins of half-brothers pairing (generation III), four brother-sister pairings (generations IV, VI, VIII, and X), and an uncle-niece relationship (generations VI and VII). Cleopatra married her brother, Ptolemy XIII, when he was 10 years old! These marriage patterns were an attempt to preserve the royal blood. **(b)** In contrast to the Egyptian pedigree, a family with polydactyly (extra fingers and toes) extends laterally, with many children. **(c)** The most common form of consanguinity is marriage of first cousins. They share one set of grandparents, and therefore risk passing on the same recessive alleles to offspring.

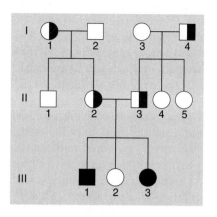

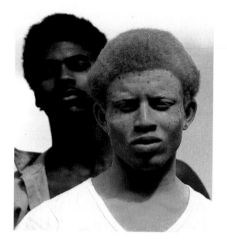

Figure 4.15 A pedigree for an autosomal recessive trait. Albinism affects males and females and can skip generations, as it does here in generations I and II. The homozygous recessive individual lacks an enzyme needed to produce melanin, which colors the eyes, skin, and hair.

carriers. One partner from each pair of grandparents must also be a carrier, which can sometimes be determined using a carrier test, inferred from family history, or deduced from a map of DNA sequence of the affected chromosome.

An autosomal dominant trait does not skip generations and can affect both sexes. A typical pedigree for an autosomal dominant trait has some squares and circles filled in to indicate affected individuals in each generation (**figure 4.16**).

A pedigree may be inconclusive, which means that either autosomal recessive or autosomal dominant inheritance can explain the pattern of filled-in symbols. **Figure 4.17** shows one such pedigree, for a type of hair loss called alopecia. According to the pedigree, this trait can be passed in an autosomal dominant mode because it affects both males and females and is present in every generation. However, the pedigree can also depict autosomal recessive inheritance if the individuals represented by unfilled symbols are carriers. Inconclusive pedigrees tend to arise when families are small and the trait is not severe enough to impair fertility.

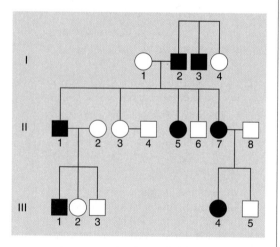

Figure 4.16 A pedigree for an autosomal dominant trait. Autosomal dominant traits do not skip generations. This trait is brachydactyly, or short fingers.

Figure 4.17 An inconclusive pedigree. This pedigree could account for an autosomal dominant trait or an autosomal recessive trait that does not prevent affected individuals from having children. (Unfilled symbols could represent carriers.)

Solving a Problem: Conditional Probability

Often genetic counselors are asked to predict the probability that a condition will occur in a particular individual, such as an offspring. Mendel's laws, pedigrees, and Punnett squares provide clues, as do logic and common sense. Consider the family depicted in **figure 4.18**.

Michael Stewart has sickle cell disease, which is inherited as an autosomal recessive condition. This means that his unaffected parents, Kate and Brad, must each be heterozygotes (carriers). Michael's sister, Ellen, also healthy, is expecting her first child. Ellen's husband, Tim, has no family history of sickle cell disease. Ellen wants to know the risk that her child will inherit the mutant allele from her and be a carrier.

Ellen's request really contains two questions. First, what is the risk that she herself is a carrier? Because Ellen is the product of a monohybrid cross, and we know that she is not homozygous recessive, she has a 2 in 3 chance of being a carrier, as the Punnett square indicates. If Ellen is a carrier, what is the chance that she will pass the mutant allele to an offspring? It is 1 in 2, because she has two copies of the gene, and according to Mendel's first law, only one goes into each gamete.

To calculate the overall risk to Ellen's child, we can apply the product rule and multiply the probability that Ellen is a carrier by the chance that, if she is, she will pass the mutant allele on. This result, following two events, is a conditional probability, because the likelihood of the second event—the child being a carrier—depends upon the first event—that Ellen is a carrier. If we assume Tim is not a carrier, Ellen's chance of giving birth to a child who carries the mutant allele is therefore 2/3 times 1/2, which equals 2/6, or 1/3. Ellen thus has a theoretical 1 in 3 chance of giving birth to a child who is a carrier for sickle cell disease.

Pedigrees can be difficult to construct and interpret for several reasons. People sometimes hesitate to supply information because they are embarrassed by symptoms affecting behavior or mental stability. Family relationships can be complicated by adoption, children born out of wedlock, serial relationships, blended families, and assisted reproductive technologies such as

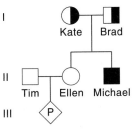

a. Ellen's brother, Michael, has sickle cell disease.

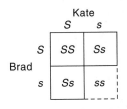

b. Probability that Ellen is a carrier: $^2/_3$

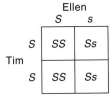

c. If Ellen is a carrier, chance that fetus is a carrier: $^1/_2$

Total probability = $^2/_3 \times ^1/_2 = ^1/_3$

Figure 4.18 Making predictions. Ellen's brother, Michael, has sickle cell disease, as depicted in this pedigree **(a).** Ellen wonders what the chance is that her fetus has inherited the sickle cell allele from her. First, she must calculate the chance that she is a carrier. The Punnett square in **(b)** shows that this risk is 2 in 3. (She must be genotype *SS* or *Ss*, but cannot be *ss* because she does not have the disease.) The risk that the fetus is a carrier, assuming that the father is not a carrier, is half Ellen's risk of being a carrier, or 1 in 3 **(c).**

surrogate mothers and artificial insemination by donor (chapter 21). Moreover, many people cannot trace their families back more than three or four generations, so they lack sufficient evidence to reveal a mode of inheritance. Still, the pedigree is perhaps the most classic genetic tool, and it remains a powerful way to see, at a glance, how a trait passes from generation to generation—just as Gregor Mendel did with peas.

Key Concepts

Pedigrees are charts that depict family relationships and the transmission of inherited traits. Squares represent males, and circles, females; horizontal lines link two partners, vertical lines show generations, and elevated horizontal lines depict siblings. Symbols for heterozygotes are half-shaded, and symbols for individuals who express the trait under study are completely shaded. • Pedigrees can reveal mode of inheritance. Along with Punnett squares, they are tools that apply Mendel's first law to predict the recurrence risks of inherited disorders or traits.

Summary

4.1 Following the Inheritance of One Gene—Segregation

1. Gregor Mendel described the two basic laws of inheritance using pea plant crosses. The laws, which derive from the actions of chromosomes during meiosis, apply to all diploid organisms.

2. Mendel used a statistical approach to investigate why some traits seem to disappear in the hybrid generation. The **law of segregation** states that alleles of a gene are distributed into separate gametes during meiosis. Mendel demonstrated this using seven traits in pea plants.

3. A diploid individual with two identical alleles of a gene is **homozygous.** A **heterozygote** has two different alleles of a gene. A gene may have many alleles.

4. A **dominant** allele masks the expression of a **recessive** allele. An individual may be homozygous dominant, homozygous recessive, or heterozygous.

5. Mendel repeatedly found that when he crossed two true-breeding types, then bred the resulting hybrids to each other, the two variants of the trait appeared in a 3:1 phenotypic ratio. Crossing these progeny further revealed a genotypic ratio of 1:2:1.

6. A **Punnett square** is a chart used to follow the transmission of alleles. It is based on probability.

4.2 Single-Gene Inheritance in Humans

7. Traits or disorders caused by single genes are called Mendelian or unifactorial traits.

8. **Modes of inheritance** enable geneticists to predict phenotypes. In **autosomal dominant** inheritance, males and females may be affected, and the trait does not skip generations. Inheritance of an **autosomal recessive** trait may affect either males or females and may skip generations. Autosomal recessive conditions are more

likely to occur in families with **consanguinity.** Recessive disorders tend to be more severe and cause symptoms earlier than dominant disorders.

9. Genetic problems can be solved by tracing alleles as gametes form and then combine in a new individual.

10. Dominance and recessiveness reflect how alleles affect the abundance or activity of the gene's protein product.

4.3 Following the Inheritance of Two Genes—Independent Assortment

11. Mendel's second law, the **law of independent assortment,** follows the transmission of two or more genes on different chromosomes. It states that a random assortment of maternally and paternally derived chromosomes during meiosis results in gametes that have different combinations of these genes.

12. The chance that two independent genetic events will both occur is equal to the product of the probabilities that each event will occur on its own. This principle, called the product rule, is useful in calculating the risk that certain individuals will inherit a particular genotype and in following the inheritance of two genes on different chromosomes.

4.4 Pedigree Analysis

13. A **pedigree** is a chart that depicts family relationships and patterns of inheritance for particular traits. A pedigree can be inconclusive.

Review Questions

1. How does meiosis explain Mendel's laws of segregation and independent assortment?

2. How was Mendel able to derive the two laws of inheritance without knowing about chromosomes?

3. Distinguish between

  a. autosomal recessive and autosomal dominant inheritance.

  b. Mendel's first and second laws.

  c. a homozygote and a heterozygote.

  d. a monohybrid and a dihybrid cross.

  e. a Punnett square and a pedigree.

4. Why would Mendel's results for the dihybrid cross have been different if the genes for the traits he followed were located near each other on the same chromosome?

5. Why are extremely rare autosomal recessive disorders more likely to appear in families in which blood relatives have children together?

6. How does the pedigree of the ancient Egyptian royal family in figure 4.14a differ from a pedigree a genetic counselor might use today?

7. People who have Huntington disease inherit one mutant and one normal allele. How would a person who is homozygous dominant for the condition arise?

8. What is the probability that two individuals with an autosomal recessive trait, such as albinism, will have a child with the same genotype and phenotype as they do?

Applied Questions

1. Achondroplasia is a common form of hereditary dwarfism that causes very short limbs, stubby hands, and an enlarged forehead. Below are four pedigrees depicting families with this specific type of dwarfism. What is the most likely mode of inheritance? Cite a reason for your answer.

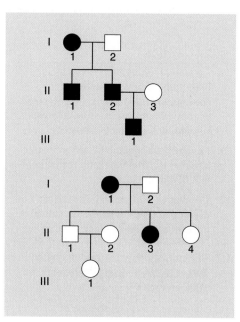

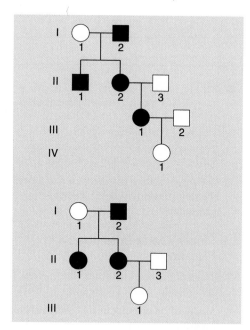

3. Chands syndrome is an autosomal recessive condition characterized by very curly hair, underdeveloped nails, and abnormally shaped eyelids. In the following pedigree, which individuals must be carriers?

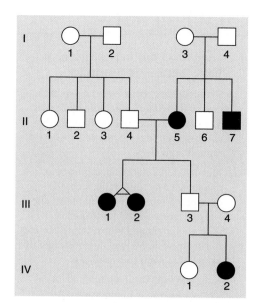

2. Draw a pedigree to depict the following family:

One couple has a son and a daughter with normal skin pigmentation. Another couple has one son and two daughters with normal skin pigmentation. The daughter from the first couple has three children with the son of the second couple. Their son and one daughter have albinism; their other daughter has normal skin pigmentation.

4. Caleb has a double row of eyelashes, which he inherited from his mother as a dominant trait. His maternal grandfather is the only other relative to have the trait. Veronica, a woman with normal eyelashes, falls madly in love with Caleb, and they marry. Their first child, Polly, has normal eyelashes. Now Veronica is pregnant again and hopes they will have a child who has double eyelashes. What chance does a child of Veronica and Caleb have of inheriting double eyelashes? Draw a pedigree of this family.

5. Congenital insensitivity to pain with anhidrosis is an extremely rare autosomal recessive condition that causes fever, inability to sweat (anhidrosis), mental retardation, inability to feel pain, and self-mutilating behavior. Researchers compared the following three families with this condition. What do these families have in common that might explain the appearance of this rare illness?

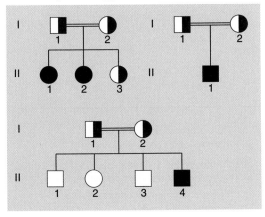

6. The child in figure 4.12 who has red urine after eating beets, colored eyelids, and short fingers, is of genotype *bbHhEe*. The genes for these traits are on different chromosomes. If he has children with a woman who is a trihybrid for each of these genes, what are the expected genotypic and phenotypic ratios for their offspring?

7. In this pedigree, individual III-1 died at age two of Tay-Sachs disease, an autosomal recessive disorder. Which other family members must be carriers, and which could be?

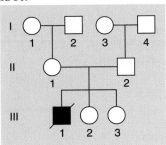

8. Recall Mackenzie, the young woman from chapter 1 who underwent genetic testing. The tests revealed that she has a 1 in 10 chance of developing lung cancer, and a 2 in 1,000 chance of developing colon cancer. What is the probability that she will develop both cancers?

9. Sclerosteosis causes overgrowth of the skull and jaws that produces a characteristic face, gigantism, facial paralysis, and hearing loss. The overgrowth of skull bones can cause severe headaches and even sudden death. In this pedigree for a family afflicted by sclerosteosis:

   a. What is the relationship between the individuals who are connected by slanted double lines?

   b. Sclerosteosis is an autosomal recessive condition. Which individuals in the pedigree must be carriers?

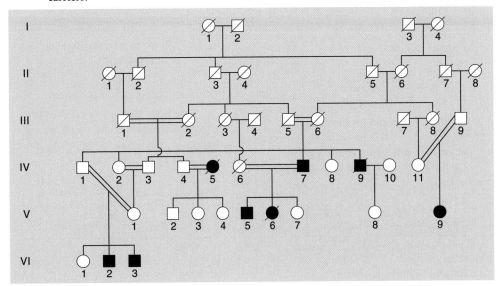

10. According to this pedigree from the soap opera "All My Children," is Charlie the product of a consanguineous relationship? The trait being tracked is freckles.

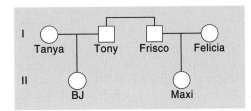

11. On "General Hospital," six-year-old Maxi suffered from Kawasaki syndrome, an inflammation of the heart. She desperately needed a transplant, and received one from BJ, who died in a bus accident. Maxi and BJ had the same unusual blood type, which is inherited. According to this pedigree, how are Maxi and BJ related?

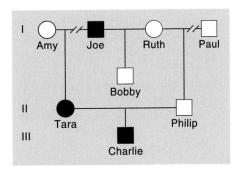

12. A man has a blood test for Tay-Sachs disease and learns that he is a carrier. His body produces half the normal amount of the enzyme hexoseaminidase A. Why doesn't he have symptoms? (This disease causes degeneration of the nervous system in early childhood.)

Web Activities

13. Go to the website for the National Organization for Rare Disorders (http://www.rarediseases.org/). Identify an autosomal recessive disorder and an autosomal dominant disorder. Create a family for each one, and describe transmission of the disease over three generations.

14. Go to the website for Gene Gateway—Exploring Genes and Genetic Disorders (http://www.ornl.gov/TechResources/Human_Genome/posters/chromosome/chooser.html). Select two disorders or traits that would demonstrate independent assortment if present in the same family, and two that would not.

Case Studies

15. On the soap opera "The Young and the Restless," several individuals suffer from a rapid aging syndrome in which a young child is sent off to boarding school and returns three months later an angry teenager. In the Newman family, siblings

Nicholas and Victoria aged from ages 6 and 8 years, respectively, to 16 and 18 years within a few months. Their parents, Victor and Nikki, are not affected; in fact, they never seem to age at all.

a. What is the mode of inheritance of the rapid aging disorder affecting Nicholas and Victoria?

b. How do you know what the mode of inheritance is?

c. Draw a pedigree to depict this portion of the Newman family.

16. Sam Fitzgerald is a carpet salesman who, at age 46, begins to slur his speech and stagger slightly when he walks. His speech worsens, he develops a shuffling gait to avoid falling, and he loses his job, because customers complain that he is intoxicated. His children, who know he does not drink alcohol, become alarmed and urge him to seek medical care. Eventually, after much counseling and thinking, he is tested and learns that he has HD. As his symptoms worsen, his sister Pam, who is tested and is free of the mutation, provides care—something she also did as a child when their parents, Ruth and Alan, died in a car crash in their thirties. Another sister, Sue, refuses to be tested.

a. Draw a pedigree for this family.

b. What is the risk that Sam's daughter has inherited HD?

c. What is the risk that Sue's son has inherited HD?

d. When Sue hears that Pam was tested and is free of the mutation, she assumes that this raises the risk that she has inherited the disease. Is she correct? Explain your answer in terms of Mendel's first law.

Learn to apply the skills of a genetic counselor with these additional cases found in the *Case Workbook in Human Genetics:*

Acrocephalosyndactyly

Carnosinemia

Huntington-like disorder

Restless leg syndrome

Schneckenbecken dysplasia

Suggested Readings

Bhattacharyya, Madan K., et al. January 12, 1990. The wrinkled-seed character of pea described by Mendel is caused by a transposon-like insertion in a gene encoding starch-branching enzyme. *Cell* 60:115–27. A description of one of the traits that Mendel studied, at the molecular level.

Gustafsson, A. February 1979. Linnaeus' Peloria: The history of a monster. *Theoretical Applied Genetics* 54:241–48. Charles Darwin demonstrated Mendel's first law using mutant flowers, but he didn't realize it.

Henig, Robin Marantz. 2000. *The Monk in the Garden: The Lost and Found Genius of Gregor Mendel, the Father of Genetics.* Boston: Houghton Mifflin Co. A complete biography of the "father of genetics."

Lester, Diane R., et al. August 1997. Mendel's stem length gene (*Le*) encodes a gibberellin 3β-hydroxylase. *Plant Cell* 9:1435–43. The molecular and cellular basis of Mendel's short and tall traits involves regulation of a growth hormone.

Lewis, Ricki. October 20, 2003. Genetic testing timeline. *The Scientist* 17(20):23. A history of four single-gene disorders.

Lewis, Ricki. October 20, 2003. A genetic check-up: Lessons from Huntington disease and cystic fibrosis. *The Scientist* 17(20):24–26. We are on the brink of many new genetic tests.

Lewis, Ricki. December 1994. The evolution of a classic genetic tool. *BioScience* 44:5–8. Pedigrees may include molecular information.

Mendel, Gregor. March 1866. Experiments in plant hybridization. *Journal of the Royal Horticultural Society,* pp. 3–47. Mendel's original paper is surprisingly understandable.

Mysliwiec, Tami H. January 2003. The genetic blues: Understanding genetic principles using a practical approach and a historical perspective. *The American Biology Teacher* 65(1):42–46. Tracing the inheritance of "the blue people of Kentucky" demonstrates Mendel's laws.

Orel, Vitězslav. 1996. *Gregor Mendel: The First Geneticist.* New York: Oxford University Press. A detailed account of Gregor Mendel and his work.

Rothenberg, Laura. 2003. *Breathing for a Living: A memoir.* New York: Hyperion. This young woman chronicles her slow death from CF, a single-gene disorder.

Tassicker, Ross, et al. February 8, 2003. Prenatal diagnosis requests for Huntington's disease when the father is at risk and does not want to know his genetic status: Clinical, legal, and ethical viewpoints. *British Medical Journal* 326:331–33. Genetic testing raises complex issues when repercussions extend beyond the individual being tested.

Weekly updates of current news related to human genetics are available through Power Web on your Online Learning Center.

VISIT YOUR ONLINE LEARNING CENTER

Visit your online learning center for additional resources and tools to help you master this chapter. See us at

www.mhhe.com/lewisgenetics6.

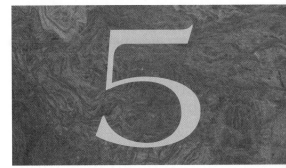

Extensions and Exceptions to Mendel's Laws

CHAPTER CONTENTS

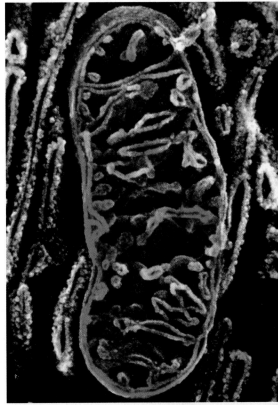

Genes in mitochondria do not follow Mendel's laws. They are present in many copies per cell, and are transmitted only from a female.

The transmission of inherited traits is not always as straightforward as Mendel's pea experiments indicated. Variations in gene expression and in allele and gene interactions can alter expected phenotypic ratios. In some situations, such as when genes are in mitochondria or are "linked" on the same chromosome, Mendel's laws do not apply. This chapter examines extensions and exceptions to Mendel's laws.

5.1 When Gene Expression Appears to Alter Mendelian Ratios

Mendel's crosses yielded offspring that were easily distinguished from each other. A pea is either yellow or green; a plant tall or short. For some characteristics, though, offspring classes do not occur in the proportions that Punnett squares or probabilities predict. In other cases, transmission patterns of a visible trait are not consistent with the mode of inheritance. In these instances, Mendel's laws operate, and the underlying genotypic ratios persist, but either the nature of the phenotype or influences from other genes or the environment alter phenotypic ratios. Following are several circumstances that appear to contradict Mendel's laws—although the laws actually still apply.

Lethal Allele Combinations

"Lethal" means deadly, so any genotype (allele combination) that causes the death of an individual is literally lethal. In a population and evolutionary sense, though, a lethal genotype has a more specific meaning—it causes death before the individual can reproduce, which prevents passage of his or her genes to the next generation. Huntington disease, which is ultimately fatal and begins in middle age, is lethal to the individual, but not lethal in a population sense because it does not typically cause death or even symptoms until after a person has had children.

In organisms used in experiments, such as fruit flies, pea plants, or mice, lethal allele combinations remove an expected progeny class following a specific cross. For example, a cross of two heterozygotes in which the homozygous recessive progeny die as embryos would leave only heterozygotes and homozygous dominant individuals as survivors.

In humans, early-acting lethal alleles cause many spontaneous abortions (technically called "miscarriages" if they occur after the embryonic period). When a man and woman each carries a recessive lethal allele for the same gene, each pregnancy has a 25 percent chance of spontaneously aborting—a proportion representing the homozygous recessive class. Sometimes a double dose of a dominant allele is lethal, as is the case for Mexican hairless dogs. Inheriting one dominant allele confers the coveted hairlessness trait, but inheriting two dominant alleles is lethal to the unlucky embryo. Breeders cross hairless to hairy ("powderpuff") dogs, rather than hairless to hairy, to avoid losing the lethal homozygous dominant class—a quarter of the pups, as **figure 5.1** indicates.

Multiple Alleles

A person has two alleles for any autosomal gene (one allele on each homolog), but a gene can exist in more than two allelic forms in a population because it can mutate in many ways. Different allele combinations can produce variations in phenotype.

Correlations between genotypes and phenotypes would enable physicians to predict

Figure 5.1 Lethal alleles.
(a) This Mexican hairless dog has inherited a dominant allele that makes it hairless. Inheriting two such dominant alleles is lethal during embryonic development.
(b) Breeders cross Mexican hairless dogs to hairy ("powderpuff") dogs to avoid dead embryos and stillbirths that represent the *HH* genotypic class.

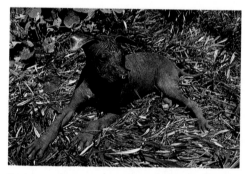

a.

Alleles	Genotypes	Phenotypes
h = hair (wild type)	HH	lethal
H = hairless (mutant)	Hh	Mexican hairless
	hh	hairy

Cross 1

Mexican hairless *Hh* × Mexican hairless *Hh*

1 : 2 : 1
hh : *Hh* : *HH*
hairy : Mexican hairless : dead

	H	h
H	HH	Hh
h	Hh	hh

$1/4$ die as embryos (*HH*)
Of survivors:
$2/3$ = Mexican hairless (*Hh*)
$1/3$ = hairy (*hh*)

Cross 2

hairy *hh* × Mexican hairless *Hh*

1 : 1
hh : *Hh*
hairy : Mexican hairless

	H	h
h	Hh	hh
h	Hh	hh

All survive:
$1/2$ = Mexican hairless
$1/2$ = hairy

b.

the course of a particular illness following a genetic test, but often other genes and environmental effects modify a disease-causing gene's expression, making this difficult. One disorder for which genotype does predict phenotype is phenylketonuria (PKU), an inborn error of metabolism. When the implicated enzyme is completely absent, the individual is profoundly mentally retarded. The amino acid phenylalanine that the enzyme normally breaks down builds up in brain cells. However, eating a special diet extremely low in phenylalanine from birth to at least 8 years of age, and possibly much longer, allows normal brain development. The more than 300 mutant alleles known for this gene combine to form four basic phenotypes: classic PKU with profound mental retardation; moderate PKU; mild PKU; and simply excreting excess of the amino acid in the urine, without symptoms. Knowing the allele combination can give parents an idea of how strict the diet need be, and how long it must continue.

The existence of multiple alleles—several hundreds of them—has greatly complicated carrier testing for cystic fibrosis (CF), as well as the ability to predict phenotypes from genotypes. When the CF gene was discovered in 1989, researchers identified one mutant allele, called ΔF508, that causes about 70 percent of cases in many populations (see figure 2.1b). Researchers were soon adding more alleles to the list, and finding that not all allele combinations cause the exact same symptoms.

People homozygous for ΔF508 have a classic combination of severe symptoms, including frequent serious respiratory infections, very sticky mucus in the lungs, and poor weight gain due to insufficient pancreatic function. Another genotype increases one's susceptibility to bronchitis and pneumonia, and another causes only absence of the vas deferens. Genetic tests for CF include panels of mutations that are the most common in a patient's particular ethnic group, maximizing the likelihood of detecting carriers.

Different Dominance Relationships

In complete dominance, one allele is expressed, while the other isn't. Alternatively, in **incomplete dominance**, the heterozygous phenotype is intermediate between that of either homozygote. (Technically, this is a lack of dominance.)

In a sense, enzyme deficiencies in which a threshold level is necessary for health illustrate both complete and incomplete dominance—depending upon how one evaluates the phenotype. For example, on a whole-body level, Tay-Sachs disease displays complete dominance because the heterozygote (carrier) is as healthy as a homozygous dominant individual. However, if phenotype is based on enzyme level, then the heterozygote is intermediate between the homozygous dominant (full enzyme level) and homozygous recessive (no enzyme). Half the normal amount of enzyme is sufficient for health.

A more obvious example of incomplete dominance occurs in the snapdragon plant. A red-flowered plant of genotype *RR* crossed to a white-flowered *rr* plant can give rise to a *Rr* plant—which has pink flowers. This intermediate color is presumably due to an intermediate amount of pigment.

Familial hypercholesterolemia (FH) is an example of incomplete dominance in humans that can be observed on the molecular and whole-body levels. A person with two disease-causing alleles lacks receptors on liver cells that take up cholesterol from the bloodstream. A person with one disease-causing allele has half the normal number of receptors. Someone with two wild type (the most common) alleles has the normal number of receptors. **Figure 5.2** shows how measurement of plasma cholesterol reflects these three genotypes. The phenotypes parallel the number of receptors—those with two mutant alleles die as children of heart attacks, those with one mutant allele may suffer heart attacks in young adulthood, and those with two wild type alleles do not develop this inherited form of heart disease.

Different alleles that are both expressed in a heterozygote are **codominant.** The ABO blood group is based on the expression of codominant alleles. Blood types are determined by the patterns of cell surface molecules on red blood cells. Most of these molecules, called antigens, are proteins embedded in the plasma membrane with attached sugars that poke out from the cell surface. People who belong to blood group A have an allele that encodes an enzyme that adds a certain final piece to a certain sugar. The final sugar is called antigen A. In people with blood type

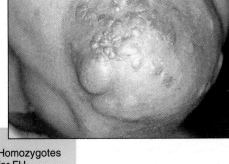

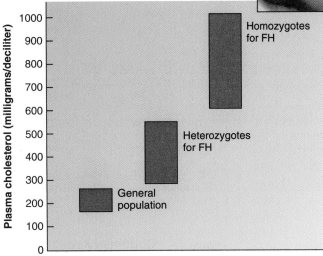

Figure 5.2 Incomplete dominance. A heterozygote for familial hypercholesterolemia (FH) has approximately half the normal number of cell surface receptors in the liver for LDL cholesterol. An individual with two mutant alleles, has the severe form of FH, with liver cells that totally lack the receptors. Serum cholesterol level is very high. The photograph shows cholesterol deposits on the elbow of an affected young man.

B, the allele and its encoded enzyme are slightly different, which causes a different piece to attach to the sugar, producing antigen B. Blood group O reflects yet a third allele of this gene. It is missing just one DNA nucleotide, but this drastically changes the encoded enzyme in a way that robs the sugar chain of its final piece (**figure 5.3**).

ABO blood types in the past have been described as variants of a gene called "*I*," although OMIM now abbreviates the designations. The older "*I*" system makes the codominance easier to understand (**table 5.1**). The three alleles are I^A, I^B, and i. People with blood type A have antigen A on the surfaces of their red blood cells, and may be of geno-

type I^A/I^A or I^Ai. People with blood type B have antigen B on their red blood cell surfaces, and may be of genotype I^B/I^B or I^Bi. People with the rare blood type AB have both antigens A and B on their cell surfaces, and are genotype I^A/I^B. People with blood type O have neither antigen, and are genotype ii.

Television program plots often misuse ABO blood type terminology, assuming that a child's ABO type must match that of one parent. This is not true, because a person with type A or B blood can be heterozygous. A person who is genotype I^Ai and a person who is I^Bi can jointly produce offspring of any ABO genotype or phenotype, as **figure 5.4** illustrates.

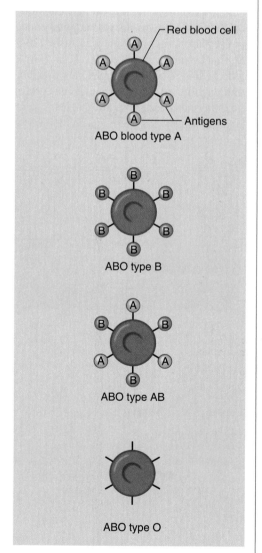

Figure 5.3 ABO blood types illustrate codominance. ABO blood types are based on antigens on red blood cell surfaces. The size of the A and B antigens is greatly exaggerated in this drawing.

Table 5.1

The ABO Blood Group

Genotypes	Phenotypes	
	Antigens on Surface	ABO Blood Type
I^A/I^A	A	Type A
I^Ai	A	
I^B/I^B	B	Type B
I^Bi	B	
I^A/I^B	AB	Type AB
ii	None	Type O

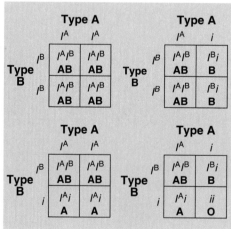

Figure 5.4 Codominance. The I^A and I^B alleles of the I gene are codominant, but they follow Mendel's law of segregation. These Punnett squares follow the genotypes that could result when a person with type A blood produces offspring with a person with type B blood.

Epistasis—When One Gene Affects Expression of Another

Mendel's laws can appear to not operate when one gene masks or otherwise affects the expression of a different gene, a phenomenon called **epistasis.** (Do not confuse this with dominance relationships between alleles of the *same* gene.) The Bombay phenotype, for example, is a result of two interacting genes: the *I* and *H* genes. The relationship of these two genes affects the expression of the ABO blood type.

The normal *H* allele encodes an enzyme that inserts a sugar molecule, called antigen H, onto a particular glycoprotein on the surface of an immature red blood cell. The recessive *h* allele produces an inactive form of the enzyme that cannot insert the sugar. (The *H* gene's product is fucosyltransferase 1, and in OMIM the *H* gene is called *FUT*1.) The A and B antigens are attached to the *H* antigen. As long as at least one *H* allele is present, the ABO genotype dictates the ABO blood type. However, in a person with genotype *hh*, there is no *H* antigen to bind to the A and B antigens, and they fall away. The person has blood type O based on phenotype (a blood test), but may have any ABO genotype. For example, Mendel's laws predict that each child of a man who has type B blood and genotype I^B/I^B and a woman who has type A blood with genotype I^A/I^A (like the upper left Punnett square in figure 5.4) must be type AB. But if the parents are each also *Hh*, then each offspring has a 25 percent chance of being *hh*, and therefore having a phenotype of type O blood, because the A and B antigens cannot bind to the red blood cells. The child's genotype, however, would be I^A/I^B, *hh*. The predicted Mendelian phenotypic ratios change because of the action of the second gene.

Individuals with the *hh* genotype are very rare with one notable exception—residents of Reunion Island, in the Indian Ocean east of Madagascar. Apparently the settlers of this isolated island included at least one *hh* or *Hh* individual, and, with time, large families, and some consanguinity, the allele multiplied in the population.

Sometimes epistasis is just a matter of common sense. For example, a hairless gene in dogs and mice, and a spineless gene in cucumbers, prevent genes that color the hairs and spines from acting. This is similar to the Bombay phenotype in that the two genes affect related structures.

Penetrance and Expressivity

The same allele combination can produce different degrees of a phenotype in different individuals because a gene does not act alone. Nutrition, toxic exposures, other illnesses, and actions of other genes may influence the expression of most genes. Cystic fibrosis illustrates how other genes can modify a gene's expression. Consider two individuals who have the most severe genotype for this illness. One is much sicker than the other because she also inherited genes predisposing her to develop asthma and respiratory allergies.

Many Mendelian traits and illnesses have distinctive phenotypes, despite all of these influences. The terms *penetrance* and *expressivity* describe degrees of gene expression. **Penetrance** refers to the all-or-none expression of a genotype; **expressivity** refers to severity or extent.

An allele combination that produces a phenotype in everyone who inherits it is considered completely penetrant. Huntington disease (see Bioethics: Choices for the Future in chapter 4) is completely penetrant—all who inherit the mutant allele will develop symptoms if they live long enough, although symptoms may not begin until late in life. A genotype is incompletely penetrant if some individuals do not express the phenotype (have no symptoms). Polydactyly (see figure 1.3) is incompletely penetrant. Some people who inherit the dominant allele have more than five digits on a hand or foot, yet others who must have the allele (because they have an affected parent and child) have the normal number of fingers and toes. The penetrance of a gene is described numerically. If 80 of 100 people who have inherited the dominant polydactyly allele have extra digits, the genotype is 80 percent penetrant.

A phenotype is variably expressive if symptoms vary in intensity in different people. One person with polydactyly might have an extra digit on both hands and a foot, but another might have just one extra fingertip. Therefore, polydactyly is both incompletely penetrant and variably expressive.

It is hard to imagine how other genes or the environment can influence the numbers of fingers or toes. For familial hypercholesterolemia, variable expressivity reflects greater influence of other genes and the environment (see figure 5.2). FH heterozygotes develop heart disease due to high serum cholesterol in middle adulthood. Healthful diet and exercise habits can delay symptom onset.

Pleiotropy—One Gene, Many Effects

A Mendelian disorder with many symptoms, or a gene that controls several functions or has more than one effect, is termed **pleiotropic.** Such conditions can be difficult to trace through families because people with different subsets of symptoms may appear to have different disorders. This is the case for porphyria variegata, an autosomal dominant, pleiotropic, inborn error of metabolism. The disease affected several members of the royal families of Europe (**figure 5.5**).

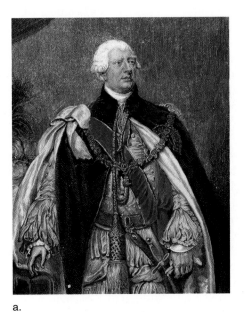

Abdominal pain
Constipation
Limb weakness
Fever
Racing pulse
Hoarseness
Dark red urine
Insomnia
Headache
Visual problems
Restlessness
Delirium
Convulsions
Stupor

a.

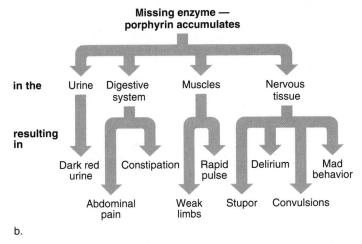

b.

Figure 5.5 Pleiotropy. King George III **(a)** suffered from the autosomal dominant disorder porphyria variegata—and so did several other family members. Because of pleiotropy, the family's varied illnesses and quirks appeared to be different, unrelated disorders. In King George, symptoms appeared every few years in a particular order **(b).**

King George III ruled England during the American Revolution. At age 50, he first experienced abdominal pain and constipation, followed by weak limbs, fever, a fast pulse, hoarseness, and dark red urine. Next, nervous system symptoms began, including insomnia, headaches, visual problems, restlessness, delirium, convulsions, and stupor. His confused and racing thoughts, combined with actions such as ripping off his wig and running about naked while at the peak of a fever, convinced court observers that the king was mad. Just as Parliament was debating his ability to rule, he recovered.

But George's ordeal was far from over. He relapsed thirteen years later, then again three years after that. Always the symptoms appeared in the same order, beginning with abdominal pain, fever, and weakness, and progressing to nervous system symptoms. Finally, an attack in 1811 placed George in a prolonged stupor, and the Prince of Wales dethroned him. George III lived for several more years, experiencing further episodes.

In George III's time, doctors were permitted to do very little to the royal body, and they simply made their diagnoses based on what the king told them. Twentieth-century researchers found that porphyria variegata caused George's red urine. In the absence of a particular enzyme, a part of the blood pigment hemoglobin called a porphyrin ring is routed into the urine instead of being broken down and metabolized by cells. Porphyrin builds up and attacks the nervous system, causing many of the symptoms. An examination of physicians' reports on George's relatives—easy to obtain for a royal family—showed that several of them also had symptoms. Before anyone realized that porphyria variegata is pleiotropic, the royal disorder appeared to be several different illnesses. Today, porphyria variegata remains rare, and people who have it are often misdiagnosed as having a seizure disorder. Unfortunately, some seizure medications and anesthetics worsen the symptoms.

Pleiotropy occurs when a single protein affects different parts of the body or participates in more than one type of biochemical reaction. Consider Marfan syndrome, an autosomal dominant defect in an elastic connective tissue protein called fibrillin.

The protein is abundant in the lens of the eye, in the aorta (the largest artery in the body, leading from the heart), and in the bones of the limbs, fingers, and ribs. Once researchers knew this, the Marfan syndrome symptoms of lens dislocation, long limbs, spindly fingers, and a caved-in chest made sense. The most serious symptom is a life-threatening weakening in the aortic wall, sometimes causing the vessel to suddenly burst. However, if the weakening is detected early, a synthetic graft can be inserted to replace the section of artery wall.

Pleiotropy can be confusing even to medical doctors. *The New England Journal of Medicine* ran a contest to see if its physician readers could identify the cause of three seemingly unrelated symptoms, illustrated in the figure in "In Their Own Words" on page 99. These symptoms are characteristic of the inborn error of metabolism alkaptonuria.

Phenocopies—When It's Not in the Genes

An environmentally caused trait that appears to be inherited is a **phenocopy.** Such a trait can either produce symptoms that resemble a Mendelian disorder's symptoms or mimic inheritance patterns by occurring in certain relatives. For example, the limb birth defect caused by the drug thalidomide, discussed in chapter 3, is a phenocopy of the inherited illness phocomelia. Physicians realized that an environmental disaster had occurred when they began seeing many children born with what looked like the very rare phocomelia. A birth defect caused by exposure to a teratogen was a more likely explanation than a sudden increase in incidence of a rare inherited disease.

An infection can be a phenocopy. Children who have AIDS may have parents who also have the disease, but these children acquired AIDS by viral infection, not by inheriting a gene. A phenocopy caused by a highly contagious infection can seem to be inherited if it affects more than one family member.

Sometimes, common symptoms may resemble those of an inherited condition until medical tests rule heredity out. For example, an underweight child who has frequent colds may show some signs of cystic fibrosis, but may instead suffer from malnu-

trition. A negative test for several CF alleles would alert a physician to look for another cause. Similarly, the lung condition emphysema may be caused by lack of an enzyme (the genetic disorder) or by smoking (the phenocopy).

Genetic Heterogeneity— More than One Way to Inherit a Trait

Different genes can produce the same phenotype, a phenomenon called **genetic heterogeneity.** This redundancy of function can make it appear that Mendel's laws are not operating. For example, 132 forms of hearing loss are transmitted as autosomal recessive traits. If a man who is heterozygous for a hearing loss gene on one chromosome has a child with a woman who is heterozygous for another hearing loss gene on a different chromosome, then that child faces only the same risk as anyone in the general population of inheriting either form of the condition. He or she *doesn't* face the 25 percent risk that Mendel's law predicts for a monohybrid cross because the parents are heterozygous for *different* genes whose encoded proteins affect hearing. Cleft palate and albinism are other traits that are genetically heterogeneic—that is, different genes can cause them.

Genetic heterogeneity can occur when genes encode different enzymes that participate in the same biochemical pathway, or different proteins involved in the same process. For example, eleven biochemical reactions lead to blood clot formation. Clotting disorders may result from mutations in the genes that specify any of the enzymes that catalyze these reactions, leading to several types of bleeding disorders. The fatal heart rhythm disorder long-QT syndrome (see Reading 2.2) can be caused by an abnormality in the potassium channel protein or in the ankyrin protein that holds the channel open in a heart muscle cell's plasma membrane.

The Human Genome Sequence Adds Perspective

Sequencing of the human genome has modified and in some cases clarified the

Alkaptonuria

Alkaptonuria was one of the first inborn errors of metabolism to be identified. Ironically, many people who have it probably never realize that the disease symptoms arise from a single metabolic abnormality **(figure 1)**. Here, Pat Wright describes her experience with the condition.

Alkaptonuria symptoms started when I was 15 years old and struggling to sit all day in high school classes. An osteopath manipulated my spine and treated the back spasms with heat and medication, which enabled me to weather the frequent flare-ups throughout high school and college. We did not relate my back problems to the metabolic disorder until many years later. These back problems persisted through five pregnancies and 26 years of teaching special education. My seriously degenerated spine, coupled with the disappearance of the cartilage in my left knee, forced me to retire on disability at the age of 57.

The first symptoms of alkaptonuria, however, began even earlier than high school. When I was a baby, my parents noticed that my diapers turned brown if not washed immediately, and even then they became stained. The doctor sent a wet diaper to a teaching hospital, and they told my parents I had a "harmless" metabolic disorder.

Fast forward sixty years.

In February 1997 I had a total knee replacement, and the surgeon was amazed to find the joint surrounded by blackened cartilage. It was the first time he had ever seen such a thing, after years of surgery. This rediscovery of alkaptonuria has answered many questions that arose over the years. It explains the dark blue-gray ears, the degenerated spine, knees, and shoulder joints. It may also explain the steadily increasing aortic stenosis and hearing loss, and perhaps the kidney stones and gallstones.

I was told I had degenerative disc disease, fibromyalgia, osteoarthritis, or degenerative joint disease. Over the years I have tried every known treatment for these conditions, with little or no success. I do recommend a regular exercise routine. I attended arthritis water aerobics classes and worked with a personal

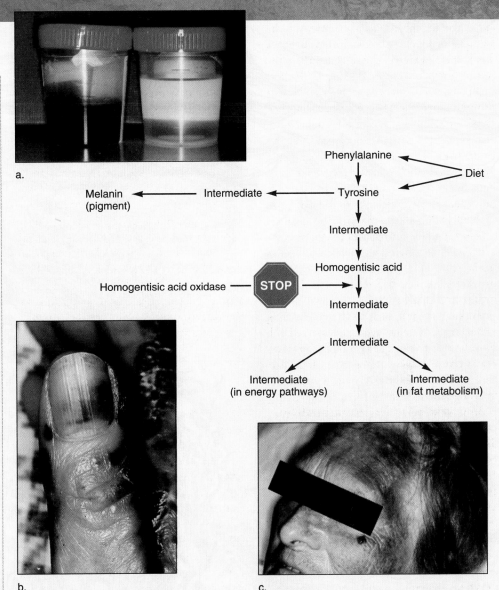

Figure 1 **Pleiotropy in alkaptonuria.** Alkaptonuria, the first recognized inborn error of metabolism, was described by Archibald Garrod in 1902. Deficiency of the enzyme homogentisic acid oxidase, discovered in 1958, leads to buildup of melanin pigment in urine when it is allowed to stand for several hours **(a)**, in nails and cartilage **(b)**, and in the skin **(c)**. The disorder is inherited as an autosomal recessive trait, and the gene is on chromosome 3. Researchers discovered a form of alkaptonuria in lab mice whose cages needed changing—the wood shavings, soaked in urine and left too long, turned blue-black!

trainer for three years before and after the knee replacement, to improve my strength, range of motion, and mobility. I think this was vital, because, though I could not do much about the condition of the joints, I could improve my muscle tone, strength, and endurance.

In January of 2000, I had my aortic valve replaced so that I might withstand further joint surgery. The following April I began aquatic physical therapy to both rehabilitate the heart and ready my body for a hip replacement in July. On June 15, 2001, I had a total left shoulder replacement and I returned to an aquatic therapy maintenance program to help with mobility and pain. Three more major joints to go! The left hip is complaining the loudest.

Pat Wright

extensions to Mendel's laws. Knowing each of the DNA bases of a protein-encoding gene, for example, greatly increases the number of known alleles—previously, we were only aware of those that affect the phenotype in an observable way.

Epistasis may not be as rare as previously thought—many genes influence each other. Gene interactions also underlie penetrance and expressivity, once thought to be strictly a characteristic of a particular gene. Similarly, DNA microarrays that reveal gene expression patterns in different tissues are painting detailed portraits of pleiotropy—which, like epistasis, may not be unusual after all. Finally, more cases of genetic heterogeneity are being discovered as genes with redundant or overlapping functions are identified.

Table 5.2 summarizes several of the phenomena that appear to alter Mendelian inheritance. Gregor Mendel derived the two laws of inheritance working with traits conferred by genes located on different chromosomes in the nucleus. When genes do not conform to these conditions, however, the associated traits may not appear in Mendelian ratios. The remainder of this chapter considers two types of gene transmission that do not fulfill the requirements for Mendelian inheritance.

Key Concepts

A lethal allele combination is never seen as a progeny class. • In incomplete dominance, the heterozygote phenotype is intermediate between those of the homozygotes; in codominance, two different alleles for the same gene are each expressed. • In epistasis, one gene influences expression of another. • Genotypes vary in penetrance (percent of individuals affected) and expressivity (intensity of symptoms) of the phenotype. A gene with more than one expression is pleiotropic. • A trait caused by the environment but resembling a known genetic trait or occurring in certain family members is a phenocopy. • Genetic heterogeneity occurs when different genes cause the same phenotype. • Examination of the human genome sequence reveals that several "exceptions" to Mendel's laws are actually more common than we thought.

5.2 Maternal Inheritance and Mitochondrial Genes

The basis of the law of segregation is that both parents contribute genes equally to offspring. This is not the case for genes in mitochondria, the organelles that house the biochemical reactions that provide energy. Mitochondria in human cells contain several copies of a "mini-chromosome" that carries just 37 genes. Sometimes it is called the twenty-fifth chromosome.

The inheritance patterns and mutation rates for mitochondrial genes differ from those for genes in the nucleus. Mitochondrial genes are maternally inherited. They are passed only from an individual's mother because sperm almost never contribute mitochondria when they fertilize an oocyte. In the rare instances when mitochondria from sperm enter an oocyte, they are usually selectively destroyed early in development. Pedigrees that follow mitochondrial genes show a woman passing the trait to all her children, while a male cannot pass the trait to any of his. The pedigree in **figure 5.6** illustrates maternal transmission of a mutation in a mitochondrial gene.

Unlike DNA in the nucleus, mitochondrial DNA does not cross over. Mitochondrial DNA also mutates faster than nuclear DNA for two reasons: it lacks DNA repair enzymes (discussed in chapter 9), and the mitochondrion is the site of the energy reactions that produce oxygen free radicals that damage DNA. Also unlike nuclear DNA, mitochondrial DNA is not wrapped in histone proteins, nor are genes "interrupted" by

Table 5.2

Factors That Alter Mendelian Phenotypic Ratios

Phenomenon	Effect on Phenotype	Example
Lethal alleles	A phenotypic class dies very early in development.	Spontaneous abortion
Multiple alleles	Many variants or degrees of a phenotype occur.	Cystic fibrosis
Incomplete dominance	A heterozygote's phenotype is intermediate between those of two homozygotes.	Familial hypercholesterolemia
Codominance	A heterozygote's phenotype is distinct from and not intermediate between those of the two homozygotes.	ABO blood types
Epistasis	One gene masks or otherwise affects another's phenotype.	Bombay phenotype
Penetrance	Some individuals with a particular genotype do not have the associated phenotype.	Polydactyly
Expressivity	A genotype is associated with a phenotype of varying intensity.	Polydactyly
Pleiotropy	The phenotype includes many symptoms, with different subsets in different individuals.	Porphyria variegata
Phenocopy	An environmentally caused condition has symptoms and a recurrence pattern similar to those of a known inherited trait.	Infection
Genetic heterogeneity	Different genotypes are associated with the same phenotype.	Hearing impairment

DNA sequences called introns that do not encode protein. Finally, inheritance of mitochondrial genes differs from inheritance of nuclear genes simply because a cell has one nucleus but many mitochondria—and each mitochondrion harbors several copies of its chromosome (**figure 5.7** and **table 5.3**). Mitochondria with different alleles for the same gene can reside in the same cell.

Mitochondrial Disorders

Mitochondrial genes encode proteins that participate in protein synthesis and energy production. Twenty-four of the 37 genes encode RNA molecules (22 transfer RNAs and 2 ribosomal RNAs) that help assemble proteins. The other 13 mitochondrial genes encode proteins that function in cellular respiration, the biochemical reactions that use energy from digested nutrients to synthesize ATP, the biological energy molecule.

In diseases resulting from mutations in mitochondrial genes, symptoms arise from tissues whose cells have many mitochondria, such as skeletal muscle. It isn't surprising that a major symptom is often great fatigue. Inherited illnesses called mitochondrial myopathies, for example, produce weak and flaccid muscles and intolerance to exercise. Skeletal muscle fibers appear red and ragged when stained and viewed under a light microscope, their abundant abnormal mitochondria visible beneath the plasma membrane. When the first case of a mitochondrial illness was recognized in 1962, it was viewed as a rarity. Today researchers suspect that mitochondrial disorders could be as common as cancer.

A defect in an energy-related gene can produce symptoms other than fatigue. This is the case for Leber's hereditary optic neuropathy (LHON), which impairs vision. First described in 1871, with its maternal transmission noted, LHON was not associated with a mitochondrial mutation that impairs cellular energy reactions until 1988. Symptoms of LHON usually begin in early adulthood with a loss of central vision. Eyesight worsens and color vision vanishes as the central portion of the optic nerve degenerates.

A mutation in a mitochondrial gene that encodes a tRNA or rRNA can be devastating because it impairs the cell's ability to manufacture proteins. Consider what happened

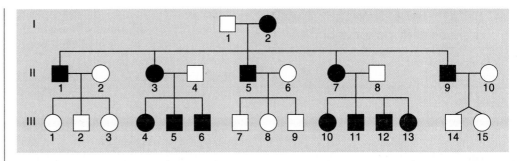

Figure 5.6 Inheritance of mitochondrial genes. Mothers pass mitochondrial genes to all offspring. Fathers do not transmit mitochondrial genes because sperm only very rarely contribute mitochondria to fertilized ova.

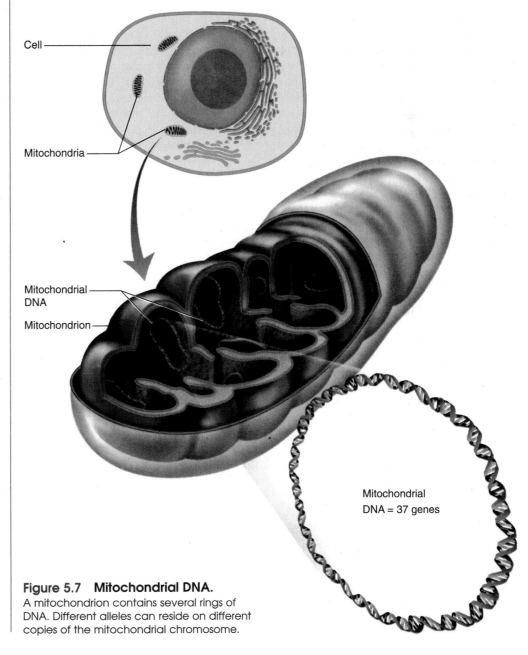

Figure 5.7 Mitochondrial DNA.
A mitochondrion contains several rings of DNA. Different alleles can reside on different copies of the mitochondrial chromosome.

Table 5.3

Features of Mitochondrial DNA

No crossing over

No DNA repair

Maternal inheritance

Many copies per mitochondrion and per cell

High exposure to oxygen free radicals

No histones

No introns

to Linda Schneider, a once active and articulate dental hygienist and travel agent. In her forties, Linda gradually began to slow down at work. She heard a buzzing in her ears and developed difficulty talking and walking. Then her memory began to fade in and out, she became lost easily in familiar places, and her conversation made no sense. Her condition worsened, and she developed diabetes, seizures, and pneumonia and became deaf and demented. She was finally diagnosed with MELAS, which stands for "mitochondrial myopathy encephalopathy lactic acidosis syndrome." Linda died. Her son and daughter will likely develop the condition because they inherited her mitochondria.

A new technique called ooplasmic transfer can enable a woman to avoid transmitting a mitochondrial disorder. Mitochondria from a healthy woman's oocyte are injected into the oocyte of a woman who is infertile. Then, the bolstered oocyte is fertilized in a laboratory dish by the partner's sperm, and the zygote is implanted in her uterus. Several dozen children, apparently free of mitochondrial disease, have been born from this technique. Headlines sensationalized the fact that, technically, the children each have three parents and were born as a result of genetic manipulation.

Heteroplasmy Complicates Mitochondrial Inheritance

The fact that a cell contains many mitochondria makes possible a rare condition called **heteroplasmy,** in which a particular mutation may be present in some mitochondrial chromosomes, but not others. At each cell division, the mitochondria are dis-

tributed at random into daughter cells. Over time, the chromosomes within a mitochondrion tend to be all wild type or all mutant for any particular gene.

Heteroplasmy has several consequences for the inheritance of mitochondrial phenotypes. Expressivity may vary widely among siblings, depending upon how many mutation-bearing mitochondria were in the oocyte that became each brother or sister. Severity of symptoms is also affected by which tissues have cells whose mitochondria bear the mutation. This is the case for a family with Leigh syndrome, which affects the enzyme that directly produces ATP. Two boys died of the severe form of the disorder because the brain regions that control movement rapidly degenerated. Another child in the family was blind and had central nervous system degeneration. Several relatives, however, suffered only mild impairment of their peripheral vision. The more severely affected family members had more brain cells that received the mutation-bearing mitochondria.

The most severe mitochondrial illnesses are heteroplasmic. This is because homoplasmy—all mitochondria bearing the mutant allele—too severely impairs protein synthesis or energy production for embryonic development to complete. Often, severe heteroplasmic mitochondrial disorders do not produce symptoms until adulthood because it takes many cell divisions, and therefore much time, for a cell to receive enough mitochondria bearing mutant alleles to cause symptoms. For this reason, LHON usually does not affect vision until adulthood. Reading 9.1 relates how investigators used detection of heteroplasmy to solve a crime of historic import.

Mitochondrial DNA Studies Clarify the Past

Interest in mitochondrial DNA extends beyond the medical. Mitochondrial DNA provides a powerful forensic tool used to link suspects to crimes, identify war dead, and support or challenge historical records. The technology, for example, identified the son of Marie Antoinette and Louis XVI, who supposedly died in prison at age 10. In 1845, the boy was given a royal burial, but some people thought the buried child was an imposter. The boy's heart had been

stolen at the autopsy, and through a series of bizarre events, wound up, dried out, in the possession of the royal family. Recently, researchers compared mitochondrial DNA sequences from cells in the boy's heart to corresponding sequences in heart and hair cells from Marie Antoinette (her decapitated body identified by her fancy underwear), two of her sisters, and the still-living Queen Anne of Romania and her brother. The genetic evidence showed that the unfortunate boy was indeed the prince, Louis XVII.

Key Concepts

Mitochondrial genes are maternally inherited and mutate rapidly. A cell contains many mitochondria, which have many copies of the mitochondrial genome. • Mitochondrial genes encode RNAs that function in protein synthesis or proteins that are part of energy metabolism. • In heteroplasmy, cells contain mitochondria that have different alleles of a gene.

5.3 Linkage

Most of the traits that Mendel studied in pea plants were conferred by genes on different chromosomes. (Some were actually at opposite ends of the same chromosome.) When genes are located close to each other on the same chromosome, they usually do not separate during meiosis. Instead, they are packaged into the same gametes (**figure 5.8**). **Linkage** refers to the transmission of genes on the same chromosome. Linked genes do not assort independently and do not result in the predicted Mendelian ratios for crosses tracking two or more genes. Understanding linkage has been critical in identifying disease-causing genes, and paved the way for sequencing the human genome.

Linkage Was Discovered in Pea Plants

William Bateson and R. C. Punnett first observed the unexpected ratios indicating linkage in the early 1900s, again in pea plants. Bateson and Punnett crossed true-breeding plants with purple flowers and long pollen grains (genotype *PPLL*) to true-breeding plants with red flowers and round pollen grains (genotype *ppll*). The plants in the next

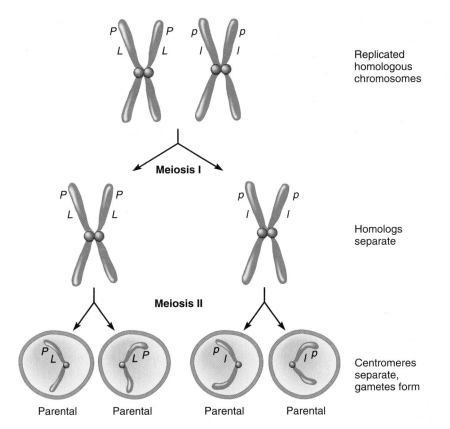

Figure 5.8 **Inheritance of linked genes.** Genes linked closely to one another on the same chromosome are usually inherited together when that chromosome is packaged into a gamete.

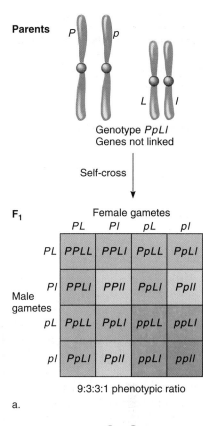

9:3:3:1 phenotypic ratio

a.

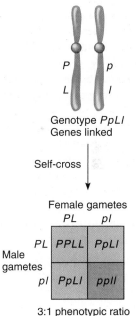

3:1 phenotypic ratio

b.

Figure 5.9 **Expected results of a dihybrid cross.** **(a)** When genes are not linked, they assort independently. The gametes then represent all possible allele combinations. The expected phenotypic ratio of a dihybrid cross would be 9:3:3:1. **(b)** If genes are linked on the same chromosome, only two allele combinations are expected in the gametes. The phenotypic ratio would be 3:1, the same as for a monohybrid cross.

generation, of genotype *PpLl*, were then self-crossed. But this dihybrid cross did not yield the expected 9:3:3:1 phenotypic ratio that Mendel's second law predicts (**figure 5.9**).

Bateson and Punnett noticed that two types of third-generation peas—those with the parental phenotypes *P_L_* and *ppll*—were more abundant than predicted, while the other two progeny classes—*ppL_* and *P_ll*—were less common (the blank indicates that the allele can be dominant or recessive). The more prevalent parental allele combinations, Bateson and Punnett hypothesized, could reflect genes that are transmitted on the same chromosome and that therefore do not separate during meiosis (see figure 5.8). The two less common offspring classes could also be explained by a meiotic event—crossing over. Recall that this is an exchange between homologs that mixes up maternal and paternal gene combinations without disturbing the sequence of genes on the chromosome (**figure 5.10**).

Progeny that exhibit this mixing of maternal and paternal alleles on a single chromosome are called **recombinant.** *Parental* and *recombinant* are relative terms. Had the parents in Bateson and Punnett's crosses been of genotypes *ppL_* and *P_ll*, then *P_L_* and *ppll* would be recombinant rather than parental classes.

Two other terms describe the configurations of linked genes in dihybrids. Consider a pea plant with genotype *PpLl*. These alleles can be arranged on the chromosomes in either of two ways. If the two dominant alleles are on one chromosome and the two recessive alleles are transmitted on the other, the genes are in "cis." In the opposite configuration, the genes are in "trans" (**figure 5.11**). Whether alleles in a dihybrid are in cis or trans is important in distinguishing recombinant from parental progeny classes in specific crosses.

Linkage Maps

As Bateson and Punnett were discovering linkage in peas, geneticist Thomas Hunt Morgan and his coworkers at Columbia University were doing the same using the fruit fly *Drosophila melanogaster,* taking the

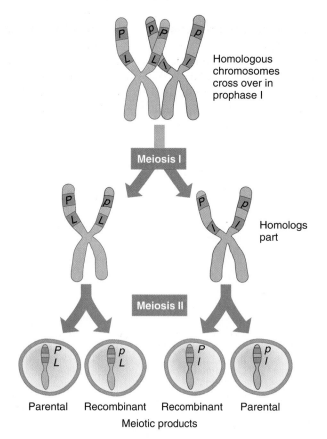

Figure 5.10 **Crossing over disrupts linkage.** The linkage between two genes may be interrupted if the chromosome they are located on crosses over with its homolog at a point between the two genes. Crossing over packages recombinant arrangements of the genes into gametes.

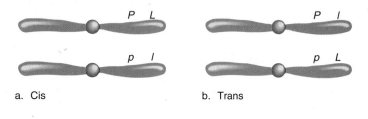

a. Cis   b. Trans

P = Purple flowers
p = Red flowers
L = Long pollen grains
l = Round pollen grains

Figure 5.11 **Allele configuration is important.** Parental chromosomes can be distinguished from recombinant chromosomes only if the allele configuration of the two genes is known—they are either in cis **(a)** or in trans **(b).**

concept of linkage further by relating genes to relative positions on chromosomes. These researchers compared progeny class sizes to assess whether various combinations of two traits were linked. They soon realized that the pairs of traits fell into four groups. Within each group, crossed dihybrids did not produce offspring according to the proportions Mendel's second law predicts. Not coincidentally, the number of these linkage groups—four—is exactly the

number of chromosome pairs in the fly. The traits fell into four groups based on progeny class proportions because the genes controlling traits that are inherited together are transmitted on the same chromosome.

Morgan wondered why the size of the recombinant classes varied depending upon which genes were studied. Might the differences reflect the physical relationship of the genes on the chromosome? Exploration of this idea fell to an undergraduate, Alfred

Sturtevant. In 1911, Sturtevant developed a theory and technique that would profoundly affect genetics. He proposed that the farther apart two genes are on a chromosome, the more likely they are to cross over simply because more physical distance separates them (**figure 5.12**).

The correlation between crossover frequency and the distance between genes is used to construct **linkage maps,** diagrams that show the order of genes on chromosomes and the relative distances between them. The distance is represented using "map units" called centimorgans (cm), where 1 cm equals 1 percent recombination (see figure 22.3). The frequency of a crossover between any two linked genes is inferred from the proportion of offspring that are recombinant. Genes at opposite ends of the same chromosome often cross over, generating a large recombinant class. Genes lying very close on the chromosome would only rarely be separated by a crossover.

As the twentieth century progressed, geneticists in Columbia University's "fly room" mapped several genes on all four chromosomes of the insect, and in other labs many genes were assigned to the human X chromosome. Localizing genes on the X chromosome was easier than doing so on the autosomes, because in human males, with their single X chromosome, recessive alleles on the X are expressed, a point we will return to in the next chapter.

By 1950, geneticists had begun to contemplate the daunting task of mapping genes on the 22 human autosomes. To start, a gene must be matched to its chromosome. Gene mapping began with the association of a particular chromosome abnormality

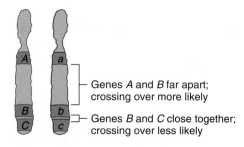

Genes *A* and *B* far apart; crossing over more likely

Genes *B* and *C* close together; crossing over less likely

Figure 5.12 **Breaking linkage.** Crossing over is more likely to occur between the widely spaced linked genes *A* and *B*, or between *A* and *C*, than between the more closely spaced linked genes *B* and *C*, because there is more room for an exchange to occur.

with a physical trait. Matching phenotypes to chromosomal variants, a field called **cytogenetics,** is the subject of chapter 13.

In 1968, researchers assigned the first human gene to an autosome. R. P. Donohue was observing chromosomes in his own white blood cells when he noticed a dark area consistently located near the centromere of one member of his largest chromosome pair (chromosome 1). He then examined chromosomes from several family members for the dark area, noting also whether each family member had a blood type called Duffy. (Recall that blood types refer to the patterns of proteins on red blood cell surfaces.) Donohue found that the Duffy blood type was linked to the chromosome variant. He could predict a relative's Duffy blood type by whether or not the chromosome had the telltale dark area.

Finding a chromosomal variation and using it to detect linkage to another gene is a valuable but rare achievement. More often, researchers must rely on the sorts of experiments Sturtevant conducted on his flies—calculating percent recombination (crossovers) between two genes whose locations on the chromosome are known. However, because humans do not have hundreds of offspring, as fruit flies do, obtaining sufficient data to establish linkage relationships requires observing the same traits in many families and pooling the information.

Solving a Problem: Linked Genes in Humans

As an idealized example of determining the degree of linkage by percent recombination, consider the traits of Rh blood type and a form of anemia called elliptocytosis (**figure 5.13**). An Rh$^+$ phenotype corresponds to genotypes RR or Rr. (This is simplified.) The anemia corresponds to genotypes EE or Ee.

Suppose that in 100 one-child families, one parent is Rh negative with no anemia (*rree*), and the other parent is Rh positive with anemia (*RrEe*), and the R and E (or r and e) alleles are in cis. Of the 100 offspring, 96 have parental genotypes (*re/re* or *RE/re*) and four individuals are recombinants for these two genes (*Re/re* or *rE/re*). Percent recombination is therefore 4 percent, and the two linked genes are 4 cm (centimorgans) apart.

Consider another pair of linked genes in humans. Nail-patella syndrome is an auto-

somal dominant trait that causes absent or underdeveloped fingernails and toenails, and painful arthritis, especially in the knee and elbow joints. It was identified in 1897, and affects only 1 in 50,000 people. The gene is located 10 map units from the I gene that determines the ABO blood type, on chromosome 9. Geneticists determined the map distance by pooling information from many families. The information can be used to predict genotypes and phenotypes in offspring, as in the following example.

Greg and Susan each have nail-patella syndrome. Greg has type A blood, and Susan has type B blood. They want to know what the chance is that a child of theirs would inherit normal nails and knees and type O blood. Because information is available on Greg and Susan's parents, a genetic counselor can deduce their allele configurations (**figure 5.14**).

	Parent 1		Parent 2	
Phenotype	Rh$^-$, no anemia		Rh$^+$, anemia	
Genotype	*rree*		*RrEe*	
Allele configuration	$\dfrac{r\ e}{r\ e}$		$\dfrac{R\ E}{r\ e}$	
Gametes:	sperm	frequency	oocytes	Progeny:
Parental	(re)	48%	(RE)	Rh$^+$, anemia
		48%	(re)	Rh$^-$, no anemia
Recombinants	(re)	2%	(Re)	Rh$^+$, no anemia
		2%	(rE)	Rh$^-$, anemia

Figure 5.13 **Tracing the inheritance of linked genes.** If we know the allele configurations of the parental generation, we can calculate the parental and recombinant class frequencies by pooling family data. In this case, the gamete frequencies correspond to the progeny class frequencies because the sperm are all the same genotype for these two genes, even if crossing over occurs.

		Greg		Susan
Phenotype		nail-patella syndrome, type A blood		nail-patella syndrome, type B blood
Genotype		$NnI^A\_\_$		$NnI^B\_\_$
Allele configuration		$\dfrac{N\quad I^A}{n\quad i}$		$\dfrac{N\quad i}{n\quad I^B}$
Gametes:		sperm	frequency	oocytes
Parental		(N I^A)	45%	(N i)
		(n i)	45%	(n I^B)
Recombinants		(N i)	5%	(N I^B)
		(n I^A)	5%	(n i)

N = nail-patella syndrome
n = normal

Figure 5.14 **Inheritance of nail-patella syndrome.** Greg inherited the N and I^A alleles from his mother; that is why the alleles are on the same chromosome. His n and i alleles must therefore be on the homolog. Susan inherited alleles N and i from her mother, and n and I^B from her father. Population-based probabilities are used to calculate the likelihood of phenotypes in the offspring of this couple.

Greg's mother has nail-patella syndrome and type A blood. His father has normal nails and type O blood. Therefore, Greg must have inherited the dominant nail-patella syndrome allele (N) and the I^A allele from his mother, on the same chromosome. We know this because Greg has type A blood and his father has type O blood—therefore, he couldn't have gotten the I^A allele from his father. Greg's other chromosome 9 must carry the alleles n and i. His alleles are therefore in cis.

Susan's mother has nail-patella syndrome and type O blood, and so Susan inherited N and i on the same chromosome. Because her father has normal nails and type B blood, her homolog bears alleles n and I^B. Her alleles are in trans.

Determining the probability that their child could have normal nails and knees and type O blood is the easiest question the couple could ask. The only way this genotype can arise from theirs is if an ni sperm (which occurs with a frequency of 45 percent, based on pooled data) fertilizes an ni oocyte (which occurs 5 percent of the time). The result—according to the product rule—is a 2.25 percent chance of producing a child with the $nnii$ genotype.

Calculating other genotypes for their offspring is more complicated, because more combinations of sperm and oocytes could account for them. For example, a child with nail-patella syndrome and type AB blood could arise from all combinations that include I^A and I^B as well as at least one N allele (assuming that the NN genotype has the same phenotype as the Nn genotype).

The Rh blood type and elliptocytosis, and nail-patella syndrome and ABO blood type, are examples of linked gene pairs. A linkage map begins to emerge when percent recombination is known between all possible pairs of three or more linked genes, just as a road map with more landmarks provides more information on distance and direction. Consider genes x, y, and z (**figure 5.15**). If the percent recombination between x and y is 10, between x and z is 4, and between z and y is 6, then the order of the genes on the chromosome is x-z-y (figure 5.15). This is the only order of the three genes that accounts for the percent recombination data.

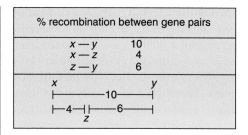

Figure 5.15 Recombination mapping. If we know the percent recombination between all possible pairs of three genes, we can determine their relative positions on the chromosome.

Knowing the percent recombination between linked genes was useful in ordering them on genetic maps in a crude sense. Understanding the structure of DNA, and then sequencing the human genome, revealed an unexpected complexity in linkage mapping: crossing over is not equally likely to occur throughout the genome. Some DNA sequences are nearly always inherited together, more often than would be predicted from their frequency in the population. This nonrandom association between DNA sequences is called **linkage disequilibrium** (LD). The human genome consists of many "LD" blocks interspersed with areas where crossing over is prevalent. Understanding LD can reveal how populations interacted in historical and evolutionary time, and LD is being used to predict disease, discussed in chapter 7.

The Evolution of Gene Mapping

Linkage mapping has had an interesting history. In the first half of the twentieth century, gene maps for nonhuman organisms, such as fruit flies, were constructed based on recombination frequencies between pairs of visible traits. In the 1950s, linkage data on traits in humans began to accumulate. At first, it was mostly a few visible or measurable traits linked to blood types or blood proteins.

In 1980 came a great stride in linkage mapping. Researchers began using DNA sequences near genes of interest as landmarks called genetic markers. These markers do not necessarily encode a protein

that causes a phenotype—they might be differences that alter where a DNA cutting enzyme cuts, or differing numbers of short repeated sequences of DNA with no obvious function, or single nucleotide polymorphisms (SNPs) (see figures 7.11 and 14.4).

Computers tally how often genes and markers are inherited together. Gene mappers express the "tightness" of linkage between a marker and the gene of interest as a **LOD score,** which stands for "logarithm of the odds." A LOD score indicates the likelihood that particular crossover frequency data indicate linkage.

A LOD score of 3 or greater signifies linkage. It means that the observed data are 1,000 (10^3) times more likely to have occurred if the two DNA sequences (a disease-causing allele and its marker) are linked than if they reside on different chromosomes and just happen to often be inherited together by chance. It is somewhat like deciding whether two coins tossed together 1,000 times always come up both heads or both tails by chance, or because they are taped together side by side in that position, as linked genes are. If the coins land with the same side up in all 1,000 trials, it indicates they are very likely linked.

Before many disease-causing genes were discovered and the human genome sequence known, genetic markers were used to predict which individuals in some families were most likely to have inherited a particular disorder, before symptoms began. Such tests are no longer necessary.

Today, genetic markers are still used to distinguish parts of chromosomes. In pedigrees, marker designations are sometimes placed beneath the traditional symbols to further describe chromosomes. Such a panel of markers, called a **haplotype,** is a set of DNA sequences inherited together on the same chromosome due to linkage disequilibrium.

Haplotypes can look complicated, because markers are often given names that have meaning only to their discoverers. They read like license plates, bearing labels such as D9S1604. The haplotypes in the pedigree in **figure 5.16,** for a family with cystic fibrosis, are simplified. Each number beneath a symbol represents a "license plate" haplotype. Haplotypes make it possible to track which parent transmits which genes and

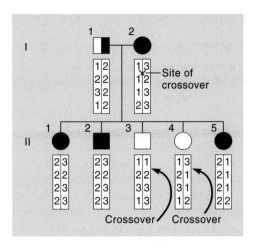

Figure 5.16 Haplotypes.
The numbers in bars beneath pedigree symbols enable researchers to track specific chromosome segments with markers. Disruptions of a marker sequence indicate crossover sites.

chromosomes to offspring. In figure 5.16, knowing the haplotype of individual II-2 reveals which chromosome in parent I-1 contributes the mutant allele. Because Mr. II-2 received haplotype 3233 from his affected mother, his other haplotype, 2222, comes from his father. Since Mr. II-2 is affected and his father is not, the father must be a heterozygote, and 2222 must be the haplotype linked to the mutant CFTR allele.

It has been interesting and exciting to watch gene mapping evolve, from the initial crude associations between blood types and chromosomal quirks, to today's maps with their millions of signposts along the sequenced genome. Throughout the 1990s, each October, *Science* magazine published a human genome map. The number of identified genes steadily grew as chromosome depictions became ever more packed with information. From that information, during your lifetime, will spring a revolution in health care and in how we understand ourselves.

Key Concepts

Genes on the same chromosome are linked, and they are inherited in patterns that differ from the patterns of the unlinked genes Mendel studied. Crosses involving linked genes produce a large parental class and a small recombinant class (caused by crossing over). • The farther apart two genes are on a chromosome, the more likely they are to recombine. Linkage maps are based on this relationship between crossover frequency and the distance between genes on the same chromosome. Linkage disequilibrium is a linkage combination that is stronger than that predicted by gene frequencies in a population. Cytogenetics can be used to associate a phenotype to a chromosomal aberration. • Linkage maps reflect the percent recombination between linked genes. LOD scores describe the tightness of linkage and thereby the proximity of a gene to a marker. Haplotypes indicate linked DNA sequences.

Summary

5.1 When Gene Expression Appears to Alter Mendelian Ratios

1. Homozygosity for lethal recessive alleles stops development before birth, eliminating an offspring class.

2. A gene can have multiple alleles because its sequence can be altered in many ways. Different allele combinations produce different variations of the phenotype.

3. Heterozygotes of **incompletely dominant** alleles have phenotypes intermediate between those associated with the two homozygotes. **Codominant** alleles are both expressed.

4. In **epistasis,** one gene affects the expression of another.

5. An incompletely **penetrant** genotype is not expressed in all individuals who inherit it. Phenotypes that vary in intensity among individuals are variably expressive.

6. **Pleiotropic** genes have several expressions.

7. A **phenocopy** is a characteristic that appears to be inherited but is environmental.

8. In **genetic heterogeneity,** two or more genes specify the same phenotype.

9. The human genome sequence is revealing that some "extensions" to Mendel's laws are not as rare as once thought.

5.2 Maternal Inheritance and Mitochondrial Genes

10. Only females transmit mitochondrial genes; males can inherit such a trait but cannot pass it on.

11. Mitochondrial genes do not cross over, do not repair DNA, and lack introns.

12. The 37 mitochondrial genes encode tRNA, rRNA, or proteins involved in protein synthesis or energy reactions.

13. Many mitochondrial disorders are **heteroplasmic,** with mitochondria in a single cell harboring different alleles.

5.3 Linkage

14. Genes on the same chromosome are **linked** and, unlike genes that independently assort, produce a large number of individuals with parental genotypes and a small number of individuals with **recombinant** genotypes.

15. **Linkage maps** are developed from studies of linked genes. Researchers can examine a group of known linked DNA sequences (a **haplotype**) to follow the inheritance of certain chromosomes.

16. Knowing whether linked alleles are in cis or trans, and using crossover frequencies determined by pooling data, one can predict the probabilities that certain genotypes will appear in progeny.

17. Genetic linkage maps assign distances to linked genes based on crossover frequencies.

Review Questions

1. Explain how each of the following phenomena can disrupt Mendelian phenotypic ratios.

   a. lethal alleles

   b. multiple alleles

   c. incomplete dominance

   d. codominance

   e. epistasis

   f. incomplete penetrance

   g. variable expressivity

   h. pleiotropy

   i. a phenocopy

   j. genetic heterogeneity

2. How does the relationship between dominant and recessive alleles of a gene differ from epistasis?

3. Why can transmission of an autosomal dominant trait with incomplete penetrance look like autosomal recessive inheritance?

4. How does inheritance of ABO blood type exhibit both complete dominance and codominance?

5. How has knowledge of the human genome sequence altered our views on "extensions" to Mendel's laws?

6. Describe why inheritance of mitochondrial DNA and linkage are exceptions to Mendel's laws.

7. How does a pedigree for a maternally inherited trait differ from one for an autosomal dominant trait?

8. What might be a confounding factor in attempting to correlate different genotypes with different expressions of a Mendelian illness?

9. If researchers could study pairs of human genes as easily as they can study pairs of genes in fruit flies, how many linkage groups would they detect?

Applied Questions

1. For each of the diseases described in situations a through i, indicate which of the following phenomena (A–H) is at work. A disorder may result from more than one of these causes.

   A. lethal alleles

   B. multiple alleles

   C. epistasis

   D. incomplete penetrance

   E. variable expressivity

   F. pleiotropy

   G. a phenocopy

   H. genetic heterogeneity

   a. A woman has severe neurofibromatosis type 1. She has brown spots on her skin and several large tumors beneath her skin. A gene test shows that her son has inherited the disease-causing autosomal dominant allele, but he has no symptoms.

   b. A man and woman have six children. They also had two stillbirths—fetuses that died shortly before birth.

   c. Most children with cystic fibrosis have frequent lung infections and digestive difficulties. Some people have mild cases, with onset of minor respiratory problems in adulthood. Some men have cystic fibrosis, but their only symptom is infertility.

   d. In Labrador retrievers, the B allele confers black coat color and the b allele brown coat color. The E gene controls expression of the B gene. If a dog inherits the E allele, the coat is golden no matter what the B genotype is. A dog of genotype ee expresses the B (black) phenotype.

   e. Two parents are heterozygous for genes that cause albinism, but each gene specifies a different enzyme in the biochemical pathway for skin pigment synthesis. Their children thus do not face a 25 percent risk of having albinism.

   f. Alagille syndrome, in its most severe form, prevents the formation of ducts in the gallbladder, causing liver damage. Affected children also usually have heart murmurs, unusual faces, a line in the eye, and butterfly-shaped vertebrae. Such children often have one seemingly healthy parent who, when examined, proves to also have a heart murmur, unusual face, and butterfly vertebrae.

   g. Two young children in a family have terribly decayed teeth. Their parents think it is genetic, but the true cause is a babysitter who puts them to sleep with juice bottles in their mouths.

   h. A woman develops dark patches on her face. Her family physician suspects that she may have alkaptonuria. However, a dermatologist discovers that the woman has been using a facial cream containing hydroquinone, which causes dark skin patches in dark-skinned people.

   i. An apparently healthy 24-year-old basketball player dies suddenly during a game when her aorta, the largest artery, ruptures. A younger brother is nearsighted and has long and thin fingers, and an older sister is extremely tall, with long arms and legs. The older sister, too, has a weakened aorta. All of these siblings have Marfan syndrome.

2. If many family studies for a particular autosomal recessive condition reveal fewer affected individuals than Mendel's law predicts, the explanation may be either incomplete penetrance or lethal alleles. How might you use haplotypes to determine which of these two possibilities is the causative factor?

3. A man who has type O blood has a child with a woman who has type A blood. The woman's mother has AB blood, and her father, type O. What is the probability that the child has each of the following blood types?

   a. type O

   b. type A

   c. type B

   d. type AB

4. Two people who are heterozygous for familial hypercholesterolemia are concerned that a child might inherit the severe form of the illness. What is the probability that this will happen?

5. Enzymes are used in blood banks to remove the A and B antigens from blood types A and B. This makes the blood type O.

   a. Does this alter the phenotype or the genotype?

   b. Removing the A and B antigens from red blood cells is a phenocopy of what genetic phenomenon?

6. Friedreich's ataxia, which impairs the ability to feel and move the limbs, usually begins in early adulthood. The molecular basis of the disease is impairment of ATP production in mitochondria, but the mutant gene is in the nucleus of the cells. Would this disorder be inherited in a Mendelian fashion? Explain your answer.

7. What is the chance that Greg and Susan, the couple with nail-patella syndrome, could have a child with normal nails and type AB blood?

8. A gene called secretor is located 1 map unit from the H gene that confers the Bombay phenotype on chromosome 19. Secretor is dominant, and a person of either genotype *SeSe* or *Sese* secretes the ABO and H blood type antigens in saliva and other body fluids. This secretion, which the person is unaware of, is the phenotype. A man has the Bombay phenotype and is not a secretor. A woman does not have the Bombay phenotype and is a secretor. She is a dihybrid whose alleles are in cis. What is the chance that a child of theirs will have the same genotype as the father?

9. A Martian creature called a gazook has 17 chromosome pairs. On the largest chromosome are genes for three traits— round or square eyeballs (R or r); a hairy or smooth tail (H or h); and 9 or 11 toes (T or t). Round eyeballs, hairy tail, and 9 toes are dominant to square eyeballs, smooth tail, and 11 toes. A trihybrid male has offspring with a female who has square eyeballs, a smooth tail, and 11 toes on each of her three feet. She gives birth to 100 little gazooks, who have the following phenotypes:

   • 40 have round eyeballs, a hairy tail, and 9 toes

   • 40 have square eyeballs, a smooth tail, and 11 toes

   • 6 have round eyeballs, a hairy tail, and 11 toes

   • 6 have square eyeballs, a smooth tail, and 9 toes

   • 4 have round eyeballs, a smooth tail, and 11 toes

   • 4 have square eyeballs, a hairy tail, and 9 toes

   a. Draw the allele configurations of the parents.

   b. Identify the parental and recombinant progeny classes.

   c. What is the crossover frequency between the R and T genes?

Web Activities

10. Go to http://www.familyvillage.wisc.edu/index.htmlx. Family Village is a clearinghouse for disease information. Click on library. Explore the diseases, and identify one that exhibits pleiotropy.

11. Go to the United Mitochondrial Disease Foundation website (http://www.umdf.org/index_mainframe.html) and describe the phenotype of a mitochondrial disorder.

12. Go to http://www.ncbi.nlm.nih.gov/mapview/map_search.cgi?chr=hum_chr.inf&query. Browse the site, and list three sets of linked genes. Consult OMIM to describe the trait or disorder that each specifies.

Case Studies

13. Connie Winslow is deaf. When she was old enough to attend school, she began having fainting spells, which her teachers and parents noticed happened when she became excited. One Christmas, she was so thrilled with her gifts that she promptly fainted. Her parents took her to the emergency room, where doctors assured them, as they had in the past, that there wasn't a problem. The spells continued, and Connie became able to predict the attacks, telling her parents that her head hurt before the spells occurred. Her parents took her to a neurologist, who checked Connie's heart and diagnosed long-QT syndrome with deafness, also known as Jervell and Lange-Nielsen syndrome (see OMIM 220400 and Reading 2.2). The physician explained that this is a severe form of long-QT syndrome, which is an inherited heartbeat irregularity that can be fatal. Seven different genes can cause long-QT syndrome. The doctor told them of a case described in a textbook from 1856: a young girl, called at school to face the headmaster for an infraction, became so agitated that she dropped dead. When the parents were summoned, they were not surprised; they had lost two other children to great excitement.

The Winslows visited a medical geneticist, who discovered that each had a mild heartbeat irregularity that did not produce symptoms. Connie's parents had normal hearing. Connie's younger brother Jim was also hearing-impaired and suffered night terrors, but had so far not fainted during the day. Like Connie, he had the full syndrome. A younger sister, Tina, was still a baby, and was tested. She did not have either form of the family's illness; her heartbeat was normal.

Today, Connie and Jim are treated with beta blocker drugs, and each has a pacemaker to regulate heartbeat. Connie may receive an implantable defibrillator to automatically correct her heartbeat when it veers out of control. Diagnosing her may have saved her brother's life.

1. Which of the following applies to the condition in this family?

   a. genetic heterogeneity

   b. pleiotropy

   c. variable expressivity

   d. incomplete dominance

   e. a phenocopy

2. How is the inheritance pattern of Jervell and Lange-Nielsen syndrome similar to that of familial hypercholesterolemia?

3. How is it possible that Tina did not inherit either the serious or asymptomatic form of the illness?

4. Do the treatments for the condition affect the genotype or the phenotype?

Learn to apply the skills of a genetic counselor with these additional cases found in the *Case Workbook in Human Genetics*:

Enamel hypoplasia

Epidermolysis bullosa

Hair and eye color

Thrombocytopenia and absent radius syndrome

Suggested Readings

Ferriman, Annabel. May 12, 2001. First cases of human germline genetic modification announced. *The British Medical Journal* 322:1144. People object to ooplasmic transfer because the resulting children have three genetic parents.

Seashore, Margretta R. December 26, 2002. Tetrahydrobiopterin and dietary restriction in mild phenylketonuria. *The New England Journal of Medicine* 347(26):2094–95. Nearly all cases of PKU are due to an enzyme deficiency, but a few result from an abnormal cofactor that the enzyme requires to function. Therefore, PKU is genetically heterogeneic.

Sijbrands, Eric J. G., et al. April 28, 2001. Mortality over two centuries in large pedigree with familial hypercholesterolemia: Family tree mortality study. *The British Medical Journal* 322:1019–23. Variable expressivity in FH reflects diet and exercise habits and the effects of other genes.

Smeitink, Jan, and Lambert van den Heuvel. June 1999. Human mitochondrial complex I in health and disease. *The American Journal of Human Genetics* 64:1505–9. Many inherited diseases affecting muscles stem from mutations in mitochondrial genes.

Weekly updates of current news related to human genetics are available through Power Web on your Online Learning Center.

VISIT YOUR ONLINE LEARNING CENTER

Visit your online learning center for additional resources and tools to help you master this chapter. See us at

www.mhhe.com/lewisgenetics6.

Matters of Sex

6

CHAPTER CONTENTS

6.1 Sexual Development

Whether we develop as female or male is determined when two X chromosomes, or an X and a Y chromosome, come together at fertilization. Our sexual selves depend further upon whether one key gene—the *SRY* gene—is present and active six weeks after fertilization. The hormone-guided events of development, and possibly our feelings and experiences, also help to mold our sexual identities.

6.2 Traits Inherited on Sex Chromosomes

The tiny Y chromosome passes few traits, while the gene-packed X carries many. Understanding Mendel's laws and the mechanism of sex chromosome distribution at fertilization enables us to follow traits controlled by the actions of proteins encoded by genes on the sex chromosomes.

6.3 X Inactivation Equalizes the Sexes

To make the number of genes on the two X chromosomes of a female equivalent to that of the single X of males, one X in each cell of a female is inactivated early in prenatal development. The female is a mosaic of gene expression for this chromosome. X inactivation has noticeable effects when a female is heterozygous for certain genes.

6.4 Sex-Limited and Sex-Influenced Traits

Some genes—autosomal as well as X- or Y-linked—are expressed in one sex but not the other, or may be inherited as a dominant trait in one but a recessive in the other.

6.5 Genomic Imprinting

In genomic imprinting, gene expression depends upon which parent transmits a particular gene.

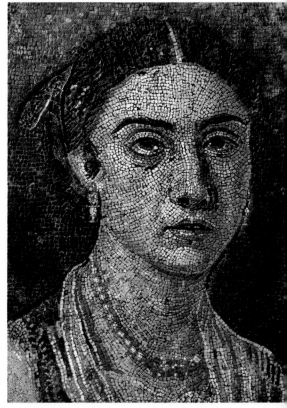

Females are mosaics. Each cell has one X chromosome inactivated. The mosaicism arises because either the X inherited from the father or that from the mother is turned off.

Whether we are male or female is enormously important in our lives, affecting our relationships, how we think and act, and how others perceive us. Gender is ultimately a genetic phenomenon, but is also layered with psychological and sociological components.

Maleness or femaleness is determined at conception, when he inherits an X and a Y chromosome, or she inherits two X chromosomes. Another level of sexual identity comes from the control that hormones exert over the development of reproductive structures. Finally, both biological factors and social cues influence sexual feelings, including the strong sense of whether we are male or female.

6.1 Sexual Development

In prenatal humans, the sexes look alike until the ninth week of prenatal development. During the fifth week, all embryos develop two unspecialized gonads, organs that will develop as either testes or ovaries. Each such "indifferent" gonad forms near two sets of ducts that give it two developmental options. If one set of tubes, called the Müllerian ducts, continue to develop, they eventually form the sexual structures characteristic of a female. If the other set, the Wolffian ducts, persist, male sexual structures form. The choice of one of these developmental pathways occurs during the sixth week, depending upon the sex chromosome constitution. If a gene on the Y chromosome called *SRY* (for "sex-determining region of the Y") is activated, hormones steer development along a male route. In the absence of *SRY* activation, a female develops (**figure 6.1**). Femaleness was long considered a "default" option in development, but sex determination is more accurately described as a fate imposed on ambiguous precursor structures.

Sex Chromosomes

Human males and females have equal numbers of autosomes, but males have one X chromosome and one Y chromosome, and females have two X chromosomes (**figure 6.2**). The sex with two different sex chromosomes is called the **heterogametic sex,** and the other, with two of the same sex chromosomes, is the **homogametic sex.** In humans, this makes males heterogametic and females homogametic. Some other species are different. In birds and snakes, for example, males are ZZ (homogametic) and females are ZW (heterogametic).

The X chromosome in humans contains more than 1,500 genes. The much smaller Y chromosome has 90 protein-encoding genes, although this is not certain. In meiosis in a male, the X and Y chromosomes act as if they are a pair of homologs. We introduce the Y chromosome here, then consider the X in section 6.2.

Identifying genes on the human Y chromosome has been extremely difficult. Before the human genome sequence became available, researchers inferred the functions and locations of Y-linked genes by examining men who are missing parts of the chromosome and determining how they differ from normal. Creating linkage maps, which was possible for the other chromosomes, didn't work for the Y because it does not have a

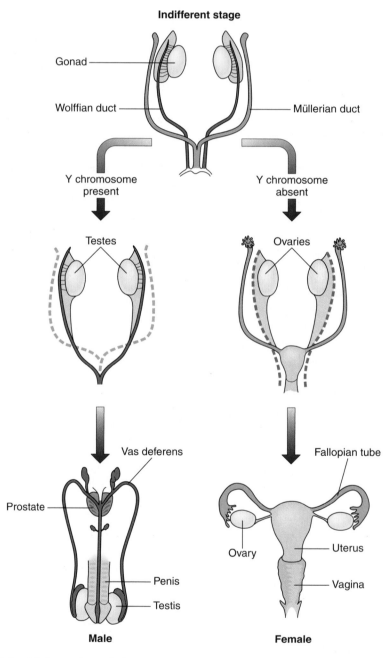

Figure 6.1 Male or female? The paired duct systems in the early human embryo may develop into male *or* female reproductive organs.

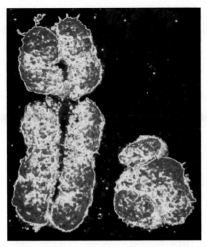

Figure 6.2 The X and Y chromosomes. In humans, females are the homogametic sex (XX) and males are the heterogametic sex (XY). (The chromosomes are in the replicated form because they were dividing when photographed.)

homolog with which to cross over (although its tips cross over with the X chromosome).

Analysis of the genome sequence has revealed one source of the difficulty in mapping the Y chromosome: It has a most unusual organization. In the 95 percent of the chromosome that harbors male-specific genes, many DNA segments are palindromes, which in written languages are sequences of letters that read the same in both directions, such as "Madam, I'm Adam." This symmetry of DNA sequence, described by Y chromosome researchers as "a hall of mirrors," destabilizes the enzymes that replicate DNA. As a result, during meiosis, sections of a Y chromosome attract each other, which can loop out parts in between and may account for many cases of male infertility caused by missing parts of the Y. Yet this organization may also provide a way for the chromosome to recombine with itself, essentially sustaining its structure. Two researchers—one an XX, one an XY—take a lighthearted look at the curious structure of the human Y chromosome in "In Their Own Words" on page 114.

The Y chromosome has a distinctive overall structure (**figure 6.3**) with a short arm and a long arm. At both tips of the Y chromosome are areas called **pseudoautosomal**

regions, termed PAR1 and PAR2. They comprise only 5 percent of the chromosome. The 63 pseudoautosomal genes are so-called because they have counterparts on the X chromosome and can cross over with them. These genes encode a variety of proteins that function in both sexes, participating in or controlling such activities as bone growth, cell division, immunity, signal transduction, the synthesis of hormones and receptors, fertility, and energy metabolism.

The bulk of the Y chromosome is termed the male-specific region, or MSY. (Until the Y chromosome was sequenced in 2003, this portion was called the nonrecombining region.) The MSY lies between the two pseudoautosomal regions, and it consists of three classes of DNA sequences. About 10 to 15 percent of the MSY consists of X-transposed sequences that are 99 percent identical to counterparts on the X chromosome. Protein-encoding genes are scarce here. Another 20 percent of the MSY consists of X-degenerate DNA sequences, which bear some similarity to X chromosome sequences, and may be remnants of an ancient autosome that long ago gave rise to the X chromosome. The remainder of the MSY includes the palindrome-ridden regions, called amplicons. The entire MSY encodes 27 proteins, but the genes include many repeats and encode protein segments that combine in different ways—another reason why counting the number of protein-encoding genes on the Y chromosome has been so difficult. Many of the genes in the MSY are essential to fertility, including *SRY.*

The Y chromosome was first seen under a light microscope in 1923, and researchers soon recognized its association with maleness. For many years, they sought to identify the gene or genes that determine sex. Important clues came from two very interesting types of people—men who have two X chromosomes (XX male syndrome), and women who have one X and one Y chromosome (XY female syndrome). A close look at their sex chromosomes revealed that the XX males actually had a small piece of a Y chromosome, and the XY females lacked a small part of the Y chromosome. The part of the Y chromosome present in the XX males was the same part that was missing in the XY females. This critical area accounted for half a percent of the Y chromosome. Finally, in 1990, two groups of

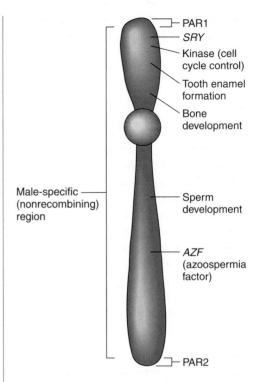

Figure 6.3 Anatomy of the Y chromosome. The Y chromosome has two pseudoautosomal regions and a large central area that comprises about 95 percent of the chromosome. The pseudoautosomal regions' genes match genes on the X chromosome and can recombine with them. The large central area does not recombine and is called the male-specific region. A few of the genes are indicated here. *SRY* determines sex. *AZF* encodes a protein essential to producing sperm; mutations in it cause infertility. "PAR" stands for pseudoautosomal region.

researchers isolated and identified the *SRY* gene in this implicated area.

The Phenotype Forms

The *SRY* gene encodes a type of protein called a **transcription factor,** which controls the expression of other genes. The *SRY* transcription factor stimulates male development by sending signals to the indifferent gonads. In response, sustentacular cells in the developing testis secrete anti-Müllerian hormone, which destroys female structures (uterus, fallopian tubes, and upper vagina). At the same time, interstitial cells in the testis secrete testosterone, which stimulates development of male structures (the epididymides, vas deferentia, seminal vesicles, and ejaculatory ducts).

The Y Wars

In 2002, researcher Jennifer Marshall-Graves struck fear in the hearts of males everywhere with a series of articles that predicted that the Y chromosome will "self-destruct" within the next 10 million years. Her comparison of Y chromosomes in a wide variety of mammals indicates that, gradually, important genes are being transferred to other chromosomes. David Page, who has led the mapping of the Y chromosome, has a more optimistic view—perhaps because he has a Y. Each researcher spoke out, in jest, at two scientific conferences. Here is some of what they had to say:

The Rise and Fall of the Human Y Chromosome

Jennifer A. Marshall-Graves,
Australian National University

The Y chromosome is unique in the human genome. It is small, gene-poor, prone to deletion and loss, variable among species, and useless. You can lack a Y and not be dead, just female. It is impossible to understand why this chromosome is so weird without understanding where it came from. It is a sad decline, and I predict its imminent loss.

The X is a decent sort of chromosome. It accounts for 5 percent of the genome, with about 1,500 perfectly normal genes. The Y is a pathetic little chromosome that has few genes interspersed with lots of junk. And those genes are a weird lot. They are particularly concerned with male sexual development, so they are rather specialized. There are a number of important genes, but some are quite bizarre and many inactive. The Y shares a lot of sequence with the X, and a lot of homology elsewhere, so the Y clearly diverged from the X.

There are several models of the Y (**figure 1**). The dominant Y model of a macho Y reflects the fact that the Y contains the male-determining *SRY* gene. The selfish Y model predicts that the Y kidnapped genes from elsewhere. The wimp Y model says that the Y is just a relic of the once glorious X chromosome. This model was first proposed by biologist Susumo Ohno in 1967 in the theory that the X and Y originated as a pair of autosomes. Then the Y acquired the male-determining locus, and other genes that are required for spermatogenesis gathered nearby. This led to suppressed recombination in this region of the Y, which allowed all sorts of horrible genetic accidents to occur that could not be repaired. Mutations, deletions, and insertions accumulated until almost nothing was left, except bits at the top and bottom that still pair with the X. A few genes survived because they found a useful male-specific function, and many of these have made copies of themselves in a desperate race to stave off disappearing altogether.

The Y is degrading fast, losing genes at the rate of 5 per million years. I predict that it will be completely gone in 5 to 10 million

Professor Jennifer A. Marshall-Graves, and friend, of Australian National University.

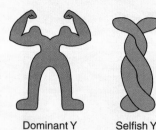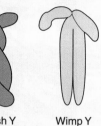

Models of the Human Y

Dominant Y   Selfish Y   Wimp Y

Figure 1 Models of the human Y chromosome. Researcher Jennifer Marshall-Graves offers a tongue-in-cheek look at the Y chromosome, but her research findings are serious—the chromosome is shrinking.

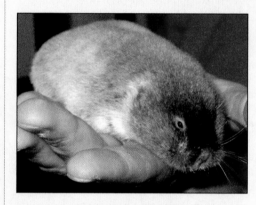

Figure 2 Life without a Y? Males of all known mammals, with the exception of two species of mole voles, have Y chromosomes. Birds and reptiles do not. Evolutionary biologists think that the Y chromosome arose from an X chromosome about 310 million years ago, as the X lost many genes and gained a few that set their carriers on the road to maleness. This animal is a Y-less male mole vole—it reproduces just fine.

Some testosterone is also converted to dihydrotestosterone (DHT), which directs the development of the urethra, prostate gland, penis, and scrotum.

Because male prenatal sexual development is a multistep process, genetic abnormalities can intervene at several different points. The result may be an XY individual with a block in the gene- and hormone-controlled elaboration of male structures so that a chromosomal he is a phenotypic she. For example, in androgen insensitivity syndrome, caused by a mutation in a gene on the X chromosome, absence of receptors for testosterone stops cells in early reproductive structures from receiving the signal to develop as male. The person looks female, but is XY.

years. Will we have males? The males in the audience can take comfort from the mole vole *Ellobius lutescens* (**figure 2**). It has no Y, but it does have males and females. It has no *SRY*, no Y chromosome at all. Both sexes are XO. How do they do it? We don't know. Clearly another gene takes over and new sex genes start evolving. Will there be new sex chromosome evolution in humans? Maybe it will happen in different ways in different populations, and we will split into two species.

Rethinking The Rotting Y Chromosome

David Page, Massachusetts Institute of Technology and Howard Hughes Medical Institute investigator

The Y chromosome has had a public relations problem for a long time. For most of the last half of the past century, people thought that the Y chromosome was a junk heap. The genomic junkyard view was the classic model for sex chromosome evolution. We can now update that model.

Back 300 million years ago, when we were reptiles, we had no sex chromosomes, only ordinary autosomes. Shortly after our ancestors parted company with the ancestors of birds, a mutation arose on one member of a pair of ordinary autosomes to give rise to *SRY*. The process of shutting down

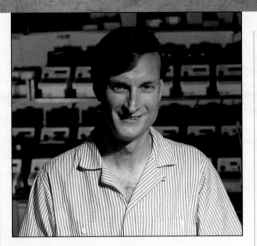

David Page, of the Massachusetts Institute of Technology and a Howard Hughes Medical Institute investigator.

XY crossing over began, first in the vicinity of *SRY*, and then in an expanding region. Once a piece of the Y was no longer able to recombine with the X, its genes began to rot. The purpose of sex (recombination in meiosis) is not just to generate new gene combinations, but to allow genes to rid themselves of mildly deleterious mutations that accumulate. Y genes are not protected, because they have lots of areas of no crossing over. Genes decayed, except for *SRY* and the tips. It wasn't a very flattering model for the Y. When Jennifer Marshall-Graves and John Aitken wrote their article in *Nature* on

the future of sex, that the Y would self-destruct in 10 million years, it truly frightened the people in my lab. We decided we needed to pick up the pace. When the popular press discovered the story of the impending death of the Y chromosome, they moved the date up to 5 million years from now.

Based on the sequencing of the Y, we've been able to rethink its evolution, and realized that the chromosome may have found a way around its seemingly inevitable problems. We looked closely at the male-specific region of the Y, reanalyzing sequences in a different way, chopped into smaller bits. And we found that each piece would find a match elsewhere on the Y. So segments on the Y are effectively functioning as alleles—30 percent have a perfect match elsewhere on the chromosome. These are not simple repeats, but highly complex sequences of tens to hundreds of kilobases. The region includes eight palindromes and one inverted repeat (**figure 3**). We propose that there is intense recombination within the palindromes. And so the Y has two forms of productive recombination: conventional routine recombination of crossing over with the X at pseudoautosomal regions, and recombination within the Y. It's not that the Y doesn't recombine, it just does it its own way. The Y does copying that preserves its identity.

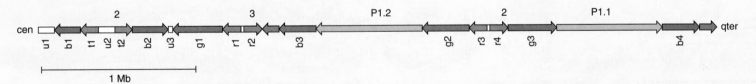

cen ——— u1 b1 t1 u2 t2 b2 u3 g1 r1 r2 b3 P1.2 g2 r3 r4 g3 P1.1 b4 qter

2 3 P1.2 2 P1.1

|—— 1 Mb ——|

Figure 3 **The Y chromosome is highly repetitive.** A section of the Y chromosome that David Page studies, called *AZFc* (for azoospermia factor c), consists of DNA sequences that read the same in either direction, an organization that can lead to instability as well as provide a mechanism to evolve new alleles. Other parts of the chromosome house similar repeats. Matching colors in this depiction represent identical sequences. Same-color arrows that point in opposite directions indicate inverted repeats, similar to palindromes in the English language.

In a group of disorders called male pseudohermaphroditism (**figure 6.4**), testes are usually present (indicating that the *SRY* gene is functioning) and anti-Müllerian hormone is produced, so the female set of tubes degenerates. However, a block in testosterone synthesis prevents the fetus from developing male structures. The child appears to be a girl. Then at puberty, the adrenal glands, which sit atop the kidneys, begin to produce testosterone (as they normally do in a male). This leads to masculinization: The voice deepens, and muscles build up into a masculine physique; breasts do not develop, nor does menstruation occur. The clitoris may enlarge so greatly under the adrenal testosterone surge that it looks like a penis. Individuals with a form of this condition in the Dominican

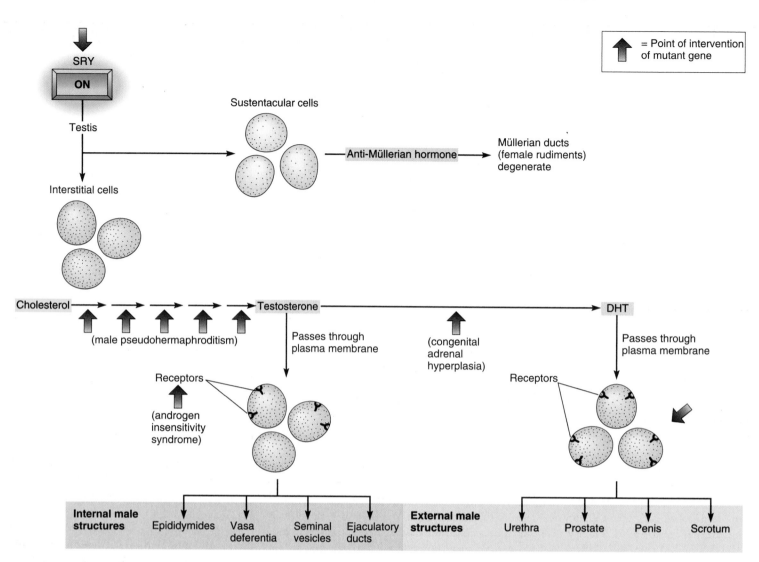

Figure 6.4 A chromosomal "he" develops as a phenotypic "she." Male pseudohermaphroditism results from mutations that disrupt differentiation and development of reproductive structures. Before puberty, the person appears female, although the sex chromosomes are XY. At puberty, the adrenal glands produce testosterone, which belatedly turns on some of the genes that control the development of male structures and secondary sex characteristics such as a deepening voice, hair growth, and muscle growth.

Republic are called *guevedoces,* for "penis at age 12." In the more common congenital adrenal hyperplasia due to 21-hydroxylase deficiency, an enzyme block leads to excess testosterone production, causing overgrowth of the clitoris or penis, so that a girl may appear to be a boy.

A hermaphrodite is an individual with both male and female sexual structures. The word comes from the Greek god of war, Hermes, and the goddess of love, Aphrodite. "Pseudohermaphroditism" refers to the presence of both types of structures, but at different stages of life. Prenatal tests that detect chromosomal sex have changed the way that pseudohermaphroditism is diagnosed. Before these tests were available, the condition was detected only after puberty, when masculinization occurred in a person who looked female. Today, pseudohermaphroditism is indicated when a prenatal chromosome check reveals an X and a Y chromosome, but the newborn is a phenotypic girl. Transgendered individuals have the phenotype and sex chromosomes of one gender, but feel extremely strongly that they are the other. The genetic or physical basis is not known.

Is Homosexuality Inherited?

No one really knows why we have feelings of belonging to one gender or the other, but these feelings are intense. Bioethics: Choices for the Future describes people whose gender identity persists even after surgery alters their phenotype in a way that contradicts their sex chromosome constitution.

In homosexuality, a person's phenotype and genotype are consistent, and physical attraction is toward members of the same sex. Homosexuality is seen in all cultures and has been observed for thousands of years.

Evidence is accumulating that homosexuality is at least partially inherited. Earlier studies cite the feelings that homosexual individuals have as young children, well before they know of the existence or the meaning of the term. Studies with twins suggest a genetic influence. A 1991 study found that identical twins are more likely to

Sex Reassignment: Making a Biological "He" into a Social "She"

Identical twins Bruce and Brian Reimer were born in 1965. At age eight months, most of Bruce's penis was accidentally burned off during a botched circumcision. After much agonizing, and on the advice of physicians and psychologists, the parents decided that it would be best to "reassign" Bruce's gender as female. At 22 months of age, corrective surgery created Brenda from Bruce. The prominent psychologist in charge hailed the transformation a resounding success, and the case came to serve as a precedent for early surgical intervention for children born with "ambiguous genitalia" or structures characteristic of both sexes, a condition termed intersex. About 1 in 2,000 newborns are intersexes, with a few others the result of a surgical accident.

Gender Identity Can't Be Changed

Sex reassignment may not be the best treatment for some intersexual individuals. Reassessment of sex reassignment began when the Reimer case came to public attention. Reality for young Brenda was far different from the published descriptions.

Always uneasy in her dress-clad body, Brenda suffered relentless ridicule and confusion, because it was always obvious to her and others that she was more than a "tomboy"—she was a boy, despite her surgically altered appearance. Comparison to twin Brian worsened matters. When confronted with the truth at age 14, "Brenda" threatened suicide unless allowed to live as the correct gender. And so she became David Reimer. He eventually married, adopted stepchildren, and is today a grandfather. He told his story to *Rolling Stone* magazine. At about the same time, 1997, a groundbreaking paper by Keith Sigmundson, David's psychiatrist in his hometown of Winnipeg, and Milton Diamond of the University of Hawaii, supported David's contention that gender identity is due more to nature than nurture.

A study published in 2000 added more evidence. William Reiner, then at Johns Hopkins University, investigated fourteen children with a form of intersex called cloacal exstrophy. They were all XY, and had normal testicles and hormone levels, but no penis. Twelve of them were reassigned as female—and all behaved as boys throughout childhood. Six of them declared themselves male between the ages of 5 and 12 years. The two children who were not surgically converted into female are normal males who lack penises, something that surgery later in life may be able to correct. Since then, other studies have confirmed Reiner's findings.

The Surgical Yardstick

In the past, physicians decided to remove a small or damaged penis and reassign sex as female using a literal yardstick: If a newborn's stretched organ exceeded an inch, he was deemed a he. If the protrusion was under three-eighths of an inch, she was deemed a she. Organs that fell in between were shortened into a clitoris during the first week of life, and girlhood officially began. Further plastic surgeries and hormone treatments during puberty completed the superficial transformation, with external female tissue sculpted from scrotal tissue. The reverse, creating a penis, is much more difficult and was therefore usually delayed several months. These surgeries can destroy fertility and sexual sensation.

Easier to surgically treat are babies with congenital adrenal hyperplasia (CAH) due to 21-hydroxylase deficiency, the most common cause of intersex. The individual is XX, but overproduces masculinizing hormones (androgens). The result is a girl with a clitoris so large that it looks like a small penis. Thirty years ago, surgeons would cut away most of the extra tissue and create a vagina from skin flaps. Recently, with the discovery that these females needed a second surgery in adolescence anyway, treatment is being postponed, giving these young women the chance to take part in decisions affecting their bodies.

Delaying surgery until a person can decide for him or herself may be the best approach for intersex individuals. Sex reassignment surgery is a bioethical issue that involves paternalism, confidentiality, the doctor-patient relationship, and the promise of physicians to "do no harm." Sums up Alice Dreger of Michigan State University, who has researched and written extensively on intersexuality, "Gender identity is very complicated, and it looks from the evidence like the various components interact and matter in different ways for different individuals. That's why unconsenting children and adults should never be subjected to cosmetic, medically unnecessary surgeries designed to alter their sexual tissue. We cannot predict what parts they may want later."

---

both be homosexual than are both members of fraternal same-sex twin pairs. Specifically, in 52 percent of identical twin pairs in which one or both were homosexual, both brothers were homosexual, but this was true for only 22 percent of fraternal twin pairs. Also, two brain areas are of different sizes in homosexual versus heterosexual men.

In 1993, National Cancer Institute researcher Dean Hamer traced the inheritance of five genetic markers on the X chromosome in 40 pairs of homosexual brothers. Although these DNA sequences are highly variable in the general population, they were identical in 33 of the sibling pairs. Hamer interpreted the finding to mean that genes causing or predisposing a male to homosexuality reside on the X chromosome. However, the work never identified a causative gene. Hamer's report is still controversial. One research group confirmed and extended the work, finding that when two brothers are homosexual and have another brother who is heterosexual, the heterosexual brother does not share the X chromosome markers. This study also did not find the X chromosome markers between pairs of lesbian sisters. Several research groups have refuted Hamer's findings. But a gene controlling homosexuality need not reside on a sex chromosome, where Hamer looked. Ongoing studies are searching among the autosomes for such genes.

In yet another approach to understanding the biological basis of homosexuality, researchers have genetically manipulated male fruit flies to display what looks like homosexual behavior. A mutant allele of an eye color gene called *white* causes the flies to have white eyes when expressed in cells of the eye only. Wild type eye color is red. Researchers altered male fly embryos so that the resulting adult insects expressed the *white* gene in every cell. The altered male flies displayed what appears to be mating behavior with each other (**figure 6.5**), presumably as a result of the altered gene expression.

The ability to genetically induce homosexual behavior suggests genetic control. The biochemical basis of the phenotype makes sense; the *white* gene's product, an enzyme that controls eye color, enables cells to use the amino acid tryptophan, which is required to manufacture the hormone sero-

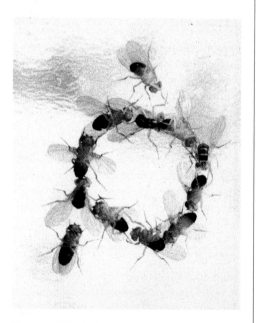

Figure 6.5 Is homosexuality inherited?   The ability to genetically alter male fruit flies, causing them to display mating behavior toward each other, adds to evidence that homosexuality is at least partially inherited.

Table 6.1

Sexual Identity

Level	Events	Timing
Chromosomal/ genetic	XY = male XX = female	Fertilization
Gonadal sex	Undifferentiated structure becomes testis or ovary	9–16 weeks after fertilization
Phenotypic sex	Development of external and internal reproductive structures continues as male or female in response to hormones	8 weeks after fertilization, puberty
Gender identity	Strong feelings of being male or female develop	From childhood, possibly earlier
Sexual orientation	Attraction to same or opposite sex	From childhood

tonin. When all the fly's cells express the mutant *white* gene, instead of just eye cells, serotonin levels in the brain drop, and this may cause the unusual behavior. In other animals, lowered brain serotonin is associated with homosexual behavior.

Table 6.1 summarizes the several components of sexual identity.

Key Concepts

The human female is homogametic, with two X chromosomes, and the male is heterogametic, with one X and one Y chromosome. The Y chromosome has about 90 protein-encoding genes, and includes two small pseudoautosomal regions and a large area that does not recombine, the male-specific region. Most of this region consists of palindromic sequences that lead to gene loss but also may provide a way to maintain the chromosome's structure. Other DNA sequences in the male-specific region are similar to sequences on the X chromosome. • Activation of the *SRY* gene on the Y chromosome causes the undifferentiated gonad to develop into a testis. Then, sustentacular cells in the testis secrete anti-Müllerian hormone, which stops development of female structures. Interstitial cells in the testis secrete testosterone, which stimulates development of male internal structures. Testosterone is also converted to DHT, which directs development of external structures. • Genes likely contribute to homosexuality.

6.2 Traits Inherited on Sex Chromosomes

Genes carried on the Y chromosome are said to be **Y-linked,** and those on the X chromosome are **X-linked.** Y-linked traits are rare, because the chromosome has few genes, and many have counterparts on the X chromosome. These traits are passed from male to male, because a female does not have a Y chromosome. No other Y-linked traits besides infertility (which obviously can't be passed on) are yet clearly defined, although certain gene products have been identified. Claims that "hairy ears" is a Y-linked trait did not hold up—it turned out that families hid their affected female members!

Genes on the X chromosome have different patterns of expression in females and males, because a female has two X chromosomes and a male just one. In females, X-linked traits are passed just like autosomal traits—that is, two copies are required for expression of a recessive allele, and one copy for a dominant allele. In males, however, a single copy of an X-linked allele causes expression of the trait or illness, because there is no copy of the gene on a second X chromosome to mask the other's effect. A man inherits an X-linked trait only from his mother, because he gets his Y chromosome from his father. The human male is considered **hemizygous** for X-linked traits, because he has only one set of X-linked genes.

Understanding how sex chromosomes are inherited is important in predicting phenotypes and genotypes in offspring. A male inherits his Y chromosome from his father and his X chromosome from his mother (**figure 6.6**). A female inherits one X chromosome from each parent. If a mother is heterozygous for a particular X-linked gene, her son or daughter has a 50 percent chance of inheriting either allele from her. X-linked traits are always passed on the X chromosome from mother to son or from either parent to daughter, but there can be no direct male-to-male transmission of X-linked traits.

X-Linked Recessive Inheritance

An X-linked recessive trait is expressed in females if the causative allele is present in two copies. Many times, an X-linked trait passes from an unaffected heterozygous mother to an affected son. **Table 6.2** summarizes the transmission of an X-linked recessive trait.

If an X-linked condition is not lethal, a man may be healthy enough to transmit it to offspring. Consider the small family depicted in **figure 6.7**, an actual case. A middle-aged man who had rough, brown, scaly skin did not realize his condition was inherited until his daughter had a son. By a year of age, the boy's skin resembled his grandfather's. In the condition, called

ichthyosis, an enzyme deficiency blocks removal of cholesterol from skin cells. The upper skin layer cannot peel off as it normally does, causing a brown, scaly appearance. A test of the daughter's skin cells revealed that she produces half the normal amount of the enzyme, indicating that she is a carrier.

Colorblindness is another X-linked recessive trait that does not hamper the ability of a man to have children. About 8 percent of males of European ancestry are colorblind, as are 4 percent of males of African descent. Only 0.4 percent of females in both groups are colorblind. Reading 6.1, on page 122, takes a closer look at this interesting trait.

Figure 6.8 shows part of a very extensive pedigree for another X-linked recessive trait, the blood-clotting disorder hemophilia A. Note the combination of pedigree symbols and a Punnett square to trace transmission of the trait. Dominant and recessive alleles are indicated by superscripts to the X and Y chromosomes.

In Their Own Words in chapter 1 vividly describes one man's experience with hemophilia. In the royal families of England, Germany, Spain, and Russia, the mutant allele arose in one of Queen Victoria's X chromosomes; it was either a new mutation or she inherited it. In either case, she passed it on through carrier daughters and one mildly affected son.

The transmission pattern of hemophilia A is consistent with the criteria for an X-linked recessive trait listed in table 6.2. A daughter can inherit an X-linked recessive disorder or trait if her father is affected and her mother is a carrier, because the daughter inherits one affected X chromosome

from each parent. Without a biochemical test, though, an unaffected woman would not know she is a carrier for an X-linked recessive trait unless she has an affected son. A genetic counselor can estimate a potential carrier's risk using probabilities derived from Mendel's laws, combined with knowledge of X-linked inheritance patterns.

Consider a woman whose brother has hemophilia A. Both her parents are healthy, but her mother is a carrier because her brother is affected. The woman's chance of being a carrier is 1/2 (or 50 percent), which is the chance that she has inherited the X chromosome bearing the hemophilia allele from her mother. The chance of the woman conceiving a son is 1/2, and of that son inheriting hemophilia is 1/2. Using the product rule, the risk that she will have a son with hemophilia, out of all the possible children she can conceive, is $1/2 \times 1/2 \times 1/2$, or 1/8.

Table 6.3 lists several X-linked disorders. Most genes on the X chromosome are not actually related to sex determination, and are necessary for normal development or physiology in both sexes.

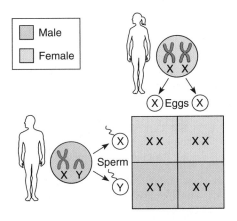

Figure 6.6 Sex determination in humans. An oocyte has a single X chromosome. A sperm cell has either an X or a Y chromosome. If a Y-bearing sperm cell with a functional *SRY* gene fertilizes an oocyte, the zygote is a male (XY). If an X-bearing sperm cell fertilizes an oocyte, then the zygote is a female (XX).

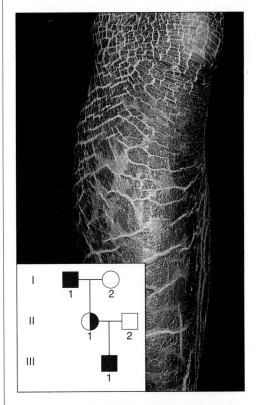

Figure 6.7 An X-linked recessive trait. Ichthyosis is transmitted as an X-linked recessive trait. A grandfather and grandson were affected in this family.

X-Linked Dominant Inheritance

Dominant X-linked conditions and traits are rare. Again, gene expression differs between the sexes (**table 6.4**). A female who inherits a dominant X-linked allele has the associated trait or illness, but a male who inherits the allele is usually more severely affected because he has no other allele to offset it. The children of a normal man and a woman with a dominant, disease-causing gene on the X chromosome face the risks summarized in **figure 6.9**.

An example of an X-linked dominant condition is incontinentia pigmenti (IP), another inborn error that Archibald Garrod described in 1906 (see In Their Own Words in chapter 5). The name reflects the major sign in affected females—swirls of skin pigment that arise when melanin penetrates the deeper skin layers. A newborn girl with IP has yellow, pus-filled vesicles on her limbs that come and go over the first few weeks. Then the lesions become warty and eventually give way to brown splotches that may remain for life, although they fade with

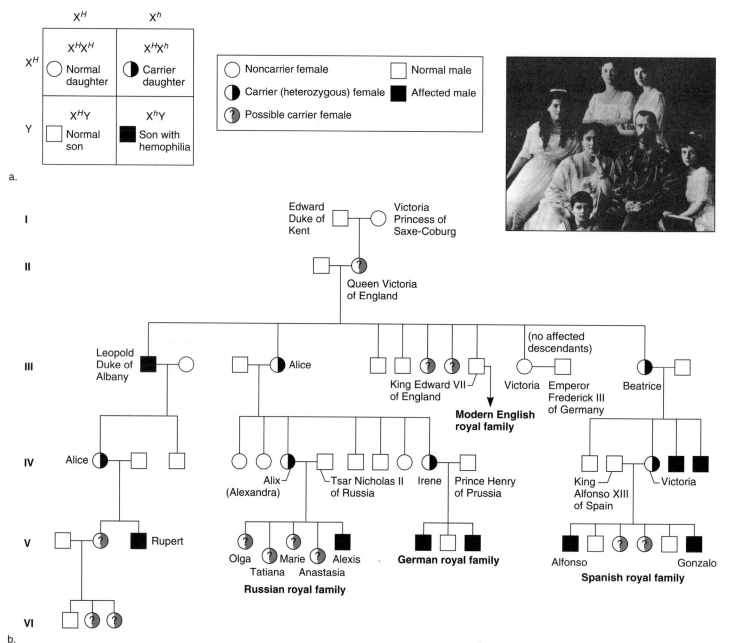

Figure 6.8   Hemophilia A.   (a) This X-linked recessive disease usually passes from a heterozygous woman (designated $X^H X^h$, where X^h is the hemophilia-causing allele) to heterozygous daughters or hemizygous sons. **(b)** The disorder has appeared in the royal families of England, Germany, Spain, and the former Soviet Union. The mutant allele apparently arose in Queen Victoria, who was either a carrier or produced oocytes in which the gene mutated. She passed the alleles to Alice and Beatrice, who were carriers, and to Leopold, who had a mild enough case that he fathered children. In the fourth generation, Alexandra was a carrier who married Nicholas II, Tsar of Russia. Alexandra's sister Irene married Prince Henry of Prussia, passing the allele to the German royal family, and Beatrice's descendants passed it to the Spanish royal family. This figure depicts only part of the enormous pedigree. The modern royal family in England does not carry hemophilia.

Table 6.3

Some Disease-Related Genes on the Human X Chromosome* (r = recessive, D = dominant)

Condition	Description
Megalocornea (r)	Enlarged cornea
Norrie disease (r)	Abnormal growth of retina, eye degeneration
Retinitis pigmentosa (r)	Constriction of visual field, night blindness, clumps of pigment in eye
Agammaglobulinemia (r)	Lack of certain antibodies
Chronic granulomatous disease (r)	Skin and lung infections, enlarged liver and spleen
Diabetes insipidus (r)	Copious urination
Fabry disease (r)	Abdominal pain, skin lesions, kidney failure
Hypophosphatemia (D and r)	Vitamin D-resistant rickets
Ornithine transcarbamylase deficiency (r)	Mental deterioration, ammonia accumulation in blood
Severe combined immune deficiency (r)	Lack of immune system cells
Wiskott-Aldrich syndrome (r)	Bloody diarrhea, infections, rash, too few platelets
Lesch-Nyhan syndrome (r)	Mental retardation, self-mutilation, urinary stones, spastic cerebral palsy
Menkes disease (r)	Kinky hair, abnormal copper transport, brain atrophy
Muscular dystrophy, Becker and Duchenne forms (r)	Progressive muscle weakness
Amelogenesis imperfecta (D)	Abnormal tooth enamel
Alport syndrome (r)	Deafness, inflamed kidney tubules
Anhidrotic ectodermal dysplasia (r)	Absence of teeth, hair, and sweat glands
Rett syndrome (D)	Mental retardation, neurodegeneration

*Some of these conditions may be inherited through genes on the autosomes as well.

Table 6.4

Criteria for an X-Linked Dominant Trait

1. Expressed in female in one copy.
2. Expressed much more severely in male.
3. High rates of miscarriage due to early lethality in males.

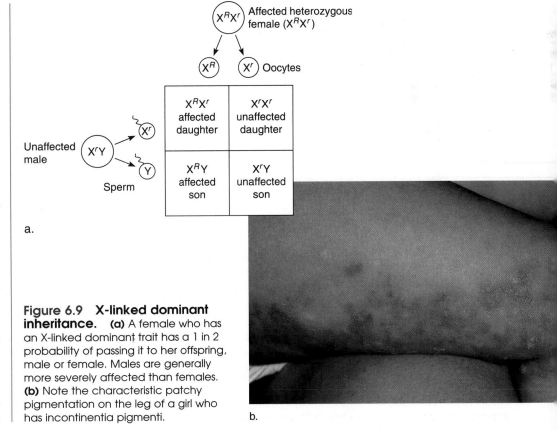

time. Other symptoms include patches of hair loss; visual problems due to abnormal and scarred blood vessels in the retina; missing, peg-shaped, or underdeveloped teeth, and seizures. Rarely, mental retardation, paralysis, and developmental delay occur. Males with the condition are so severely affected that they do not survive to be born. This is why women with the disorder have a miscarriage rate of about 25 percent.

The gene that causes IP (called *NEMO*) encodes a transcription factor that activates genes that carry out the immune response and apoptosis in tissues that

Figure 6.9 X-linked dominant inheritance. **(a)** A female who has an X-linked dominant trait has a 1 in 2 probability of passing it to her offspring, male or female. Males are generally more severely affected than females. **(b)** Note the characteristic patchy pigmentation on the leg of a girl who has incontinentia pigmenti.

Of Preserved Eyeballs and Duplicated Genes—Colorblindness

English chemist John Dalton saw things differently than most people. In a 1794 lecture, he described his visual world. Sealing wax that appeared red to other people was as green as a leaf to Dalton and his brother. Pink wildflowers were blue, and Dalton perceived the cranesbill plant as "sky blue" in daylight, but "very near yellow, but with a tincture of red," in candlelight. He concluded, "that part of the image which others call red, appears to me little more than a shade, or defect of light." The Dalton brothers had X-linked recessive colorblindness.

Curious about the cause of his colorblindness, Dalton asked his personal physician, Joseph Ransome, to dissect his eyes after he died. Ransome snipped off the back of one eye, removing the retina, where the cone cells that provide color vision are nestled among the more abundant rod cells that impart black-and-white vision. Because Ransome could see red and green normally when he peered through the back of his friend's eyeball, he concluded that it was not an abnormal filter in front of the eye that altered color vision. He stored the eyes in dry air, enabling researchers at the London Institute of Ophthalmology to analyze DNA in Dalton's eyeballs in 1994. Dalton's remaining retina lacked one of the three types of photopigments that enable cone cells to capture certain wavelengths of light.

Color Vision Basics

Cone cells are of three types, defined by the presence of any of three types of photopigments. An object appears colored because it reflects certain wavelengths of light, and each cone type captures a particular range of wavelengths with its photopigment. The brain then interprets the incoming information as a visual perception, much as an artist mixes the three primary colors to create many hues and shadings.

Each photopigment has a vitamin A-derived portion called retinal and a protein portion called an opsin. The presence of reti-

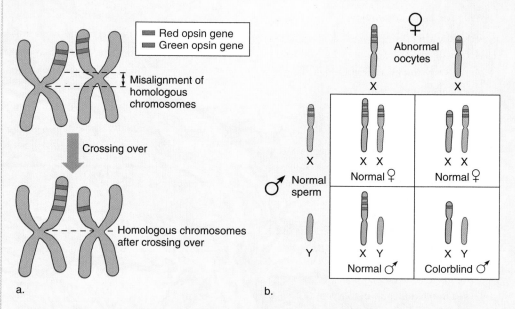

Figure 1 How colorblindness arises. **(a)** The sequence similarities among the opsin genes responsible for color vision may cause chromosome misalignment during meiosis in the female. Offspring may inherit too many, or too few, opsin genes. A son inheriting an X chromosome missing an opsin gene would be colorblind. A daughter, unless her father is colorblind, would be a carrier. **(b)** A missing gene causes X-linked colorblindness.

derive from ectoderm, such as skin, hair, nails, eyes, and the brain. Genetic tests can detect the deletion that causes most cases. Before such tests became available, children with IP were sometimes incorrectly diagnosed with severe skin infections, and then treated inappropriately with antibiotics. The genetic test can also identify women with very mild cases, whose only symptoms are abnormal teeth and bald patches.

Another X-linked dominant condition, congenital generalized hypertrichosis (CGH), produces many extra hair follicles, and hence denser and more abundant hair. Unlike hirsutism, which is caused by a hormonal abnormality that makes a woman grow hair in places where it is usually more pronounced in males, CGH causes excess facial and upper body hair that covers extensive areas of skin (**figure 6.10**). Hair growth is milder and patchier in females with CGH than in males with CGH because of hormonal differences and the mitigating presence of a second X chromosome.

Researchers studied a large Mexican family that had 19 members with CGH. The pattern of inheritance was distinctive for X-linked dominant inheritance. In one portion of the pedigree, depicted in figure 6.10b, an affected man passed the trait to all four daughters, but to none of his nine sons. Because sons inherit the X chromosome from their mother, and only the Y from their father, they could not inherit CGH from their affected father.

The mutant gene that causes CGH is atavistic, which means that it controls a trait also present in ancestral species. Some version of the gene is probably present in

nal in photopigments explains why eating carrots, rich in vitamin A, promotes good vision. The presence of opsins—because they are controlled by genes—explains why colorblindness is inherited. The three types of opsins correspond to short, middle, and long wavelengths of light. Mutations in opsin genes cause three different types of colorblindness.

A gene on chromosome 7 encodes short-wave opsins, and mutations in it produce the rare autosomal "blue" form of colorblindness. Dalton had deuteranopia (green colorblindness), which means his eyes lacked the middle-wavelength opsin. In the third type, protanopia (red colorblindness), long-wavelength opsin is absent. Deuteranopia and protanopia are X-linked.

Molecular Analysis

Jeremy Nathans of Johns Hopkins University is another researcher who has personally contributed to understanding color vision. First, he used a cow version of a protein called rhodopsin that provides black-and-white vision to identify the human counterpart of this gene. Hypothesizing that the DNA sequence in the rhodopsin gene would be similar to that in the three opsin genes, and therefore able to bind to them, Nathans used the human rhodopsin gene as a "probe" to search his own DNA for genes with similar sequences. He found three. One was on chromosome 7, the other two on the X chromosome.

Although Nathans can see colors, his opsin genes are not entirely normal, which

provided a big clue to how colorblindness arises and why it is so common. On his X chromosome, Nathans has one red opsin gene and two green genes, instead of the normal one of each. Because the red and green genes have similar sequences, Nathans reasoned, they can misalign during meiosis in the female (**figure 1**). The resulting oocytes would then have either two or none of one opsin gene type. An oocyte lacking either a red or a green opsin gene would, when fertilized by a Y-bearing sperm, give rise to a colorblind male.

People who are colorblind must get along in a multicolored world. To help them overcome the disadvantage of not seeing important color differences, computer algorithms can convert colored video pictures into shades they can see. **Figure 2** shows one of the tests typically used to determine whether someone is colorblind. Absence of one opsin type prevents affected individuals from seeing a different color in certain circles in the figure. These individuals cannot perceive a particular embedded pattern that other people can see.

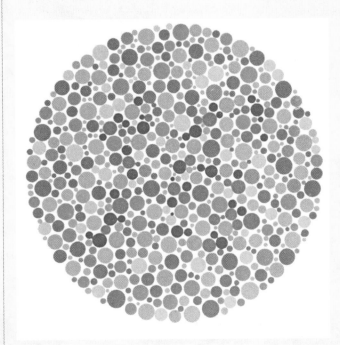

Figure 2   A test for color-blindness.   Males with red-green colorblindness cannot see the number 16 within this pattern of circles, as a person with normal color vision can. Reproduced from *Ishihara's Tests for Colour Blindness,* published by Kanehara & Co. Ltd, Tokyo, Japan. Tests for colorblindness cannot be conducted with this material. For accurate testing, the original plates should be used.

chimpanzees and other hairy primates. At some time in our distant past, the functional form of the gene must have mutated in a way that enables humans to grow dense hair only on their heads and in areas dictated by sex hormones.

Solving a Problem: X-Linked Inheritance

Mendel's first law (segregation) applies to genes on the X chromosome. Therefore, the same logic is used to solve problems as to

trace traits transmitted on autosomes, with the added step of considering the X and Y chromosomes in Punnett squares. Follow these steps:

1. Determine the mode of inheritance (recessive or dominant).
   For an X-linked recessive trait:
   • An affected male has a carrier mother.
   • An unaffected female with an affected brother has a 50 percent (1 in 2) chance of being a carrier.

• An affected female has a carrier or affected mother *and* an affected father.
• A carrier (female) has a carrier mother *or* an affected father.

For an X-linked dominant trait:
• There may be no affected males, because they die early.
• An affected female has an affected mother.

2. List all genotypes and phenotypes and their probabilities.

Figure 6.10 An X-linked dominant condition.
(a) This six-year-old child has congenital generalized hypertrichosis (CGH). **(b)** In this partial pedigree of a large Mexican family with CGH, the affected male in the second generation has passed the condition to all of his daughters and none of his sons. This is because he transmits his X chromosome only to females.

a.

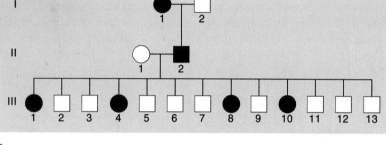

b.

6.3 X Inactivation Equalizes the Sexes

Females have two alleles for every gene on the X chromosome, whereas males have only one. In mammals, a mechanism called **X inactivation** balances this inequality. Early in the development of the female embryo, most of the genes on one X chromosome in each cell are inactivated. Which X chromosome is turned off in each cell—the one inherited from the mother or the one from the father—is random. As a result, a female mammal expresses the X chromosome genes inherited from her father in some cells and those from her mother in others (**figure 6.11**).

By studying rare human females who have lost a small part of one X chromosome, researchers identified a specific region, the **X inactivation center,** that shuts off much of the chromosome. A few genes on the chromosome, however, remain active. (Genes in the PARs and some others escape inactivation.) A gene called *XIST* controls X inactivation. It encodes an RNA that binds to a specific site on the same (inactivated) X chromosome. From this point to the chromosome tip, the X chromosome is inactivated. In mice, *XIST* RNA applied to an autosome inactivates that chromosome.

Once an X chromosome is inactivated in one cell, all its daughter cells have the same X chromosome inactivated. Because the inactivation occurs early in development, the adult female has patches of tissue that differ in their expression of X-linked genes. With each cell in her body having only one active X chromosome, she is chromosomally equivalent to the male.

3. Assign genotypes and phenotypes to the parents in the problem. Look for clues in the phenotypes of relatives. In X-linkage problems, often the phenotype of a male, such as a brother, provides a clue, because X-linked recessive traits, unlike autosomal recessive traits, are expressed in males.
4. Determine how alleles might separate into gametes for the genes of interest on the X and Y chromosomes.
5. Unite the gametes in a Punnett square.
6. Determine the phenotypic and genotypic ratios for the F_1 generation.
7. To extend predictions to further generations, use the genotypes of the F_1 individuals and repeat steps 4 through 6.

As an example, consider the X-linked recessive Kallmann syndrome, which causes very poor or absent sense of smell and small gonads (testes or ovaries). Tanisha does not have Kallmann syndrome, but her brother Jamal and her maternal cousin Malcolm (her mother's sister's child) have it. Tanisha's and Malcolm's parents are unaffected, as is Tanisha's husband Sam. Tanisha and Sam wish to know the risk that a son of theirs would inherit the condition. Sam has no affected relatives.

Solution

1. Mode of inheritance: The trait is X-linked recessive because males are affected through carrier mothers.

2. K = wild type k = Kallmann syndrome

Genotypes	Phenotypes
$X^K X^K, X^K X^k, X^K Y$	normal
$X^k X^k, X^k Y$	affected

3.

Individual	Genotype	Phenotype	Probability
Tanisha	$X^K X^k$ or $X^K X^K$	normal (carrier)	50% each
Jamal	$X^k Y$	affected	100%
Malcolm	$X^k Y$	affected	100%
Sam	$X^K Y$	normal	100%

4. Tanisha's gametes if she is a carrier: X^K X^k
   Sam's gametes: X^K Y

5. Punnett Square

	X^K	X^k
X^K	$X^K X^K$	$X^K X^k$
Y	$X^K Y$	$X^k Y$

6. Interpretation: The probability that their son will have Kallmann syndrome is 50 percent, or 1 in 2. (Note that this is a conditional probability. The chance that any particular son will have the condition is actually 1 in 4, because Tanisha also has a 50 percent chance of being genotype $X^K X^K$ and therefore not a carrier.)

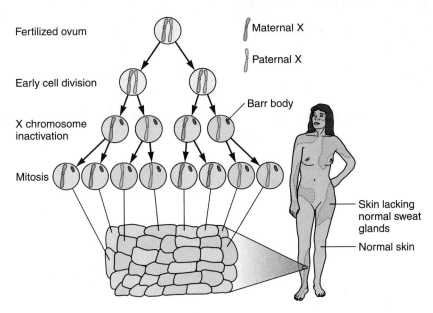

Figure 6.11 **X inactivation.** A female is a mosaic for expression of genes on the X chromosome because of the random inactivation of either the maternal or paternal X in each cell early in prenatal development. In anhidrotic ectodermal dysplasia, a woman has patches of skin that lack sweat glands and hair. (Colors are meant to distinguish cells with the inactivated X, not to depict skin color.)

X inactivation can alter the phenotype (gene expression), but not the genotype. It is not permanent, because the inactivation is reversed in germline cells destined to become oocytes. Therefore, a fertilized ovum does not have an inactivated X chromosome. We can observe X inactivation at the cellular level because the turned-off X chromosome absorbs a stain much faster than the active X. This differential staining occurs because inactivated DNA has chemical methyl groups (CH_3) that prevent it from being transcribed into RNA and also enable it to absorb stain.

The nucleus of a cell in a female, during interphase, has one dark-staining X chromosome called a **Barr body.** This structure is named after Murray Barr, a Canadian researcher who noticed these dark bodies in 1949 in the nerve cells of female cats. In humans, a cell from a male has no Barr body because his one X chromosome remains active (**figure 6.12**).

In 1961, English geneticist Mary Lyon proposed that the Barr body is the inactivated X chromosome and that the turning off occurs early in development. She reasoned that for homozygous X-linked genotypes, X inactivation would have no effect. No matter which X chromosome is turned off, the same allele is left to be expressed. For heterozygotes, however, X inactivation leads to expression of one allele or the other. Usually this doesn't affect health, because enough cells express the functional gene product. However, some traits reveal striking evidence of X inactivation. For example, the swirls of skin color in incontinentia pigmenti (IP) patients reflect patterns of X inactivation in cells in the skin layers. In cells where the normal allele for melanin pigment is shut off, pale swirls develop. In cells where pigment is produced, brown swirls result.

The mosaic nature of the female due to X inactivation is also seen in the expression of the X-linked recessive condition anhidrotic ectodermal dysplasia. In heterozygous females, patches of skin in which the normal allele is inactivated lack sweat glands, while patches descended from cells in which the mutant allele is inactivated do have sweat glands (see figure 6.11).

Sometimes a female who is heterozygous for an X-linked recessive gene expresses the associated condition because the tissues that the illness affects happen to have the normal version of the allele inactivated. This can happen in a carrier of hemophilia A. If the X chromosome carrying the normal allele for the clotting factor is turned off in many immature blood platelet cells, then the woman's blood will take longer than normal to clot—causing mild hemophilia. Luckily for her, slowed clotting time also greatly reduces her risk of cardiovascular disease caused by blood clots blocking circulation! A carrier of an X-linked

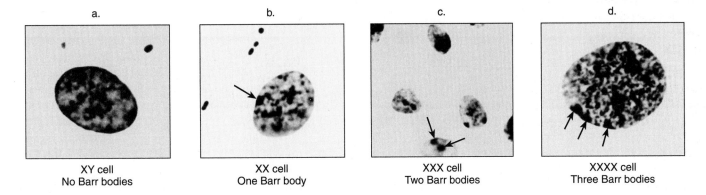

Figure 6.12 **Barr body.** One X chromosome is inactivated in each cell of a female mammal. The turned-off X chromosome absorbs a stain faster than the active X chromosome, forming a dark spot called a Barr body. A normal male cell has no Barr body **(a)**, and a normal female cell has one **(b)**. Individual **(c)** has two Barr bodies and three X chromosomes. She is normal in appearance, behavior, and intellect, but has a lower IQ than her siblings. Rarely, a female has two extra X chromosomes, as in **(d)**.

trait who expresses the phenotype is called a **manifesting heterozygote.** In IP, X-inactivation is skewed in the opposite direction: The mutation-bearing X chromosome is preferentially silenced. Perhaps females in whom the normal X chromosome is silenced in most cells are so severely affected that they do not survive to be born.

A familiar example of X inactivation appears in the coat colors of tortoiseshell and calico cats. An X-linked gene confers brownish-black (dominant) or yellowish-orange (recessive) color. A female cat heterozygous for this gene has patches of each color, forming a tortoiseshell pattern that reflects different cells expressing either of the two alleles (**figure 6.13**). The earlier the X inactivation, the larger the patches, because more cell divisions can occur afterward. White patches may also occur due to epistasis by an autosomal gene that shuts off pigment synthesis. A cat with patches against such a white background is a calico. These cats are nearly always female, because a male can have these coat color patterns only if he inherits an extra X chromosome.

X inactivation can be used to detect carriers of some X-linked disorders. This is the case for Lesch-Nyhan syndrome, in which an affected boy has cerebral palsy, bites his or her fingers and lips to the point of mutilation, is mentally retarded, and passes painful urinary stones. Mutation results in defective or absent HGPRT, an enzyme. A woman who carries Lesch-Nyhan syndrome can be detected when hairs from widely separated parts of her head are tested for HGPRT. (Hair is used for the test because it is accessible and produces the enzyme.) If some hairs contain HGPRT but others do not, she is a carrier. The hair cells that lack the enzyme have turned off the X chromosome that carries the normal allele; the hair cells that manufacture the normal enzyme have turned off the X chromosome that carries the disease-causing allele. The woman is healthy because her brain has enough HGPRT, but each son has a 50 percent chance of inheriting the disease.

Key Concepts

In female mammals, X inactivation compensates for differences between males and females in the numbers of gene copies on the X chromosome. Early in development, one X chromosome in each cell of the female is turned off. The effects of X inactivation can be noticeable when heterozygous alleles are expressed in certain tissues.

6.4 Sex-Limited and Sex-Influenced Traits

An X-linked recessive trait generally is more prevalent in males than females. Other situations, however, can affect gene expression in the sexes differently.

Sex-Limited Traits

A **sex-limited trait** affects a structure or function of the body that is present in only males or only females. Such a gene may be X-linked or autosomal.

Understanding sex-limited inheritance is important in animal breeding. In cattle, for example, milk yield and horn development are traits that affect only one sex each, but the genes controlling them can be transmitted by either parent. In humans, beard growth and breast size are sex-limited traits. A woman does not grow a beard because she does not manufacture the hormones required for facial hair growth. She can, however, pass to her sons the genes specifying heavy beard growth.

An inherited medical condition that arises during pregnancy is by definition a sex-limited trait, since males do not become pregnant. Preeclampsia is a sudden increase in blood pressure in the pregnant woman as the birth nears. It is fatal to 50,000 women worldwide each year. Obstetricians have routinely asked their patients if their mothers had preeclampsia, because it has a tendency to occur in women whose mothers were affected. However, a study of 1.7 million pregnancies in Norway revealed that if a man's first wife had preeclampsia, his second wife had double the relative risk of developing the condition, too. The Norway study led to the hypothesis that a male can transmit a tendency to develop preeclampsia.

Another study on 298 men and 237 women in Utah supports the hypothesis that preeclampsia risk is sex-limited. This investigation found that women whose mothers-in-law had experienced preeclampsia when pregnant with the womens' husbands had approximately twice the relative risk of developing the condition themselves. One hypothesis to explain the results of the two studies is that a gene from the male affects the placenta in a way that elevates the pregnant woman's blood pressure. Genes that may confer the increased risk include those whose protein products participate in

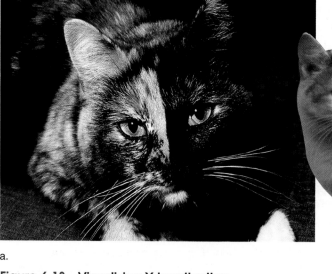

a.

Figure 6.13 Visualizing X inactivation.
X inactivation is obvious in tortoiseshell **(a)** and calico **(b)** cats. X inactivation is rarely observable in humans because most cells do not remain together during development, as a cat's skin cells do.

b.

blood clotting, blood glucose control, and blood pressure. An alternative explanation might be that an infection transmitted by the male causes preeclampsia. Further investigations are warranted.

Sex-Influenced Traits

In a **sex-influenced trait,** an allele is dominant in one sex but recessive in the other. Such a gene may be X-linked or autosomal. The difference in expression can be caused by hormonal differences between the sexes. For example, an autosomal gene for hair growth pattern has two alleles, one that produces hair all over the head and another that causes pattern baldness (**figure 6.14**). The baldness allele is dominant in males but recessive in females, which is why more men than women are bald. A heterozygous male is bald, but a heterozygous female is not. A bald woman is homozygous recessive. Even a bald woman tends to have some wisps of hair, whereas an affected male may be completely hairless on the top of his head.

Key Concepts

A sex-limited trait affects body parts or functions present in only one gender.
• A sex-influenced allele is dominant in one sex but recessive in the other.

6.5 Genomic Imprinting

In Mendel's pea experiments, it didn't matter whether a trait came from the male or female parent. For some genes in mammals, however, parental origin does influence the phenotype. In a poorly understood process called **genomic imprinting,** methyl groups cover a gene or several linked genes and prevent them from being accessed to synthesize protein. For a particular imprinted gene, the copy from either the father or the mother is always imprinted, even in different individuals. The result: a disease may be more severe, or different, depending upon which parent transmitted the gene.

Silencing the Contribution from One Parent

Imprinting is an **epigenetic alteration,** in which a layer of meaning is stamped upon

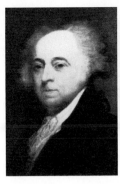
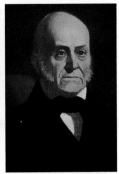

a.   b.

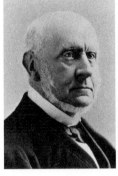
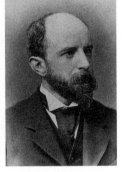

c.   d.

Figure 6.14 Pattern baldness.
This sex-influenced trait was seen in the Adams family. John Adams (1735–1826) **(a)** was the second president of the United States and the father of John Quincy Adams (1767–1848) **(b)**, the sixth president. John Quincy was the father of Charles Francis Adams (1807–1886) **(c)**, a diplomat and the father of historian Henry Adams (1838–1918) **(d)**.

---

a gene without changing its DNA sequence. The imprinting pattern is passed from cell to cell in mitosis, but not from individual to individual through meiosis. When silenced DNA is replicated during mitosis, the pattern of blocked genes is exactly placed, or imprinted, on the new DNA, covering the same genes as in the parental DNA (**figure 6.15**). In this way, the "imprint" of inactivation is perpetuated, as if each such gene "remembers" which parent it came from. In meiosis, however, imprints are removed and reset. As oocyte and sperm form, the protective groups shielding their imprinted genes are stripped away, and new patterns are set down, depending upon whether the fertilized ovum is male or female. This is how women can have sons and men can have daughters without passing on their sex-specific parental imprints.

The function of genomic imprinting isn't known. Because many imprinted genes take part in early development, it may be a way to finely regulate the amounts of key proteins in the embryo. The fact that some genes lose their imprints after birth supports this idea of early importance. Also, imprinted genes occur in clusters, which are under the control of other regions of DNA called imprinting centers. Perhaps one gene in a cluster is essential for early development, and the others become imprinted simply because they are nearby.

In addition to its confusing effects on the inheritance of diseases, genomic imprinting has implications for understanding early human development and for artificial conception technologies such as cloning (see Bioethics: Choices for the Future, chapter 3) and *in vitro* fertilization. Imprinting means that for mammals, it takes two opposite-sex parents to produce a healthy embryo and placenta. This was discovered in the early 1980s, through experiments on early mouse embryos and examination of certain rare pregnancy problems in humans. To investigate the roles of the genomes passed from the male and the female to the fertilized ovum in mice, researchers created cells that contained two male pronuclei or two female pronuclei. The results were bizarre. When the fertilized ovum contained two male genomes, a normal placenta developed, but the embryo was tiny and quickly stopped developing. A zygote with two female pronuclei, on the other hand, developed into an embryo, but the placenta was grossly abnormal. It appeared that the male genome controls placenta development, and the female genome, embryo development.

The mouse results were consistent with abnormalities of human development. When two sperm fertilize an oocyte, abnormal growths of placenta-like tissue form. When a sperm fertilizes an oocyte that has two female genomes, the embryo is normal, but the placenta is malformed. However, if a fertilized ovum contains only two female genomes but no male genome, a mass of random differentiated tissue, called a teratoma, grows. No embryo develops.

These abnormalities indicate that, early in development, genes from a female parent direct different activities than genes from a male parent. The requirement that both male and female contribute to a zygote may

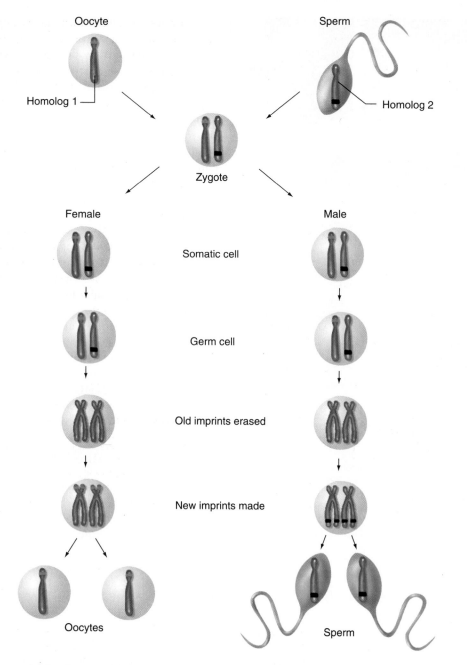

Figure 6.15 **Genomic imprinting.** Imprints are erased during meiosis, then reinstituted according to the sex of the new individual.

Labels on figure: Oocyte, Homolog 1, Sperm, Homolog 2, Zygote, Female, Male, Somatic cell, Germ cell, Old imprints erased, New imprints made, Oocytes, Sperm

causes more than thirty disorders. The effects of genomic imprinting are revealed only when an individual has one copy of a normally imprinted gene and the other copy is inactivated or deleted (absent). This chapter concludes with compelling examples of the effects of genomic imprinting gone awry.

A striking example of genomic imprinting involves two different syndromes that arise from small deletions in the same region of chromosome 15 (**figure 6.16**). A child with Prader-Willi syndrome is obese, has small hands and feet, eats uncontrollably, and does not mature sexually. The other condition, Angelman syndrome, causes mental retardation, an extended tongue, large jaw, poor muscle coordination, and convulsions that make the arms flap. In many cases of Prader-Willi syndrome, only the mother's chromosome 15 region is expressed; the father's chromosome is deleted in that region. In Angelman syndrome, the reverse occurs: the father's gene (or genes) is expressed, and the mother's chromosome has the deletion.

Symptoms of Prader-Willi arise because several paternal genes that are not normally imprinted (that is, that are normally active) are missing. In Angelman syndrome, a normally active single maternal gene is deleted. This part of chromosome 15 is especially unstable because it includes highly repetitive DNA sequences, which bracket the genes that cause the symptoms.

Imprinting gone awry can cause rare forms of diabetes mellitus, autism, and tumor syndromes. Clues that indicate a condition is associated with genomic imprinting include increased severity depending on whether it is inherited from the father or mother and also a phenomenon called uniparental disomy. This term literally means "two bodies from one parent," and refers to an offspring who inherits both copies of a gene from one parent. (Chapter 13 discusses uniparental disomy further.)

A Sheep With a Giant Rear End

Genomic imprinting is easier to observe in species that can be bred, so that traits can be followed over several generations. This is the case for Solid Gold, a ram with an overmuscled rear end (**figure 6.17a**), and his many offspring. Solid Gold was born in 1983 in Oklahoma, and by three weeks of age, his hefty hindquarters were attracting attention.

explain why cloned mammals are almost always unhealthy.

In vitro fertilization and a variation of the procedure in which a sperm pronucleus is injected into an oocyte are associated with increased incidence of two imprinting disorders, Angelman syndrome and Beckwith-Wiedemann syndrome. This finding suggests that manipulation of gamete nuclei may alter imprinting.

Genomic imprinting can explain incomplete penetrance, in which an individual is known to have inherited a genotype associated with a particular phenotype, but has no signs of the trait him or herself—such as a person with normal fingers whose parent and child have polydactyly. An imprinted gene that silences the mutant allele could explain these cases: The predicted genotype is present, but not expressed.

Imprinting Disorders in Humans

About 1 percent of human genes are imprinted, and disruption of imprinting

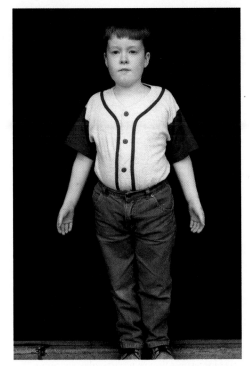

a.

With visions of extra-meaty lamb chops, the breeder, instead of shipping Solid Gold to market, mated him to see if the trait was inherited. Sure enough, at three weeks of age, some of the lambs started to grow giant rears. Solid Gold became a favorite in the show ring. When a biology graduate student in search of a research project became interested in him, the ram's story continued in the genetics journals. Researchers named the mutation *callipyge*, which is Greek for "beautiful buttocks."

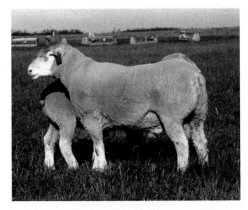

a.

Figure 6.17 Genomic imprinting in a sheep's rear. **(a)** Solid Gold astounded breeders with his overly muscled hindquarters. **(b)** Only callipyge males can pass on the trait, and only if the ewe is wild type.

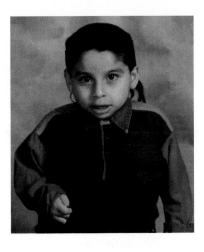

b.

Figure 6.16 Prader-Willi and Angelman syndromes. Two syndromes result from missing genetic material in the same chromosomal region. **(a)** Tyler has Prader-Willi syndrome. Note his small hands and feet. **(b)** Angelman syndrome also causes mental retardation, but the other symptoms differ from those of Prader-Willi syndrome.

The trait was autosomal dominant, but people who tried to breed a stock from Solid Gold's lambs ran into a problem. The sheep seemed to be resisting Mendel's first law—the trait was passed only if it came from the father! In other words, a callipyge ewe did not yield a callipyge lamb (figure 6.17b). The situation turned

out to be even more complex than straight genomic imprinting—not only must the ram be callipyge, but the ewe must be wild type to transmit the trait to all offspring.

Researchers eventually identified the callipyge gene, and also discovered that when it is overexpressed in the big-reared sheep, so are seven neighboring genes on sheep chromosome 18. (These other genes control wool quality and which muscles overgrow.) The involvement of several genes was another clue pointing to imprinting, which can affect a chromosome segment as well as an individual gene. Yet other researchers traced the entire suite of silenced genes to a single DNA base change which disrupts imprinting. Alas, the curious callipyge mutation did not turn out to be valuable to breeders—the meat was tough—but the same set of genes is found in humans, prompting coverage in several popular magazines.

Key Concepts

In genomic imprinting, the phenotype differs depending on whether a gene is inherited from the mother or the father. Methyl groups may bind to DNA and temporarily suppress gene expression in a pattern determined by the individual's sex. • Imprinting may be a normal process in mammalian embryos.

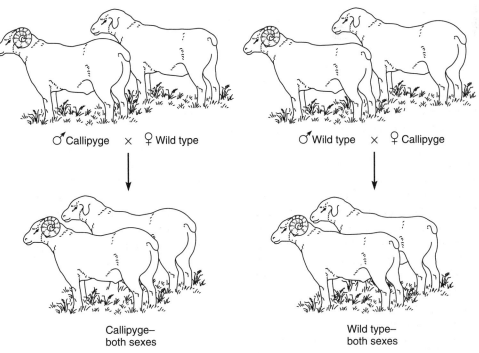

♂Callipyge × ♀ Wild type

Callipyge—
both sexes

♂ Wild type × ♀ Callipyge

Wild type—
both sexes

b.

Summary

6.1 Sexual Development

1. Sexual identity includes sex chromosome makeup; gonadal specialization; phenotype (reproductive structures); and gender identity.

2. The human male is the **heterogametic sex,** with an X and a Y chromosome. The female, with two X chromosomes, is the **homogametic sex.** The *SRY* gene on the Y chromosome determines sex.

3. The human Y chromosome includes two **pseudoautosomal regions** and a large, male-specific region that does not recombine. Y-linked genes may correspond to X-linked genes, be similar to them, or be unique to the Y chromosome. Palindromic DNA sequences can cause gene loss on the Y.

4. If the *SRY* gene is expressed, undifferentiated gonads develop as testes. If *SRY* is not expressed, the gonads develop as ovaries.

5. Starting about eight weeks after fertilization, sustentacular cells in the testes secrete anti-Müllerian hormone, which prevents development of female structures, and interstitial cells produce testosterone, which triggers development of the epididymides, vasa deferentia, seminal vesicles, and ejaculatory ducts.

6. Testosterone converted to DHT controls development of the urethra, prostate gland, penis, and scrotum. If *SRY* is not turned on, the Müllerian ducts continue to develop into female reproductive structures.

7. Evidence points to an inherited component to homosexuality.

6.2 Traits Inherited on Sex Chromosomes

8. Y-linked traits are rare. They are passed from fathers to sons only.

9. Males are **hemizygous** for genes on the X chromosome and express such genes because they do not have another allele on a homolog. An X-linked trait passes from mother to son because he inherits his X chromosome from his mother and his Y chromosome from his father.

10. An X-linked allele may be dominant or recessive. X-linked dominant traits are more devastating to males than to females.

6.3 X Inactivation Equalizes the Sexes

11. **X inactivation** shuts off one X chromosome in each cell in female mammals, making them mosaics for heterozygous genes on the X chromosome. This phenomenon evens out the dosages of genes on the sex chromosomes between the sexes.

12. A female who expresses the phenotype corresponding to an X-linked gene she carries is a **manifesting heterozygote.**

6.4 Sex-Limited and Sex-Influenced Traits

13. **Sex-limited traits** may be autosomal or sex-linked, but they only affect one sex because of anatomical or hormonal gender differences.

14. A **sex-influenced gene** is dominant in one sex but recessive in the other.

6.5 Genomic Imprinting

15. In **genomic imprinting,** the phenotype corresponding to a particular genotype differs depending on whether the parent who passes the gene is female or male. Imprints are erased during meiosis and reassigned based on the sex of a new individual. Methyl groups that temporarily suppress gene expression are the physical basis of genomic imprinting.

Review Questions

1. How is sex expressed at the chromosomal, gonadal, phenotypic, and gender identity levels?

2. How do genes in the pseudoautosomal region of the Y chromosome differ from genes in the male-specific region?

3. What are the phenotypes of the following individuals?

   a. a person with a mutation in the *SRY* gene, rendering it nonfunctional

   b. a normal XX individual

   c. an XY individual with a block in testosterone synthesis

4. List the cell types and hormones that contribute to the development of male reproductive structures.

5. List the events that must take place for a fetus to develop as a female.

6. Cite evidence that may point to a hereditary component to homosexuality.

7. Why would it be extremely unlikely to see a woman who is homozygous dominant for an X-linked dominant disease?

8. Why are male calico cats very rare?

9. How might X inactivation cause patchy hairiness on women who have congenital generalized hypertrichosis (CGH), even though the disease-causing allele is dominant?

10. How does X inactivation even out the "doses" of X-linked genes between the sexes?

11. Traits that appear more frequently in one sex than the other may be caused by genes that are inherited in an X-linked, sex-limited, or sex-influenced fashion. How might you distinguish among these possibilities in a given individual?

12. Cite evidence that genetic contributions from both parents are necessary for normal prenatal development.

Applied Questions

1. In Hunter syndrome, lack of the enzyme iduronate sulfate sulfatase leads to buildup of carbohydrates called mucopolysaccharides. In severe cases, this may swell the liver, spleen, and heart. In mild cases, deafness may be the only symptom. A child with this syndrome is deaf and has unusual facial features. Hunter syndrome is X-linked recessive. Intellect is usually unimpaired and life span can be normal. Suppose a man who has mild Hunter syndrome has a child with a carrier.

   a. What is the probability that a male child would inherit Hunter syndrome?

   b. What is the chance that a female child would inherit Hunter syndrome?

   c. What is the chance that a girl would be a carrier?

   d. How might a carrier of this condition experience symptoms?

2. Coffin-Lowry syndrome causes short, tapered fingers; abnormal finger and toe bones; puffy hands; soft, elastic skin; curved fingernails; facial anomalies; and sometimes hearing loss and heart problems. Evidence suggests that the syndrome is X-linked recessive, but girls are affected to a much lesser degree than boys. Suggest two explanations for why girls tend to have milder cases.

3. Amelogenesis imperfecta is an X-linked dominant condition that affects tooth enamel. Affected males have extremely thin enamel layers all over each tooth. Female carriers have grooved teeth from the uneven deposition of enamel. Explain the difference in phenotype between the sexes.

4. A prenatal test finds that cells of a fetus have two Barr bodies. What sex is the fetus?

5. Huntington disease (see Bioethics: Choices for the Future, Chapter 4) begins earlier and symptoms progress faster if the affected person inherits the disorder from his or her father. Explain this observation.

Web Activities

6. Identify an X-linked disorder at http://www.ncbi.nlm.nih.gov/disease/chr21-Y.html, then find it in OMIM and describe it.

7. From the Imprinted Gene Catalogue at http://cancer.otago.ac.nz/IGC/web/home.html, click on "search by species name" and then click on "complete list." Find two disorders that involve imprinting, one transmitted from the mother and one from the father, and use OMIM to describe them.

Case Studies

8. Reginald has mild hemophilia A that he can control by taking a clotting factor. He marries Lydia, whom he met at the hospital where he and Lydia's brother, Marvin, receive their treatment. Lydia and Marvin's mother and father, Emma and Clyde, do not have hemophilia. What is the probability that Reginald and Lydia's son will inherit hemophilia A?

9. Harold works in a fish market, but the odor does not bother him because he has anosmia, an X-linked recessive lack of sense of smell. Harold's wife, Shirley, has a normal sense of smell. Harold's sister, Maude, also has a normal sense of smell, as does her husband, Phil, and daughter, Marsha, but their identical twin boys, Alvin and Simon, cannot detect odors. Harold and Maude's parents, Edgar and Florence, can smell normally. Draw a pedigree for this family, indicating people who must be carriers of the anosmia gene.

10. Metacarpal 4–5 fusion is an X-linked recessive condition in which certain finger bones are fused. It occurs in many members of the Flabudgett family, depicted in the pedigree to the left:

    a. Why are three females affected, considering that this is an X-linked condition?

    b. What is the risk that individual III-1 will have an affected son?

    c. What is the risk that individual III-5 will have an affected son?

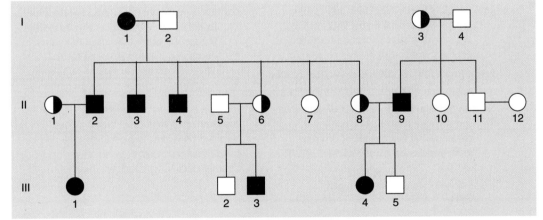

11. Herbert is 58 years old and bald. His wife, Sheri, also has pattern baldness. What is the risk that their son, Frank, will lose his hair?

12. The Addams family knows of three relatives who had kinky hair disease, an X-linked recessive disorder in which a child does not grow, has brain degeneration, and dies by age two. Affected children have peculiar white stubby hair, from which the disorder takes its name.

Wanda Addams is hesitant about having children because her two sisters have each had sons who died from kinky hair disease. Her mother had a brother who died of the condition, too. The pedigree for the family is shown here.

a. Fill in the symbols for the family members who must be carriers of kinky hair disease.

b. What is the chance that Wanda (III-7) is a carrier?

c. If Wanda is a carrier, what is the chance that a son of hers would inherit kinky hair disease?

d. Why don't any women in the family have kinky hair disease?

Learn to apply the skills of a genetic counselor with these additional cases found in the *Case Workbook in Human Genetics*:

Anhidrotic ectodermal dysplasia
Blue diaper syndrome
Chronic granulomatous disease
Congenital muscular dystrophies
Intersex

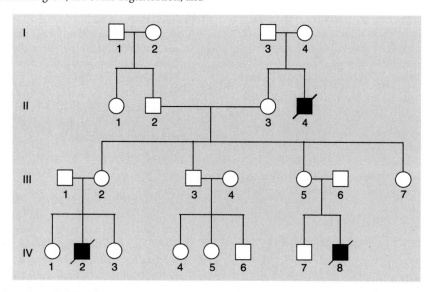

Suggested Readings

Aitken, R. John, and Jennifer A. Marshall-Graves. February 28, 2002. The future of sex. *Nature* 415:963. Is the human Y chromosome doomed?

Boylan, Jennifer Finney. 2003. *She's Not There: A Life in Two Genders.* New York: Broadway Books. Jennifer Boylan, an English professor in Maine, was once Jim. She is transgendered.

Colapinto, J. 2000. *As Nature Made Him.* New York: HarperCollins. The true story of David Reimer, whose sex reassignment surgery was a tragic failure.

Hunt, David M., et al. February 17, 1995. The chemistry of John Dalton's colorblindness. *Science,* vol. 267. The famous chemist requested that his eyeballs be examined after his death to localize the cause of his colorblindness.

Lewis, Ricki. July 10, 2000. Reevaluating sex reassignment. *The Scientist* 14:14. Research supports anecdotal evidence that sex reassignment is often unsuccessful.

Lewis, Ricki. October 28, 2002. Solid Gold sheepstakes. *The Scientist* 16(21):16. A sheep with a huge rear end illustrates genomic imprinting.

Lewis, Ricki. July 28, 2003. Y envy. *The Scientist* 17(15):64. The author laments lacking a Y.

Skaletsky, Helen et al. June 19, 2003. The male-specific region of the human Y chromosome is a mosaic of discrete sequence classes. *Nature* 423:825–37. The DNA sequence of the Y chromosome is revealed.

Tilford, Charles A. February 15, 2001. A physical map of the human Y chromosome. *Nature* 409:943–45. The Y chromosome carries very few protein-encoding genes.

Zimmer, Carl. September 2002. The once and future male: Men will survive even after the pivotal genes that make them men disappear. *Natural History* 111(9):22–26. The Y chromosome may be on the way out, but the human male is here to stay.

Weekly updates of current news related to human genetics are available through Power Web on your Online Learning Center.

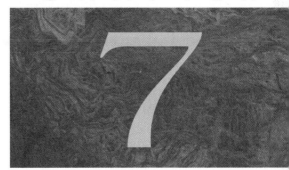

CHAPTER 7

Multifactorial Traits

CHAPTER CONTENTS

7.1 Genes and the Environment Mold Most Traits
Environmental influences mold many human traits. Genes and the environment combine to influence fingerprint pattern, skin color, disease susceptibilities, and even intelligence and behavior.

7.2 Methods Used to Investigate Multifactorial Traits
Separating genetic from environmental influences on phenotype is enormously difficult. Observations of how common a trait is in a population, combined with theoretical predictions of the percentages of genes that certain relatives should share, enable us to calculate heritability. This is an estimate of genetic contribution to individual variations in a trait. Adopted individuals and twins have been important in studying multifactorial traits, but recent investigations use association studies that correlate complex phenotypes to sets of genetic markers, delineating genome regions where causative genes may lie.

7.3 Some Multifactorial Traits
Cardiovascular health and body weight are two common characteristics that the interactions of specific predisposing genes and environmental factors influence.

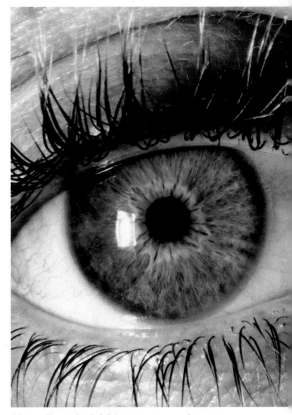

More than just blue or green, brown or black, eye color is perhaps the most purely polygenic human trait.

A woman who is a prolific writer has a daughter who becomes a successful novelist. An overweight man and woman have obese children. A man whose father suffers from alcoholism has the same problem. Are these characteristics—writing talent, obesity, and alcoholism—inherited or learned? Or are they a combination of nature (genetics) and nurture (the environment)?

Most of the traits and medical conditions mentioned so far in this book are single-gene characteristics, inherited according to Mendel's laws, or linked on the same chromosome. Many single-gene disorders are very rare, each affecting one in hundreds or even thousands of individuals. Using Mendel's laws, geneticists can predict the probability that certain family members will inherit single-gene conditions. Most more common traits and diseases, though, can seem to "run in families" with no apparent pattern, or they occur sporadically, with just one case in a family.

Genes rarely act completely alone. Even single-gene disorders are modified by environmental factors or other genes. This chapter discusses the nature of non-Mendelian characteristics, and the tools used to study them. Chapter 8 focuses on the most difficult traits to assess for their inherited components—behaviors.

7.1 Genes and the Environment Mold Most Traits

On the first page of the first chapter of *On the Origin of Species,* Charles Darwin noted that two factors are responsible for variation among organisms—"the nature of the organism and the nature of the conditions." Darwin's thoughts were a nineteenth-century musing on "heredity versus the environment." Though this phrase might seem to indicate that genes and the environment are adversaries, they are actually two forces that interact, and they do so in ways that mold many of our characteristics.

A trait can be described as either Mendelian or **polygenic.** A single gene is responsible for a Mendelian trait. A polygenic trait, as its name implies, reflects the activities of more than one gene, and the effect of these multiple inputs is often additive, although the individual inputs are not necessarily equal. Both Mendelian and polygenic traits can also be **multifactorial,** which means they are influenced by the environment (multifactorial traits are also called complex traits). Pure polygenic traits—those not influenced by the environment—are very rare.

Multifactorial traits include common characteristics such as height and skin color, illnesses, and behavioral conditions and tendencies. Behavioral traits are not inherently different from other types of traits; they simply involve the functioning of the brain, rather than another organ. **Figure 7.1** depicts the relative contributions of genes and the environment to several disorders and events.

In contrast to a single-gene disorder, a complex multifactorial condition may be caused by the additive contributions of several genes, each of which confers some degree of susceptibility. For example, we know that multiple sclerosis (MS) has a genetic component, because siblings of an affected individual are 25 times as likely to

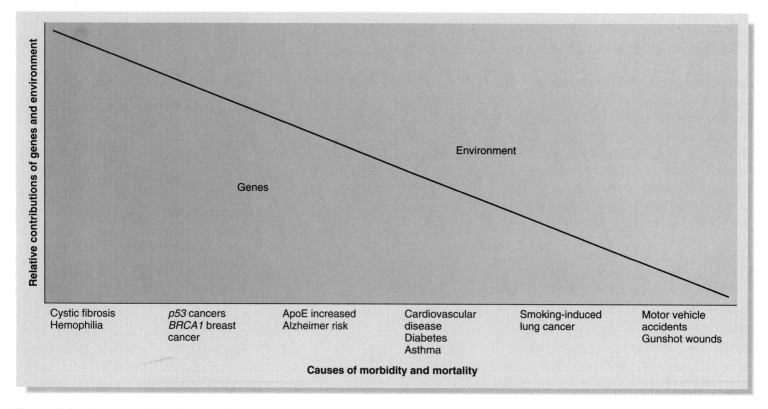

Figure 7.1   Genes and environment.   The relative contributions of genes and the environment in causing traits and disorders fall on a continuum. In this schematic representation, the examples toward the left are caused mostly by genes; those to the right are caused more by environmental effects. The classic multifactorial conditions are in the middle—these are polygenic and influenced by the environment.

develop MS as siblings of people who do not have MS. One model of MS origin suggests that five susceptibility genes have alleles, each of which increases the risk of developing the condition. Those risks add up, and, in the presence of an appropriate (and unknown) environmental trigger, the disease begins.

Polygenic Traits Are Continuously Varying

For a polygenic trait, the combined action of many genes often produces a continuum of the phenotype, making this a continuously varying or quantitative trait. The parts of chromosomes that contribute to polygenic traits are therefore called quantitative trait loci, or QTLs. A multifactorial trait is continuously varying only if it is also polygenic. That is, it is the genetic component of the trait that contributes the continuing variation of the phenotype. The individual genes that confer a polygenic trait follow Mendel's laws (if they are unlinked), but together they do not produce Mendelian ratios. They all contribute to the phenotype, without showing dominance or recessiveness with respect to each other. For example, the multiple genes that regulate height and skin color result in continuously varying traits that exhibit a range of possible phenotypes. Mendelian traits are instead discrete or qualitative, often providing an all-or-none phenotype such as "affected" versus "normal."

A polygenic trait varies in populations, as the many nuances of hair color, body weight, and cholesterol levels demonstrate. Some genes contribute more to a polygenic trait than others. Within genes, alleles can have differing impacts depending upon exactly how they alter an encoded protein, as well as upon how common they are in a particular population. For example, a mutation in the gene that encodes the receptor that takes low-density lipoproteins (LDL cholesterol) into cells drastically raises a person's blood serum cholesterol level. But because fewer than 1 percent of the individuals in most populations have this mutation, it contributes very little to the variation in cholesterol level seen at the population level.

Although the expression of a polygenic trait is continuous, we can categorize individuals into classes and calculate the frequencies of the classes. When we do this and plot the frequency for each phenotype class, a bell-shaped curve results. This curve indicating continuous variation of a polygenic trait is strikingly similar for any trait. Even when different numbers of genes affect the trait, the curve takes the same shape, as is evident in the following examples.

Fingerprint Patterns

The skin on the fingertips folds into patterns of raised skin called dermal ridges that in turn align to form loops, whorls, and arches. A technique called dermatoglyphics ("skin writing") compares the number of ridges that comprise these patterns to identify and distinguish individuals (**figure 7.2**). Dermatoglyphics is part of genetics because certain disorders (such as Down syndrome) are characterized by unusual ridge patterns, and of course it is also part of forensics in fingerprint analysis. Fingerprint pattern is a multifactorial trait.

The number of ridges in a fingerprint pattern is largely determined by genes, but also responds to the environment. During weeks 6 through 13 of prenatal development, the ridge pattern can alter as the fetus touches the finger and toe pads to the wall of the amniotic sac. This early environmental effect explains why the fingerprints of identical twins, who share all genes, are not exactly alike.

We can quantify a fingerprint with a measurement called a total ridge count, which tallies the number of ridges comprising a whorl, loop, or arch part of the pattern for each finger. The average total ridge count in a male is 145, and in a female, 126. Plotting total ridge count reveals the bell curve characteristic of a continuously varying trait.

Height

The effect of the environment on height is obvious—people who do not have enough to eat do not reach their genetic potential for height. Students lined up according to height, but raised in two different decades and under different circumstances, vividly reveal the effects of genes and the environment on this continuously varying trait. Part *a* of **figure 7.3** depicts students from 1920, and part *b*, students from 1997. The similarity of the bell curve reflects the inherited component of the trait. But also note that the tallest people in the old photograph are 5'9", whereas the tallest people in the more recent photograph are 6'5". The difference is attributed to such environmental factors as improved diet and better overall health.

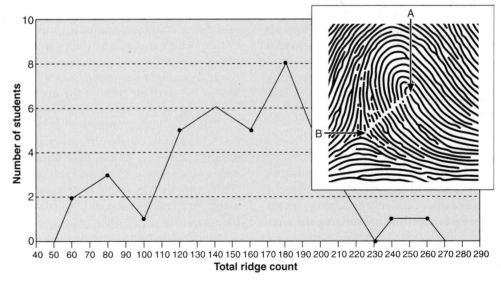

Figure 7.2 Anatomy of a fingerprint. Total ridge counts for a number of individuals, plotted on a bar graph, form an approximate bell-shaped curve, signaling a multifactorial trait. The number of ridges between landmark points A and B on this loop pattern is 12. Total ridge count includes the number of ridges on all fingers.

Data and print from Gordon Mendenhall, Thomas Mertens, and Jon Hendrix, "Fingerprint Ridge Count," in *The American Biology Teacher*, vol. 51, no. 4, April 1989, pp. 204–6.

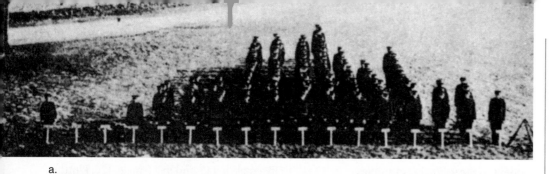

a.

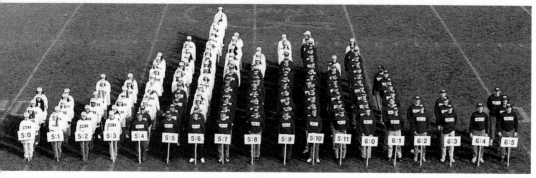

b.

Figure 7.3 **The inheritance of height.** Previous editions of this (and other) textbooks have used the photograph in **(a)** to illustrate the continuously varying nature of height. In the photo, taken around 1920, 175 cadets at the Connecticut Agricultural College lined up by height. In 1997, professor Linda Strausbaugh asked her genetics students at the school, today the University of Connecticut at Storrs, to recreate the scene **(b)**. They did, and confirmed the continuously varying nature of human height. But they also elegantly demonstrated how height has increased during the twentieth century. Improved nutrition has definitely played a role in expressing genetic potential for height. The tallest people in the old photograph (a) are 5'9" tall, whereas the tallest people in the more recent photograph (b) are 6'5" tall.

We usually do not know exactly how many genes contribute to multifactorial traits that are also polygenic. However, geneticists can suggest models for a certain number of genes contributing to a trait based on the number of variants that can be discerned—although this is limited by what we can perceive.

Eye Color

Eye color is probably a pure polygenic trait—one with no environmental input. But eye color isn't only a matter of brown, blue, green, or hazel. Overlying the common tones are specks and flecks, streaks and rings, and regions of dark versus light. These modifications arise from the way pigment is laid down onto the distinctive peaks and valleys at the back of the iris, the colored portion of the eye.

Two genes specify greenish-blue pigments called lipochromes, and two or more other genes encode the brownish melanins. These genes interact in a hierarchy, with the brown genes masking the green/blues, and everything masking pure blue. Unlike the browns, which are caused by chemical pigments, pure blue is a "spectral color" that results from light scattering, much as the blue of the sky is an effect of the sun's rays penetrating the atmosphere. Hazel eyes have a mixture of lipochromes and melanins. Blue-eyed parents can have brown-eyed children if the parents do not have pure blue eyes—which few people do. Each parent contributes a slight ability to produce pigment, which adds in the child to color the irises a pale brown. Unlike pigment in the skin, melanin in the iris stays in the cell that produces it.

The topography at the back of the iris is as distinctive as fingerprints, and is an inherited trait. Thicker parts of this area darken the appearance of the pigments, rendering brown eyes nearly black in some parts, or blue eyes closer to purple. The bluest of blue eyes have thin irises with very little pigment. The effect of the iris surface on color is a little like the visual effect of a rough-textured canvas on paint.

For many years, eye color was thought to arise from two genes with two alleles each, as depicted in **figure 7.4**. Although this is a gross oversimplification, it does illustrate the bell curve that describes the phenotypes resulting from gene interaction. These alleles interact additively to produce five eye colors—light blue, deep blue or green, light brown, medium brown, and dark brown/black. If each allele contributes a certain amount of pigment, then the greater the number of such alleles, the darker the eye color. If eye color is controlled by two genes, A and B, each of which comes in two allelic forms—A and a and B and b—then the lightest color would be genotype $aabb$; the darkest, $AABB$. The bell curve arises because there are more ways to inherit light brown eyes, the midrange color, with any two contributing dominant alleles, than there are ways to inherit the other colors.

Analysis of the human genome will likely reveal additional eye color genes—the mouse has more than 60! Recognizing that there may be dozens of variations of eye color, with distinctions perhaps beyond our perception, one company has analyzed 300 sites within the two lipochrome and two melanin genes in hundreds of individuals. From this information, their researchers have developed a forensic tool called the "retinome," which is a database of eye colors that goes well beyond the standard four that appear on a driver's license.

A Closer Look at Skin Color

Melanin pigment colors the skin to different degrees in different individuals. Cells called melanocytes in skin have long extensions that snake between the other, tile-like skin cells, distributing pigment granules through the skin layers. Some melanin exits the melanocytes and enters the hardened cells in the skin's upper layers. Here the melanin breaks into pieces, and as the skin cells are pushed up toward the skin's surface, the melanin bits provide color. The pigment protects against DNA damage from ultraviolet radiation, and exposure to the sun increases melanin syn-

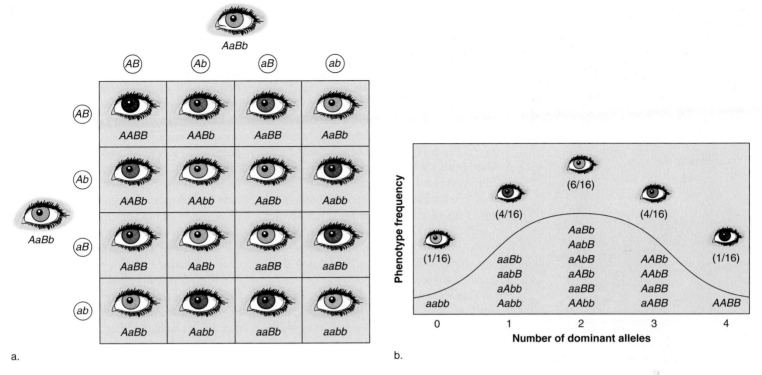

Figure 7.4 **Variations in eye color.** **(a)** A model of two genes, with two alleles each, can explain the existence of five eye colors in humans. **(b)** The frequency distribution of eye colors forms the characteristic bell-shaped curve for a polygenic trait.

thesis. **Figure 7.5** shows a three-gene model for human skin color—an oversimplification of this highly variable trait.

Although people come in a wide variety of hues, we all have about the same number of melanocytes per unit area of skin. Differences in skin color arise from the number and distribution of melanin pieces in the skin cells in the uppermost layers. People with albinism cannot manufacture melanin (see figure 4.15).

The definition of race based on skin color is more a social construct than a biological concept, for skin color is but one of thousands of traits. From a genetic perspective, when referring to other types of organisms, races are groups within species that are distinguished by different allele frequencies. Although we tend to classify people by skin color because it is an obvious visible way to distinguish individuals, skin color is not a reliable indicator of heritage. Golfer Tiger Woods, for example, is African American, Caucasian, Asian, and Native American. He illustrates that skin color alone hardly indicates a person's ethnic and genetic background (**figure 7.6**). The case of Thomas Jefferson and his dark-skinned descendants described in chapter 1 also illustrates how the traditional definition of

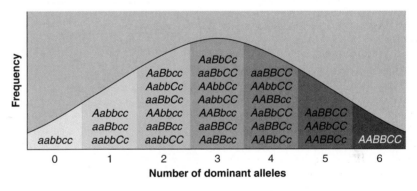

Figure 7.5 **Variations in skin color.** A model of three genes, with two alleles each, can explain broad hues of human skin. In actuality, this trait likely involves many more than three genes.

race based on skin color considers only one trait—the distribution of melanin. When many genes are examined, two people with black skin may be less alike than either is to another person with white skin. On a population level, sub-Saharan Africans and Australian aborigines have dark skin, but they are very dissimilar in other inherited characteristics. Their dark skins may reflect the same adaptation (persistence of a valuable genetic trait) to life in a sunny, tropical climate. Overall, 93 percent of inherited traits that vary are no more common in people of one skin color than any other.

Although in a genetic sense the concept of race based on skin color has little meaning, in a practical sense, such groups do have different incidences of certain diseases. This reflects the tendency to choose partners from within the group, thereby retaining certain alleles, but also may result from social inequalities, such as limited access to good nutrition or health care. Observations that particular races have a higher incidence of certain illnesses have influenced medical practice; at least one drug company markets hypertension drugs to African Americans, who have a higher incidence of

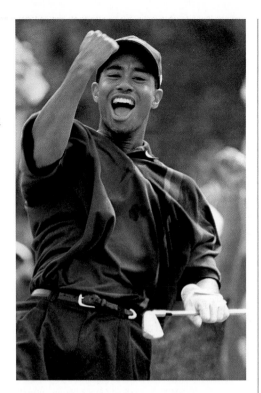

Figure 7.6 Skin color is only one way humans differ from each other.
Golfer Tiger Woods objects to being called black; he is actually African American, Caucasian, Asian, and Native American.

this condition than do people in other populations. Offering medical treatments based on skin color may make sense on a population level, but on the individual level it may lead to errors. A white person might be denied a drug that would work, or a black person given one that doesn't, if the treatment decision is based on a superficial trait not directly related to how the body responds to a particular drug.

Genetics and genomics may address the problems inherent in race-based medicine. In one study, researchers identified variants of a gene called *MDR* (for multidrug resistance) in four population groups. This gene encodes a protein that pumps poisons out of certain white blood cells and intestinal lining cells. When a variant results in a pump that works too well, the protein recognizes drugs that treat cancer, AIDS, and other conditions as toxins, blasting them out of the cell. Researchers found this protein variant in 83 percent of West Africans, 61 percent of African Americans, 26 percent of Caucasians, and 34 percent of Japanese. MDR variant status could be used to pre-scribe certain drugs only for individuals whose cells would not pump the drugs out. MDR genotype is a more biologically meaningful basis for prescribing a drug than skin color.

In an even more compelling study, researchers cataloged 23 markers for genes that control drug metabolism in 354 people representing eight classically defined races: black (Bantu, Ethiopian, and Afro-Caribbean,), white (Norwegian, Armenian, and Ashkenazi Jews), and Asian (Chinese and New Guinean). The genetic markers fell into four very distinct groups that predict which of several blood thinners, chemotherapies, and painkillers will be effective—and these drug response groups did not at all match the traditional racial groups.

Fingerprint pattern, height, eye color, and skin color are "normal" polygenic, multifactorial traits. Illnesses, too, may result from the interplay of a gene or genes with environmental influences. Reading 7.1 presents three interesting examples of environmental influences on illness.

Key Concepts

Polygenic traits are determined by more than one gene and vary continuously in expression. Multifactorial traits are determined by a combination of a gene or genes and the environment. ● A bell curve describes the distribution of phenotypic classes of a polygenic trait, such as fingerprint pattern, height, eye color, and skin color.

7.2 Methods Used to Investigate Multifactorial Traits

It is much more challenging to predict recurrence risks for polygenic traits and disorders than it is for Mendelian traits. Geneticists evaluate the input of genes, using information from population and family studies.

Empiric Risk

Using Mendel's laws, it is possible to predict the risk that a single-gene trait will recur in a family if one knows the mode of inheritance—such as autosomal dominant or recessive. To predict the chance that a multifactorial trait will occur in a particular individual, geneticists use **empiric risks,** which are based on incidence in a specific population. Incidence is the rate at which a certain event occurs, such as the number of new cases of a particular disorder diagnosed per year in a population of known size.

Empiric risk is not a calculation, but an observation, a population statistic. The population might be broad, such as an ethnic group or community, or genetically more well-defined, such as families that have a particular disease. Empiric risk increases with the severity of the disorder, the number of affected family members, and how closely related a person is to affected individuals.

Empiric risk may be used to predict the likelihood of a neural tube defect (NTD). In the United States, the overall population risk of carrying a fetus with an NTD is about 1 in 1,000 (0.1 percent). For people of English, Irish, or Scottish ancestry, the risk is about 3 in 1,000. However, if a sibling has an NTD, no matter what the ethnic group, the risk of recurrence increases to 3 percent, and if two siblings are affected, the risk to a third child is even greater. By determining whether a fetus has any siblings with NTDs, a genetic counselor can predict the risk to that fetus, using the known empiric risk.

If a trait has an inherited component, then it makes sense that the closer the relationship between two individuals, one of whom has the trait, the greater the probability that the second individual has the trait, too, because they have more genes in common. Studies of empiric risk support this logic. **Table 7.1** summarizes empiric risks for cleft lip (**figure 7.7**).

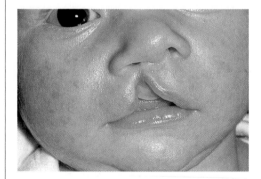

Figure 7.7 Cleft lip. Cleft lip is more likely to occur in a person who has a relative with the condition.

Reading 7.1

Disentangling Genetic from Environmental Effects

Sometimes it is difficult to determine whether individual differences for a trait are caused by genes, the environment, or both. The following examples illustrate how important it can be to understand effects on gene expression. Even a Mendelian (single-gene) disorder can be influenced by the actions of other genes or environmental factors.

Cystic Fibrosis

When researchers discovered that different allele combinations produce varying degrees of symptom severity in cystic fibrosis (CF), they attempted to correlate genotypes to phenotypes to predict the course of illness. But they could not establish a direct correlation. Apparently, other genes influence the expression of the cystic fibrosis alleles.

CF held another surprise. In many disorders, an environmental input influences the course of an inherited illness; in CF, it was the other way around. The thick mucus that builds up along airway linings provides a very attractive environment for bacteria, most notably a highly transmissible and quick-killing species called *Burkholderia cepacia*. Bacterial infection is familiar to people with CF, but in the past, they have usually been infected by *Pseudomonas aeruginosa*. Unlike a *Pseudomonas* infection, which can be present, on and off, for two decades before it kills, a *B. cepacia* infection can do so in weeks. *B. cepacia* have appendages called cable pili that enable them to cling to the mucus-covered cells lining the airway. The bacteria resist most antibiotic drugs.

Epidemics of *B. cepacia* were first reported a few years ago from Toronto and Edinburgh, under tragic circumstances. Because the infection is transferred so easily from person to person, it swept through summer camps for children with CF. Patients and their families were not prepared for such deadly bacterial infections. The camps and other support services are vitally important to affected families, but suddenly any patient with a *B. cepacia* diagnosis was isolated to avoid spread of the infection to others with CF. Today, doctors can type the DNA of the bacteria, and isolate only patients with the more virulent strains of *B. cepacia*.

Type I Diabetes Mellitus

Type I or juvenile diabetes mellitus runs in families, but in no particular pattern of recurrence. The reason for the unpredictability may be environmental. In this inborn error in glucose (sugar) metabolism, the immune system attacks the pancreas. As a result, the pancreas does not produce the insulin required to route blood glucose into cells for use.

When studying the pancreases of young people who died suddenly just weeks after being diagnosed with diabetes, researchers observed severe infection of the pancreas plus an unusually strong immune response to the infection. They concluded that certain individuals may inherit a susceptibility to that type of infection or a strong immune response to it, but not develop diabetes unless such an infection occurs.

Neural Tube Defects

Sometimes the same symptoms can be genetic or acquired. This is the case for neural tube defects (NTDs), which are openings in the brain or spinal cord that occur at the end of the first month of prenatal development. The causes are unclear. A woman who has one affected child has an increased risk of having another, but this could be due to genetics or to an environmental exposure. Many women who have had affected children have low levels of folic acid and vitamin B_{12} in their blood serum. On a population level, taking folic acid supplements diminishes the risk of recurrence of a NTD by 70 percent.

Sorting out the contributing genes is complex—mutation in one gene may set the stage for failure of the neural tube to close, or effects of several gene variants may add up. Defects in the metabolism of the amino acid methionine seem to be at the root of many inherited cases. Of the 56 single-gene defects behind NTDs listed in Online Mendelian Inheritance in Man, several implicate this pathway, and the genetic and environmental evidence is consistent. For example, many women who have children with NTDs have low levels of folic acid and vitamin B_{12}, both of which are necessary to metabolize methionine. Some women with affected children have normal blood levels of folic acid and B_{12}, but have low levels of, or lack, the enzyme necessary to catalyze the only biochemical reaction known to require both of these vitamins. That is, dietary vitamin deficiencies may be phenocopies of specific enzyme deficiencies. As with any phenocopy, the dietary route tends to be far more common than the inherited phenotype it mimics. For this reason, doctors advise all pregnant women to take folic acid supplements. (Vitamin B_{12} supplementation offers no protective effect). Genetic testing will soon be able to determine which women have variants in the genes whose products contribute to the methionine and other relevant pathways in ways that put their embryos at increased risk for a NTD, and supplementation can become targeted.

Table 7.1

Empiric Risk of Recurrence for Cleft Lip

Relationship to Affected Person	Empiric Risk of Recurrence
Identical twin	40.0%
Sibling	4.1%
Child	3.5%
Niece/nephew	0.8%
First cousin	0.3%
General population risk (no affected relatives)	0.1%

Table 7.2

Heritabilities for Some Human Traits

Trait	Heritability
Clubfoot	0.8
Height	0.8
Blood pressure	0.6
Body mass index	0.5
Verbal aptitude	0.7
Mathematical aptitude	0.3
Spelling aptitude	0.5
Total fingerprint ridge count	0.9
Intelligence	0.5–0.8
Total serum cholesterol	0.6

Because empiric risk is based solely on observation, we can use it to derive risks for disorders with poorly understood transmission patterns. For example, certain multifactorial disorders affect one sex more often than the other. Pyloric stenosis is an overgrowth of muscle at the juncture between the stomach and the small intestine. It is five times more common among males than females. The condition must be corrected surgically shortly after birth, or the newborn will be unable to digest foods. Empiric data show that the risk of recurrence for the brother of an affected brother is 3.8 percent, but the risk for the brother of an affected sister is 9.2 percent. An empiric risk, then, is based on real-world observations—the mechanism of the illness or its cause need not be known.

Heritability—The Genetic Contribution to a Multifactorial Trait

As Charles Darwin observed, some of the variation of a trait is due to heredity, and some to environmental influences. A measurement called **heritability,** designated H, estimates the proportion of the phenotypic variation for a particular trait that is due to genes in a certain population at a certain time. Empiric risk could result from nongenetic influences, whereas heritability focuses on the genetic component of a trait.

Figure 7.8 outlines the factors that contribute to observed variation in a trait. Heritability equals 1.0 for a trait that is completely the result of gene action, and 0 if it is entirely caused by an environmental influence. Most traits lie in between. For example, height has a heritability of 0.8. **Table 7.2** lists some traits and their heritabilities.

Heritability changes as the environment changes. For example, the heritability of skin color would be higher in the winter months, when sun exposure is less likely to increase melanin synthesis.

Researchers use several statistical methods to estimate heritability. One way is to compare the actual proportion of pairs of people related in a certain manner who share a particular trait, to the expected proportion of pairs that would share it if it were inherited in a Mendelian fashion. The expected proportion is derived by knowing the blood relationships of the individuals and using a measurement called the **correlation coefficient,** which is the proportion of genes that two people related in a certain way share (**table 7.3**). (It is also called the coefficient of relatedness.) A parent and child, for example, share 50 percent of their genes, because of the mechanism of meiosis. Siblings share on average 50 percent of their genes, because they have a 50 percent chance of inheriting each allele for a gene from each parent. The designations of primary (1°), secondary (2°), and tertiary (3°) relatives are useful in genetic counseling when empiric risks are consulted.

If the heritability of a trait is very high, then of a group of 100 sibling pairs, nearly 50 would be expected to have it, because siblings share on average 50 percent of their genes. Height is a trait for which heritability

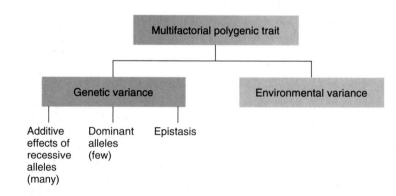

Figure 7.8 Heritability estimates the genetic contribution to a trait. Observed variance in a polygenic, multifactorial trait or illness reflects genetic and environmental contributions. Genetic variants are mostly determined by the additive effects of recessive alleles of different genes, but they can also be influenced by the effects of a few dominant alleles and by epistasis (interactions between alleles of different genes).

Table 7.3

Correlation Coefficients for Pairs of Relatives

Relationship	Degree of Relationship	Percent Shared Genes (Correlation Coefficients)
Sibling to sibling	1°	50% (1/2)
Parent to child	1°	50% (1/2)
Uncle/aunt to niece/nephew	2°	25% (1/4)
Grandparent to grandchild	2°	25% (1/4)
First cousin to first cousin	3°	12 1/2% (1/8)

reflects the environmental influence of nutrition. Of 100 sibling pairs in a population, for example, 40 might be the same number of inches tall. Heritability for height among this group of sibling pairs is .40/.50, or 80 percent, which is the observed phenotypic variation divided by the expected phenotypic variation if environment had no influence.

Genetic variance for a polygenic trait is mostly due to the additive effects of recessive alleles of different genes. For some traits, a few dominant alleles can greatly influence phenotype, but because they are rare, they do not contribute greatly to heritability. This is the case for heart disease caused by a faulty LDL receptor, a rare dominant condition that is also influenced by many other genes. Epistasis (interaction between alleles of different genes) can also influence heritability. Geneticists calculate a "narrow" heritability that considers only additive recessive effects, and a "broad" heritability that also considers the effects of rare dominant alleles and epistasis. For LDL cholesterol level, for example, the narrow heritability is 0.36, but the broad heritability is 0.96, reflecting the fact that a rare dominant allele can have a large impact on LDL level. The ability to taste bitter substances is another trait that is largely determined by one gene, on chromosome 7, but influenced by several others with much lesser, but additive effects.

Multifactorial inheritance has many applications in agriculture, where a breeder needs to know whether heredity or the environment mostly determines such traits as birth weight, milk yield, length of wool fiber, and egg hatchability. It is also valuable to know whether the genetic influences are additive or epistatic. The breeder can con-trol the environmental input by adjusting the conditions under which animals are raised, and the inherited input by setting up matings between particular individuals.

Studying multifactorial traits in humans is difficult, because information must be obtained from many families. Two special types of people, however, can help geneticists to tease apart the genetic and environmental components of multifactorial traits—adopted individuals and twins.

Adopted Individuals

A person adopted by people who are not blood relatives shares environmental influences, but typically not many genes, with his or her adoptive family. Conversely, adopted individuals share genes, but not the exact environment, with their biological parents. Therefore, biologists assume that similarities between adopted people and adoptive parents reflect mostly environmental influences, whereas similarities between adoptees and their biological parents reflect mostly genetic influences. Information on both sets of parents can reveal how heredity and the environment each contribute to the development of a trait.

Many early adoption studies used the Danish Adoption Register, a database of all adopted Danish children and their families from 1924 to 1947. One study examined correlations between causes of death among biological and adoptive parents and adopted children. If a biological parent died of infection before age 50, the adopted child was five times more likely to die of infection at a young age than a similar person in the general population. This may be because inherited variants in immune system genes increase susceptibility to certain infections. In support of this hypothesis, the risk that an adopted individual would die young from infection did not correlate with adoptive parents' death from infection before age 50. Although researchers concluded that length of life is mostly determined by heredity, they did find evidence of environmental influences. For example, if adoptive parents died before age 50 of cardiovascular disease, their adopted children were three times as likely to die of heart and blood vessel disease as a person in the general population. What environmental factor might account for this correlation?

Twins

Studies that use twins to separate the genetic from the environmental contribution to a phenotype provide more meaningful information than studying adopted individuals. In fact, twin studies have largely replaced adoption methods.

Using twins to study genetic influence on traits dates to 1924, when German dermatologist Hermann Siemens compared school transcripts of identical versus fraternal twins. Noticing that grades and teachers' comments were much more alike for identical twins than for fraternal twins, he proposed that genes contribute to intelligence.

A trait that occurs more frequently in both members of identical (monozygotic or MZ) twin pairs than in both members of fraternal (dizygotic or DZ) twin pairs is at least partly controlled by heredity. Geneticists calculate the **concordance** of a trait as the percentage of pairs in which both twins express the trait.

In one study, 142 MZ twin pairs and 142 DZ twin pairs took a "distorted tunes test," in which 26 familiar songs were played, each with at least one note altered. A person was considered to be "tune deaf" if he or she failed to detect three or more of the mistakes. Concordance for "tune deafness" was 0.67 for MZ twins, but only 0.44 for DZ twins, indicating a considerable inherited component in the ability to accurately perceive musical pitch. **Figure 7.9** compares twin types for a variety of hard-to-measure traits. (Figure 3.16 shows how DZ and MZ twins arise.)

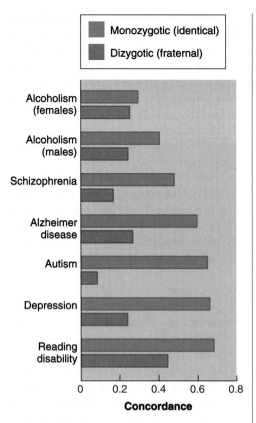

Figure 7.9 Twin studies. A trait more often present in both members of MZ twin pairs than in both members of DZ twin pairs presumably has a significant inherited component.

Source: Robert Plomin, et al., "The Genetic Basis of Complex Human Behaviors," *Science,* 17 June 1994, vol. 264, pp. 1733–39. Copyright 1994 American Association for the Advancement of Science.

Diseases caused by single genes that are 100 percent penetrant, whether dominant or recessive, are 100 percent concordant in MZ twins. If one twin has the disease, so does the other. However, among DZ twins, concordance generally is 50 percent for a dominant trait and 25 percent for a recessive trait. These are the Mendelian values that apply to any two siblings. For a polygenic trait with little environmental input, concordance values for MZ twins are significantly greater than for DZ twins. A trait molded mostly by the environment exhibits similar concordance values for both types of twins.

An ongoing investigation called the Twins Early Development Study shows how concordance values indicate the degree to which heredity contributes to a trait.

Headed by Robert Plomin of the Institute of Psychiatry in London, this project is following 7,756 pairs of twins born in England and Wales in 1994. One experiment looked at 2-year-olds whose language skills place them in the lowest 5 percent of children that age. With the parents' help, researchers recorded the number of words in the vocabularies of 1,044 pairs of identical twins, 1,006 pairs of same-sex fraternal twins, and 989 pairs of opposite-sex twins. The results clearly indicated a large genetic influence for children lagging behind in language skills—the concordance for the identical twins was 81 percent, but it was 42 percent for the fraternal twins. Put another way, if an identical twin fell into the lowest 5 percent of 2-year-olds for language acquisition, the chance that her identical twin would, too, was 81 percent. But if a fraternal twin was in this category, the chance that her twin would also be was only 42 percent. When similar assessments were done on twin pairs of all abilities, the differences between the concordance values were not nearly as great. This indicates that the environment plays a larger role in most children's adeptness at learning vocabulary than it does for the 5 percent who struggle to do so.

Comparing twin types has a limitation—the technique assumes that both types of twins share similar experiences. In fact, identical twins are often closer than fraternal twins. This discrepancy between the closeness of the two types of twins led to misleading results in twin studies conducted in the 1940s. One study concluded that tuberculosis is inherited because concordance among identical twins was higher than among fraternal twins. Actually, part of the reason for the difference in concordance was that the infectious disease was more readily passed between identical twins because their parents kept them in close physical contact.

A more informative way to assess the genetic component of a multifactorial trait is to study identical twins who were separated at birth, then raised in very different environments. Hermann Siemens suggested this in 1924, but much of the work using this "twins reared apart" approach has taken place at the University of Minnesota. Here, since 1979, hundreds of sets of identical/fraternal twins and triplets who were

separated at birth have visited the laboratories of Thomas Bouchard. For a week or more, the twins and triplets undergo tests that measure physical and behavioral traits, including 24 different blood types, handedness, direction of hair growth, fingerprint pattern, height, weight, functioning of all organ systems, intelligence, allergies, and dental patterns. Researchers videotape facial expressions and body movements in different circumstances and probe participants' fears, vocational interests, and superstitions.

Twins and triplets separated at birth provide natural experiments for distinguishing nature from nurture. Many of their common traits can be attributed to genetics, especially if their environments have been very different (**figure 7.10**). By contrast, their differences tend to reflect differences in upbringing, since their genes are identical (MZ twins and triplets) or similar (DZ twins and triplets).

The researchers have found that identical twins and triplets separated at birth and reunited later are remarkably similar, even when they grow up in very different adoptive families. Idiosyncrasies are particularly striking. For example, twins who met for the first time when they were in their thirties responded identically to questions; each paused for 30 seconds, rotated a gold necklace she was wearing three times, and then answered the question. Coincidence, or genetics?

The "twins reared apart" approach is not a perfectly controlled way to separate nature from nurture. Identical twins and other multiples share an environment in the uterus and possibly in early infancy that may affect later development. Siblings, whether adoptive or biological, do not always share identical home environments. Differences in sex, general health, school and peer experiences, temperament, and personality affect each individual's perception of such environmental influences as parental affection and discipline.

Adoption studies, likewise, are not perfectly controlled experiments. In the past, adoption agencies tended to search for adoptive families with ethnic, socioeconomic, or religious backgrounds similar to those of the biological parents. Thus, even when different families adopted and raised separated twins, their environments were not as different as they might have been for

7.3 S
Trait

Multifac
conditio
diovascu
harder-t
gence an
behavior

Heart

Arthur A
er who s
early thii
tion and
inheritec
on the in
a heart a
which he
during h

In coi
year-old
For years
healthy
level. Th
orchestra
large loa
ferent he
the elder
erful infl
preventa
attack; tl
with cho
vascular
do affect

Genes
lipids in
clots; blc

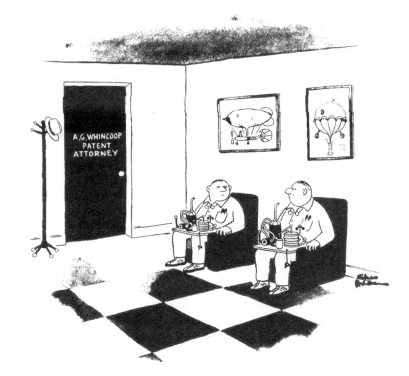

Separated at birth, the Mallifert twins meet accidentally.

Figure 7.10
Copyright *The New Yorker* Collection 1981, Charles Addams from cartoonbank.com. All Rights Reserved.

two unrelated adoptees. However, twins and triplets reared apart are still providing intriguing insights into the number of body movements, psychological quirks, interests, and other personality traits that seem to be rooted in our genes.

Association Studies

Empiric risk, heritability, and adoptee and twin studies are traditional ways of estimating the degree to which genes contribute to the variability of a trait or illness. With the availability of more types of genetic markers and genome sequence data, researchers have more refined tools to identify DNA sequences that contribute directly to pathogenesis, or confer susceptibility to disease.

Identification of the single genes behind Mendelian traits and disorders has largely relied on linkage analysis, discussed in chapter 5. Researchers compiled data on families with more than one affected member, determining whether a section of chromosome (a genetic marker) was inherited along with a disease-causing gene by inferring whether alleles of the two genes were in cis or trans (see figure 5.11). Linkage analysis in humans

is difficult to do because the rarity of single-gene disorders makes it hard to find enough families and individuals to compare. Because detecting linkage to one gene is so difficult, using the approach to identify the several genes that contribute to a polygenic trait is even more daunting. Fortunately, another, related method can detect DNA sequences that are inherited with, and therefore may contribute to, a polygenic trait—SNP mapping. Because SNP mapping tracks large populations, it is easier to find subjects for study than for classic linkage studies based on extended families with rare conditions. SNP studies are also better suited to track polygenic disorders.

Recall from chapter 1 that a SNP, or single nucleotide polymorphism, is a site within a DNA sequence that varies in at least 1 percent of a population. The human genome has about 12 to 16 million SNPs among the nearly 3 billion bases, and researchers have identified several million of them. The number of SNPs is derived from an analysis of linkage disequilibrium (LD), which is the tendency for certain SNPs to be inherited together. Linkage disequilibrium generally occurs over areas that are 5,000 to 50,000

bases long. Several million SNPs, spread out over the genome, will enable researchers to pair specific SNPs with specific genes that cause or contribute to a particular disease or trait, because the distance between the SNPs will be less than the average length of a DNA sequence in linkage disequilibrium. Several SNPs that are transmitted together constitute a haplotype, which is short for "haploid genotype."

SNPs are useful in **association studies,** in which researchers compare SNP patterns between a group of individuals who have a particular disorder and a group who do not. An association study may use a case-control design, which means that each individual in one group is matched to an individual in the other group who shares as many characteristics as possible, such as age, sex, activity level, and environmental exposures. SNP differences then correlate to presence or absence of the particular medical condition. If 500 individuals with hypertension (high blood pressure) have particular DNA bases at six sites in the genome, and 500 matched individuals who do not have hypertension have different bases at only these six sites, then further investigation can probe these genome regions for genes whose protein products could control blood pressure. When many SNPs are considered, many susceptibility genes can be tracked, and patterns may emerge that can then be used to predict the course of the illness.

An association study achieves greater power if it borrows from the older technique of looking at family members. In the "affected sibling pair" strategy, researchers scan genomes for markers that most siblings who have the same condition share, but that siblings who do not have the condition do not often share. Such genome regions may harbor genes that contribute to the condition. The underlying logic is that because siblings share 50 percent of their genes, a trait or condition that many siblings share is likely to be inherited. Returning to the hypertension example, an affected sibling pair analysis would include 500 pairs of siblings who both have hypertension, and 500 pairs of siblings who do not. Genome regions for which all (or most) of the 500 affected siblings have the same SNP, but few of the other group do, are areas where researchers might search for genes that might contribute to the trait.

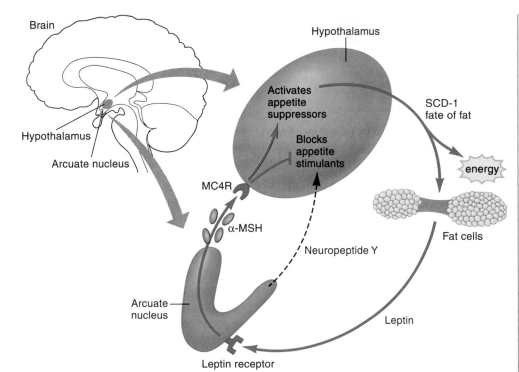

α-MSH	α-melanocyte stimulating hormone
MC4R	melanocortin-4 receptor
SCD-1	stearoyl-CoA desaturase-1

Figure 7.13 Genes control body weight. Fat cells (adipocytes) secrete leptin, which binds to receptors in the arcuate nucleus of the hypothalamus, triggering appetite suppressors and blocking appetite stimulants. The melanocortin-4 receptor stifles appetite, whereas neuropeptide Y stimulates it. Ghrelin and PYY are made in the stomach and provide short-term appetite control. Ghrelin activates neuropeptide Y, and PYY suppresses appetite.

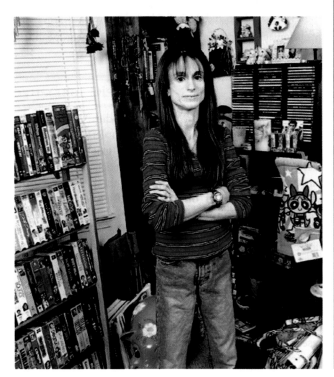

Figure 7.14 Leptin to the rescue. Shots of leptin have enabled Christina Vena, who has lipodystrophy, to lead a near-normal existence.

skin suddenly shrink away, leaving the person extremely skinny, yet constantly hungry. Adipocytes disappear, but fats are laid down beneath the skin in painful lesions. Triglycerides enter the blood so swiftly that they must be cleansed from it often. Within days of receiving leptin shots, Christina and eight others in a study began to gain weight and feel less hungry. At least two different genes are known to cause lipodystrophy, and their connection to leptin isn't yet understood.

Researchers are tracing other causes of obesity to proteins that interact with leptin. For example, most people who are heterozygotes (carriers) for a mutation in the gene that encodes the melanocortin-4 receptor are obese, and individuals lacking both functional alleles are morbidly obese. Melanocortin-4 receptor mutations account for about 6 percent of very obese children, and so far these mutations are the most common single-gene cause of obesity—much more common than leptin deficiency.

Microarray experiments are useful for discovering new weight-related genes. Researchers applied leptin to a DNA microarray containing 12,000 genes expressed in the liver. Leptin had the greatest effect on expression of the gene encoding an enzyme, stearoyl-CoA desaturase-1 (SCD-1), which determines whether the body stores fat or metabolizes it to release its energy.

The stomach is another source of obesity-related proteins. Ghrelin is a peptide (small protein) hormone produced in the stomach that responds to hunger, telling the hypothalamus to produce more neuropeptide Y, which stimulates appetite. PYY is another peptide made in the stomach. Its action opposes ghrelin, signaling satiety to the brain. While leptin acts in the long term to maintain weight, ghrelin and PYY function in the short term. All of these hormonal signals impinge on the arcuate nucleus, where they are integrated to finely control appetite in a way that maintains weight.

Environmental Influences on Obesity

Many studies on adopted individuals and twins suggest that obesity has a heritability of 75 percent. Because the heritability for BMI is lower than this, the discrepancy suggests that genes play a larger role in those

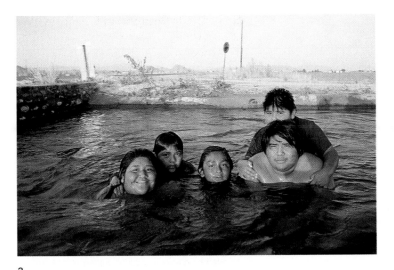 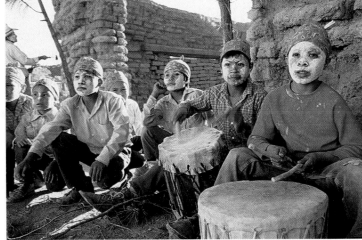

a.   b.

Figure 7.15 **The environment influences gene expression.**   Comparison of average body weights among the Arizona population of Pima Indians **(a)** and the Mexican population **(b)** reveals the effects of the environment.

who tend to gain weight easily. This becomes obvious when populations that have a genetic tendency to obesity experience a drastic and sudden change in diet.

On the tiny island of Naura, in Western Samoa, the residents' lifestyles changed drastically when they found a market for the tons of bird droppings on their island as commercial fertilizer. The influx of money translated into inactivity and a high-fat diet, replacing an agricultural lifestyle and a diet of fish and vegetables. Within just a generation, two-thirds of the population had become obese, and a third suffered from diabetes.

The Pima Indians offer another example of environmental effects on body weight (**figure 7.15**). These people separated into two populations during the Middle Ages, one group settling in the Sierra Madre mountains of Mexico, the other in southern Arizona. By the 1970s, the Arizona Indians no longer farmed nor ate a low-fat diet, but instead consumed 40 percent of their calories from fat. With this drastic change in lifestyle, they developed the highest prevalence of obesity of any population on earth. (Prevalence is the total number of individuals with a certain condition in a particular population at a given time.) Half of the Arizona group had diabetes by age 35, weighing, on average, 57 pounds (26 kilo-

grams) more than their southern relatives, who still eat a low-fat diet and are very active.

The Pima Indians demonstrate that the tendency to gain weight is not sealed in the genes at conception, but instead is much more likely to occur if the environment provides fatty foods. They illustrate what geneticist James Neel termed the "thrifty gene hypothesis" in 1962. He suggested that long ago, the hunter-gatherers who survived famine had genes that enabled them to efficiently conserve fat stores. Leptin would have played a pivotal role in providing such an advantage. Today, with plenty of food available, the genetic tendency to retain fat is no longer healthful, but harmful.

A corollary to the thrifty gene hypothesis is the "fertile crescent" hypothesis. This refers to the area where agriculture—and therefore more abundant food—originated. In these societies, those who put on weight experienced higher rates of associated disorders, and were not as likely to survive as those with genes that promoted leanness. People who can eat a lot and stay thin inherited these genes, but those who tend toward obesity may have inherited more "thrifty" genes. Unfortunately, for many of us, our genomes hold an energy-conserving legacy that works too well—it is much easi-

er to gain weight than to lose it, for sound evolutionary reasons.

Interactions and contributions of genes and the environment provide some of the greatest challenges in studying human genetics. Why does one heavy smoker develop lung cancer, but another does not? Why can one person consistently overeat and never gain weight, while another puts weight on easily? Because we exist in an environment, no gene functions in a vacuum. Subtle interactions of nature and nurture profoundly affect our lives and make us all—even identical twins—unique individuals.

Key Concepts

Genes that affect lipid metabolism, blood clotting, leukocyte adhesion, and blood pressure influence cardiovascular health. ● Genes that encode leptin, the leptin receptor, and proteins that transmit or counter leptin's signals affect body weight. Studies on adopted individuals and twins indicate a heritability of 75 percent for obesity. Populations that suddenly became sedentary and switched to a fatty diet reflect environmental influences on body weight.

Summary

7.1 Genes and the Environment Mold Most Traits

1. **Multifactorial traits** are attributable to both the environment and genes. A **polygenic trait** is determined by more than one gene and varies continuously in its expression. The frequency distribution of phenotypes for a polygenic trait forms a bell curve.

7.2 Methods Used to Investigate Multifactorial Traits

2. **Empiric risk** measures the likelihood that a multifactorial trait will recur based on its prevalence in a population. The risk rises as genetic closeness to an affected individual increases, as the severity of the phenotype increases, and as the number of affected relatives rises.

3. **Heritability** estimates the proportion of variation in a multifactorial trait that is attributable to genetics. It describes a trait in a particular population at a particular time. Heritability is estimated by comparing the actual incidence of a shared trait among people related in a certain way to the expected incidence (**correlation coefficient**). Rare dominant alleles can contribute to heritability.

4. Characteristics shared by adopted people and their biological parents are mostly inherited, whereas similarities between adopted people and their adoptive parents reflect environmental influences.

5. **Concordance** measures the frequency of expression of a trait in both members of MZ or DZ twin pairs. The more influence genes exert over a trait, the higher the concordance.

6. **Association studies** correlate SNP patterns to increased risk of developing a disorder.

7.3 Some Multifactorial Traits

7. Genes that control lipid metabolism and blood clotting contribute to cardiovascular health.

8. Leptin, its receptor, its transporter, neuropeptide Y, and the melanocortin-4 receptor are proteins that affect body weight. Fat cells secrete leptin in response to starvation, and the protein acts in the hypothalamus. Populations that switch to a fatty diet and a less-active lifestyle reveal the effects of the environment on weight.

Review Questions

1. Consider the traits of eye color and body weight. Which is more likely to be inherited as a Mendelian trait, and which is multifactorial? Cite reasons for your answer.

2. Cite two examples from the chapter of a rare illness that helped researchers understand a process that could be applied to treat or help more people.

3. What is the difference between a Mendelian multifactorial trait and a polygenic multifactorial trait?

4. Which has a greater heritability—eye color or height? State a reason for your answer.

5. How can skin color have a different heritability at different times of the year?

6. How can the environment influence the course of cystic fibrosis, which is a Mendelian (single-gene) disorder?

7. Describe the type of information in a(n)
   a. empiric calculation.
   b. twin study.
   c. adoption study.
   d. association study.

8. Why does SNP mapping require enormous amounts of data?

9. Name three types of proteins that affect cardiovascular functioning and three that affect body weight.

10. In a large, diverse population, why are medium brown skin colors more common than very white or very black skin?

11. Describe or sketch the circuitry for appetite control during starvation, based on figure 7.13.

Applied Questions

1. Attention deficit hyperactivity disorder (ADHD) affects 5 percent of children and adolescents and 3 percent of adults. Individuals with ADHD have difficulty learning in a classroom situation where they must remain still and controlled. Heritability ranges from .6 to .9 in different populations, and the relative risk to someone with an affected sibling ranges from .4 to .8. An adopted person is more likely to develop ADHD if a biological parent has the condition. An affected sibling pair association study using 270 pairs from the United States identified areas of chromosomes 16 and 17 that might harbor susceptibility genes. A study of 164 sib pairs in the Netherlands, however, pointed to sites on chromosomes 7 and 15.

   a. Explain how the data indicate that ADHD is either more likely caused by inherited factors or environmental factors.

   b. Why might the results differ for different populations?

   c. What should the next step be in understanding the biological basis of ADHD?

   d. Drug treatment is widely used for ADHD. What would be an advantage of knowing which genes predispose a person to the condition?

   e. Suggest a possible danger in developing a genetic test for ADHD.

2. Using figure 7.13, propose a drug treatment for obesity and explain how it would work.

3. The incidence of obesity in the United States has doubled over the past two decades. Is this due more to genetic or environmental factors? Cite a reason for your answer.

4. Association studies often produce negative results—that is, they may *not* find an association between a haplotype and a phenotype. Do you think it is important to publish such results? (Many researchers do not.) Cite a reason for your answer.

5. One way to calculate heritability is to double the difference between the concordance values for MZ versus DZ twins. For multiple sclerosis, concordance for MZ twins is 30 percent, and for DZ twins, 3 percent. What is the heritability? What does the heritability suggest about the relative contributions of genes and the environment in causing MS?

6. In chickens, weight gain is a multifactorial trait. Heritability accounts for several genes that contribute a small effect additively, as well as a few genes that exert a great effect. Is this an example of narrow or broad heritability?

7. In a given population at a particular time, a researcher examines 200 parent-child pairs for bushy eyebrows. In 50 pairs, both parent and child have the trait. Another researcher examines 100 sibling pairs for the trait of selfishness, as assessed by the parents. In 10 of the sibling pairs, the parents rate both children as selfish.

   a. What is the heritability of bushy eyebrows for this population?

   b. What is the heritability of selfishness?

   c. What are some problems with calculating the heritability for selfishness?

Web Activities

8. Locate a website that deals with breeding show or farm animals or crops for specific traits, such as litter size, degree of meat marbling, milk yield, or fruit ripening rate. Identify three traits with heritabilities that indicate a greater contribution from genes than the environment.

9. From the leading causes of death at http://www.cdc.gov/nchs/Default.htm, list three that have high heritabilities, and three that do not. Base your decisions on common sense or data, and explain your selections.

Case Studies

10. Lydia and Reggie Parker grew up poor in New York City in the 1960s. Both took advantage of the City University of New York, then free, and went to medical school in Boston, where they met. Today, each has a thriving medical practice, and they are the parents of 18-year-old Jamal and 20-year-old Tanya.

    Jamal, taking a genetics class, wonders why he and Tanya do not resemble each other, or their parents, for some traits. The family is African American. Lydia and Reggie are short, 5'2" and 5'7" respectively, and each has medium brown eyes and skin, and dark brown hair. Tanya and Jamal are 5'8" and 6'1", respectively, and were often in the highest height percentiles since they were toddlers. Jamal has very dark skin, darker than his parents' skin, while Tanya's skin is noticeably lighter than that of either parent. Tanya's eyes are so dark that they appear nearly black.

    a. Give two explanations for why Tanya's eyes appear darker than those of her parents or brother.

    b. How can Jamal's skin be darker than that of his parents, and Tanya's skin be lighter?

    c. Which of the four traits considered—height, and eye, skin, and hair color—is most influenced by environmental factors?

    d. What is the evidence that Jamal and Tanya's height is due to environmental and genetic factors?

    e. Which of the four traits has the highest heritability?

Learn to apply the skills of a genetic counselor with additional cases found in the *Case Workbook in Human Genetics.*

> *Cleft lip with or without cleft palate*
>
> *Complex traits among the Hutterites*

Suggested Readings

Deng, Hone-Wen, et al. May 2002. A genomewide linkage scan for quantitative trait loci for obesity phenotypes. *The American Journal of Human Genetics,* 70: 1138–51. More than thirty regions of the human genome probably include genes that control body weight.

Farooqi, I. Sadaf, et al. March 20, 2003. Clinical spectrum of obesity and mutations in the melanocortin-4 receptor gene. *The New England Journal of Medicine,* 348(12): 1085–95.

Friedman, Jeffrey M. February 7, 2003. A war on obesity, not the obese. *Science,* 299: 856–58. The tendency to gain weight is largely a legacy of ancient "thrifty" genes.

Glazier, Anne M., et al. December 20, 2002. Finding genes that underlie complex traits. *Science,* 298:2345–48. Complex traits are difficult to analyze because they have multiple genetic and environmental causes.

Korner, Judith and Rudolph L. Leibel. September 4, 2003. To eat or not to eat— how the gut talks to the brain. *The New England Journal of Medicine,* 349(10): 926–28. A small study found that giving people PYY makes them eat less.

Lewis, Ricki. June 3, 2003. The bitter truth about PTC tasting. *The Scientist* 17(11): 32. One gene controls most of our ability to taste certain bitter substances.

Lewis, Ricki. February 18, 2002. Race and the clinic: Good science? *The Scientist* 16(3):16–18. Genotypes are better predictors of drug response than skin color.

Lewis, Ricki. July 20, 1998. Unraveling leptin pathways identifies new drug targets. *The Scientist* 12:1. Leptin, its receptor, and other proteins may inspire development of new weight-control drugs.

Mathew, Christopher. April 28, 2001. Postgenomic technologies: Hunting the genes for common disorders. *The British Medical Journal* 322:1031–34. The focus of genetics is shifting from rare to common disorders.

Pray, Leslie. February 10, 2003. Researchers put linkage disequilibrium on the map. *The Scientist,* 17(3):30–31. A review of the association and linkage studies used to identify a gene that causes Crohn disease.

Pritchard, Jonathan. July 2001. Are rare variants responsible for susceptibility to complex diseases? *The American Journal of Human Genetics* 69:124–37. Not all genes contribute equally to multifactorial traits.

The Editors. February 1, 2003. In search of genetic precision. *The Lancet,* 361:357. Should researchers report negative associations?

Weekly updates of current news related to human genetics are available through Power Web on your Online Learning Center.

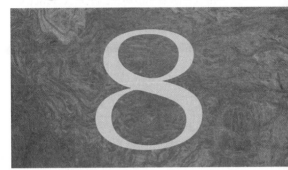

C H A P T E R

8

The Genetics of Behavior

CHAPTER CONTENTS

8.1 Genes Contribute to Most Behavioral Traits
Several genes and environmental factors contribute to most behavioral traits and disorders. Researchers associate patterns of gene expression in specific brain regions with particular behaviors.

8.2 Eating Disorders
Anorexia and bulimia are common in affluent nations. Heritability is high, yet the behavior may be a response to powerful societal pressures. Candidate genes control appetite or regulate the neurotransmitters dopamine or serotonin. Psychological factors are harder to study.

8.3 Sleep
Sleep habits are largely inherited. A Utah family with many members who have a highly unusual sleep-wake cycle led researchers to discover the first "clock" gene in humans.

8.4 Intelligence
Heritability for intelligence is high, but environmental influences are profound, particularly early in life. Psychologists measure "general intelligence," whereas geneticists search for genes whose protein products can explain variations in intelligence.

8.5 Drug Addiction
Genes whose protein products affect the brain's limbic system influence variations in susceptibility to addiction. Candidate genes affect neurotransmission and signal transduction.

8.6 Mood Disorders
Deficits of the neurotransmitters serotonin or norepinephrine cause major depressive disorder. Less common are the mood swings of bipolar disorder, whose genetic roots are many and difficult to isolate.

8.7 Schizophrenia
A condition like no other, schizophrenia devastates the ability to think and perceive clearly. Several candidate genes and environmental associations contribute to causing this disorder.

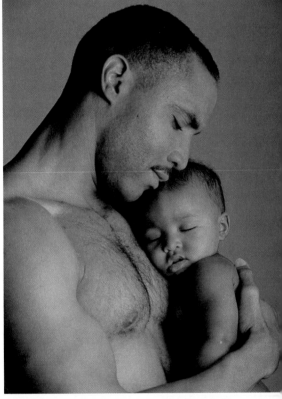

Genes influence whether a person is a night owl or an early riser.

In 2001, a tennis promoter offered Steffi Graf and Andre Agassi, expecting a baby, $10 million if they would promise that their child would play a tennis match in the year 2017 against the offspring of another tennis great. *People* magazine called the child "the most DNA-advantaged prodigy in tennis" and quoted Agassi as saying, "I've got genetics on my side" when asked if Junior would win the match. Once Jaden was born, speculation about his future athletic abilities continued.

The idea that children of athletes will grow up to be athletes themselves illustrates the popular but flawed idea of genetic determinism, that a gene dictates every imaginable trait, even the ability to whack a ball over a net. Jaden Agassi may indeed have inherited fortuitous muscle anatomy, quick reflexes, athletic grace, and a competitive spirit from his parents. He will also experience powerful environmental cues, and, judging by his father's comment, will probably have a racquet in his hands before kindergarten. Still, whether or not he chooses to follow in his parents' footsteps—or how he will react if his athletic prowess does not match people's expectations—depends upon an unpredictable combination of many factors, both genetic and environmental.

This chapter explores how researchers are disentangling the genetic and environmental threads that contribute to several familiar behaviors and disorders.

8.1 Genes Contribute to Most Behavioral Traits

Behavioral traits include abilities, feelings, moods, personality, intelligence, and how a person communicates, copes with rage, and handles stress. Disorders with behavioral symptoms are wide-ranging and include phobias, anxiety, dementia, psychosis, addiction, and mood alteration. Very few medical conditions with behavioral components can be traced to a single gene—Huntington disease, with its characteristic anger, is a rare example. Most behavioral disorders fit the classic complex disease profile: they affect more than 1 in 1,000 individuals and are caused by several genes and the environ-

ment—that is, they are common, polygenic and multifactorial.

Until recently, geneticists and social scientists studying behavior were limited to such tools as empiric risk estimates and adoptee and twin studies, discussed in chapter 7. These approaches clearly indicate that nearly all behaviors have inherited influences. Two powerful new approaches to understanding the biological basis of behavioral traits are:

1. Association studies that correlate genetic markers such as SNP (single nucleotide polymorphism) patterns with particular symptoms

2. Analysis of mutations in specific candidate genes that are present exclusively in individuals with the behavior

Behavioral genetics is, by definition, a study of nervous system variation and

function. Genes control the synthesis, levels, and distribution of neurotransmitters, which are the chemical messengers that connect nerve cells (neurons) into networks. **Figure 8.1** indicates the points of gene control over the sending and receiving of nervous system information—neurotransmission. Enzymes oversee the synthesis of neurotransmitters and their transport from the sending (presynaptic) neuron across a space called the synapse to receptors on the plasma membrane of the receiving (postsynaptic) neuron. Genes also control the synthesis of myelin, a fatty substance that coats neuron extensions called axons, insulating the neuron and thereby speeding neurotransmission. Signal transduction is also a key part of the function of the nervous system (see figure 2.20). Therefore, candidate genes for the inherited components of a variety of mood disorders and mental illnesses—as well as of normal variations in

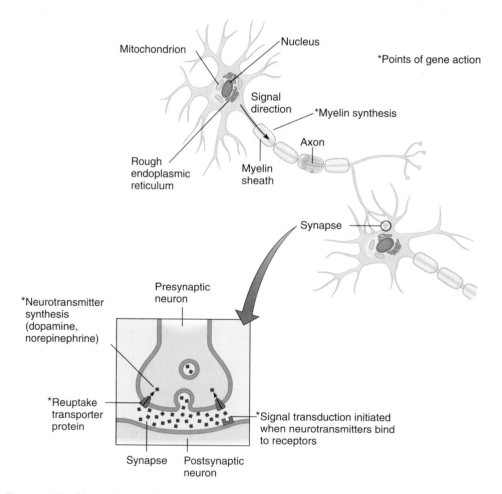

Figure 8.1   Neurotransmission. Many genes that affect behavior produce proteins that affect neurotransmission (the sending of a signal from one neuron to another across a synapse via a neurotransmitter molecule) and/or signal transduction.

temperament and personality—affect neurotransmission and signal transduction.

Traditional methods identify a large inherited component to a behavior, and further studies identify and describe candidate genes. Consider attention deficit hyperactivity disorder (ADHD). Applied Question 1 in chapter 7 presents evidence for an inherited component to ADHD. Linkage analysis on families with more than one affected member implicates the neurotransmitter dopamine. A "transporter" protein shuttles dopamine between neurons, and the dopamine D(4) receptor protein binds dopamine on the postsynaptic neuron. Development of drugs to treat ADHD focus on dopamine and the molecules that control its functioning.

Deciphering genetic components of most behavioral disorders is not as straightforward as ADHD analysis appears to be. Investigating the causes of autism illustrates the difficulty of reconciling empiric, adoptee, and twin data with molecular methods.

Autism is a disorder of communication—the individual does not speak or interact with others and is comfortable only with restricted or repetitive behaviors. Asperger syndrome is a related condition that does not impair language ability and may be a mild form of autism. The general population incidence of autism is only 10 to 12 per 10,000 (<0.1 percent), but for a sibling of a person with the condition, risk of recurrence is 2 to 4 percent. Twin studies indicate high heritability. Yet the search for causative genes so far has yielded many candidates with weak linkage, rather than a few compelling candidate genes. Four whole genome scans, using many markers and hundreds of families that have more than one affected member, point to possible risk-raising genes on 14 different chromosomes! Perhaps autism is actually several different disorders that have similar symptoms.

Investigating the genetics of behavior is more challenging, for several reasons, than understanding a disorder in which an abnormal protein disrupts physiology in a clear way. Many behavioral disorders have symptoms in common, which can delay or obscure accurate diagnosis. However, many symptoms also fall within the range of normal behavior. Whether extreme anxiety is warranted, or not, depends upon the situation, and different individuals may react with different intensity to the same situation. Another complication of studying the genetics of behavior is that self-reporting of symptoms may be highly subjective. A person can also unintentionally copy someone's unusual behavior, because he or she does not realize it is unusual. Such sources of confusion do not crop up in a strictly physical condition such as sickle cell disease. However, being too quick to assign a genetic cause to a behavior can be dangerous, as Bioethics: Choices for the Future, "Blaming Genes" discusses.

The examples that follow begin with the traditional approaches of evaluating siblings, adoptees, and twins, and conclude with a look at genes that underlie, contribute to, or influence certain behaviors. The eventual impact of human genome information on the study of behavior promises to be great. Wrote one psychologist, "Ultimately, the human genome sequence will revolutionize psychology and psychiatry." Identifying human behavioral genes may reveal the causes of disease and make it possible to subtype mental disorders so that individualized treatment can begin early. **Table 8.1** lists some of the more common behavioral disorders.

Key Concepts

Most behavioral traits and disorders are fairly common, polygenic, and multifactorial. Traditional methods to estimate the genetic contribution to a behavior include empiric risk estimates and adoptee and twin studies. Association studies and candidate gene analyses are now extending these data. Behavioral disorders are difficult to study because symptoms overlap and behaviors can be imitated.

8.2 Eating Disorders

When gymnast Christy Henrich was buried on a Friday morning in July 1994, she weighed 61 pounds and was 22 years old (**figure 8.2**). Three weeks earlier, she had weighed an unbelievable 47 pounds. Christy suffered from anorexia nervosa, a psychological disorder that is fairly common among professional athletes. The person perceives herself or himself as obese, even when obviously not, and starves intentionally. Christy's decline began in 1988, when a judge at a gymnastics competition told her that at 90

Table 8.1

Prevalence of Behavioral Disorders in the U.S. Population

Condition	Prevalence (%)
Alzheimer disease	4.0
Anxiety	8.0
Phobias	2.5
Posttraumatic stress disorder	1.8
Generalized anxiety disorder	1.5
Obsessive compulsive disorder	1.2
Panic disorder	1.0
Attention deficit hyperactivity disorder	2.0
Autism	0.1
Drug addiction	4.0
Eating disorders	3.0
Mood disorders	7.0
Major depression	6.0
Bipolar disorder	1.0
Schizophrenia	1.3

Source: Psychiatric Genomics Inc., Gaithersburg, MD. The information was collated from the Surgeon General's 1999 Report on Mental Health.

Blaming Genes

It has become fashionable to blame genes for our shortcomings. A popular magazine's cover shouts "Infidelity: It May Be in Our Genes," advertising an article that actually has little to do with genetics. When researchers identify a gene that plays a role in fat metabolism, people binge on chocolate and forsake exercise, because, after all, if obesity is in their genes, there's nothing they can do to prevent it. Some behaviors have even been blamed on a gene for "thrill seeking" (**figure 1**).

Behavioral genetics has a checkered past. Early in the twentieth century, it was part of eugenics, the attempt to improve a population's collection of genes, or gene pool. The horrific experiments and exterminations the Nazis performed in the name of eugenics turned many geneticists away from studying the biology of behavior. Social scientists then dominated the field, attributing many behavioral disorders to environmental influences. For example, autism and schizophrenia were at one time blamed on "adverse parenting." By the 1960s, with a clearer concept of the gene, biologists reentered the debate. Today, researchers apply knowledge from biochemistry and neurobiology to identify specific genotypes that predispose a person to developing a clearly defined behavior.

Untangling the causes of human behavior remains highly controversial. One scientific conference to explore genetic aspects of violence was cancelled after a noted psychiatrist objected that "behavioral genetics is the same old stuff in new clothes. It's another way for a violent, racist society to say people's problems are their own fault, because they carry 'bad' genes." Genetic researchers on the trail of physical explanations for behaviors counter that their work

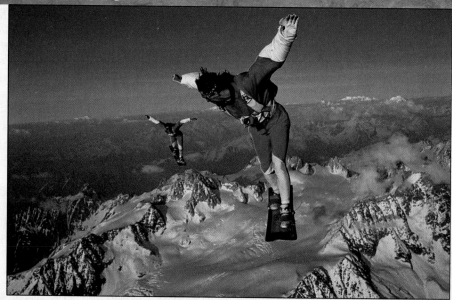

Figure 1   A thrill-seeking gene?   These air surfers were dropped from a helicopter over a mountain. Does a gene variant make them seek thrills?

can help uncover ways to alter or prevent dangerous behaviors. Attempts to hold meetings that discuss the genetics of violence still elicit public protests.

Even in the rare instances when a behavior is associated with a particular DNA variant, environmental influences remain important. Consider a 1993 study of a Dutch family that had "a syndrome of borderline mental retardation and abnormal behavior." Family members had committed arson, attempted rape, and engaged in exhibitionism. Researchers found a mutation in a gene that made biological sense. Alteration of a single DNA base in the X-linked gene encoding an enzyme, monoamine oxidase A (MAOA), rendered the enzyme nonfunctional. This enzyme normally catalyzes reactions that metabolize dopamine, serotonin, and norepinephrine, and it is therefore important in conducting nerve messages. Other studies confirmed that some combinations of alleles

of the MAOA gene correlate with highly aggressive behavior, and others with calmer temperaments. The direct effect of mutations in the MAOA gene still isn't known. Perhaps the inherited enzyme deficiency causes slight mental impairment, and this interferes with the person's ability to cope with certain frustrating situations, resulting in violence. Hence, the argument returns once again to how genes interact with the environment.

The study on the Dutch family was publicized and applied to other situations. An attorney tried to use the "MAOA deficiency defense" to free a client from a scheduled execution for committing murder. A talk-show host suggested that people who had inherited the "mean gene" be sterilized so they couldn't pass on the tendency. This may have been meant as a joke, but it is frighteningly close to the eugenics practiced early in the last century.

pounds, she was too heavy to make the U.S. Olympic team. From then on, her life consisted of starving, exercising, and taking laxatives to hasten weight loss.

For economically advantaged females in the United States, the lifetime risk of developing anorexia nervosa is 0.5 percent. Anorexia has the highest risk of death of

any psychiatric disorder—15 to 21 percent. The same population group has a lifetime risk of 2.5 percent of developing another eating disorder, bulimia. A person with bulimia eats huge amounts but exercises and vomits to maintain weight.

About 10 percent of people with eating disorders are male. One survey of 8-year-

old boys revealed that more than a third of them had attempted to lose weight. In an eating disorder called muscle dysmorphia, or, more coloquially, bigorexia, boys and young men take amino acid food supplements to bulk themselves up. Just as the person with anorexia looks in a mirror and sees herself as too large, a person

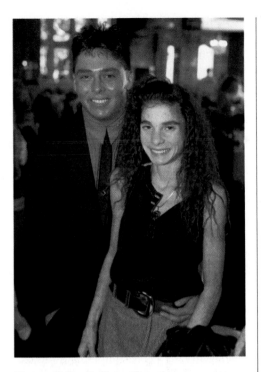

Figure 8.2 Eating disorders.
World-class gymnast Christy Henrich died of complications of anorexia nervosa in July 1994. In this photo, taken eleven months before her death, she weighed under 60 pounds. Concern over weight gain propelled her down the path of this deadly psychiatric illness.

with muscle dysmorphia sees himself as too small.

Because eating disorders were once associated almost exclusively with females, most available risk estimates exclude males. Twin studies reveal a considerable genetic component to eating disorders. Heritability ranges from 0.5 to 0.8. Studies of eating disorders that recur in families without twins are more difficult to interpret. It's hard to determine whether a young girl is imitating her older sister by starving herself because she has inherited genes that predispose her to develop an eating disorder or because she wants to be like her sister.

Genes that encode proteins that control appetite are candidate genes for eating disorders (see table 7.6). Genes that regulate the neurotransmitters dopamine and serotonin may also contribute to the risk of developing an eating disorder. It will be interesting to learn which genes affect body image, and how they do so.

Whole genome scans associate SNP patterns with eating disorders in association studies, as described in chapter 7. One biotechnology company is cataloging 60 SNP sites among the genomes of 2,000 individuals representing 600 families where more than one member has anorexia nervosa. The researchers are searching for a SNP pattern—if there is one—that appears disproportionately among individuals who have anorexia. Once the SNP maps highlight chromosome regions that seem to mark a predisposition to develop anorexia, researchers will look for genes in those regions whose protein products might affect appetite.

Key Concepts

Eating disorders are common. Twin and heritability studies indicate a high genetic contribution. Genes whose products control appetite or regulate the neurotransmitters dopamine and serotonin may cause or raise the risk of developing an eating disorder.

8.3 Sleep

Sleep has been called "a vital behavior of unknown function," and, indeed, without sleep, animals die. We spend a third of our lives in this mysterious state.

Genes influence sleep characteristics. When asked about sleep duration, schedule, quality, nap habits, and whether they are "night owls" or "morning people," MZ twins report significantly more in common than do DZ twins, even MZ twins separated at birth. Twin studies of brain wave patterns through four of the five stages of sleep confirm a hereditary influence. The fifth stage, REM sleep, is associated with dreaming and therefore may reflect more the input of experience rather than genes.

Narcolepsy

Researchers discovered the first gene related to sleep in 1999, for a condition called "narcolepsy with cataplexy" in dogs. Humans have the disorder, but it is rarely inherited as a single-gene trait—it is more often polygenic requiring an environmental trigger, or due to an autoimmune condition (the immune system attacking the body) that also involves a genetic susceptibility.

A person (or dog) with narcolepsy falls asleep suddenly several times a day. Extreme daytime sleepiness greatly disrupts ability to attend classes or work. People with narcolepsy have a tenfold higher rate of car accidents than others. Another symptom is sleep paralysis, the inability to move for a few minutes after awakening. The most dramatic manifestation of narcolepsy is cataplexy. During these short and sudden episodes of muscle weakness, the jaw sags, the head drops, knees buckle, and the person falls to the ground. This often occurs during a bout of laughter or excitement—which can be quite disturbing both for the affected individual and bystanders. People with narcolepsy and cataplexy cannot participate in even the most mundane of activities for fear of falling and injuring themselves. Narcolepsy with cataplexy affects only 0.02 to 0.06 of the general populations of North America and Europe, but the fact that it is much more common in certain families suggests a genetic component.

Dogs led the way to discovery of the narcolepsy gene. In 1999, Emmanuel Mignot and his team at Stanford University identified mutations in a gene that encodes a receptor for a neuropeptide called hypocretin. In Doberman pinschers and Labrador retrievers, the receptor does not arrive at the cell surfaces of certain brain cells, which, as a result, cannot receive signals to stay awake. Dachshunds have their own mutation—they make a misshapen, nonfunctional receptor. **Figure 8.3** shows a still frame of a film that Mignot made of narcoleptic dogs playing. Suddenly, they all collapse! A minute later, they get up and resume their antics. "You can't make dogs laugh, but you can make them so happy that they have attacks," jokes Mignot. All he needs to do to induce a narcoleptic episode in puppies is to let them play with each other. He feeds older dogs meat, which excites them so much that they can take a while to finish a meal because they fall down in delight so often. Getting dogs to breed was difficult, too—sex proved even more exciting than play or food!

A year earlier, Masahi Yanagisawa, at the University of Texas Southwestern Medical Center in Dallas, discovered a protein called orexin, but thought it only sent signals to eat. Yanagisawa's orexin turned out to bind Mignot's hypocretin receptor. Yanagisawa bred mice that lacked the orexin gene, and then noticed something

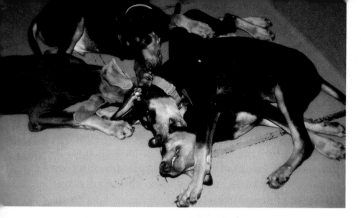

Figure 8.3 Letting sleeping dogs lie. These Doberman pinschers have inherited narcolepsy. They suddenly fall into a short but deep sleep while playing. Research on dogs with narcolepsy led to discovery of a version of the gene in humans.

odd while watching the animals feed at night—the rodents suddenly fell down fast asleep! Researchers are now trying to figure out how one molecule can apparently control feeding as well as wakefulness. The hypocretin/orexin receptor gene, found on dog chromosome 12, is on human chromosome 6. The brains of humans with narcolepsy and cataplexy are remarkably deficient in hypocretin/orexin. Pharmaceutical researchers are trying to synthesize a drug that can mimic the missing neuropeptide to treat narcolepsy.

Familial Advanced Sleep Phase Syndrome

A multigenerational Utah family with many members who have an unusual sleep pattern has enabled researchers to identify the first "biological clock" gene in humans that controls sleep. The subjects have familial advanced sleep phase syndrome (FASPS) and the effect is striking—they promptly fall asleep at 7:30 each night and awaken with a jolt each morning at 4:30. The family is a geneticist's dream—a distinctive behavioral phenotype, many affected individuals, and a clear mode of inheritance (autosomal dominant) **(figure 8.4).**

An analysis of the Utah family followed the standard approach to gene identification that chapter 7 described. A whole genome scan for short repeated DNA sequences revealed a variant area at the tip of the long arm of chromosome 2 that is found exclusively in the affected family members. Within that

defined area is a gene, called *period,* that has a counterpart in golden hamsters and fruit flies that causes the same disrupted sleep-wake cycle phenotype. The humans with the condition have a single DNA base substitution in the gene. This mutation prevents the encoded protein from binding a phosphate chemical group, which it must do to pass on the signal that synchronizes the sleep-wake cycle with daily sunrise and sunset.

Despite the clear connection between sleep behavior and a specific gene in the Utah family, this gene is just one influence on this behavior. In others of the 50 known families with FASPS, linkage analysis did not point to this gene, meaning that the condition is genetically heterogeneic. Environmental influence is great, too. Daily rhythms such as the sleep-wake cycle are set by cells that form a "circadian pacemaker" in a part of the brain called the suprachiasmatic nuclei. Genes are expressed in these cells in response to light or dark in the environment. Other environmental effects on sleeping and waking are more subtle. Knowing that the hour is late may trigger an "I should go to sleep" or, if early, "yikes, I have to get up for

class" response. Culture also affects the times that we retire and rise. Understanding how the *period* gene and others control the sleep-wake cycle may lead to new treatments for jet lag, insomnia, and the form of advanced sleep phase syndrome that is common among older individuals.

Key Concepts

Twin studies on sleep habits indicate a high heritability for sleep characteristics. A single gene causes narcolepsy in dogs, and, more rarely, in humans. A Utah family with a very unusual sleep-wake cycle led researchers to identify the first "clock" gene in humans.

8.4 Intelligence

Intelligence is a vastly complex and variable trait that is subject to many genetic and environmental influences, and also to intense subjectivity. Consider the work of Sir Francis Galton, a half first cousin of Charles Darwin. Galton investigated genius, which he defined as "a man endowed with superior faculties," by first identifying successful and prominent people in Victorian-era English society, and then assessing success among their relatives.

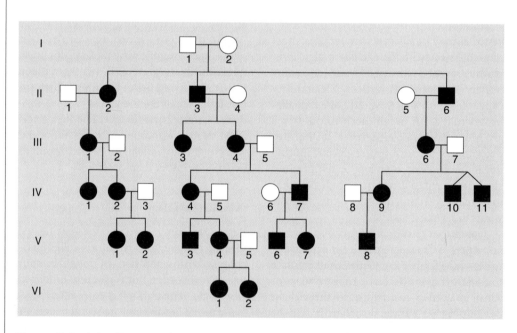

Figure 8.4 Inheritance of a disrupted sleep-wake cycle. This partial pedigree depicts a large family with familial advanced sleep phase syndrome. The condition is genetically heterogeneic—that is, different families have causative mutations in different genes. In this family from Utah, the condition is autosomal dominant.

In his 1869 book, *Hereditary Genius*, Galton wrote that relatives of eminent people were more likely to also be successful than people in the general population. The closer the blood relationship, he concluded, the more likely the person was to succeed. This, he believed, established a hereditary basis for intelligence as he measured it.

Definitions of intelligence vary. In general, intelligence refers to the ability to reason, learn, remember, connect ideas, deduce, and create. The first intelligence tests, developed in the late nineteenth century, assessed sensory perception and reaction times to various stimuli. In 1904, Alfred Binet at the Sorbonne developed a test with verbal, numerical, and pictorial questions. Its purpose was to predict the success of developmentally disabled youngsters in school. The test was subsequently modified at Stanford University to assess white, middle-class Americans. An average score on this "intelligence quotient," or IQ test, was 100, with two-thirds of all people scoring between 85 and 115 in a bell curve or normal distribution (**figure 8.5**). An IQ between 50 and 70 is considered mild mental retardation, and below 50, severe mental retardation.

Over the years, IQ has been a fairly accurate predictor of success in school and work. However, low IQ also correlates with many societal situations, such as poverty, a high divorce rate, failure to complete high school, incarceration (males), and having a child out of wedlock (females). In 1994, a book called *The Bell Curve* asserted that because certain minorities are overrepresented in these groups, they must be of genetically inferior intelligence and that is why they are prone to suffering social ills. It was a controversial thesis, to put it mildly.

The IQ test consists of short exams that measure verbal fluency, mathematical reasoning, memory, and spatial visualization skills. Because people tend to earn similar scores in all these areas, psychologists hypothesized that a general or global intelligence ability, called "g," must underlie the four basic skills that IQ encompasses. Statistical analysis indeed reveals one factor that accounts for general intelligence. In contrast, similar analysis of personality reveals five contributing factors. The g value is the part of IQ that accounts for differences between individuals based on a generalized intelligence, rather than on enhanced opportunities such as attending classes to boost test-taking skills.

Environment does not seem to play too great a role in IQ differences. Evidence includes the observation that IQ scores of adoptees, with time, become closer to those of their biological parents than to those of their adoptive parents. Heritability studies also reveal a declining environmental impact with age (**table 8.2**). This makes sense. As a person ages, he or she has more control over the environment, so genetic contributions to intelligence become more prominent.

Researchers have long realized there must be a genetic explanation for intelligence differences because nearly all syndromes that result from abnormal chromosomes include some degree of mental retardation. Down syndrome and fragile X syndrome (see figure 13.1 and Reading 12.1) are two of the more common chromosomal causes of mental retardation. Down syndrome is usually caused by an extra chromosome, and fragile X syndrome by an expanding gene on the X chromosome. The human genome sequence revealed that mutations in genes located next to the tips of chromosomes—the subtelomeric regions—also account for many cases of mental retardation.

The search for single genes that contribute to intelligence differences focuses on proteins that control neurotransmission. For example, a certain SNP pattern in a gene encoding neural cellular adhesion molecule (N-CAM) correlates strongly with high IQ. Perhaps this gene variant facilitates certain neural connections that enhance an individual's learning ability.

Identifying the N-CAM variant illustrates the candidate gene approach—relating a gene with a known function to intelligence. In another approach, whole genome scans are locating other genes whose protein

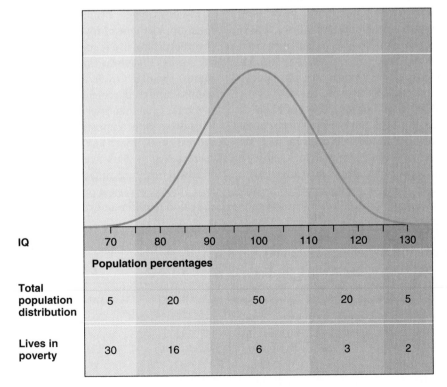

Figure 8.5   Success and IQ. IQ scores predict success in school and the workplace in U.S. society. The bell curve for IQ indicates that most people fall in the 85 to 115 range, shown in the total population distribution. However, when the population is stratified economically, those living in poverty tend to have lower IQs. Cause and effect are unclear.

IQ	70	80	90	100	110	120	130
Population percentages							
Total population distribution		5	20	50	20	5	
Lives in poverty		30	16	6	3	2	

Table 8.2	
Heritability of Intelligence Changes Over Time	
Age Group	**Heritability**
Preschoolers	0.4
Adolescents	0.6
Adults	0.8

products affect neural connections. For example, a section of chromosome 4 harbors intelligence-related genes. Researchers identified three candidate genes here by comparing 147 markers in one group of children with very high IQ scores to controls who had average scores.

8.5 Drug Addiction

Drug addiction is compulsively seeking and taking a drug despite knowing its adverse effects. Drug addiction has two identifying characteristics: tolerance and dependence. Tolerance is the need to take more of the drug to achieve the same effects as time goes on; dependence is the onset of withdrawal symptoms when a person ceases taking the drug. Both tolerance and dependence contribute to the biological and psychological components of craving the drug. The behavior associated with drug addiction can be extremely difficult to break.

Drug addiction produces long-lasting, rather than temporary, brain changes, because the craving and high risk of relapse remain even after a person has abstained for years. Heritability is 0.4 to 0.6, with a two- to threefold increase in risk among adopted individuals who have one affected biological parent. Twin studies also indicate an inherited component to drug addiction.

Brain imaging techniques have localized the "seat" of drug addiction in the brain by highlighting the cell surface receptors that bind neurotransmitters. The brain changes that contribute to addiction occur in a group of functionally related structures called the limbic system (figure 8.6). These structures are the nucleus accumbens, the prefrontal cortex, and the ventral tegmental area. The effects of cocaine seem to be largely confined to the nucleus accumbens, whereas alcohol affects the prefrontal cortex.

Although the specific genes and proteins that are implicated in addiction to different substances may vary, several general routes of interference in brain function are at play. Proteins involved in drug addiction are those that

- are part of the biosynthetic pathways of neurotransmitters, such as enzymes;

- form reuptake transporters, which remove excess neurotransmitter from the synapse;

- form receptors on the postsynaptic neuron that are activated or inactivated when specific neurotransmitters bind;

- are part of the signal transduction pathway in the postsynaptic neuron

An interesting aside is the fact that abused drugs are often plant-derived chemicals, such as cocaine, opium, and tetrahydrocannabinol (THC), the main active ingredient in marijuana. These substances bind to receptors on human neurons, which indicates that our bodies have their own versions of these substances. The human equivalents of the opiates are the endorphins and enkephalins, and the equivalent of THC is anandamide. The endorphins and enkephalins relieve pain. Anandamide modulates how brain cells respond to stimulation by binding to neurotransmitter receptors on presynaptic (sending) neurons. (This contrasts with neurotransmitters, which bind to receptors on postsynaptic neurons.)

DNA microarray technology is probing the biology of addiction by revealing the expression of many genes at a time. In the past, research focused on individual genes whose encoded proteins fit a part of the picture—such as alcohol dehydrogenase, an enzyme that is part of the pathway to metabolize ethanol. An allele of the gene that encodes the dopamine D(2) receptor has also been implicated in the predisposition to drug addiction. People who are homozygous for the A1 allele of the D(2) dopamine receptor gene are overrepresented among people with alcoholism and other addictions, though not to a clinically useful extent.

DNA microarray tests that detect expression of thousands of genes at a time before and after exposure to a particular drug reveal that 1 to 5 percent of the genes are expressed. Consider a comparison of gene expression profiles in human brain cells, 10 samples from deceased people who had alcoholism and 10 from people who died from other causes. Of 4,000 genes screened, 160 varied in expression by at least 40 percent between the two types of brains. In addition to identifying genes involved in signal transduction and neurotransmitter activity, the study also highlighted genes that function in the cell cycle and particularly in apoptosis, and other genes that help a cell survive oxidative damage. Perhaps the genes that affect neurotransmitter function and signal transduction underlie the tolerance and dependency of addiction in general, and the other activated genes reflect the body's response to the specific toxic effects of alcohol. DNA microarray tests also revealed a subset of genes whose actions are unique to brain cells, such as genes that control the synthesis of myelin, the fatty insulation on some neurons. Impairment of myelin synthesis with chronic alcohol use is consistent with imaging studies that show that the brain's white matter shrinks. Other microarray experiments compared expression of 6,000 genes in mouse brain neurons growing in culture, with or without exposure to alcohol. The expression of dozens of genes increased or decreased in the presence of alcohol.

It will be interesting to determine if and how DNA expression profiles change with addiction to different drugs.

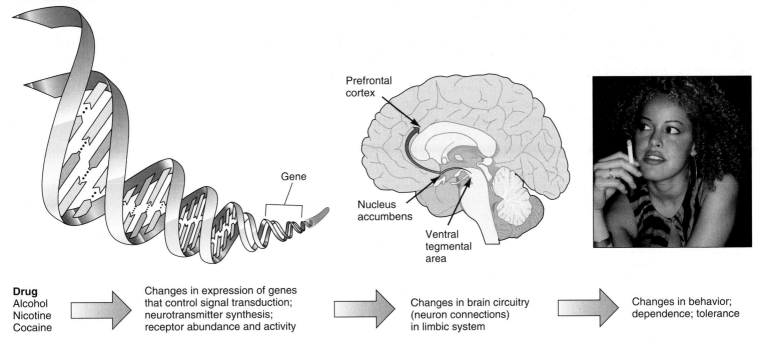

Figure 8.6 **The events of addiction.** Addiction is manifest at several levels: at the molecular level, in neuron-neuron interactions, and in behavioral responses.

8.6 Mood Disorders

Mood disorders are especially difficult to separate into genetic and environmental components because they may appear to be extremes of normal behavior. For example, a person who has previously been happy but inexplicably becomes lethargic and sad, and no longer enjoys activities that once gave pleasure, may receive a diagnosis of **major depressive disorder** (MDD), or clinical depression (**table 8.3**). A person with the exact same symptoms who can trace the onset to the death of a loved one may be the victim of extended grief and loss, not clinical depression. Context is important.

The two most prevalent mood disorders are major depressive disorder and **bipolar affective disorder** (also called bipolar disorder or manic-depression). MDD affects 6 percent of the U.S. population at any given time, and occurs in more women than men. Lifetime risk of MDD for the general population is 5 to 10 percent. Often depression is chronic, interspersed with acute episodes provoked by stress. Fifteen percent of people hospitalized for severe, recurrent depression ultimately end their lives. About half of all people who experience a depressive episode will suffer others. Half of affected individuals do not seek medical help, and among those who do, a third do not respond to drug therapy; those who do

Table 8.3
Signs of Clinical Depression

Physicians use degrees of these feelings to assess whether antidepressant therapy is effective:

1. Depressed mood (feeling hopeless, helpless, worthless, unhappy)
2. Guilt
3. Suicidal ideation
4. Insomnia
5. Loss of interest in work or activities that formerly gave pleasure
6. Difficulty concentrating, thinking, speaking, moving
7. Agitation
8. Anxiety out of proportion to the problem, with associated physical symptoms
9. Poor or absent appetite
10. Fatigue, lack of energy
11. Hypochondriasis (convinced a medical condition is present)
12. Weight loss
13. Lack of realization that he/she is depressed
14. Worsening symptoms at certain times of day, usually night
15. Paranoia
16. Obsessive-compulsive behavior
17. Feelings of unreality

Based on the Hamilton Rating Scale for Depression

may relapse when they discontinue taking an effective drug. Electroconvulsive (shock) therapy can fairly quickly help some patients who are drug-resistant.

Bipolar disorder is much rarer than MDD, affecting 1 percent of the population and with a general population lifetime risk of 0.5 to 1.0 percent. With this disorder, weeks or months of depression alternate with periods of mania, when the person is hyperactive and restless, and may experience a rush of ideas and excitement. Ideas may be fantastic, and behavior reckless. For example, a person who is normally quiet and frugal might, when manic, suddenly make large monetary donations and spend lavishly—very out-of-character behavior. In one subtype of bipolar disorder, the "up" times are termed hypomania, and they seem more a temporary reprieve from the doldrums than the starkly aberrant behavior of a full manic period. Bipolar disorder and hypomania may appear to be depression.

At the root of depression, and possibly of bipolar disorder too, is deficiency of the neurotransmitter serotonin, which affects mood, emotion, appetite, and sleep. Levels of norepinephrine, another type of neurotransmitter, are important as well. The abnormality appears to occur in transporter proteins that ferry neurotransmitters from the synapse to "reuptake pumps" in the presynaptic neuron. Overactive or overabundant transporters deplete neurotransmitter levels. Millions of people take drugs called selective serotonin reuptake inhibitors (SSRIs) to prevent presynaptic neurons from admitting serotonin from the synapse. This leaves more of the neurotransmitter available to stimulate the postsynaptic cell (**figure 8.7**), which apparently offsets the neurotransmitter deficit. Older antidepressants called tricyclics target norepinephrine, and newer drugs affect both serotonin and norepinephrine levels.

The SSRIs and dual drugs may begin to produce effects after one week, often enabling a person with moderate or severe depression to return to some activities, but full response can take six weeks. Other older drugs take longer to work. Evidence suggests that people with mild depression may seem to respond to drugs due to a placebo effect. DNA microarray tests can predict which drugs are most likely to help a particular patient, with the most tolerable or least number of side effects.

Researchers do not know how the distribution of serotonin deficiency in the brain of a depressed person differs from normal. One study of the brains of 220 people who had died while clinically depressed revealed a generalized decrease in serotonin activity in many brain regions, but a concentrated area of poor activity in the prefrontal cortex of those individuals who had been suicidal.

Assigning specific genes or even chromosomal regions to bipolar disorder has lagged behind such efforts for depression. Over the past thirty years, linkage studies in large families, or association studies in very isolated populations such as the Amish, have indicated genome regions that may harbor genes that predispose to bipolar disorder, such as parts of chromosomes 4, 10, 18, 22, and mitochondrial DNA (because in some families only females pass on the trait). Evidence is more specific for depression, pointing strongly toward malfunction of the serotonin transporter coupled with a precipitating environmental trigger. For bipolar disorder, evidence is insufficient to support either a polygenic model of many genes, each with an additive effect; roles for several genes, each with a large and independent effect (genetic heterogeneity); or epistasis, where different genes interact and control each other's expression.

The National Institute of Mental Health has formed a consortium of nine U.S. centers to search the human genome sequence for the causes of bipolar disorder among more than 1,800 people in 500 families with more than one affected member. Researchers are also looking for variants of known genes that are more common in individuals who have subtypes of bipolar disorder. For example, one experiment found sequence variants associated with the serotonin transporter in people with bipolar disorder who had many episodes of psychosis, and associated variants of monoamine oxidase A, another neurotransmitter, in people with bipolar disorder who were also suicidal. Another candidate gene for bipolar disorder encodes one of six types of serotonin receptors. In addition, abundant evidence rules out certain neurotransmitters from having a role in bipolar disorder. The fact that groups of patients with similar symptoms have polymorphisms in the same candidate genes is evidence that the condition is genetically heterogeneic—that is, it may be several disorders with similar and overlapping symptoms.

Key Concepts

Major depressive disorder is common compared to bipolar disorder, and is likely caused by deficits of serotonin, norepinephrine, or both. Bipolar disorder is associated with several chromosomal sites, and its genetic roots are difficult to isolate.

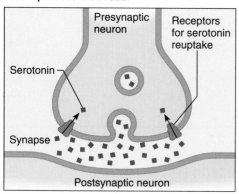
Nondepressed individual

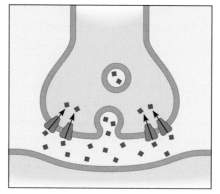
Depressed individual, untreated

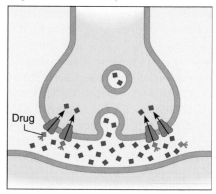
Depressed individual, treated with SSRI

Figure 8.7 Anatomy of an antidepressant. Selective serotonin reuptake inhibitors (SSRIs) are antidepressant drugs that act as their name states—they block the reuptake of serotonin, making more of the neurotransmitter available in the synapses. This corrects a neurotransmitter deficit that presumably causes the symptoms. Overactive or overabundant reuptake receptors can cause the deficit. The precise mechanism of SSRIs is not well understood.

8.7 Schizophrenia

Schizophrenia is a debilitating loss of the ability to organize thoughts and perceptions, which leads to a withdrawal from reality. Various forms of the condition affect 1 percent of the world's population, and 10 percent of affected individuals commit suicide.

Identifying genetic contributions to schizophrenia illustrates the difficulties in analyzing a behavioral condition. Some of the symptoms are also associated with other illnesses; many genes cause or contribute to it; and several environmental factors may be phenocopies.

The first signs of schizophrenia often are cognitive, affecting thinking. In late childhood or early adolescence, a person might suddenly have trouble paying attention in school, and learning may become difficult as memory falters and information-processing skills lag. Symptoms of psychosis begin between ages 17 and 27 for males and 20 and 37 for females, including delusions and hallucinations—sometimes heard, sometimes seen. A person with schizophrenia may hear a voice giving instructions. What others perceive as irrational fears, such as being followed by monsters, are very real to the person with schizophrenia. Meanwhile, cognitive skills continue to decline. Speech reflects the garbled thought process; the person skips from topic to topic with no obvious thread of logic, or displays inappropriate emotional responses, such as laughing at sad news. Artwork by a person with schizophrenia can display the characteristic fragmentation of the mind (**figure 8.8**). (Schizophrenia means "split mind," but it does not cause a split or multiple personality.)

The course of schizophrenia often plateaus (evens out) or becomes episodic. It is not a continuous decline, as is the case for dementia. Schizophrenia is frequently misdiagnosed as depression or bipolar affective disorder. However, schizophrenia primarily affects thinking; these other conditions mostly affect mood. It is a very distinctive mental illness.

A heritability of 0.8 and empiric risk values indicate a strong role for genes in causing schizophrenia (**table 8.4**). Because most of the symptoms are behavioral, however, it is possible to develop some of them—such as disordered thinking—from living with and imitating people who have schizophrenia. Although concordance is high, a person who has an identical twin with schizophrenia has a 54 percent chance of *not* developing schizo-

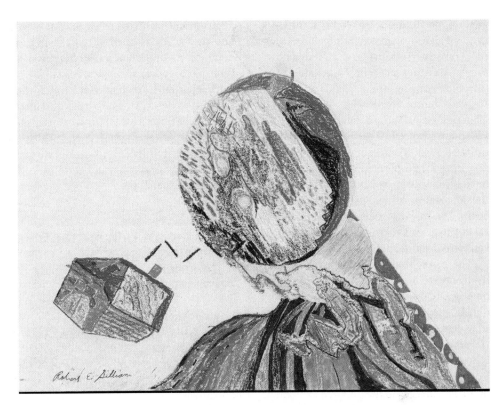

Figure 8.8   Schizophrenia alters thinking.   People with schizophrenia communicate the disarray of their thoughts in characteristically disjointed drawings.

phrenia. Therefore, the condition has a significant environmental component, too.

One environmental hypothesis for the cause of schizophrenia is that influenza in a woman during the second trimester of pregnancy predisposes offspring to developing schizophrenia. The evidence is that people with schizophrenia are more likely than the general population to have been born in the spring, with the second trimester spanning the winter months. During this time, the influenza virus can cross the placenta and alter brain cells. **Table 8.5** lists other environmental factors associated with schizophrenia.

Early investigations on the inheritance of schizophrenia focused on affected individuals who also had visible chromosome abnormalities, such as two Chinese brothers who had a duplication of part of chromosome 5. Assuming that the mental illness and the extra chromosomal material were related, researchers looked to this chromosome in other affected families, and identified five families in Iceland and two in England that had mutations in this part of the genome. But in other families, other chromosome regions or genes are associated with schizo-

Table 8.4	
Risk of Developing Schizophrenia	
Relationship to an affected individual	**Risk**
None (general population)	1%
First cousin	2%
Uncle/aunt	2%
Niece/nephew	4%
Grandchildren	5%
Half sibling	6%
One affected parent	6%
Sibling, DZ twin	9%
Child	13%
Sibling and one affected parent	17%
Two affected parents	46%
MZ twin	46%

phrenia, indicating genetic heterogeneity. For example, 30 percent of individuals missing the same small section of chromosome 22 develop schizophrenia, which is significantly greater than the 1 percent incidence in the general population. In some families, a gene on chromosome 6 that encodes a signal transduction protein called dystrobrevin binding protein 1 causes schizophrenia. Among the 80,000 citizens of Iceland being evaluated in DeCODE Genetics' population database project, (see Bioethics: Choices for the Future, chapter 1), mutation in a gene called neuregulin accounts for 30 percent of the people who have schizophrenia. This protein controls the formation of synapses in parts of the brain, and may normally control how neural connections form in response to environmental influences.

The genes that encode neuregulin and dystrobrevin binding protein 1, and predisposing DNA sequences on chromosomes 5 and 22, may be only a few of dozens of genes that can combine with an environmental trigger to cause the strange symptoms of schizophrenia. Genomewide screens of families with schizophrenia reveal at least twenty-four sites where affected siblings share alleles much more often than the 50 percent of the time that Mendel's first law predicts.

Behavioral traits have been much more difficult to describe, categorize, and attribute to genetic and/or environmental influences than other characteristics. **Table 8.6** lists the heritabilities and candidate genes for the behavioral traits and conditions discussed in this chapter.

Table 8.5

Environmental Risk Factors for Schizophrenia

Maternal malnutrition

Infection by Borna virus

Fetal oxygen deprivation

Obstetric or birth complication

Psychoactive drug use (phencyclidine)

Traumatic brain injury

Herpes infection at time of birth

Table 8.6

Review of Behavioral Traits and Disorders

Condition	Heritability	Candidate Genes
ADHD	0.80	Dopamine transporter
		Dopamine D(4) receptor (DRD4)
Eating disorders	0.50–0.80	Leptin
		Leptin transporter
		Leptin receptor
		Neuropeptide Y
		Melanocortin-4 receptor
Intelligence	0.80	Neural cellular adhesion molecule (N-CAM)
Addiction	0.40–0.60	Dopamine D(2) receptor (DRD2)
		Myelin synthesis
Depression	0.40–0.54	Serotonin synthesis, transporter, receptor
		Norepinephrine synthesis, transporter, receptor
Bipolar disorder	0.80	Serotonin transporter, receptor
		Monoamine oxidase A control
Schizophrenia	0.80	Dopamine synthesis, transporter, receptor
		Glutamate synthesis, transporter, receptor

Summary

8.1 Genes Contribute to Most Behavioral Traits

1. Most behavioral traits and conditions are multifactorial and are more common than most single-gene disorders.

2. Candidate genes for behavioral traits and disorders affect neurotransmission and signal transduction.

3. Analyzing behaviors is difficult because symptoms of different syndromes overlap, study participants can provide biased information, and behaviors can be imitated.

8.2 Eating Disorders

4. Eating disorders affect both sexes and are prevalent in the United States and Canada. Twin studies indicate high heritability.

5. Candidate genes for eating disorders include those whose protein products control appetite and the neurotransmitters dopamine and serotonin.

8.3 Sleep

6. Twin studies and single-gene disorders that affect the sleep-wake cycle reveal a large inherited component to sleep behavior.

7. A large family with familial advanced sleep phase syndrome enabled researchers to identify the first "clock" gene in humans. The *period* gene enables a person to respond to day and night environmental cues.

8.4 Intelligence

8. Intelligence is difficult to define and to measure. IQ testing predicts success in school or work, but is being replaced by the general intelligence (g) value that underlies population variance in IQ test performance.

9. Heritability for intelligence increases with age, suggesting that environmental factors are more important early in life.

10. Many chromosomal disorders affect intelligence, suggesting high heritability. An N-CAM is a candidate gene.

8.5 Drug Addiction

11. Defining characteristics of drug addiction are tolerance and dependence. Addiction produces stable brain changes, yet heritability is not as high as for some other behavioral conditions.

12. A candidate gene for drug addiction is the dopamine D(2) receptor. DNA microarray tests on gene expression in the brains of people with alcoholism help to identify genes involved in neurotransmission, signal transduction, cell cycle control, apoptosis, surviving oxidative damage, and myelination of neurons.

8.6 Mood Disorders

13. **Major depressive disorder** is relatively common and associated with deficits of serotonin and/or norepinephrine.

14. **Bipolar affective disorder,** which consists of depressive periods interspersed with times of mania or hypomania, is much rarer. Linkage and association studies implicate several chromosomal sites as housing genes that raise the risk of developing this disorder.

8.7 Schizophrenia

15. **Schizophrenia** greatly disrupts the ability to think and perceive the world. Onset is typically in early adulthood, and the course is episodic or steady but not degenerative.

16. Empiric risk estimates and heritability indicate a large genetic component, yet certain environmental associations exist, too.

17. There are many candidate genes and genome regions associated with schizophrenia.

Review Questions

1. In general, what types of gene products are responsible for variations in behaviors?

2. Why is the genetics of ADHD easier to analyze than that of autism?

3. Which behaviors are traced to altered activities in the following regions of the brain?

   a. suprachiasmatic nuclei

   b. nucleus accumbens

   c. prefrontal cortex

4. Why is identifying a candidate gene only a first step in understanding how behavior arises and varies among individuals?

5. Name a candidate gene for the following traits or disorders:

   a. intelligence

   b. cocaine addiction

   c. alcoholism

   d. bipolar affective disorder

   e. schizophrenia

6. Describe three factors that can complicate the investigation of a behavioral trait.

7. Why does the heritability of intelligence decline with age?

Applied Questions

1. Serotonin levels are implicated in eating disorders, major depressive disorder, and bipolar disorder.

   a. How can an abnormality in one type of neurotransmitter contribute to different disorders?

   b. What is another neurotransmitter that is implicated in more than one behavioral disorder?

2. How has DNA microarray technology changed the study of the genetics of behavior?

3. What might be the advantages and disadvantages of a SNP profile or other genotyping test done at birth that indicates whether a person is at high risk for developing a drug addiction?

4. The U.S. government prohibits recreational use of cocaine, marijuana, and opiates, which are physically addictive drugs, but not of alcohol and nicotine (cigarettes), also physically addictive. Do you think that the legal status of any of these drugs should be changed, and if so, how and why? What measures, if any, should the government use in deciding which drugs to outlaw?

5. Do you think that having a genotype known to predispose someone to aggressive or violent behavior should be a valid legal defense? Cite a reason for your answer.

6. In some association studies of depression and bipolar disorder, correlations to specific alleles are only evident when participants are considered in subgroups based on symptoms. What might be a biological basis for this finding?

7. Many older individuals experience advanced sleep phase syndrome. Even though this condition is probably a normal part of aging, how might research on the Utah family with an inherited form of the condition help researchers develop a drug to help the elderly sleep through the night and awaken later in the morning?

8. What alternate explanation besides genetic differences might account for the over-representation of minority groups among people with low IQ scores in the United States?

9. A study found that the risk of schizophrenia among spouses of people with schizophrenia who have no affected blood relatives is 2 percent. What does this indicate about the causes of schizophrenia?

10. Wolfram syndrome is a rare autosomal recessive disorder that causes severe diabetes, impaired vision, and neurological problems. Examinations of hospital records and self-reports reveal that blood relatives of Wolfram syndrome patients have an eightfold risk over the general population of developing serious

psychiatric disorders such as depression, violent behavior, and suicidal tendencies. Can you suggest further experiments and studies to test the hypothesis that these mental manifestations are a less severe expression of Wolfram syndrome?

11. A study of 2,685 twin pairs showed that female MZ twins are six times as likely as female DZ twins to both have alcoholism. Does this finding suggest a large genetic or environmental component to alcoholism?

Web Activities

12. Consult the Diagnostic and Statistical Manual of Mental Disorders (DSM-IV) at http://www.psychologynet.org/dsm.html. Follow links and list three disorders for which candidate genes have been identified. Discuss how those genes might cause the phenotype.

Case Studies

13. Marjorie and Joyce are mothers of pre-teen girls and survivors of eating disorders. While growing up in the 1950s and 1960s, Marjorie and Joyce were careful about what they ate, because their mother, stick thin, was always trying one diet or another and constantly worrying about putting on weight. Marjorie, like her mother, learned to control her weight by eating practically nothing. Joyce ate more, but exercised at least two hours a day. When either gave in to hunger and ate a large amount, they would induce vomiting or take laxatives. When the medical community began to recognize eating disorders and the media began to publicize them, the sisters learned that their lack of body fat could prevent them from becoming pregnant. They underwent psychotherapy and learned (slowly) how to eat normally.

Now seeing familiar behavior patterns in their daughters terrifies Marjorie and Joyce. Marjorie's daughter Sherry seems to do nothing but exercise, living on smoothies and salads. It seems, to Marjorie, a fine line

between a healthy lifestyle and obsession with weight control. Joyce's daughter binges and purges, and was so secretive that it took Joyce many months to be certain there was a problem, even though she had once engaged in the same behavior.

The sisters learn of a company offering testing for gene variants that have been associated with increased risk of developing eating disorders. Marjorie encourages Sherry to take the test, feeling guilty that she passed on the causative genes. But Joyce feels that the testing will have no benefit, and attributes the development of an eating disorder to living in a society that pressures women to be skeletal.

Do you agree with Marjorie or Joyce? Cite a reason for your answer.

Learn to apply the skills of a genetic counselor with an additional case found in the *Case Workbook in Human Genetics.*

Alcoholism

Suggested Readings

Bradbury, Jane. May 19, 2001. Teasing out the genetics of bipolar disorder. *The Lancet* 257:1596. Many genes lead to the mood swings of bipolar disorder.

Bulik, C. M., et al. January 2003. Significant linkage on chromosome 10p in families with bulimia nervosa. *The American Journal of Human Genetics* 72:200–7. Certain gene variants may set the stage for developing an eating disorder, given a permissive environment.

Cavendish, Harry. December 2001. Saved by Ezmerelda. *The Lancet,* suppl., 560. This journalist describes what it's like to live with schizophrenia.

Clayton, J. D., et al. February 15, 2001. Keeping time with the human genome. *Nature* 409:829–31. Several genes control the sleep-wake cycle.

Lesch, Peter K. December 2001. Weird world inside the brain. *The Lancet,* suppl., 559. Schizophrenia is actually several disorders.

Lewis, Ricki. June 25, 2001. Focusing on endocannabinoid. *The Scientist* 15(13):14. Marijuana exerts its effects because our brain cells have receptors for it.

McGuffin, Peter, et al. February 16, 2001. Toward behavioral genomics. *Nature* 291:1232–33. Part of the human genome project is to identify genes that affect behavior.

Nestler, Eric J. November 2000. Genes and addiction. *Nature Genetics* 26:277–80. Drug-seeking behavior reflects aberrant brain function, which reflects the actions of certain gene variants.

Peyron, C., et al. September 2000. A mutation in a case of early-onset narcolepsy and a generalized absence of hypocretin peptide

in human narcoleptic brains. *Nature Medicine* 6(9):991–97. A single-gene mutation can cause narcolepsy.

Stefansson, H., et al. October 2002. Neuregulin 1 and susceptibility to schizophrenia. *The American Journal of Human Genetics* 71:877–92. The Icelandic population database reveals a gene that can cause schizophrenia.

Wilson, Jennifer Fisher. October 15, 2001. Identifying the first sleep-related genes. *The Scientist* 15(20):20–22. A family with unusual sleep habits led to a major discovery.

Weekly updates of current news related to human genetics are available through Power Web on your Online Learning Center.

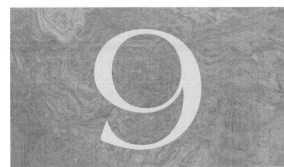

CHAPTER

9

DNA Structure and Replication

CHAPTER CONTENTS

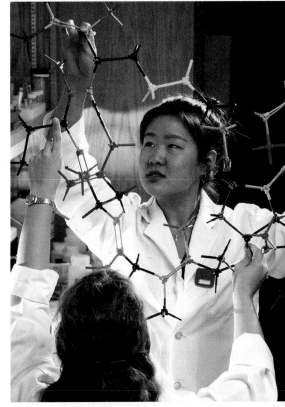

Today, DNA models are found in classrooms as well as laboratories.

A genetic material must carry out two jobs: duplicate itself and control the development of the rest of the cell in a specific way, wrote Francis Crick, codiscoverer with James Watson of the three-dimensional structure of DNA in 1953. Only DNA can do this. When geneticists celebrated the fiftieth anniversary of the discovery of the structure of DNA in 2003, they acknowledged the many experiments that provided the clues that enabled Watson and Crick to build their model of the molecule of life. Reading 9.1 is one of many essays on DNA published at the time of the anniversary. **Figure 9.1** shows one view of DNA.

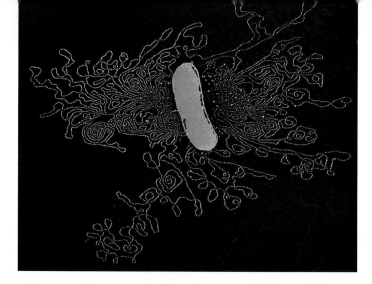

Figure 9.1 DNA is highly packaged.
DNA bursts forth from this treated bacterial cell, illustrating how tightly DNA. winds to fit into a single cell. The two copies of the human genome in a cell would each unravel to 1.8 meters, yet fit into a cell 6 millionths of a meter across.

9.1 Experiments Identify and Describe the Genetic Material

DNA was first described in the mid-eighteenth century, when Swiss physician and biochemist Friedrich Miescher isolated nuclei from white blood cells in pus on soiled bandages. In the nuclei, he discovered an unusual acidic substance containing nitrogen and phosphorus. He and others found it in cells from a variety of sources. Because the material resided in cell nuclei, Miescher called it nuclein in an 1871 paper; subsequently, it was called a nucleic acid. But few people appreciated the importance of Miescher's discovery, because at the time, the study of heredity focused on the association between inherited disease and protein.

In 1902, English physician Archibald Garrod was the first to link human inheritance and protein. He noted that people who had certain inborn errors of metabolism lacked certain enzymes. One of the first inborn errors that he described was alkaptonuria, the subject of In Their Own Words in chapter 5. Other researchers added evidence of a link between heredity and enzymes from other species, such as fruit flies with unusual eye colors and bread molds with nutritional deficiencies. Both organisms had absent or abnormal specific enzymes. As researchers wondered what, precisely, was the connection between enzymes and heredity, they returned to Miescher's discovery of nucleic acids.

DNA Is the Hereditary Molecule

In 1928, English microbiologist Frederick Griffith took the first step in identifying DNA as the genetic material. Griffith noticed that mice with a certain variety of pneumonia harbored one of two types of *Diplococcus pneumoniae* bacteria. Type R bacteria are rough in texture. Type S bacteria are smooth because they are enclosed in a polysaccharide capsule. Mice injected with type R bacteria did not develop pneumonia, but mice injected with type S did. The polysaccharide coat seemed to be necessary for infection.

When type S bacteria were heated—which killed them but left their DNA intact—they no longer could cause pneumonia in mice. However, when Griffith injected mice with a mixture of type R bacteria plus heat-killed type S bacteria—neither of which, alone, was deadly to the mice—the mice died of pneumonia (**figure 9.2**). Their bodies contained live type S bacteria, encased in polysaccharide. Griffith termed the apparent conversion of one bacterial type into another "transformation." How did it happen? What substance transformed type R to type S?

U.S. physicians Oswald Avery, Colin MacLeod, and Maclyn McCarty hypothesized that a nucleic acid might be the "transforming principle." They observed that treating type R bacteria with a protease—an enzyme that dismantles protein—did not prevent the transformation of a nonvirulent to a virulent strain, but treating it with deoxyribonuclease (or DNase), an enzyme that dismantles DNA only, did disrupt transformation. In 1944, they confirmed that DNA transformed the bacteria. They isolated DNA from heat-killed type S bacteria and injected it along with type R bacteria into mice (**figure 9.3**). The mice died, and their bodies contained active type S bacteria. The conclusion: DNA passed from type S bacteria to type R, enabling it to manufacture the smooth coat necessary for infection.

DNA Is the Hereditary Molecule—and Protein Is Not

In 1953, U.S. microbiologists Alfred Hershey and Martha Chase confirmed that DNA is the genetic material. They used *E. coli* bacteria infected with a virus that consisted of a protein "head" surrounding DNA. Viruses infect bacterial cells by injecting their DNA into them. The viral protein coats remain outside the bacterial cells.

When Hershey and Chase grew viruses with radioactive sulfur, the viral protein coats emitted radioactivity. When they repeated the experiment with radioactive phosphorus, the viral DNA emitted radioactivity.

Next, Hershey and Chase "labeled" two batches of virus by growing one in a medium containing radioactive sulfur (designated ^{35}S) and the other in a medium containing radioactive phosphorus (designated ^{32}P). The viruses grown on sulfur had their protein marked but not their DNA, because protein incorporates sulfur but DNA does not. Conversely, the viruses grown on labeled phosphorus had their DNA marked but not their protein, because this element is found in DNA but not protein. (Miescher had noted the presence of phosphorus in DNA from soiled bandages.)

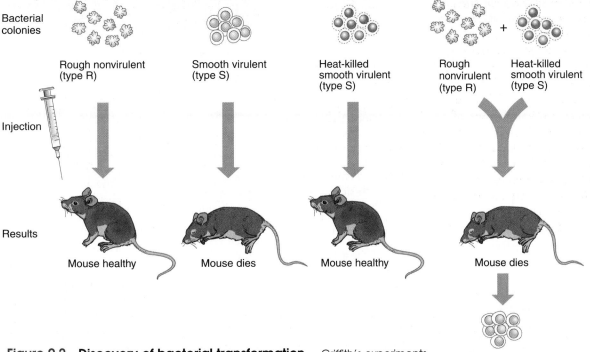

Figure 9.2 Discovery of bacterial transformation. Griffith's experiments showed that a molecule in a lethal type of bacteria can transform nonkilling (nonvirulent) bacteria into killers (virulent).

Live type S bacteria in blood sample from dead mouse

After allowing several minutes for the virus particles to bind to the bacteria and inject their DNA into them, Hershey and Chase agitated each mixture in a blender, shaking free the empty virus protein coats. The contents of each blender were collected in test tubes, then centrifuged (spun at high speed). This settled the bacteria at the bottom of each tube because virus coats drift down more slowly than bacteria.

At the end of the procedure, Hershey and Chase examined fractions containing the virus coats from the top of each test tube and the infected bacteria that had set-tled to the bottom of each tube (**figure 9.4**). In the tube containing viruses labeled with sulfur, the virus coats were radioactive, but the virus-infected bacteria, containing viral DNA, were not. In the other tube, where the virus had incorporated radioactive phosphorus, the virus coats carried no radioactive label, but the infected bacteria were radioactive. This meant that the part of the virus that could enter bacteria and direct them to mass produce more virus was the part that had incorporated phosphorus DNA. The genetic material, therefore, was DNA, and not protein.

Deciphering the Structure of DNA

In 1909, Russian-American biochemist Phoebus Levene identified the 5-carbon sugar **ribose** as part of some nucleic acids, and in 1929, he discovered a similar sugar—**deoxyribose**—in other nucleic acids. He had revealed a major chemical distinction between RNA and DNA: RNA contains ribose, and DNA contains deoxyribose.

Levene then discovered that the three parts of a nucleic acid—a sugar, a nitrogen-containing base, and a phosphorus-containing component—are present in equal proportions. He deduced that a nucleic acid building block must contain one of each component. Furthermore, although the sugar and phosphate portions were always the same, the nitrogen-containing bases were of four types. Scientists at first thought that the bases were present in equal amounts, but if this were so, DNA could not encode as much information as it could if the number of each base type varied. Imagine how much less versatile a written language would be if all the letters in a document had to occur with equal frequency.

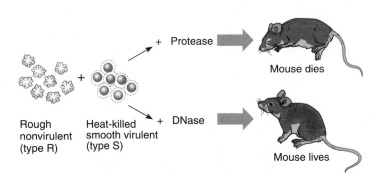

Figure 9.3 DNA is the "transforming principle." Avery, MacLeod, and McCarty identified DNA as Griffith's transforming principle. By adding enzymes that either destroy proteins (protease) or DNA (deoxyribonuclease or DNase) to the types of solutions that Griffith used in his experiments, they demonstrated that DNA transforms bacteria—and that protein does not.

Happy Anniversary, DNA!

Much was written to commemorate the fiftieth anniversary of the discovery of the DNA double helix. The author of this book contributed the following essay, which was read at celebrations and was featured on the Cold Spring Harbor "DNA at 50" website.

On the Meaning of Gene

To a biologist, *gene* has a very specific and not terribly intriguing definition—a sequence of DNA building blocks that tells a cell how to string together amino acids in a particular order to manufacture a particular protein. A collagen gene specifies the tightly entwined collagen protein that builds connective tissue; a fibrin gene specifies a key component of the blood clotting apparatus. The repertoire of proteins produced in different cells, at different times, guides our development from a fertilized ovum to a many-trillion-celled adult, distinguishing nerve from muscle, fat from bone along the journey. A missing or malfunctioning gene can alter a protein in a way that causes disease—a clotting factor is absent in hemophilia; a cell surface channel for salts is obliterated in cystic fibrosis. The effects of many genes add together to mold traits, and the environment fine-tunes the expression of nearly all genes. Because of our experiences, we are much more than the biochemical information in our genes.

Once called by such colorful names as gemmules and stirps, plastidules and idioblasts, genes are the units of inheritance, each one a packet of instructions passed from one cell generation to the next. Whatever its name, the gene has held different meanings for different individuals across the landscape of time:

To 7-year-old Molly Nash, gene means both sickness and health—an abnormal gene caused the Fanconi anemia that would have killed her, if not for the gift of the normal version of the gene from her brother, Adam, who was conceived to save her.

To Jesse Gelsinger, an 18-year-old who died in a gene therapy experiment in 1999, gene meant a risk taken—and tragically realized.

To folksinger Arlo Guthrie, gene means passing age 45 without showing signs of the Huntington disease that slowly claimed his father, legendary folksinger Woody Guthrie.

To one in seven cats in New England, gene means extra toes.

To Adolph Hitler and others who have dehumanized those not like themselves, the concept of gene was abused to justify genocide.

To a smoker, a gene may determine whether or not lung cancer develops.

To a redhead in a family of brunettes, gene means an attractive variant.

To a 39-year-old woman whose mother and sisters had breast cancer, a gene means escape from their fate—and survivor guilt.

To a lucky few, gene means a mutation that robs T cells of a surface protein that enables HIV to enter. They cannot become infected.

To defense attorneys for Richard Speck, killer of nine student nurses in the 1960s, extra genes on Speck's extra Y chromosome meant he wasn't responsible for his behavior—an association that has not held up.

To people with diabetes, gene means safer insulin.

To a child suffering from severe vitamin A deficiency, genetically modified yellow rice that produces beta carotene may mean health, even life.

To an elephant that lives on the African savannah and one that lives in the forest, gene means that they cannot mate with each other—their species diverged from a shared ancestor 2.6 million years ago.

To a forensic entomologist, gene means a clue to the identity of a victim or criminal in the guts of maggots devouring a corpse.

To scientists-turned-biotech-entrepreneurs, gene means money.

To those who inherit a particular gene variant on chromosome 4, gene means a very long life—if they can avoid accidents.

Collectively, our genes mean that we are very much more alike than different from one another.

In the early 1950s, two lines of experimental evidence converged to provide the direct clues that finally revealed DNA's structure. Austrian-American biochemist Erwin Chargaff showed that DNA in several species contains equal amounts of the bases **adenine** (A) and **thymine** (T) and equal amounts of the bases **guanine** (G) and **cytosine** (C). Next, English physicist Maurice Wilkins and English chemist Rosalind Franklin bombarded DNA with X rays using a technique called X-ray diffraction, then deduced information about the structure of the molecule from the patterns in which the X rays were deflected.

Rosalind Franklin provided a clue that would prove pivotal in revealing the structure of DNA to Watson and Crick—she distinguished two forms of DNA, a dry, crystalline "A" form, which had been well-studied, and the wetter type seen in cells, the "B" form. It took her 100 hours to obtain "photo 51" of the B form in May 1952 (**figure 9.5**). Its remarkable symmetry told Franklin that the molecule was a sleek helix, and revealed the position of the phosphates. She had long thought of DNA as a

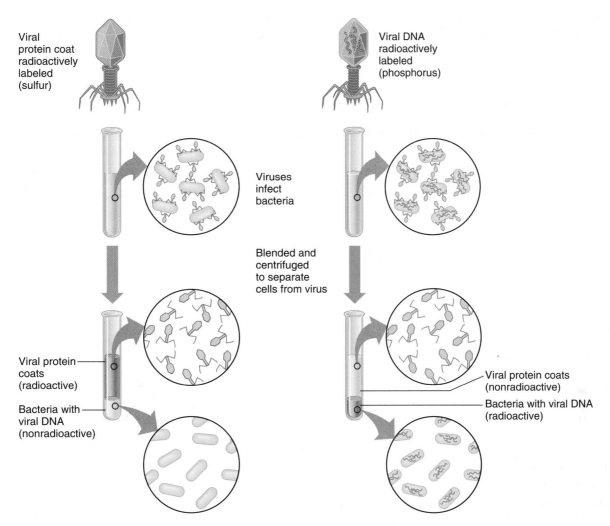

Viral protein coat radioactively labeled (sulfur)

Viral DNA radioactively labeled (phosphorus)

Viruses infect bacteria

Blended and centrifuged to separate cells from virus

Viral protein coats (radioactive)

Bacteria with viral DNA (nonradioactive)

Viral protein coats (nonradioactive)

Bacteria with viral DNA (radioactive)

Figure 9.4   DNA is the hereditary material; protein is not.   Hershey and Chase used different radioactive molecules to distinguish the viral protein coat from the genetic material (DNA). These "blender experiments" showed that the virus transfers DNA, and not protein, to the bacterium. Therefore, DNA is the genetic material. The blender experiments used particular types of sulfur and phosphorus atoms that emit detectable radiation.

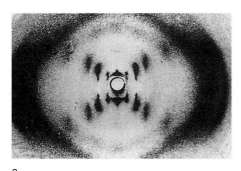

a.

Figure 9.5   Deciphering DNA structure.   (a) Rosalind Franklin's "photo 51" of B DNA was critical to Watson and Crick's deduction of the three-dimensional structure of the molecule. The "X" in the center indicates a helix, and the darkened regions reveal symmetrically organized subunits. **(b)** Franklin died very young, of cancer.

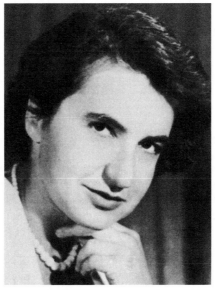

b. Rosalind Franklin 1920–1958

candidate for the genetic material. A lab notebook from her college days in 1939 bears the comment, "Geometrical basis for inheritance?" next to an illustration of a nucleic acid. By early 1953, she was very close to deducing the entire structure. On January 30, Wilkins showed Franklin's photo 51 to Watson.

The race was on. During February, famed biochemist Linus Pauling suggested a triple helix structure for DNA. Meanwhile, Watson and Crick, certain of the sugar-phosphate backbone largely from photo 51, turned their attention to the bases. Ironically, their eureka moment occurred not with sophisticated chemistry or crystallography, but while working with cardboard cutouts. On Saturday morning, February 28, Watson arrived early for a meeting with Crick. While he was waiting, he sat playing with cardboard cutouts of the four DNA bases, pairing A with A, then A with G. When he assembled A next to T, and G next to C, he noted the similar shapes, and suddenly all of the pieces fit. When Crick arrived forty minutes later, the two quickly realized they had solved the puzzle (**figure 9.6**). Watson, Crick, and Wilkins eventually received the Nobel prize. In 1958, Franklin died at the age of 37 from ovarian cancer, and the Nobel can only be awarded to a living person. In recent years, she has become a heroine for her role in deciphering the structure of DNA. **Table 9.1** summarizes some of the experiments that led to the discovery.

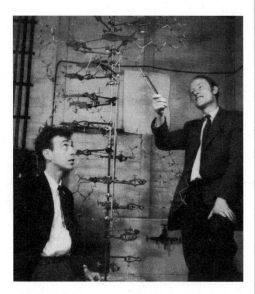

Figure 9.6 Watson and Crick.
Prints of this famed, if posed, photo fetched a high price when signed and sold at celebrations of DNA's fiftieth anniversary in 2003. Crick was told to point to the model, and picked up a slide rule.

Key Concepts

DNA replicates, and it contains the information the cell requires to synthesize protein. Miescher first isolated DNA in 1869, naming it nuclein. Garrod first linked heredity to enzymes. • DNA was chemically characterized in the 1940s. Griffith identified a substance capable of transmitting infectiousness, which Avery, MacLeod, and McCarty showed was DNA. • Hershey and Chase confirmed that DNA, and not protein, is the genetic material. • Using Chargaff's discovery that the number of adenine bases equals the number of thymines, and the number of guanines equals the number of cytosines, along with Franklin's discovery that DNA is regular and symmetrical in structure, Watson and Crick deciphered the structure of DNA.

9.2 DNA Structure

A **gene** is a section of a DNA molecule whose sequence of building blocks specifies the sequence of amino acids in a particular protein. The activity of the protein is responsible for the phenotype associated with the gene. The fact that different building blocks combine to form nucleic acids enables them to carry information, as the letters of an alphabet combine to form words. A gene may also encode RNA that does not specify a protein, but instead assists in protein synthesis or controls gene expression. These types of genes are discussed in chapters 10 and 11.

Inherited traits are diverse because proteins have diverse functions; biological proteins are extremely varied in three-dimensional shape and function. Pea color, plant height, and the chemical reactions of metabolism are all the consequence of enzyme activity. Table 10.1 lists some proteins in the human body. Proteins such as collagen and elastin provide structural support in connective tissues, and actin and myosin form muscle. Hemoglobin transports oxygen, and antibodies protect against infection. Malfunctioning or inactive proteins, which reflect genetic defects, can devastate health, as we have seen for many hereditary disorders. Most of the amino acids that are assembled into proteins ultimately come from the diet; the body synthesizes the others.

The structure of DNA is easiest to understand if we begin with the smallest components. A single building block of DNA is a **nucleotide.** It consists of one deoxyribose sugar, one phosphate group (which is a phosphorus atom bonded to four oxygen atoms), and one nitrogenous base. **Figure 9.7** shows the components of a nucleotide and the chemical structures of the four types of bases. Adenine (A) and guanine (G) are **purines,** which have a two-ring structure. Cytosine (C) and thymine (T) are **pyrimidines,** which have a single-ring structure. It was the similar shapes of the purine/pyrimidine pairs that provided Watson with the final clue to DNA's structure. Reading 9.2 explains how clues in DNA base sequences helped investigators solve a mystery of history.

Nucleotides join into long chains when chemical bonds form between the deoxyribose sugars and the phosphates, which creates a continuous **sugar-phosphate backbone**

Table 9.1		
The Road to the Double Helix		
Investigator	**Contribution**	**Timeline**
Friedrich Miescher	Isolated nuclein in white blood cell nuclei	1869
Frederick Griffith	Transferred killing ability between types of bacteria	1928
Oswald Avery, Colin MacLeod, and Maclyn McCarty	Discovered that DNA transmits killing ability in bacteria	1940s
Alfred Hershey and Martha Chase	Determined that the part of a virus that infects and replicates is its nucleic acid and not its protein	1950
Phoebus Levene, Erwin Chargaff, Maurice Wilkins, and Rosalind Franklin	Discovered DNA components, proportions, and positions	1909–early 1950s
James Watson and Francis Crick	Elucidated DNA's three-dimensional structure	1953

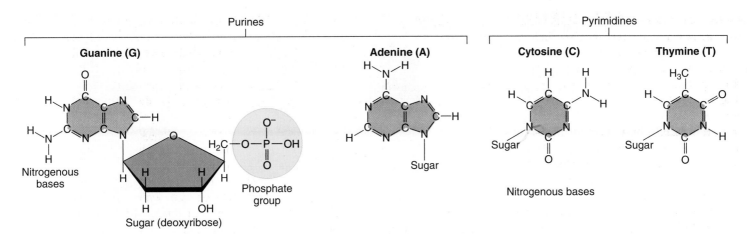

Figure 9.7 DNA bases are the informational parts of nucleotides. Each nucleotide of a nucleic acid consists of a 5-carbon sugar, a phosphate group, and an organic, nitrogenous base (G, A, C, and T). The DNA bases adenine and guanine are purines, each composed of a six-membered organic ring plus a five-membered ring. Cytosine and thymine are pyrimidines, each with a single six-membered ring. (Within the molecules, C, H, N, O, and P are atoms of carbon, hydrogen, nitrogen, oxygen, and phosphorus, respectively.)

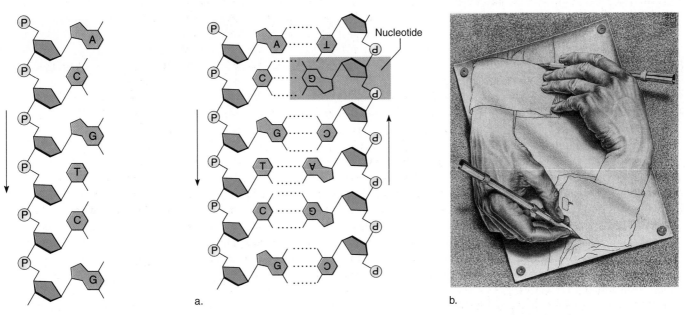

Figure 9.8 A chain of nucleotides.
A single DNA strand consists of a chain of nucleotides that forms when the deoxyribose sugars (green) and phosphates (yellow) bond to create a sugar-phosphate backbone. The bases A, C, G, and T are indicated in blue.

Figure 9.9 DNA consists of two chains of nucleotides. **(a)** The nitrogenous bases of one strand are held to the nitrogenous bases of the second strand by hydrogen bonds (dotted lines). Note that the sugars point in opposite directions—that is, the strands are antiparallel. **(b)** Artist M. C. Escher captured the essence of antiparallelism in his depiction of hands.

(**figure 9.8**). Two such chains of nucleotides align head-to-toe, as **figure 9.9** depicts. M. C. Escher's drawing of hands in figure 9.9*b* resembles the spatial relationship of the two strands of the DNA double helix.

The opposing orientation of the two nucleotide chains is called **antiparallelism.** It derives from the structure of the sugar-phosphate backbone. Antiparallelism becomes evident when the carbons of the sugars are assigned numbers to indicate their positions in the molecule. The carbons are numbered from 1 to 5, starting with the first carbon moving clockwise from the oxygen in each sugar in **figure 9.10*a*.** One chain runs from the 5 carbon (top of the figure) to the 3 carbon, but the chain aligned with it runs from the 3 to the 5 carbon. These ends are called 5′ ("5 prime") and 3′ ("3 prime").

The symmetrical double helix of DNA forms when nucleotides containing A pair with those containing T, and nucleotides containing G pair with those carrying C. Because purines have two rings and pyrimidines one, the consistent pairing of a purine with a pyrimidine ensures that the double helix has the same width throughout. These specific purine-pyrimidine couples are called **complementary base pairs.** Chemical attractions called hydrogen bonds hold the base pairs together. Two hydrogen bonds join A and T, and three hydrogen

DNA Makes History

One night in July 1918, Tsar Nicholas II of Russia and his family met gruesome deaths at the hands of Bolsheviks in a Ural mountain town called Ekaterinburg (**figure 1**). Captors led the tsar, tsarina, three of their daughters, the family physician, and three servants to a cellar and shot them, bayoneting those whose diamond jewelry deflected the bullets. The executioners then stripped the bodies and loaded them onto a truck, planning to hurl them down a mine shaft. But the truck broke down, and the killers instead placed the bodies in a shallow grave, then damaged them with sulfuric acid to mask their identities.

In another July—many years later, in 1991—two Russian amateur historians found the grave. Because they were aware that the royal family had spent its last night in Ekaterinburg, they alerted the government that they might have unearthed the long-sought bodies of the Romanov family. An official forensic examination soon determined that the skeletons represented nine individuals. The sizes of the skeletons indicated that three were children, and the porcelain, platinum, and gold in some of the teeth suggested royalty. Unfortunately, the acid had so destroyed the facial bones that some conventional forensic tests were not feasible. But one type of evidence survived—DNA. Thanks to DNA amplification made possible by the polymerase chain reaction (PCR—see section 9.4), researchers obtained enough genetic material to solve the mystery.

British researchers eagerly examined DNA from cells in the skeletal remains. DNA sequences specific to the Y chromosome enabled the investigators to distinguish males from females. Then the genetic material of mitochondria, inherited from mothers only, established one woman as the mother of the children.

But a mother, her children, and companions were not necessarily a royal family. The researchers had to connect the skeletons to known relatives of Tsar Nicholas II. To do

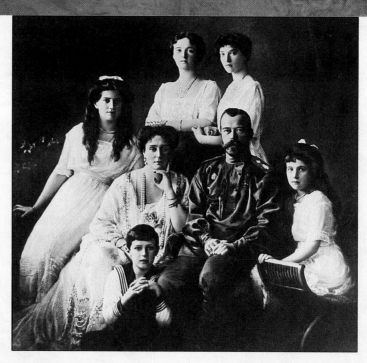

Figure 1 DNA profiling sheds light on history. DNA analysis identified the remains of the murdered Romanovs—and revealed an interesting genetic quirk.

so, they again turned to DNA. However, an inherited quirk proved, at first, to be quite confusing.

The challenge in proving that the male remains with fancy dental work were once Tsar Nicholas II centered around nucleotide position 16169 of a mitochondrial gene whose sequence is highly variable among individuals. About 70 percent of the bone cells examined from the remains had cytosine (C) at this position, while the remainder had thymine (T). Skeptics at first suspected contamination or a laboratory error, but when the odd result was repeated, researchers realized that this historical case had revealed a genetic phenomenon called heteroplasmy. The bone cells of this man apparently harbored two populations of mitochondria, one type with C at this position, the other with T.

The DNA of a living blood relative of the tsar, Countess Xenia Cheremeteff-Sfiri, had only T at nucleotide site 16169. Xenia is the great-granddaughter of Tsar Nicholas II's sister. However, mitochondrial DNA from Xenia and the murdered man matched at every other site. DNA of another living rel-

ative, the Duke of Fife, the great-grandson of Nicholas's maternal aunt, matched Xenia at the famed 16169 site. A closer relative, Nicholas's nephew Tikhon Kulikovsky, refused to lend his DNA, citing anger at the British for not assisting the tsar's family during the Bolshevik revolution.

But the story wasn't over. In yet another July, in 1994, researchers would finally solve the mystery.

Attention turned to Nicholas's brother, Grand Duke of Russia Georgij Romanov. In 1899, Georgij had died at age 28 of tuberculosis. His body was exhumed in July 1994, and researchers sequenced the troublesome mitochondrial gene in bone cells from his leg. They found a match! Georgij's mitochondrial DNA had the same polymorphic site as the man murdered in Siberia, who was, therefore, Tsar Nicholas II. The researchers calculated the probability that the remains are truly those of the tsar, rather than resembling Georgij's unusual DNA sequence by chance, as 130 million to 1. The murdered Russian royal family can finally rest in peace, thanks to DNA analysis.

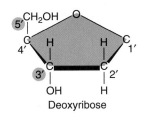

a.

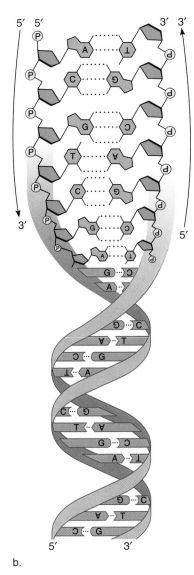

b.

Figure 9.10 DNA is directional.

(a) The antiparallel nature of the DNA double helix becomes apparent when the carbons in the sugar are numbered. **(b)** One half of the double helix runs in a 5′ to 3′ direction, and the other half runs in a 3′ to 5′ direction.

bonds join G and C, as **figure 9.11** shows. Complementary base pairing is crucial to the utilization of genetic information, and to many biotechnologies. Finally, the DNA assumes the double helix form when the

antiparallel, base-paired strands twist about one another in a regular fashion. The double-stranded, helical structure of DNA gives it great strength—50 times the strength of single-stranded DNA, which would not form a helix. The many negative charges of the phosphate groups on the outside of the molecule attract positively charged DNA binding proteins, whose interactions are critical to using genetic information.

DNA molecules are incredibly long. The DNA of the smallest human chromosome, if stretched out, would be 14 millimeters long. But it is packed into a chromosome that, during cell division, is only 2 micrometers long. This means that the DNA molecule must fold so tightly that its compacted length shrinks by a factor of 7000:

$$\left(\frac{14 \times 10^{-3} \text{ meters}}{2 \times 10^{-6} \text{ meters}} \right)$$

Various types of proteins compress the DNA without damaging or tangling it. Scaffold proteins form frameworks that guide DNA strands. Then, the DNA coils around proteins called **histones,** forming a beads-on-a-string-like structure. The bead part is called a **nucleosome.** It is a little like taking a very long, thin piece of thread, and wrapping parts of it around small spools or your fingers, to keep it from unraveling and tangling. In this way, the DNA wraps at several levels, until it is compacted into a chromosome (**figure 9.12**). A nucleosome forms around packets of eight histone proteins (a pair of each of four types of histones). A fifth type of histone anchors nucleosomes to short "linker" regions of DNA, which then tighten the nucleosomes into fibers 30 nanometers (nm) in diameter. At any given time, only small portions of the DNA double helix peek out from surrounding proteins. Chemical modification of the histones control when particular parts of the genome are exposed so that their information can be accessed. (This is discussed further in Chapter 11.) DNA also unwinds locally when it replicates.

Altogether, the chromosome substance is called **chromatin,** which means "colored material." Chromatin is much more than DNA. It is about 30 percent histone proteins, 30 percent DNA binding proteins, 30 percent DNA, and 10 percent RNA. Points along the chromatin attach it, in great

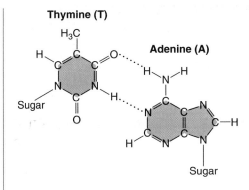

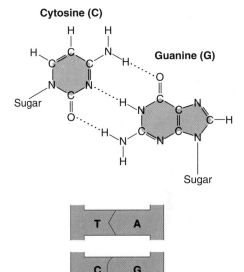

Figure 9.11 DNA base pairs.
The key to the constant width of the DNA double helix is the pairing of purines with pyrimidines. Two hydrogen bonds join adenine and thymine; three hydrogen bonds link cytosine and guanine.

loops, to nuclear matrix material on the inner face of the nuclear membrane. Without the proteins that are part of chromatin, it is unlikely that DNA would be biologically useful.

Key Concepts

The DNA double helix is a spiral ladder-like structure, its backbone comprised of alternating deoxyribose and phosphate groups and its rungs formed by complementary pairs of A-T and G-C bases. A and G are purines; T and C are pyrimidines. The DNA double helix is antiparallel, its strands running in an opposite head-to-toe manner. DNA winds tightly about histone proteins, forming nucleosomes, which in turn wind into a tighter structure to form chromatin.

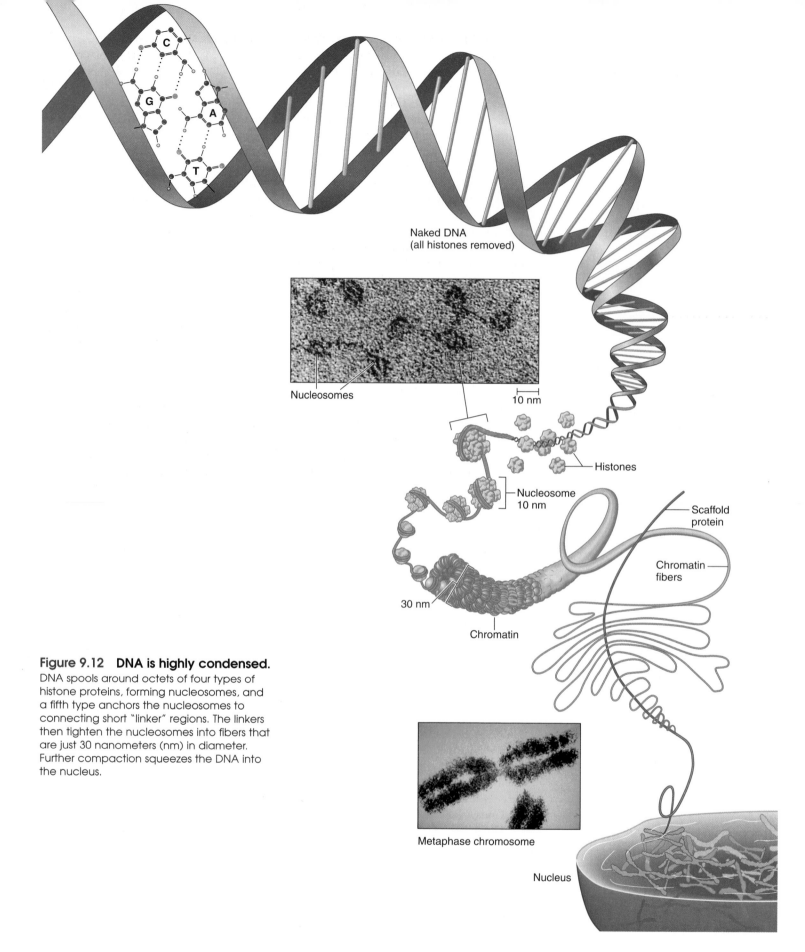

Naked DNA
(all histones removed)

Nucleosomes

10 nm

Histones

Nucleosome
10 nm

Scaffold
protein

Chromatin
fibers

30 nm

Chromatin

Metaphase chromosome

Nucleus

Figure 9.12 DNA is highly condensed.
DNA spools around octets of four types of histone proteins, forming nucleosomes, and a fifth type anchors the nucleosomes to connecting short "linker" regions. The linkers then tighten the nucleosomes into fibers that are just 30 nanometers (nm) in diameter. Further compaction squeezes the DNA into the nucleus.

9.3 DNA Replication—Maintaining Genetic Information

As soon as Watson and Crick deciphered the structure of DNA, its mechanism for replication became obvious. They ended their report on the structure of DNA with the oft-quoted statement, "It has not escaped our notice that the specific pairing we have postulated immediately suggests a possible copying mechanism for the genetic material."

Replication Is Semiconservative

Watson and Crick envisioned DNA as an immense molecule unwinding and exposing unpaired bases that would attract their complements, and form two double helices from one. This route to replication is called **semiconservative,** because each new DNA molecule conserves half of the original double helix. But separating the long strands posed a huge physical challenge. Wrote Max Delbrück, another of the founders of molecular biology, "For a DNA molecule of molecular weight 3,000,000 there would be about 500 turns around each other. These would have to be untwiddled to separate the strands." Although "untwiddled" is hardly a scientific term, the problem at hand was clear—separating the DNA strands was like having to keep two pieces of thread the length of a football field from tangling.

Some researchers suggested that DNA replicated some other way. Gunther Stent, another early molecular biologist, named three possible mechanisms of DNA replication: semiconservative; **conservative,** with one double helix specifying creation of a second double helix; or **dispersive,** with a double helix shattering into pieces that would then join with newly synthesized DNA pieces to form two molecules (**figure 9.13**).

An experimental approach to reveal how DNA replicates was first suggested in 1941, when English geneticist J. B. S. Haldane wrote, "How can one distinguish between model and copy? Perhaps you could use heavy nitrogen atoms in the food supplied to your cell, hoping that the 'copy' genes would contain it while the models did not."

Delbrück suggested using radioactivity to distinguish new and old DNA, but the results were fuzzy. In 1957, two young researchers, Matthew Meselson and Franklin Stahl, tried the very experiment that Haldane had suggested, without knowing he had done so. Meselson and Stahl looked at DNA replication in bacteria. Their experiments were an excellent illustration of scientific inquiry, because they not only supported one hypothesis, but disproved the other two.

Meselson and Stahl labeled newly synthesized DNA with heavy nitrogen (^{15}N), which could then be distinguished from older DNA that had been synthesized with the more common lighter form, ^{14}N. The idea was that DNA that incorporated the heavy nitrogen could be separated from newly synthesized DNA that incorporated the normal lighter nitrogen by its greater density. DNA in which one half of the double helix was light and one half heavy would be of intermediate density.

In their **density shift experiments,** Meselson and Stahl grew cells on media with heavy nitrogen and then shifted the cells to media with light nitrogen. In this way they traced replicating DNA through several cell divisions. The researchers grew cells, broke them open, extracted DNA, and spun it in a centrifuge. The heavier DNA

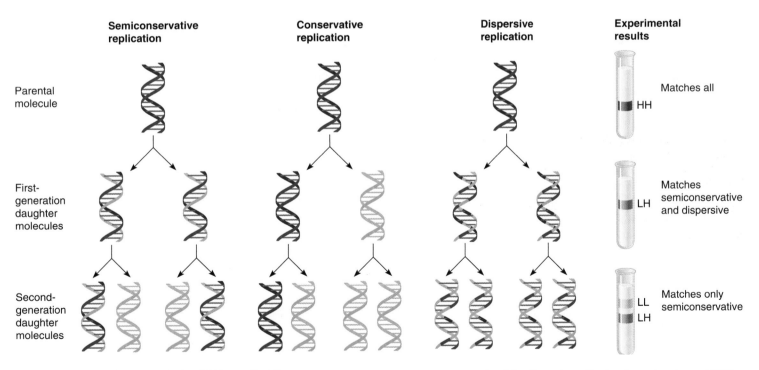

Figure 9.13   Three models for DNA replication.   Density shift experiments distinguished the three hypothesized mechanisms of DNA replication. DNA molecules containing light nitrogen are designated "LL" and those with heavy nitrogen, "HH." Molecules containing both isotopes are designated "LH." These experiments established that DNA replication is semiconservative.

sank to the bottom of the centrifuge tube, the light DNA rose to the top, and the heavy-light double helices settled in the middle area of the tube.

Meselson and Stahl grew *E. coli* on media containing ^{15}N for several generations, making all of the DNA heavy. They knew this because only "heavy-heavy" molecules appeared in the tube after centrifugation. They then shifted the bacteria to media containing ^{14}N, allowing enough time for the bacteria to divide only once (about 30 minutes).

When Meselson and Stahl collected the DNA after one generation and centrifuged it, the double helices were all of intermediate density, occupying a region in the middle of the tube, indicating that they contained half ^{14}N and half [15]N. This pattern was consistent with semiconservative DNA replication—but it was also consistent with a dispersive mechanism. In contrast, the result of conservative replication would have been one band of material in the tube completely labeled with ^{15}N, corresponding to one double helix, and another totally "light" band containing ^{14}N only, corresponding to the other double helix. This did not happen.

To definitively distinguish among the three routes to DNA replication, supporting the semiconservative mode and disproving the others, Meselson and Stahl extended the experiment one more generation. If the semiconservative mechanism held up, each hybrid (half ^{14}N and half ^{15}N) double helix present after the first generation following the shift to ^{14}N medium would part and assemble a new half from bases labeled only with [14]N. This would produce two double helices with one [15]N (heavy) and one [14]N (light) chain, plus two double helices containing only [14]N. The tube would have one heavy-light band and one light-light band. This is indeed what Meselson and Stahl saw.

The conservative mechanism would have yielded two bands in the tube in the third generation, indicating three completely light double helices for every completely heavy one. The third generation for the dispersive model would have been a single large band, somewhat higher than the second-generation band because additional ^{14}N would have been randomly incorporated.

Steps and Participants in DNA Replication

After experiments demonstrated the semiconservative nature of DNA replication, the next challenge was to decipher the steps of the process.

When DNA replicates, it must unwind, break, build a new nucleotide chain, and mend (**figure 9.14**). A contingent of enzymes carries out the process. Enzymes called **helicases** unwind and hold apart replicating DNA so that other enzymes can guide the assembly of a new DNA strand. A helicase looks like a bagel through which replicating DNA is threaded. One DNA strand shoots through the bagel's hole, at the rate of 300 nucleotides per second, while the other strand is moved out of the way. Helicases can also repair errors in replicated DNA.

Human DNA replicates at a rate of about 50 bases per second. To get the job done, a human chromosome replicates simultaneously at hundreds of points along its length, and the individual pieces join. A site where DNA is locally opened, resembling a fork, is called a **replication fork.**

DNA replication begins when a helicase breaks the hydrogen bonds that connect a base pair (**figure 9.15**). This first step occurs at a region called an origin of replication site. Binding proteins hold the two strands apart. Another enzyme, **primase,** then attracts complementary RNA nucleotides to build a short piece of RNA, called an **RNA primer,** at the start of each segment of DNA to be replicated. The RNA primer is required because the major replication enzyme, **DNA polymerase** (DNAP), can only add bases to an existing strand. (A polymerase is an enzyme that builds a polymer, which is a chain of chemical building blocks.) Next, the RNA primer attracts DNA polymerase, which brings in DNA nucleotides complementary to the exposed bases on the parental strand; this strand serves as a mold, or template. New bases are added one at a time, starting at the RNA primer, and the new DNA strand grows as hydrogen bonds form between the complementary bases.

DNA polymerase (DNAP) works directionally, adding new nucleotides to the exposed 3′ end of the sugar in the growing strand. Replication proceeds in a 5′ to 3′

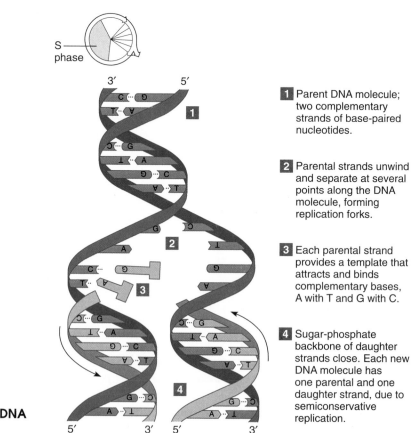

Figure 9.14
Overview of DNA replication.

1. Parent DNA molecule; two complementary strands of base-paired nucleotides.

2. Parental strands unwind and separate at several points along the DNA molecule, forming replication forks.

3. Each parental strand provides a template that attracts and binds complementary bases, A with T and G with C.

4. Sugar-phosphate backbone of daughter strands close. Each new DNA molecule has one parental and one daughter strand, due to semiconservative replication.

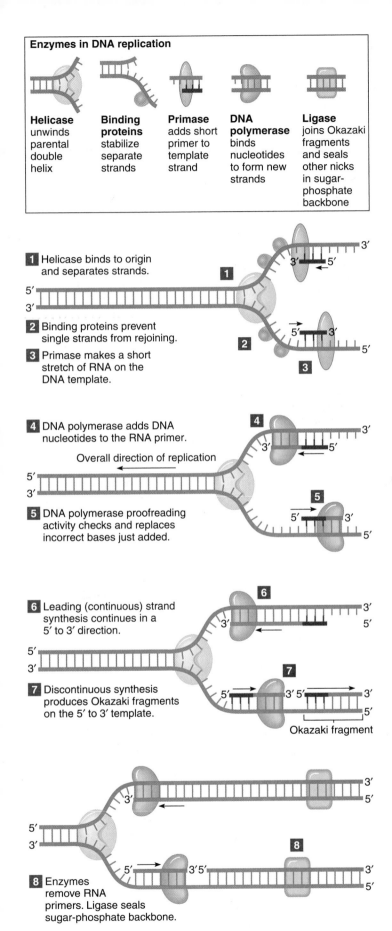

direction, because this is the only chemical configuration in which DNAP can add bases. How can the growing fork proceed in one direction, when 5′ to 3′ elongation requires movement in both directions? The answer is that on at least one strand, replication is discontinuous. It is accomplished in small pieces from the inner part of the fork outward in a pattern similar to backstitching. **Ligase** is an enzyme that then seals the sugar-phosphate backbones of the pieces, building the new strand. These pieces, up to 150 nucleotides long, are called Okazaki fragments, after their discoverer (see figure 9.15).

DNA polymerase also "proofreads" as it goes, excising mismatched bases and inserting correct ones. At the same time, another enzyme, a type of **exonuclease,** removes the RNA primer and replaces it with the correct DNA bases. Finally, ligases seal the sugar-phosphate backbone. Ligase comes from a Latin word meaning "to tie."

Key Concepts

Experiments that followed the distribution of labeled DNA showed that DNA replication is semiconservative, not conservative or dispersive.
  Enzymes orchestrate DNA replication. DNA replication occurs simultaneously at several points on each chromosome, and the pieces then join. At each initiation site, primase directs synthesis of a short RNA primer. DNA eventually replaces this RNA primer. DNA polymerase adds complementary DNA bases to the RNA primer, building a new half of a helix against each template. Finally, ligase joins the sugar-phosphate backbone. DNA is synthesized in a 5′ to 3′ direction, discontinuously on one strand.

Figure 9.15 DNA replication takes many steps.
Because DNA can only be replicated in a 5′ to 3′ direction, the process occurs continuously on one strand (called the leading strand) and discontinuously, similar to backstitching, as Okazaki fragments form against the other strand of parental DNA (called the lagging strand). Enzymes replicate DNA. First, a helicase opens the initiation site. Then primase adds a short RNA primer, which is later removed by an enzyme and replaced with DNA. DNA polymerase extends the new strands and proofreads the base sequences, and ligase seals the sugar-phosphate backbone and joins Okazaki fragments.

9.4 PCR—Directing DNA Replication

Every time a cell divides, it replicates all of its DNA. A technology called the **polymerase chain reaction** (PCR) uses DNA polymerase to rapidly produce millions of copies of a specific DNA sequence of interest.

Applications of PCR are eclectic. In forensics, it is used routinely to establish blood relationships, to identify remains, and to help convict criminals or exonerate the falsely accused. When used to amplify the nucleic acids of microorganisms, viruses, and other parasites, PCR is useful in agriculture, veterinary medicine, environmental science, and human health care. In genetics, PCR is both a crucial laboratory tool to identify genes as well as the basis of many diagnostic tests. **Table 9.2** lists some uses of PCR.

PCR was born in the mind of Kary Mullis on a moonlit night in northern California in 1983. As he drove the hills, Mullis was thinking about the incredible precision and power of DNA replication and, quite suddenly, a way to tap into that power popped into his mind. He excitedly explained his idea to his girlfriend and then went home to think it through further. "It was difficult for me to sleep with deoxyribonuclear bombs exploding in my brain," he wrote much later.

The idea behind PCR was so simple that Mullis had trouble convincing his superiors at Cetus Corporation that he was really onto something. He spent the next year using the technique to amplify a well-studied gene. One by one, other researchers glimpsed Mullis's vision of that starry night. After winning over his colleagues at Cetus, Mullis published a landmark 1985 paper and filed patent applications, launching the field of gene amplification. Mullis received only a $10,000 bonus from Cetus for his invention, which the company sold to another for $300 million. Mullis did, however, win a Nobel prize.

PCR rapidly replicates a selected sequence of DNA in a test tube (**figure 9.16**). The requirements include:

1. Knowing parts of a target DNA sequence to be amplified.

2. Two types of lab-made, single-stranded, short pieces of DNA called primers. These are complementary in sequence to opposite ends of the target sequence.

3. A large supply of the four types of DNA nucleotide building blocks.

4. Taq1, a DNA polymerase produced by *Thermus aquaticus,* a microbe that inhabits hot springs. This enzyme is adapted to its host's hot surroundings and makes PCR easy because it does not fall apart when DNA is heated.

In the first step of PCR, heat is used to separate the two strands of the target DNA, and the two short DNA primers and Taq1 DNA polymerase are added. Next, the temperature is lowered. The primers bind by complementary base pairing to the separated target strands. In the third step, the Taq1 DNA polymerase adds bases to the primers and builds a sequence complementary to the target sequence. The newly synthesized strands then act as templates in the next round of replication, which is initiated immediately by raising the temperature. All of this is done in an automated device called a thermal cycler that controls the key temperature changes. The heat-resistant DNA polymerase is crucial to the process.

The pieces of DNA accumulate exponentially. The number of amplified pieces of DNA equals 2^n, where n equals the number of temperature cycles. After just 20 cycles, 1 million copies of the original sequence have accumulated in the test tube.

PCR's greatest strength is that it works on crude samples of rare, old, and minute

---

Table 9.2

Uses of PCR

PCR has been used to amplify DNA from:

- a cremated man, from skin cells left in his electric shaver, to diagnose an inherited disease in his children.
- human tissue from the site of the World Trade Center in the days following September 11, 2001, to identify victims.
- a preserved quagga (a relative of the zebra) and a marsupial wolf, both of which are extinct.
- microorganisms that cannot be cultured for study.
- the brain of a 7,000-year-old human mummy.
- the digestive tracts of carnivores, to reveal food web interactions.
- roadkills and carcasses washed ashore, to identify locally threatened species.
- products illegally made from endangered species, such as powdered rhinoceros horn, sold as an aphrodisiac.
- genetically altered bacteria that are released in field tests, to follow their dispersion.
- one cell of an 8-celled human embryo to detect a disease-related genotype.
- poached moose meat in hamburger.
- remains in Jesse James's grave, to make a positive identification.
- the guts of genital crab lice on a rape victim, which matched the DNA of the suspect.
- dried semen on a blue dress belonging to a White House intern.
- fur from Snowball, a cat used to link a murder suspect to a crime.

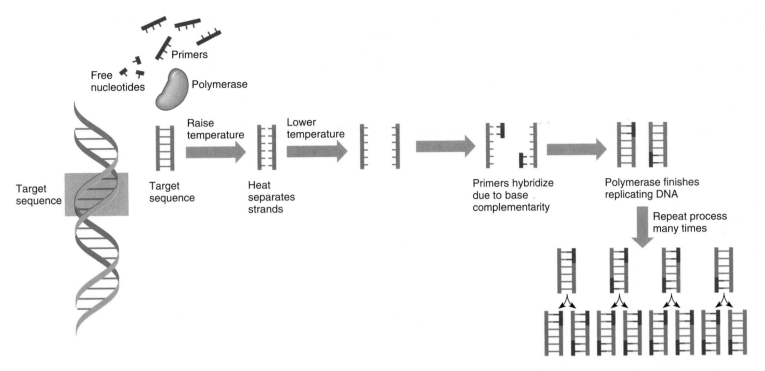

Figure 9.16 Amplifying a specific DNA sequence. In the polymerase chain reaction, specific primers along with a thermostable DNA polymerase and plenty of free nucleotides, are used to replicate a DNA sequence of interest. The reaction rapidly builds up millions of copies of the target sequence. Figure 14.6 shows an application of PCR.

sequences, as Reading 9.2 describes. PCR's greatest weakness, ironically, is its exquisite sensitivity. A blood sample submitted for diagnosis of an infection, if contaminated by leftover DNA from a previous test or a stray eyelash from the person running the reaction, can yield a false result.

PCR has revolutionized genetics research and biotechnology, impacting diverse fields, as table 9.2 shows. More philosophically, PCR illustrates how a natural process can be understood and applied, with long-lasting, practical, and even life-saving results.

Key Concepts

PCR is a technique that induces rapid DNA replication of a small, selected part of an organism's genome. It has many uses in forensics, agriculture, and medicine.

Summary

9.1 Experiments Identify and Describe the Genetic Material

1. DNA encodes information that the cell uses to synthesize protein. DNA can also replicate, so that its information is passed on.

2. Many experimenters described DNA and showed it to be the hereditary material. Miescher identified DNA in white blood cell nuclei. Garrod conceptually connected heredity to symptoms caused by enzyme abnormalities. Griffith identified a substance that transmits infectiousness in pneumonia-causing bacteria; Avery, MacLeod, and McCarty discovered that the transforming principle is DNA; and

Hershey and Chase confirmed that the genetic material is DNA and not protein.

3. Levene described the three components of a DNA building block and found that they appear in DNA in equal amounts. Chargaff discovered that the amount of **adenine** (A) equals the amount of **thymine** (T), and the amount of **guanine** (G) equals that of **cytosine** (C). Rosalind Franklin's photo 51 depiction of B DNA showed that the molecule is a certain type of helix. Watson and Crick put all these clues together to deduce DNA's double helix structure.

9.2 DNA Structure

4. A **nucleotide** is a DNA building block. It consists of a **deoxyribose**, a phosphate, and a nitrogenous base.

5. The rungs of the DNA double helix consist of hydrogen-bonded complementary base pairs (A with T, and C with G). The rails are chains of alternating sugars and phosphates that run **antiparallel** to each other. DNA is highly coiled, and complexed with protein to form **chromatin.**

9.3 DNA Replication—Maintaining Genetic Information

6. Meselson and Stahl demonstrated the **semiconservative** nature of DNA replication with **density shift experiments.**

7. During replication, the DNA unwinds locally at several origin of replication sites. **Replication forks** form as the hydrogen bonds break between initial base pairs. **Primase** builds short RNA primers, which DNA sequences eventually replace. Next, **DNA polymerase** fills in DNA bases, and **ligase** seals the sugar-phosphate backbone.

8. Replication proceeds in a 5′ to 3′ direction, so the process must be discontinuous in short stretches on one strand.

9.4 PCR—Directing DNA Replication

9. Gene amplification techniques, such as **PCR,** utilize the power and specificity of DNA replication enzymes to selectively amplify certain sequences.

10. In PCR, primers corresponding to a gene of interest direct the polymerization of supplied nucleotides to construct many copies of the gene.

Review Questions

1. DNA specifies and regulates the cell's synthesis of protein. If a cell contains all the genetic material required to carry out protein synthesis, why must its DNA be replicated?

2. Match the experiment described in the left column to the concept it illustrates in the right column.

   1. Density shift experiments

   2. Discovery of an acidic substance that includes nitrogen and phosphorus on dirty bandages

   3. "Blender experiments" that showed that the part of a virus that infects bacteria contains phosphorus, but not sulfur

   4. Determination that DNA contains equal amounts of guanine and cytosine, and of adenine and thymine

   5. Discovery that bacteria can transfer a "factor" that transforms a harmless strain into a lethal one

   a. DNA is the hereditary material

   b. Complementary base pairing is part of DNA structure and maintains a symmetrical double helix

   c. Identification of nuclein

   d. DNA, not protein, is the hereditary material

   e. DNA replication is semiconservative, not conservative or dispersive

3. What part of the DNA molecule encodes information?

4. Explain how DNA is a directional molecule in a chemical sense.

5. Place the following enzymes in the order in which they begin to function in DNA replication.

   ligase   primase
   exonuclease   helicases
   DNA polymerase

6. Write the sequence of a strand of DNA replicated from each of the following base sequences:

   a. T C G A G A A T C T C G A T T

   b. C C G T A T A G C C G G T A C

   c. A T C G G A T C G C T A C T G

7. Place in increasing size order:

   nucleosome

   histone protein

   chromatin

8. Define:

   a. antiparallelism

   b. semiconservative replication

   c. complementary base pairing

9. Describe two experiments that supported one hypothesis while also disproving another.

10. List the steps in DNA replication.

11. Why wouldn't PCR work if DNA replication were conservative or dispersive?

Applied Questions

1. In Bloom syndrome, ligase malfunctions. As a result, replication forks move too slowly. Why?

2. DNA contains the information that a cell uses to synthesize a particular protein. How do proteins assist in DNA replication?

3. To diagnose a rare form of encephalitis (brain inflammation), a researcher needs a million copies of a viral gene. She decides to use the polymerase chain reaction on a sample of the patient's cerebrospinal fluid, which bathes his infected brain. If one cycle of PCR takes two minutes, how long will it take the researcher to obtain her millionfold amplification?

4. Why would a DNA structure in which each base type could form hydrogen bonds with any of the other three base types not produce a molecule that is easily replicated?

5. A person with deficient or abnormal ligase may have an increased cancer risk and chromosomes that cannot heal breaks. The person is, nevertheless, alive. Why are there no people who lack DNA polymerase?

6. HIV infection was formerly diagnosed by detecting antibodies in a person's blood or documenting a decline in the number of the type of white blood cell that HIV initially infects. Why is PCR detection of HIV more sensitive?

7. Which do you think was the more far-reaching accomplishment, determining the structure of DNA, or sequencing the human genome? State a reason for your answer.

Web Activities

8. Go to http://www.genet.sickkids.on.ca/cftr/CFTRseq.html. Select twenty contiguous bases of the sequence for the cystic fibrosis gene and write the complementary sequence.

Case Studies

9. Researchers in Belgium discovered a new form of abnormal bone growth (a skeletal dysplasia), in two families with extensive consanguinity. Affected individuals have short limbs and fingers, a large head, and a narrow, malformed chest. The condition resembles dwarfism in the most extreme cases. It is autosomal recessive, and linkage mapping established chromosome 2 as the site of the causative gene. Examining the human genome sequence implicated a gene called IHH (for Indian hedgehog). The IHH gene produces a protein involved in signaling in growing bone tissue.

Examination of the gene in the affected families revealed the following substituted base in a part of the DNA sequence:

wild type ... C G T G C C G C T C G ...
mutant ... C G T G C T G C T C G

Hans and Eva Brinker are first cousins. Their first child, Peter, is normal, but their daughter Anna has the skeletal dysplasia. When Anna was diagnosed, geneticists examined Peter's gene and discovered that unlike his parents, he is not a carrier (heterozygote). Write the DNA sequence for this part of the IHH gene, in both copies of chromosome 2, for Hans, Eva, Peter, and Anna.

Learn to apply the skills of a genetic counselor with this additional case found in the *Case Workbook in Human Genetics:*

DNA replication

Suggested Readings

Holmes, Frederic Lawrence. 2001. *Meselson, Stahl, and the Replication of DNA: A History of the Most Beautiful Experiment in Biology.* New Haven: Yale University Press. The story of "untwiddling" DNA.

Kennedy, Don. April 11, 2003. DNA: One teacher's reflection. *Science* 300:213. A one-page history of the discovery of DNA structure and function.

Kilesnikov, Lev L., et al. February 15, 2001. Anatomical appraisal of the skulls and teeth associated with the family of Tsar Nicolay Romanov. *Anatomical Record* 265:15–32. Forensic analysis of skeletal remains supports DNA evidence that the royal Romanovs were brutally murdered.

Maddox, Brenda. 2002. *Rosalind Franklin: The Dark Lady of DNA.* New York: HarperCollins. A moving account of the tragically short life of Rosalind Franklin.

McElheny, Victor K. 2003. *Watson and DNA: Making a Scientific Revolution.* Cambridge, MA: Perseus Publishing. One of the best books on the discovery of the DNA double helix and the aftermath.

Pennisi, Elizabeth. April 11, 2003. DNA's cast of thousands. *Science* 300:282–85. Many researchers before and after Watson and Crick learned DNA's secrets.

Sherwood, Peter. April 24, 2003. DNA from Alberts to Zinder. *Nature* 422:806–7. Doodlings of DNA, from a who's who of geneticists.

Strasser, Bruno J. April 24, 2003. Who cares about the double helix? *Nature* 422:803–4. It wasn't until the 1990s, with the onset of the human genome project, that interest in the deciphering of DNA's structure peaked.

Watson, James. 2003. *DNA: The Secret of Life.* New York: Alfred A. Knopf. The codiscoverer of DNA's structure looks back on half a century of DNA science.

Weekly updates of current news related to human genetics are available through Power Web on your Online Learning Center.

Gene Action: From DNA to Protein

C H A P T E R

10

CHAPTER CONTENTS

10.1   Transcription—The Link Between Gene and Protein
The proteins that a particular type of cell manufactures constitute its proteome. The information in the nucleotide base sequence of a protein-encoding gene is transcribed into mRNA, which is then translated into the amino acid sequence of a protein.

10.2   Translation of a Protein
The genetic code is the correspondence between RNA base triplets and particular amino acids. It is universal—the same messenger RNA codons specify the same amino acids in humans, hippos, herbs, and bacteria. Ribosomes provide structural support and enzyme activity for transfer RNA molecules to align the designated amino acids against a messenger RNA. The amino acids are linked, building proteins.

10.3   Protein Folding
A protein must fold into a particular three-dimensional shape to function. The cell has a quality control system to ensure this. Misfolded proteins cause disease.

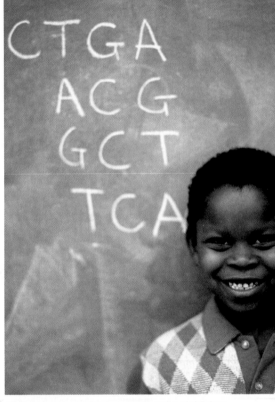

DNA sequences are familiar to schoolchildren.

DNA replication preserves genetic information by giving each new cell a complete set of operating instructions. A cell uses some of the information to manufacture proteins, which have a great variety of functions (**table 10.1**). First the process of **transcription** copies a particular part of the DNA sequence of a chromosome into an RNA molecule that is complementary to one strand of the DNA double helix. Then the process of **translation** uses the information copied into three types of RNA to manufacture a protein by aligning and joining the specified amino acids.

Cells replicate their DNA only during S phase of the cell cycle. In contrast, transcription and translation occur continuously, except during M phase, to supply the proteins essential for life as well as those that give a cell its specialized characteristics. This chapter considers the steps of transcription and translation (the utilization of genetic information), and the next chapter discusses control of these processes during development and under different circumstances (gene expression).

Watson and Crick, shortly after publishing their structure of DNA in 1953, described the relationship between nucleic acids and proteins as a directional flow of information called the "central dogma" (**figure 10.1**). As Francis Crick explained in 1957, "The specificity of a piece of nucleic acid is expressed solely by the sequence of its bases, and this sequence is a code for the amino acid sequence of a particular protein." This simple statement led to more than a decade of intense research to identify the participants in protein synthesis and discover how they interact. At center stage: RNA.

10.1 Transcription— The Link Between Gene and Protein

RNA is the bridge between gene and protein. RNA and DNA share an intimate relationship, as **figure 10.2** depicts. RNA is synthesized against (is complementary to) one side of the double helix, called the **template strand,** with the assistance of an enzyme, **RNA polymerase.** The other side of the DNA double helix is the **coding strand.**

RNA Structure and Types

RNA and DNA have similarities and differences (**figure 10.3** and **table 10.2**). They are both nucleic acids, consisting of sequences of nitrogen-containing bases joined by sugar-phosphate backbones. However, RNA

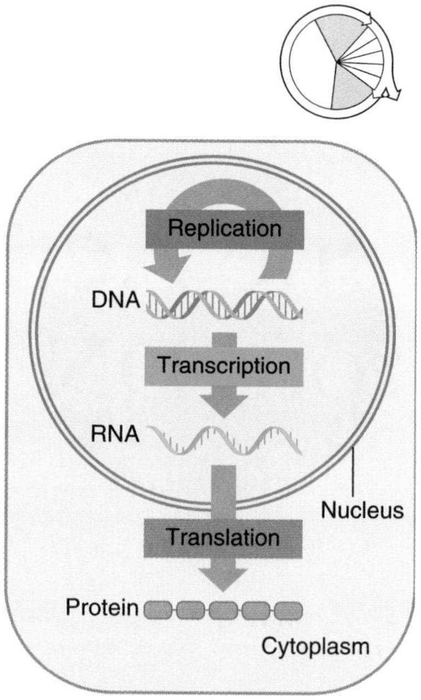

Figure 10.1 DNA to RNA to protein.
The central dogma of molecular biology states that information stored in DNA is copied to RNA (transcription), which is used to assemble proteins (translation). DNA replication perpetuates genetic information. This figure repeats within the chapter, with the part under discussion highlighted.

is usually single-stranded, whereas DNA is double-stranded. Also, RNA has the pyrimidine base **uracil** in place of DNA's thymine. As their names imply, RNA nucleotides include the sugar ribose, rather than DNA's deoxyribose. Functionally, DNA stores genetic information, whereas RNA controls how that information is used.

As RNA is synthesized along DNA, it folds into a three-dimensional shape, or **conformation,** that is determined by complementary base pairing within the same RNA molecule. These shapes are very important for RNA's functioning. The three major types of RNA are messenger RNA, ribosomal RNA, and transfer RNA (**table 10.3**). Table 11.2 describes other types of RNA molecules.

Messenger RNA (mRNA) carries the information that specifies a particular protein product. Each three mRNA bases in a row form a genetic code word, or **codon,** that specifies a certain amino acid. Recall that a protein is built of a chain of amino acids. Because genes vary in length, so do mature mRNA molecules. Most such mRNAs are 500 to 4,500 bases long. Specialized cells can carry out particular functions because they "express" certain

Table 10.1

Protein Diversity in the Human Body

Protein	Function
Actin, myosin, dystrophin	Muscle contraction
Antibodies, antigens, cytokines	Immunity
Carbohydrases, lipases, proteases, nucleases	Digestion (digestive enzymes)
Casein	Milk protein
Collagen, elastin	Connective tissue
Colony stimulating factors	Blood cell formation
DNA and RNA polymerase	DNA replication, gene expression
Ferritin	Iron transport in blood
Fibrin, thrombin	Blood clotting
Growth factors, kinases, cyclins	Cell division
Hemoglobin, myoglobin	Oxygen transport
Insulin, glucagon	Control of blood glucose level
Keratin	Hair structure
Tubulin, actin	Cell movements
Tumor suppressors	Cancer prevention

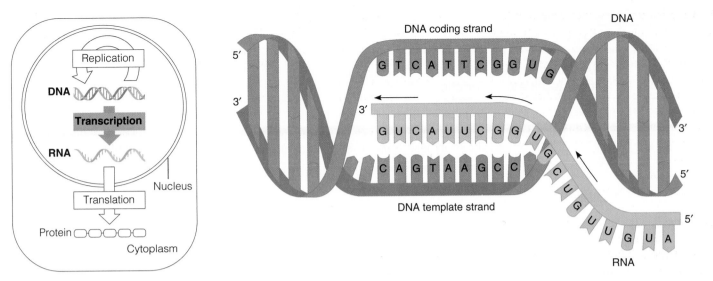

DNA coding strand

5′ G T C A T T C G G U G
DNA

3′

3′ G U C A U U C G G U G C U G U U G U A 5′

C A G T A A G C C

DNA template strand

RNA

Figure 10.2 The relationship among RNA, the DNA template strand, and the DNA coding strand. The RNA sequence is complementary to that of the DNA template strand and so is the same sequence as the DNA coding strand, with uracil (U) in place of thymine (T).

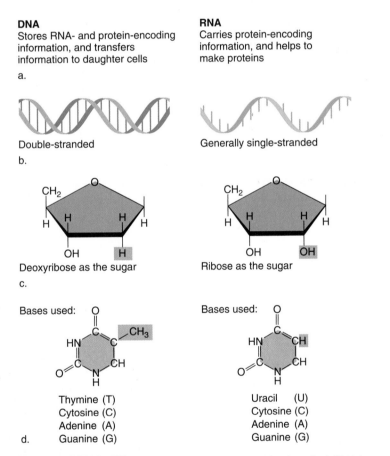

DNA
Stores RNA- and protein-encoding information, and transfers information to daughter cells

a.

Double-stranded

b.

Deoxyribose as the sugar

c.

Bases used:

Thymine (T)
Cytosine (C)
Adenine (A)
d.   Guanine (G)

RNA
Carries protein-encoding information, and helps to make proteins

Generally single-stranded

Ribose as the sugar

Bases used:

Uracil   (U)
Cytosine (C)
Adenine (A)
Guanine (G)

Figure 10.3 DNA and RNA differences. (a) DNA is double-stranded; RNA is usually single-stranded **(b)**. DNA nucleotides include deoxyribose, whereas RNA nucleotides have ribose **(c)**. Finally, DNA nucleotides include the pyrimidine thymine, whereas RNA has uracil **(d)**.

Table 10.2
How DNA and RNA Differ

DNA

Usually double-stranded

Thymine as a base

Deoxyribose as the sugar

Maintains protein-encoding information

Cannot function as an enzyme

RNA

Usually single-stranded

Uracil as a base

Ribose as the sugar

Carries protein-encoding information and
controls how information is used

Can function as an enzyme

subsets of genes—that is, they produce certain mRNA molecules, or transcripts. A muscle cell, for example, has many mRNAs that specify the abundant contractile proteins actin and myosin, whereas a skin cell contains many mRNAs that specify the scaly protein keratin.

To use the information encoded in an mRNA sequence, a cell requires two other major classes of RNA. **Ribosomal RNA** (rRNA) molecules range from 100 to nearly 3,000 nucleotides long. This type of RNA associates with certain proteins to form a ribosome. Recall from chapter 2 that a ribosome is a structural support for protein synthesis **(figure 10.4)**. A ribosome has two subunits that are separate in the cytoplasm but join at the initiation of protein synthesis. The larger ribosomal subunit has three types of rRNA molecules, and the small subunit has one. Ribosomal RNA, however, is much more than just a structural support. Certain rRNAs catalyze the formation of the peptide bonds between

Table 10.3

Major Types of RNA

Type of RNA	Size (number of nucleotides)	Function
mRNA	500–4,500+	Encodes amino acid sequence
rRNA	100–3,000	Associates with proteins to form ribosomes, which structurally support and catalyze protein synthesis
tRNA	75–80	Transports specific amino acids to the ribosome for protein synthesis.

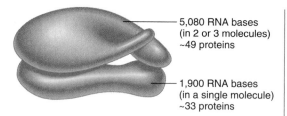

5,080 RNA bases
(in 2 or 3 molecules)
~49 proteins

1,900 RNA bases
(in a single molecule)
~33 proteins

Figure 10.4   The ribosome.   A ribosome from a eukaryotic cell, shown here, has two subunits; together, they contain 82 proteins and four rRNA molecules.

amino acids. Such an RNA with enzymatic function is called a **ribozyme.** Other rRNAs help to align the ribosome and mRNA.

The third major type of RNA molecule, **transfer RNA** (tRNA), binds an mRNA codon at one end and a specific amino acid at the other. A tRNA molecule is only 75 to 80 nucleotides long. Some of its bases weakly bond with each other, folding the tRNA into loops in a characteristic cloverleaf shape (**figure 10.5**). One loop of the tRNA has three bases in a row that form the **anticodon,** which is complementary to an mRNA codon. The end of the tRNA opposite the anticodon strongly bonds to a specific amino acid. A tRNA with a particular anticodon sequence always carries the same amino acid. (There are 20 types of amino acids in organisms.) For example, a tRNA with the anticodon sequence GAA always picks up the amino acid phenylalanine. Special enzymes attach amino acids to tRNAs that bear the appropriate anticodons.

Transcription Factors

Study of the control of gene expression began in 1961, when French biologists François Jacob and Jacques Monod described the remarkable ability of *E. coli* to produce the enzymes to metabolize the sugar lactose only when lactose is present in the cell's surroundings. What "tells" a simple bacterial cell to transcribe those proteins it needs—at exactly the right time?

Jacob and Monod discovered that a modified form of lactose "turned on" the genes whose encoded proteins break down the sugar. They named the set of genes that are coordinately controlled an operon, writing in 1961, "The genome contains not only a series of blueprints, but a coordinated program of protein synthesis and means of controlling its execution."

In bacteria, operons act like switches, turning transcription of a few genes on or off. In multicellular eukaryotes like ourselves, genetic control is more complex because different cell types express different subsets of genes. To manage such complexity, groups of proteins called **transcription factors** come together, forming an apparatus that binds DNA at certain sequences and initiates transcription at specific sites on a chromosome. The transcription factors, activated by signals from outside the cell, set the stage for transcription to begin by forming a pocket for RNA polymerase—the enzyme that actually builds an RNA chain.

Several types of transcription factors interact to transcribe a gene. Because transcription factors are proteins, they themselves are gene-encoded. The DNA sequences that transcription factors bind may be located near the genes they control, or as far as 40,000 bases away. DNA may form loops so that the genes encoding proteins that act together come near each other for transcription. Other proteins in the nucleus may help bring certain genes and their associated transcription factors in close proximity, much as books on a specialized topic might be grouped together in a library for easier access.

Many transcription factors have regions in common, called motifs, that fold into similar conformations. These motifs generally enable the transcription factor to bind DNA. They have very colorful names, such as "helix-turn-helix," "zinc fingers," and "leucine zippers," that reflect their distinctive shapes.

The human genome encodes at least 2,000 transcription factors. Overall, they control gene expression and link the genome to the environment. For example, lack of oxygen, such as from choking or smoking, sends signals that activate transcription factors to turn

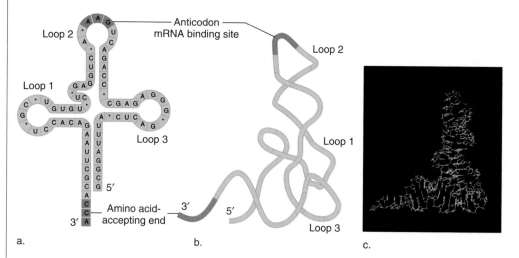

Figure 10.5   Transfer RNA.   (a) Certain nucleotide bases within a tRNA hydrogen bond with each other to give the molecule a "cloverleaf" conformation that can be represented in two dimensions. The darker bases at the top form the anticodon, the sequence that binds a complementary mRNA codon. Each tRNA terminates with the sequence CCA, where a particular amino acid covalently bonds. Three-dimensional representations of a tRNA **(b)** and **(c)** depict the loops that interact with the ribosome.

on dozens of genes that enable cells to handle the stress of low-oxygen conditions.

Mutations in transcription factor genes can have wide-ranging effects, because the factors control many genes. If the mutation is germinal, occurring in all of a person's cells, it may affect several organ systems. A mutation in a transcription factor gene that occurs in a somatic cell may cause cancer, as discussed further in chapter 18.

Steps of Transcription

How do transcription factors and RNA polymerase "know" where to bind to DNA to begin transcribing a specific gene? Transcription factors and RNA polymerase are attracted to a **promoter,** which is a special sequence that signals the start of the gene. Factors from outside the cell send signals that alter the chromatin structure in a way that exposes the promoter of a gene whose transcription is required under the particular conditions. **Figure 10.6** shows a simplified view of transcription factor binding, which sets up a site called a preinitiation complex to receive RNA polymerase. The first transcription factor to bind, called a TATA binding protein, is attracted to a DNA sequence called a TATA box—the base sequence TATA surrounded by long stretches of G and C. Once the first transcription factor binds, it attracts others in groups, and finally RNA polymerase joins the complex, binding just in front of the start of the gene sequence. The coming together of these components is **transcription initiation.**

Complementary base pairing underlies transcription, just as it does DNA replication. In the next stage, **transcription elongation,** enzymes unwind the DNA double helix locally, and RNA nucleotides bond with exposed complementary bases on the DNA template strand (see figure 10.2). RNA polymerase adds the RNA nucleotides in the sequence the DNA specifies, moving along the DNA strand in a 3′ to 5′ direction, synthesizing the RNA molecule in a 5′ to 3′ direction. A terminator sequence in the DNA indicates where the gene's RNA-encoding region ends. When it is reached **transcription termination** occurs (**figure 10.7a**). A typical rate of transcription is 20 bases per second.

RNA is transcribed using only one strand of the gene's DNA double helix as the template. The DNA strand that isn't transcribed is called the coding strand because its sequence is identical to that of the RNA, except with thymine (T) in place of uracil (U). Several RNAs may be transcribed from the same DNA template strand simultaneously (figure 10.7b). Since mRNA is relatively short-lived, with about half of it degraded every 10 minutes, a cell must constantly transcribe certain genes to maintain supplies of essential proteins. However, different genes on the same chromosome may be transcribed from different halves of the double helix.

To determine the sequence of RNA bases transcribed from a gene, write the RNA bases that are complementary to the template DNA strand, using uracil opposite adenine. For example, if a DNA template strand has the sequence

C C T A G C T A C

then it is transcribed into RNA with the sequence

G G A U C G A U G

and the coding DNA sequence is

G G A T C G A T G.

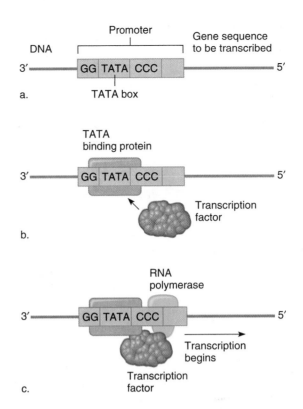

Figure 10.6 Setting the stage for transcription to begin. (a) Proteins that initiate transcription recognize specific sequences in the promoter region of a gene. **(b)** A binding protein recognizes the TATA region and binds to the DNA. This allows other transcription factors to bind. **(c)** The bound transcription factors form a pocket that allows RNA polymerase to bind and begin making RNA.

RNA Processing

In bacteria, RNA is translated into protein as soon as it is transcribed from DNA because a nucleus does not physically separate the two processes. In eukaryotic cells, mRNA must first exit the nucleus to enter the cytoplasm and organelles of the secretory pathway where protein synthesis occurs. RNA is altered before it participates in protein synthesis in these more complex cells. (Some protein synthesis may occur in the nucleus, although the evidence is controversial.)

First, after mRNA is transcribed, a short sequence of modified nucleotides, called a cap, is added to the 5′ end of the molecule. The cap consists of a backwardly inserted guanine (G), which attracts an enzyme that adds methyl groups (CH_3) both to the G and to one or two adjacent nucleotides. This methylated cap is a recognition site for protein synthesis. At the 3′ end, a special polymerase adds about 200 adenines, forming a "poly A tail." The poly A tail is necessary for protein synthesis to begin, and may also stabilize the mRNA so that it exists longer.

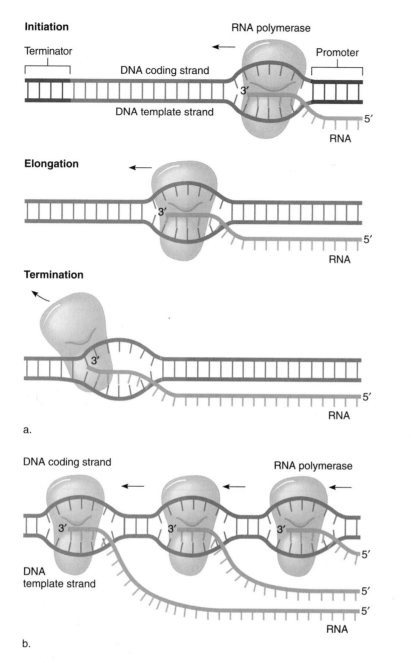

Figure 10.7 Transcription of RNA from DNA. **(a)** Transcription occurs in three stages: initiation, elongation, and termination. Initiation is the control point that determines which genes are transcribed. RNA nucleotides are added during elongation. A terminator sequence in the gene signals the end of transcription. **(b)** Many identical copies of RNA are simultaneously transcribed. Usually 100 or more DNA bases are between RNA polymerases.

Further changes occur to the capped, poly A tailed mRNA before it is translated into protein. Parts of mRNAs called **introns** (short for "intervening sequences") that were transcribed are now removed. The ends of the remaining molecule are spliced together before the mRNA is translated. The parts of mRNA that are translated are called **exons (figure 10.8).**

Once introns have been spliced out, enzymes check the remaining mRNA for accuracy. Messenger RNAs that are too short or too long may be stopped from exiting the nucleus. Such a proofreading mechanism also monitors tRNAs, ensuring that the correct conformation takes shape.

The mRNA prior to intron removal is the pre-mRNA. Introns are excised by small RNA molecules that are ribozymes, which associate with proteins to form small nuclear ribonucleoproteins (snRNPs), or "snurps." Four snurps form a structure called a spliceosome that cuts introns out and knits exons together to form the mature mRNA that exits the nucleus.

Introns range in size from 65 to 10,000 or more bases; the average intron is 3,365 bases. The average exon, in contrast, is 145 bases long. The number, size, and organization of introns vary from gene to gene. The coding portion of the average human gene is 1,340 bases, whereas the average total size of a gene is 27,000 bases. The dystrophin gene (see figure 2.1a) is 2,500,000 bases, but its corresponding mRNA sequence is only 14,000 bases! The gene contains 80 introns.

The discovery of introns surprised geneticists, who likened gene structure to a sentence in which all of the information contributes to the meaning. In the 1980s, some geneticists called introns "junk DNA," Francis Crick among them. The persistent finding of introns, however, convinced researchers that introns must have some function, or they would not have been retained through evolution. Said one speaker at a genomics conference, "Anyone who still thinks that introns have no function, please volunteer to have them removed, so we can see what they do." He had no takers.

The abundance and size of its introns distinguishes the human genome from those of our closest relatives. Introns have complicated analysis of the human genome sequence. Computer programs must hunt among strings of A, T, G, and C—raw DNA sequence—for the telltale signs of a protein-encoding gene, and then distinguish the exons from the introns. For example, a short sequence that indicates the start of a protein-encoding gene is called an open reading frame. Another clue is that dinucleotide repeats, such as CGCGCG, flank some introns, forming splice sites that signal the spliceosome where to cut and paste the RNA.

We do not know why some genes have introns and some do not. Introns may be ancient genes that have lost their original function, or they may be remnants of the DNA of viruses that once infected the cell. Combining genes in discrete pieces may be one way that our genome maximizes its informational content. Introns may enable exons to combine in different ways, even from different genes, much as many outfits can be assembled from a few basic pieces of clothing. The fact that some disease-causing mutations disrupt intron/exon splice sites suggests that this cutting and pasting of gene parts is essential to health, a subject discussed in chapter 12.

For some genes, mRNA is cut to different sizes in different tissues, which is called **alternate splicing.** The trimming of genes may explain how cell types use the same protein in slightly different ways in different tissues. This is the case for apolipoprotein B (apo B), which transports fats. In the small intestine, the mRNA that encodes apo B is short, and the protein binds and carries dietary fat. In the liver, however, the mRNA is not shortened, and the longer protein transports fats manufactured in the liver, which do not come from food.

Key Concepts

RNA differs from DNA: it is single-stranded, contains uracil instead of thymine and ribose instead of deoxyribose, and has different functions. Messenger RNA transmits information to build proteins. Each three mRNA bases in a row forms a codon that specifies a particular amino acid. Ribosomal RNA and proteins form ribosomes, which physically support protein synthesis and help catalyze bonding between amino acids. Transfer RNAs connect mRNA codons to amino acids. • Bacterial operons are simple gene control systems. In more complex organisms, transcription factors control gene expression. • Transcription proceeds as RNA polymerase inserts complementary RNA bases opposite the DNA template strand. • Messenger RNA gains a modified nucleotide cap and a poly A tail. Introns are transcribed and cut out, and exons are reattached. Introns are common, numerous, and large in human genes. Introns provide a way to maximize the information encoded in DNA. Certain genes are transcribed into different-sized RNAs in different cell types.

10.2 Translation of a Protein

Transcription copies the information encoded in a DNA base sequence into the complementary language of RNA. The next step is translating mRNA into the specified sequence of amino acids that forms a protein. Particular mRNA codons correspond to particular amino acids (**figure 10.9**). This correspondence between the chemical languages of mRNA and protein is the **genetic code.**

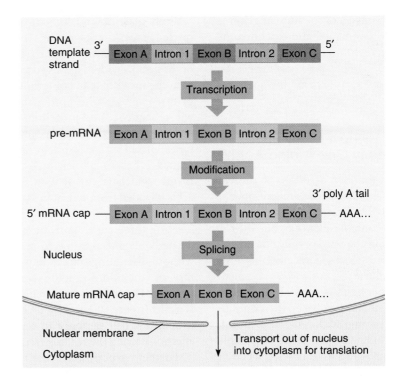

Figure 10.8   Messenger RNA processing—the maturing of the message.   Several steps are necessary to process pre-mRNA into mature mRNA. First, a large region of DNA containing the gene is transcribed. Then a modified nucleotide cap and poly A tail are added, and introns are spliced out. Finally, the mature mRNA is transported out of the nucleus.

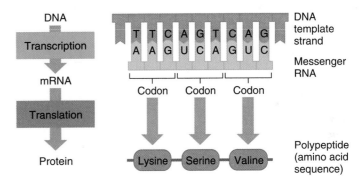

Figure 10.9   From DNA to RNA to protein.   Messenger RNA is transcribed from a locally unwound portion of DNA. In translation, transfer RNA matches mRNA codons with amino acids. Table 10.4 lists the codon-amino acid combinations that make up the genetic code.

Francis Crick hypothesized that an "adaptor" molecule would enable the RNA message to attract and link amino acids into proteins. He wrote in an unpublished paper in early 1955, "In its simplest form there would be 20 different kinds of adaptor molecule, one for each amino acid, and 20 different enzymes to join the amino acids to their adaptors." He was describing tRNAs, but the solution was more complex than originally thought. In the 1960s, many researchers deciphered the genetic code, determining which mRNA codons correspond to which amino acids.

The news media, on announcing the sequencing of the human genome in June 2000, widely reported that the "human genetic code" had been cracked. This was not the case. The genetic code is not unique to humans, and it was cracked decades ago. The code is the correspondence between nucleic acid triplet and amino acid, not the sequence itself.

Deciphering the Genetic Code

The researchers who deciphered the genetic code used logic and experiments. More recently, annotation of the human genome sequence has confirmed and extended the earlier work, revealing new nuances in the genetic code. To understand how the genetic code works, it is helpful to ask the questions that researchers asked in the 1960s.

Question 1—How Many RNA Bases Specify One Amino Acid?

Because the number of different protein building blocks (20) exceeds the number of different mRNA building blocks (4), each codon must contain more than one mRNA base. If a codon consisted of only one mRNA base, then codons could specify only four different amino acids, one corresponding to each of the four bases: A, C, G, and U. If each codon consisted of two bases, then only 16 (4^2) different amino acids could be specified, one corresponding to each of the 16 possible combinations of two RNA bases. If a codon consisted of three bases, then the genetic code could specify as many as 64 (4^3) different amino acids, sufficient to encode the 20 different amino acids that make up proteins. Therefore, the minimum number of bases in a codon is three.

Francis Crick and his coworkers conducted experiments on a type of virus called T4 that confirmed the triplet nature of the genetic code. They exposed the viruses to chemicals that add or remove one, two, or three bases, and examined a viral gene whose sequence and protein product were known. Altering the sequence by one or two bases produced a different amino acid sequence, because it disrupted the **reading frame,** which is the sequence of amino acids encoded from a certain starting point in a DNA sequence. However, adding or deleting three contiguous bases added or deleted only one amino acid in the protein without disrupting the reading frame. The rest of the amino acid sequence was retained. The code, the researchers deduced, is triplet (**figure 10.10**). Entry 4 in table 12.7 uses an English sentence to represent the effect of altering the reading frame.

Further experiments confirmed the triplet nature of the genetic code. Adding a base at one point in the gene and deleting a base at another point disrupted the reading frame only between these sites, resulting in a protein with a stretch of the wrong amino acids.

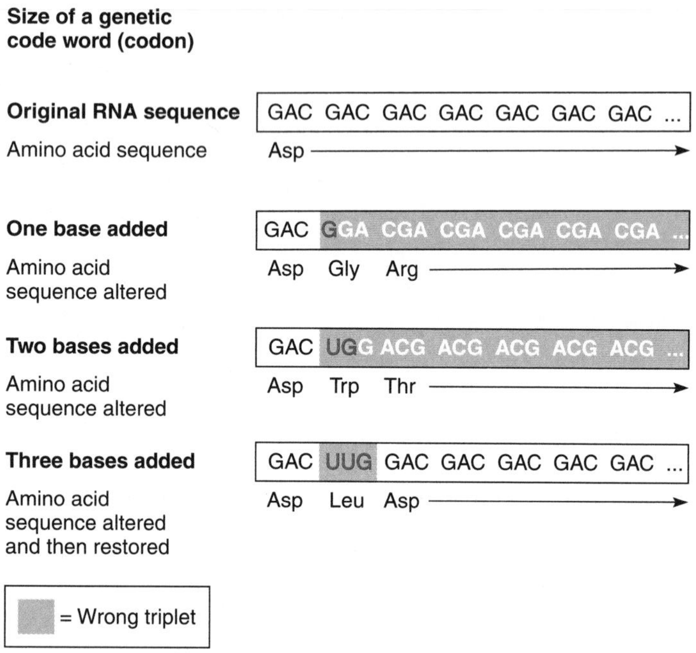

Size of a genetic code word (codon)

Original RNA sequence	GAC GAC GAC GAC GAC GAC GAC ...
Amino acid sequence	Asp ⟶
One base added	GAC GGA CGA CGA CGA CGA CGA ...
Amino acid sequence altered	Asp Gly Arg ⟶
Two bases added	GAC UGG ACG ACG ACG ACG ACG ...
Amino acid sequence altered	Asp Trp Thr ⟶
Three bases added	GAC UUG GAC GAC GAC GAC GAC ...
Amino acid sequence altered and then restored	Asp Leu Asp ⟶

☐ = Wrong triplet

Figure 10.10 Three at a time. Adding or deleting one or two nucleotides in a DNA sequence results in a frame shift and thus disrupts the encoded amino acid sequence. However, adding or deleting three bases does not disrupt the reading frame. Therefore, the code is triplet. This is a simplified representation of the Crick experiment. First a G is added, then a U, then another U so that the altered codons are GGA, UGG, and UUG, corresponding to the amino acids glycine, tryptophan, and leucine. (Table 10.4 includes the full names of the amino acids abbreviated here.)

Question 2—Does a DNA Sequence Contain Information in an Overlapping Manner?

Consider the hypothetical mRNA sequence:

AUGCCCAAG

If the genetic code is triplet and a DNA sequence is "read" in a nonoverlapping manner (that is, three bases in a row form a codon, but any one base is part of only one codon), then this sequence contains only three codons and specifies three amino acids:

AUGCCCAAG
AUG (methionine)
CCC (proline)
AAG (lysine)

If the DNA sequence is overlapping, however, the sequence contains seven codons:

AUGCCCAAG
AUG (methionine)
UGC (cysteine)
GCC (alanine)
CCC (proline)
CCA (proline)
CAA (glutamine)
AAG (lysine)

An overlapping DNA sequence seems to pack maximal information into a limited number of bases, but this would constrain protein structure because certain amino acids must always follow certain others. For example, AUG would always be followed by an amino acid whose codon begins with UG. This does not happen. Therefore, the protein-encoding DNA sequence is not overlapping. (There are a few exceptions, particularly in viruses, where the same DNA sequence can be read from different starting points.)

Question 3—Can mRNA Codons Signal Anything Other Than Amino Acids?

Chemical analysis eventually showed that the genetic code contains directions for starting and stopping translation. The codon AUG signals "start," and the codons UGA, UAA, and UAG all signify "stop." Another form of "punctuation" is a short sequence of bases at the start of each mRNA, called the leader sequence, that enables the mRNA to hydrogen bond with rRNA in a ribosome.

Question 4—Do All Species Use the Same Genetic Code?

All species use the same mRNA codons to specify the same amino acids, despite the popular idea of a "human" genetic code. This universality of the genetic code is evidence that all life evolved from a common ancestor. No other mechanism as efficient at directing cellular activities has emerged and persisted.

The only known exceptions to the "universality" of the genetic code are a few codons in mitochondria and in certain single-celled eukaryotes (ciliated protozoa). These deviations may be tolerated because they do not affect the major repositories of DNA. The mitochondrial genome is small, and the affected ciliated protozoa have a second, smaller nucleus that houses some genes with one or two alternate codon-amino acid assignments. In both cases, the major DNA sites adhere to the universal genetic code.

The ability of mRNA from one species to be translated in a cell of another species has made recombinant DNA technology possible, in which bacteria manufacture proteins normally made in the human body. Chapter 19 explains the role of biotechnology in developing protein-based drugs.

Question 5—Which Codons Specify Which Amino Acids?

In 1961, Marshall Nirenberg and Heinrich Matthaei at the National Institute of Health began deciphering which codons specify which amino acids, using a precise and logical series of experiments. First they synthesized mRNA molecules in the laboratory. Then they added them to test tubes that contained all the chemicals and structures needed for translation, extracted from *E. coli* cells. Which amino acid would each synthetic RNA specify?

The first synthetic mRNA they made had the sequence UUUUUU. . . . In the test tube, this was translated into a peptide consisting entirely of one amino acid type: phenylalanine. Thus was revealed the first entry in the genetic code dictionary: The codon UUU specifies the amino acid phenylalanine. The number of phenylalanines always equaled one-third the number of mRNA bases, con-firming that the genetic code is triplet and nonoverlapping. The next experiments revealed that AAA codes for the amino acid lysine and CCC for proline. (GGG was unstable.)

Other researchers synthesized chains of alternating bases. Synthetic mRNA of the sequence AUAUAU . . . introduced codons AUA and UAU. When translated, the mRNA yielded an amino acid sequence of alternating isoleucines and tyrosines. But was AUA the code for isoleucine and UAU for tyrosine, or vice versa? Another experiment answered the question.

The mRNA UUUAUAUUUAUA encoded alternating phenylalanine and isoleucine. Because the first experiment had showed that UUU codes for phenylalanine, the researchers deduced that AUA must code for isoleucine. If AUA codes for isoleucine, then UAU must code for tyrosine.

By the end of the 1960s, researchers had deciphered the entire genetic code (**table 10.4**). Sixty of the possible 64 codons specify particular amino acids, three indicate "stop," and one encodes both the amino

Table 10.4

The Genetic Code

First Letter		Second Letter							Third Letter
		U		**C**		**A**		**G**	
U	UUU	Phenylalanine (Phe)	UCU	Serine (Ser)	UAU	Tyrosine (Tyr)	UGU	Cysteine (Cys)	U
	UUC		UCC		UAC		UGC		C
	UUA	Leucine (Leu)	UCA		UAA	"stop"	UGA	"stop"	A
	UUG		UCG		UAG	"stop"	UGG	Tryptophan (Trp)	G
C	CUU	Leucine (Leu)	CCU	Proline (Pro)	CAU	Histidine (His)	CGU	Arginine (Arg)	U
	CUC		CCC		CAC		CGC		C
	CUA		CCA		CAA	Glutamine (Gln)	CGA		A
	CUG		CCG		CAG		CGG		G
A	AUU	Isoleucine (Ile)	ACU	Threonine (Thr)	AAU	Asparagine (Asn)	AGU	Serine (Ser)	U
	AUC		ACC		AAC		AGC		C
	AUA		ACA		AAA	Lysine (Lys)	AGA	Arginine (Arg)	A
	AUG	Methionine (Met) and "start"	ACG		AAG		AGG		G
G	GUU	Valine (Val)	GCU	Alanine (Ala)	GAU	Aspartic acid (Asp)	GGU	Glycine (Gly)	U
	GUC		GCC		GAC		GGC		C
	GUA		GCA		GAA	Glutamic acid (Glu)	GGA		A
	GUG		GCG		GAG		GGG		G

acid methionine and "start." This means that some amino acids are specified by more than one codon. For example, both UUU and UUC encode phenylalanine. Different codons that specify the same amino acid are termed synonymous, just as synonyms are words with the same meaning. The genetic code is said to be degenerate because each amino acid is not uniquely specified. Synonymous codons often differ from one another by the base in the third position. The corresponding base of a tRNA's anticodon is called the "wobble" position because it can bind to more than one type of base in synonymous codons. The degeneracy of the genetic code protects against mutation, because changes in the DNA that substitute a synonymous codon do not affect the protein's amino acid sequence.

Deciphering the genetic code revealed the "rules" that essentially govern life at the cellular level. Because genetics was still a very young science, the code breakers came largely from the ranks of chemistry, physics, and math. Some of the more exuberant personalities organized an "RNA tie club" and inducted a member whenever someone added a piece to the puzzle of the genetic code, anointing him (there were no prominent hers) with a tie and tie pin emblazoned with the structure of the specified amino acid (**figure 10.11**).

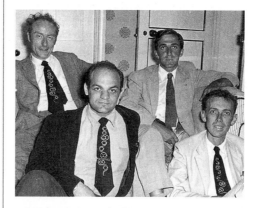

Figure 10.11 The RNA tie club. In 1953, physicist-turned-biologist George Gamow started the RNA tie club, to "solve the riddle of RNA structure and to understand the way it builds proteins." The club had 20 members, and each received a tie and tie pin bearing the name of the particular amino acid he had worked on. Francis Crick (upper left) was tyrosine; James Watson (lower right) was proline.

The human genome project picked up where the genetic code experiments of the 1960s left off by identifying the DNA sequences that are transcribed into tRNAs. That is, 61 different tRNAs could theoretically exist, one for each codon that specifies an amino acid (the 64 triplets minus 3 stop codons). However, only 49 different genes were found to encode tRNAs. This is because the same type of tRNA can detect synonymous codons that differ only in whether the wobble (third) position is U or C. The same type of tRNA, for example, binds to both UUU and UUC codons, which specify the amino acid phenylalanine. Synonymous codons ending in A or G use different tRNAs.

Building a Protein

Protein synthesis requires mRNA, tRNA molecules carrying amino acids, ribosomes, energy-storing molecules such as adenosine triphosphate (ATP) and guanosine triphosphate (GTP), and various protein factors. These pieces come together in a stage called **translation initiation (figure 10.12)**.

Translation initiation

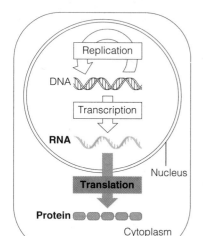

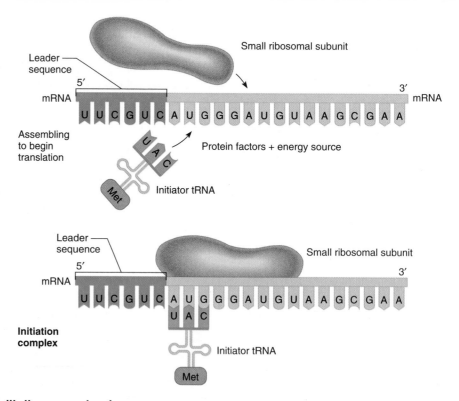

Figure 10.12 Translation begins as the initiation complex forms. Initiation of translation brings together a small ribosomal subunit, mRNA, and an initiator tRNA, and aligns them in the proper orientation to begin translation. (The 5'-3' mRNA orientation is flipped from the direction shown in figures 10.2 and 10.7.)

First, the mRNA leader sequence hydrogen bonds with a short sequence of rRNA in a small ribosomal subunit. The first mRNA codon to specify an amino acid is always AUG, which attracts an initiator tRNA that carries the amino acid methionine (abbreviated *met*). This methionine signifies the start of a polypeptide. The small ribosomal subunit, the mRNA bonded to it, and the initiator tRNA with its attached methionine form the **initiation complex.**

To start the next stage of translation, called **elongation,** a large ribosomal subunit attaches to the initiation complex. The codon adjacent to the initiation codon (AUG), which is GGA in **figure 10.13a,** then bonds to its complementary anticodon, which is part of a free tRNA that carries the amino acid glycine. The two amino acids (*met* and *gly* in the example), still attached to their tRNAs, align.

The part of the ribosome that holds the mRNA and tRNAs together can be described as having two sites. The positions of the sites on the ribosome remain the same with respect to each other as translation proceeds, but they cover different parts of the mRNA as the ribosome moves. The **P site** holds the growing amino acid chain, and the **A site** right next to it holds the next amino acid to be added to the chain. In figure 10.13, when the protein-to-be consists of only the first two amino acids, *met* occupies the P site and *gly* the A site.

With the help of rRNA that functions as a ribozyme, the amino acids link by peptide bonds (**figure 10.14**). Then the first tRNA is released. It will pick up another amino acid of the same type and be used again. The ribosome and its attached mRNA are now bound to a single tRNA, with two amino

acids extending from it at the P site. This is the start of a polypeptide.

Next, the ribosome moves down the mRNA by one codon. The region of the mRNA that was at the A site is thus now at the P site. A third tRNA enters, carrying its amino acid (*cys* in figure 10.13b). This third amino acid aligns with the other two and forms a peptide bond to the second amino acid in the growing chain, now extending from the P site. The tRNA attached to the second amino acid is released and recycled. The polypeptide continues to build, one amino acid at a time. Each piece is brought in by a tRNA whose anticodon corresponds to a consecutive mRNA codon as the ribosome moves down the mRNA (figure 10.13c).

Elongation halts when the A site of the ribosome contains a "stop" codon (UGA, UAG, or UAA), because no tRNA molecules

Translation Elongation

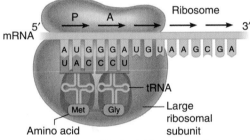

a. Second amino acid joins initiation complex.

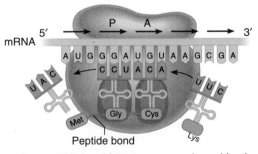

b. First peptide bond forms, as new amino acid arrives.

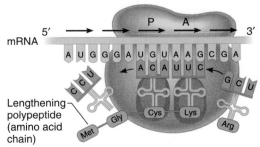

c. Amino acid chain extends.

Translation Termination

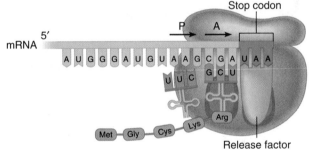

d. Ribosome reaches stop codon.

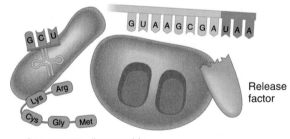

e. Components disassemble.

Figure 10.13 Building a polypeptide. **(a)** A large ribosomal subunit binds to the initiation complex, and a tRNA bearing a second amino acid (glycine, in this example) forms hydrogen bonds between its anticodon and the mRNA's second codon at the A site. The first amino acid, methionine, occupies the P site. **(b)** The methionine brought in by the first tRNA forms a peptide bond with the amino acid brought in by the second tRNA, and a third tRNA arrives, in this example carrying the amino acid cysteine. **(c)** A fourth amino acid is linked to the growing polypeptide chain, and the process continues until a termination codon is reached. **(d)** A protein release factor binds to the stop codon, releasing the completed protein from the tRNA and **(e)** freeing all of the components of the translation complex.

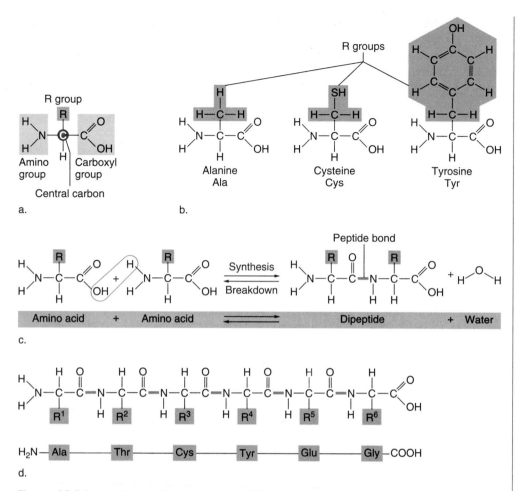

correspond to these codons. The last tRNA leaves the ribosome, the ribosomal subunits separate from each other and are recycled, and the new polypeptide is released. Ribosomes, obviously, are critical to protein synthesis. Antibiotic drugs whose names end in "mycin" destroy bacterial ribosomes, which are smaller than those in eukaryotic cells.

Protein synthesis is economical. A cell can produce large amounts of a particular protein from just one or two copies of a gene. A plasma cell in the immune system, for example, manufactures 2,000 identical antibody molecules per second. To mass-produce proteins at this rate, RNA, ribosomes, enzymes, and other proteins must be continually recycled. Transcription always produces multiple copies of a particular mRNA, and each mRNA may be bound to dozens of ribosomes, as **figure 10.15** shows. As soon as one ribosome has moved far enough along the mRNA, another ribosome attaches. In this way, many copies of the encoded protein are made from the same mRNA.

As complex as protein synthesis is, stringing together amino acids is only a first step. **Chaperone proteins** stabilize partially folded regions as the molecule assumes its conformation. Certain proteins must be altered before they can function. Insulin, which is 51 amino acids long, for example, is initially translated as the polypeptide proinsulin, which is 80 amino acids long. Enzymes cut it to 51 amino acids. Some proteins must have sugars attached for them to become functional, or must aggregate.

Figure 10.14 Amino acids join by peptide bonds. Amino acids are the building blocks of proteins. **(a)** An amino acid is composed of an amino group, an acid (carboxyl) group, and one of 20 R groups attached to a central carbon atom. **(b)** The composition of the R group contributes specific functions to the final protein. **(c)** A peptide bond forms when an OH from a carboxyl group of one amino acid combines with a hydrogen from the amino group of another amino acid, creating a water molecule (H-O-H) and linking the carboxyl carbon of the first amino acid to the nitrogen of the other. **(d)** Long chains of amino acids form proteins.

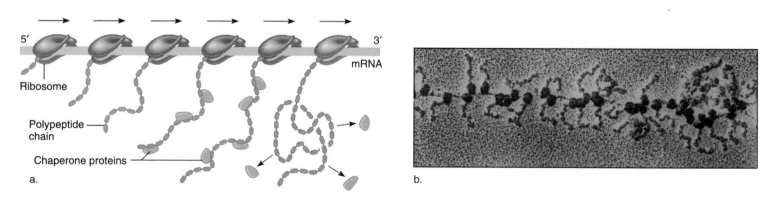

Figure 10.15 Making multiple copies of a protein. Several ribosomes can translate the same protein from a single mRNA at the same time. **(a)** These ribosomes have different-sized polypeptides dangling from them—the closer a ribosome is to the end of a gene, the longer its polypeptide. Chaperone proteins help fold the polypeptide into its characteristic conformation. **(b)** In the micrograph, the ribosomes on the left have just begun translation and the polypeptides are short. Further along in translation, the polypeptides are longer. The chaperones are not visible.

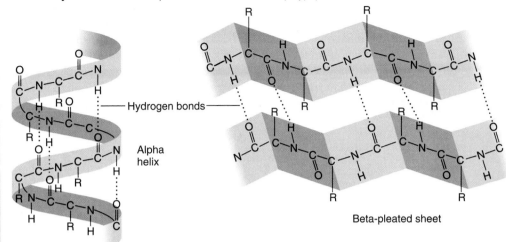

H₂N—Ala—Thr—Cys—Tyr—Glu—Gly—COOH

a. **Primary structure**—the sequence of amino acids in a polypeptide chain

Hydrogen bonds

Alpha helix

Beta-pleated sheet

b. **Secondary structure**—loops, coils, sheets or other shapes formed by hydrogen bonds between nonadjacent carboxyl and amino groups

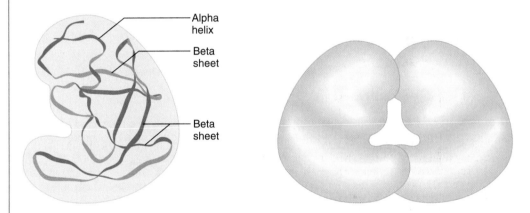

Alpha helix

Beta sheet

Beta sheet

c. **Tertiary structure**—three-dimensional forms shaped by bonds between R groups, interactions between R groups and water

d. **Quaternary structure**—proteins formed by bonds between separate polypeptides

Figure 10.16 **Four levels of protein structure.** **(a)** The amino acid sequence of a polypeptide forms the primary structure, while **(b)** hydrogen bonds between non-R groups create secondary structures such as helices and sheets. The tertiary structure **(c)** is formed when R groups interact, folding the polypeptide in three dimensions and forming a unique shape. **(d)** If different polypeptide units must interact to be functional, the protein forms a quaternary structure.

10.3 Protein Folding

Proteins must fold into one (or more) specific three-dimensional shape(s), or conformation(s), to function. This folding occurs because of attractions and repulsions between the protein's atoms. In addition, thousands of water molecules surround a growing chain of amino acids, and, because some amino acids are attracted to water and some are repelled by it, the water contorts the protein's shape. Sulfur atoms also affect overall conformation by bridging the two types of amino acids that contain them.

The conformation of a protein may be described at several levels (**figure 10.16**). The amino acid sequence of a polypeptide chain determines its **primary (1°) structure.** Chemical attractions between amino acids that are close together in the 1° structure fold the polypeptide chain into its **secondary (2°) structure,** which may form loops, coils, barrels, helices, sheets, or other distinctive shapes. Secondary structures wind into larger **tertiary (3°) structures** as more widely separated amino acids attract or repel in response to water molecules. Finally, proteins consisting of more than one polypeptide form a

quaternary (4°) structure. Hemoglobin, the blood protein that carries oxygen, has four polypeptide chains; it is depicted schematically in figure 11.1. The liver protein ferritin has 20 identical polypeptides of 200 amino acids each. In contrast, the muscle protein myoglobin is a single polypeptide chain.

So crucial is a protein's conformation that cells have evolved "quality control" systems to ensure that proteins fold correctly, and that misfolded proteins are destroyed before they can kill cells and cause disease. This surveillance begins as soon as an amino acid chain starts to fold as it emerges from the ribosome. Localized regions of shape form, and possibly break apart and form again, as translation proceeds. Experiments that isolate proteins as they are synthesized show that other proteins oversee the process of proper folding.

These accessory proteins include enzymes that foster chemical bonds and chaperone proteins (see figure 10.15).

Still other proteins can tell if a protein has folded incorrectly and add a protein "tag" called **ubiquitin** if it has. A misfolded protein bearing just one ubiquitin tag may straighten itself out and refold correctly, but a protein with more than one tag is taken to a cellular garbage disposal of sorts called a **proteasome (figure 10.17)**. A proteasome is a tunnel-like multi-protein structure. Here, the protein is stretched out, chopped up, and its peptide pieces degraded.

Misfolded proteins that are not destroyed can cause disease. Some mutations that cause cystic fibrosis, for example, prevent the encoded protein from assuming its final form and anchoring in the plasma membrane, where it normally controls the flow of chloride ions.

In several disorders that affect the brain, misfolded proteins—different proteins in different conditions—aggregate, forming masses that clog the proteasomes and block them from processing any malformed proteins. In Huntington disease, for example, extra glutamines tacked onto the protein huntingtin cause it to obstruct proteasomes, which eventually kills the cell. Misfolded proteins that clog proteasomes also occur in Alzheimer disease, amyotrophic lateral sclerosis (Lou Gehrig's disease), Parkinson disease, and Lewy body dementia.

Another type of protein folding disorder arises in glycoproteins called prions (pronounced *pree-ons*). Diseases called transmissible spongiform encephalopathies result when one conformation of the prion glycoprotein (PrP) is infectious, causing others to misfold like it (**figure 10.18**). Unlike other misfolded proteins that cause disease, the variant forms of prion protein have the same primary structure, but they can fold into at least eight conformations (**figure 10.19**). Transmissible spongiform encephalopathies are known in 85 types of mammals, including humans. They were first identified in a disease of sheep called scrapie. The affected brain is shot full of holes, resembling a sponge. Nerve cells die, and star-shaped supportive cells overgrow. Reading 10.1 describes prion disorders in humans.

The "rules" by which DNA sequences specify protein shapes are still not well understood, even as we routinely decipher the sequences of entire genomes. The straightforward linear relationship between gene and protein that emerged from the experiments of the 1960s was not all there is to the story of how a cell builds its proteins.

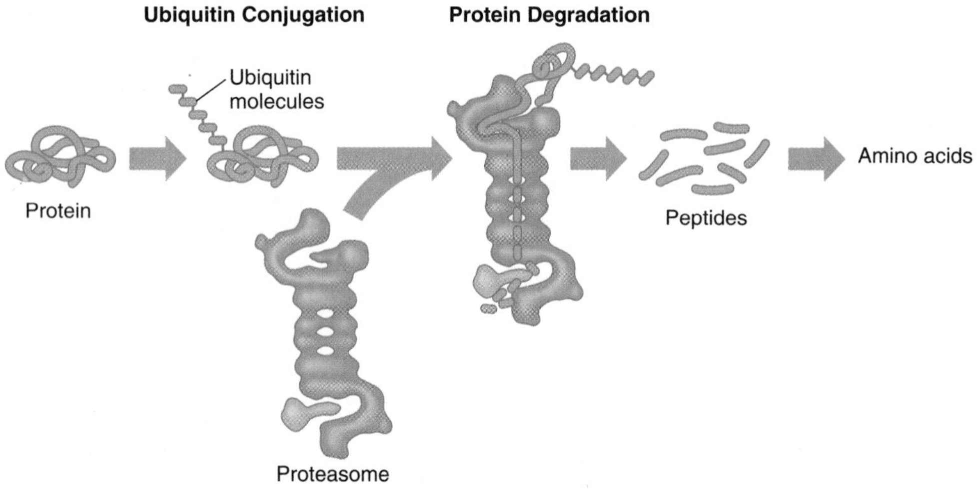

Ubiquitin Conjugation

Protein Degradation

Ubiquitin molecules

Protein

Amino acids

Peptides

Proteasome

Figure 10.17   Protein folding quality control.   Ubiquitin binds to a misfolded protein and escorts it to a proteasome. The proteasome, which is composed of several proteins, encases the misfolded protein, straightening and dismantling it.

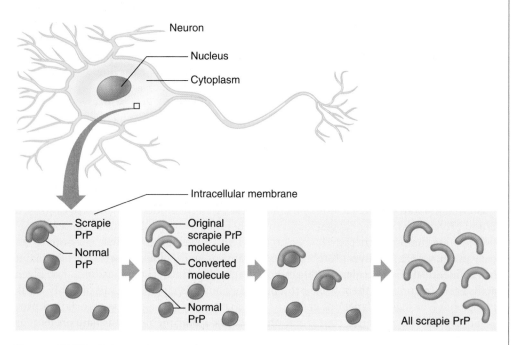

Neuron

Nucleus

Cytoplasm

Intracellular membrane

Scrapie PrP

Normal PrP

Original scrapie PrP molecule

Converted molecule

Normal PrP

All scrapie PrP

Figure 10.18   Prions change shape.   A prion disease may begin when a single scrapie PrP contacts a normal PrP and changes it into the scrapie conformation. As the change spreads, disease results, usually with accumulated scrapie prion proteins clogging brain tissue.

Key Concepts

Protein folding begins as translation proceeds, with enzymes and chaperone proteins assisting. Misfolded proteins are tagged with ubiquitin and sent through a proteasome for dismantling. A protein can fold in more than one way. Infectious conformations of prion proteins cause disease.

Considering Kuru

Prion diseases cause extreme weight loss and poor coordination, with other symptoms, such as dementia or relentless insomnia, reflecting the part of the brain that is eaten away. These diseases are typically fatal within 18 months once symptoms appear.

About 10 percent of people who suffer from prion diseases inherit the condition because they have mutations in the gene that encodes prion protein, called *PrP*. Most cases, however, are acquired. A person is exposed to prions that are in the infectious conformation, triggering conversion of their own normal prions. These rare illnesses were first discovered in sheep, which develop a disease called scrapie when they eat prion-infected brains from other sheep.

A dramatic example of a prion disease in humans was kuru, which affected the Foré people in a remote mountainous area of New Guinea (**figure 1**). In the Foré language, *kuru* means to tremble. The disease began with wobbling legs, quickly followed by trembling hands and fingers. Gradually, the entire body became wracked with uncontrollable shaking. A peculiar symptom was uncontrollable laughter, leading to the nickname "laughing disease." Speech slurred and faded, thinking slowed, and after several months, the person could no longer walk or eat. Death typically came within a year.

The fact that only women and young children developed kuru at first suggested that the disease might be inherited, but D. Carleton Gajdusek, a physician who has spent much of his lifetime studying the Foré, learned that the preparation of human brain for a cannibalism ritual probably passed on the infectious prions. When the people abandoned the ritual in the 1970s, the disease gradually vanished. Gajdusek vividly described the Foré preparation of human brains at a time when he thought the cause was viral:

> **Children participated in both the butchery and the handling of cooked meat, rubbing their soiled hands in their armpits or hair, and elsewhere on their bodies. They rarely or never washed. Infection with the kuru virus was most probably through the cuts and abrasions of the skin or from nose picking, eye rubbing, or mucosal injury.**

Although kuru vanished, other prion diseases surfaced. In the 1970s and 1980s, several people acquired Creutzfeldt-Jakob disease (CJD). This time, the route of transmission was either through corneal transplants, in which infectious prions entered the brain through the optic nerve, or from human growth hormone taken from cadavers and used to treat short stature in children. The most familiar prion disease is probably "mad cow disease" and the variant CJD it has caused in more than 120 people in the United Kingdom since 1995. People likely acquired the infectious prions by eating infected beef.

Researchers have studied the *PrP* gene in great detail, and discovered that several specific polymorphisms (variants) that affect different sites in the protein interact in ways that make some people resistant to prion

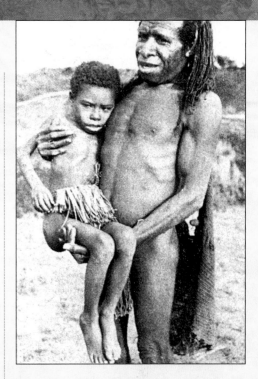

Figure 1 **Kuru.** Kuru is a prion disease that affected the Foré people of New Guinea until they gave up a cannibalism ritual that spread an infectious form of prion protein.

diseases, yet others highly susceptible. These mutations are discussed further in chapter 12. The persistence of the protective gene variants, some researchers say, is evidence that cannibalism may have been common in some of our prehistoric ancestors—protected individuals survived. This hypothesis is consistent with anthropological evidence of cannibalism, such as human bite marks on human bones. The function of normal prion protein isn't known, but it resides in the plasma membranes of brain neurons.

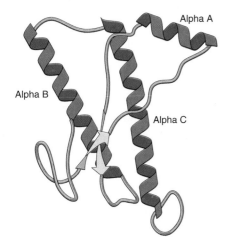

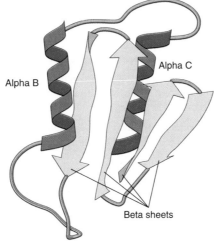

a. Cellular prion protein (noninfectious)

b. Scrapie prion protein (infectious)

Figure 10.19 **One protein, multiple conformations.** Biochemists once thought that the primary structure of a protein dictated one conformation. This is not true. A cellular form of prion protein, for example, does not cause disease **(a)**. The scrapie form is infectious—it converts the cellular form to more of itself **(b)**. Infectious prions cause scrapie in sheep, bovine spongiform encephalopathy in cows, and variant Creutzfeldt-Jakob disease in humans.

Summary

10.1 Transcription—The Link Between Gene and Protein

1. Some DNA is **transcribed** into RNA, which is then **translated** into protein.

2. RNA is transcribed from the **template strand** of DNA. The other DNA strand is called the **coding strand.**

3. RNA is a single-stranded nucleic acid similar to DNA but containing uracil and ribose rather than thymine and deoxyribose.

4. Several types of RNA participate in protein synthesis. **Messenger RNA** (mRNA) carries a protein-encoding gene's information. **Ribosomal RNA** (rRNA) associates with certain proteins to form ribosomes, which physically support protein synthesis. **Transfer RNA** (tRNA) is cloverleaf-shaped, with a three-base **anticodon** that is complementary to mRNA on one end and bonds to a particular amino acid on the other end.

5. Operons control gene expression in bacteria. In more complex organisms, **transcription factors** regulate which genes are transcribed in a particular cell type.

6. Transcription begins when transcription factors help **RNA polymerase** (RNAP) bind to a gene's **promoter.** RNAP then adds RNA nucleotides to a growing chain, in a sequence complementary to the DNA template strand.

7. After a gene is transcribed, the mRNA receives a "cap" of modified nucleotides at the 5′ end and a poly A tail at the 3′ end.

8. Many genes do not encode information in a continuous manner. After transcription, segments called **exons** are translated into protein, but segments called **introns** are removed. Introns may outnumber and outsize exons. Alternate splicing can increase protein diversity.

10.2 Translation of a Protein

9. Each three consecutive mRNA bases form a **codon** that specifies a particular amino acid. The **genetic code** is the correspondence between each codon and the amino acid it specifies. Of the 64 different possible codons, 60 specify amino acids, one specifies the amino acid methionine and "start," and three signal "stop." Because 61 codons specify the 20 amino acids, more than one type of codon may encode a single amino acid. The genetic code is nonoverlapping, triplet, universal, and degenerate.

10. In the 1960s, researchers used logic and clever experiments that used synthetic RNAs to decipher the genetic code.

11. Translation requires tRNA, ribosomes, energy-storage molecules, enzymes, and protein factors. An **initiation complex** forms when mRNA, a small ribosomal subunit, and a tRNA carrying methionine join. The amino acid chain begins to elongate when a large ribosomal subunit joins the small one. Next, a second tRNA binds by its **anticodon** to the next mRNA codon, and its amino acid bonds with the first amino acid. Transfer RNAs add more amino acids, forming a polypeptide. The ribosome moves down the mRNA as the chain grows. The P site bears the amino acid chain, and the A site holds the newest tRNA. When the ribosome reaches a "stop" codon, it falls apart into its two subunits and is released. The new polypeptide breaks free.

12. After translation, some polypeptides are cleaved, have sugars added, or aggregate. The cell uses or secretes the protein.

10.3 Protein Folding

13. A protein must fold into a particular **conformation** to be active and functional.

14. A protein's **primary structure** is its amino acid sequence. Its **secondary structure** forms as amino acids close in the primary structure attract one another. **Tertiary structure** appears as more widely separated amino acids attract or repel in response to water molecules. **Quaternary structure** forms when a protein consists of more than one polypeptide.

15. **Chaperone proteins** help mold conformation.

16. **Ubiquitin** is added to misfolded proteins, and escorts them to **proteasomes** for dismantling. Protein misfolding causes disease.

17. Some proteins can fold into several conformations, some of which can cause disease.

18. At least one conformation of prion protein is infectious, causing transmissible spongiform encephalopathies.

Review Questions

1. Explain how complementary base pairing is responsible for
   a. the structure of the DNA double helix.
   b. DNA replication.
   c. transcription of RNA from DNA.
   d. the attachment of mRNA to a ribosome.
   e. codon/anticodon pairing.
   f. tRNA conformation.

2. A retrovirus has RNA as its genetic material. When it infects a cell, it uses enzymes to copy its RNA into DNA, which then integrates into the host cell's chromosome. Is this flow of genetic information consistent with the central dogma? Why or why not?

3. Genomics is highly dependent upon computer algorithms that search DNA sequences for indications of specialized functions. Explain the significance of detecting the following sequences:
   a. a promoter
   b. a sequence of 75 to 80 bases that folds into a cloverleaf shape
   c. RNAs with poly A tails

4. Many antibiotic drugs work by interfering with protein synthesis in the bacteria that cause infections. Explain how each of the

following antibiotic mechanisms disrupts genetic function in bacteria.

   a. Transfer RNAs misread mRNA codons, binding with the incorrect codon and bringing in the wrong amino acid.

   b. The first amino acid is released from the initiation complex before translation can begin.

   c. Transfer RNA cannot bind to the ribosome.

   d. Ribosomes cannot move.

   e. A tRNA picks up the wrong amino acid.

5. How is the bacterial lactose operon similar to the transcription factor response to low-oxygen conditions?

6. List the differences between RNA and DNA.

7. Where in a cell do DNA replication, transcription, and translation occur?

8. How does transcription control cell specialization?

9. How can the same mRNA codon be at an A site on a ribosome at one time, but at a P site at another time?

10. Describe the events of transcription initiation.

11. List the three major types of RNA and their functions.

12. Describe three ways RNA is altered after it is transcribed.

13. What are the components of a ribosome?

14. Why would an overlapping genetic code be restrictive?

15. How are the processes of transcription and translation economical?

16. How does the shortening of proinsulin to insulin differ from the shortening of apolipoprotein B?

17. Explain how protein misfolding conditions and illnesses that result from abnormal transcription factors might each produce many different symptoms.

18. What factors determine how a protein folds into its characteristic conformation?

19. Why would two-nucleotide codons be insufficient to encode the number of amino acids in biological proteins?

20. Cite two ways RNA helps in its own synthesis, and two ways proteins help in their own synthesis.

Applied Questions

1. The *BRCA1* gene that, when missing several bases, causes a form of breast cancer has 24 exons and 23 introns.

   a. How many splice sites does the gene contain? (A splice site is the junction of an exon and an intron.)

   b. In a woman with *BRCA1* breast cancer, an entire exon is missing, or "skipped." How many splice sites does her affected copy of the gene have?

2. List the RNA sequences that would be transcribed from the following DNA template sequences.

   a. TTACACTTGCTTGAGAGTC

   b. ACTTGGGCTATGCTCATTA

   c. GGCTGCAATAGCCGTAGAT

   d. GGAATACGTCTAGCTAGCA

3. Given the following partial mRNA sequences, reconstruct the corresponding DNA template sequences.

   a. GCUAUCUGUCAUAAAAGAGGA

   b. GUGGCGUAUUCUUUUCCGGGUAGG

   c. GAGGGAAUUCUUUCUCAACGAAGU

   d. AGGAAAACCCCUCUUAUUAUAGAU

4. List three different mRNA sequences that could encode the following amino acid sequence:

   histidine-alanine-arginine-serine-leucine-valine-cysteine

5. Write a DNA sequence that would encode the following amino acid sequence:

   valine-tryptophan-lysine-proline-phenylalanine-threonine

6. In the film *Jurassic Park,* which is about cloned dinosaurs, a cartoon character named Mr. DNA talks about the billions of genetic codes in DNA. Why is this statement incorrect?

7. When researchers investigating the genetic code examined synthetic RNA of sequence ACACACACACACACA, they found that it encoded the amino acid sequence *thr-his-thr-his-thr-his*. How did the researchers determine the codon assignments for ACA and CAC?

8. Titin is a muscle protein named for its gargantuan size—its gene has the largest known coding sequence of 80,781 DNA bases. How many amino acids long is it?

9. An extraterrestrial life form has a triplet genetic code with five different bases. How many different amino acids can this code specify, assuming no degeneracy?

10. In malignant hyperthermia, a person develops a life-threateningly high fever after taking certain types of anesthetic drugs. In one family, the mutation deletes three contiguous bases in exon 44. How many amino acids are missing from the protein?

11. A mutation in a gene that encodes RPGR-interacting protein causes visual loss. The protein is 1,259 amino acids long. What is the minimal size of this gene?

Web Activities

12. Go to http://www.mcb.harvard.edu/ BioLinks/gencode.html Scroll down to the lists of "noncanonical" codes in organisms other than humans. (Noncanonical means it differs from the universal genetic code.) Find three examples of deviations from the universal code, and list what the codon-amino acid assignment is in most organisms. (Replace the T's on the website with the U's to correspond to the genetic code chart in the textbook.)

13. Use the Web to find out how the ubiquitin-proteasome system is overtaxed or disabled in a neurodegenerative disease such as Alzheimer disease, Parkinson disease, Huntington disease, amyotrophic lateral sclerosis, or Lewy body dementia. (Find websites for these disorders and discuss how the mechanism involves proteasomes.)

Case Studies

14. Five patients meet at a clinic for families in which several members have early-onset Parkinson disease. This condition causes rigidity, tremors, and other motor symptoms. Only 2 percent of cases of Parkinson disease are inherited. The five patients all have mutations in a gene that encodes the protein parkin, which has 12 exons. For each patient, indicate whether the mutation shortens, lengthens, or does not change the size of the protein.

   a. Manny Filipo's parkin gene is missing exon 3.

   b. Frank Myer's parkin gene has a duplication in intron 4.

   c. Theresa Ruzi's parkin gene lacks six contiguous nucleotides in exon 1.

   d. Elyse Fitzsimmon's parkin gene has an altered splice site between exon 8 and intron 8.

   e. Scott Shapiro's parkin gene is deleted.

Learn to apply the skills of genetic counselor with this additional case found in the *Case Workbook in Human Genetics*:

   Alpha-antitrypsin deficiency

Suggested Readings

Bunk, Steve. November 11, 2002. Chaperones to the rescue. *The Scientist* 16(22):21–23. Chaperone proteins suggest a new class of drugs to correct misfolded proteins.

Dahlberg, Albert. May 4, 2001. The ribosome in action. *Science* 292:868–69. A review of recent research reveals the structures of interacting ribosomes, tRNA, and mRNA in bacteria.

Gilbert, Walter. February 9, 1978. Why genes in pieces? *Nature* 271:501. A classic and insightful look at the enigma of introns.

Hoagland, Mahlon. 1990. *Toward the habit of truth.* New York: W. W. Norton. The story of the RNA tie club, by a member.

Kay, Lily E. 2001. *Who Wrote the Book of Life?* Stanford, CA: Stanford University Press. The story of how a group of mostly physicists-turned-biologists deciphered the genetic code in the 1960s.

Lewis, Ricki. February 1996. On cracked codes, cell walls, and human fungi. *The American Biology Teacher* 58:16. A funny look at errors in genetic code usage.

Pennisi, Elizabeth. April 11, 2003. Cannibalism and prion disease may have been rampant in ancient humans *Science* 300:227–28. A protein's conformation can be infectious.

Pollack, Andrew. July 24, 2001. Scientists are starting to add letters to life's alphabet. *The New York Times*, p. F1. Investigators at the Scripps Research Institute in La Jolla, California, are attempting to create life forms that use a more extensive genetic code.

Prusiner, Stanley. May 17, 2001. Shattuck lecture—Neurodegenerative diseases and prions. *The New England Journal of Medicine* 344:1516–20. The normal and pathogenic forms of prion protein have the same amino acid sequence, but different conformations.

Weekly updates of current news related to human genetics are available through Power Web on your Online Learning Center.

VISIT YOUR ONLINE LEARNING CENTER

Visit your online learning center for additional resources and tools to help you master this chapter. See us at

www.mhhe.com/lewisgenetics6.

Control of Gene Expression

CHAPTER CONTENTS

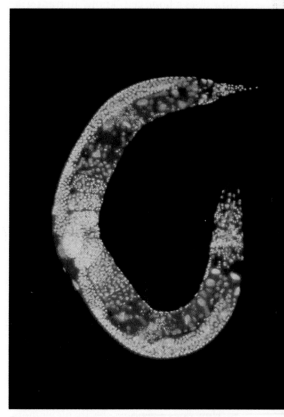

Researchers worked out many of the details of RNA interference—a mechanism of transcription regulation—in *Caenorhabditis elegans,* a tiny, transparent, well-studied roundworm. Such work on the lowly worm may lead to new treatments for obesity.

Rarely do all of the instruments in an orchestra sound at once. Instead, the musical composition dictates precisely how the instruments interact, with only some sounding at any one time, their intensity building and diminishing in a controlled manner. So it is, in a sense, with genomes. Shortly after a new genome is launched at conception, a program of gene expression begins to enfold that oversees the sculpting of the body. Yet the program is flexible enough that signals from the environment can also influence the process of building the organism.

The discoveries of the 1950s and 1960s on DNA structure and function answered some questions while raising many more. How does a bone cell "know" to transcribe the genes that control the synthesis of collagen and not to transcribe genes that specify muscle proteins? How does a bone marrow stem cell "know" when to divide and send some daughter cells on pathways to become white blood cells, red blood cells, or platelets? How does the balance of blood cell types shift when a person has leukemia or sickle cell disease?

Watson and Crick's depiction of DNA inspired the idea that a single gene specifies a single protein. But the neat one-gene-one-protein picture is a great oversimplification. The diverse proteins in the body outnumber the genes that encode them. Moreover, genes not only encode proteins, but they control each other's functioning, in sometimes complex hierarchies. Much of the human genome does not encode protein at all. Just as the discovery of the genetic code answered certain old questions while it raised new ones, the sequencing of the human genome today has posed new questions:

- How does a genome specify many more proteins than there are genes?

- If only a tiny portion of the genome encodes protein, what does the rest of it do?

This chapter addresses these compelling questions that are at the forefront of genomic research. We begin, however, with a question that has brewed as genetic discoveries have accrued—how does a multicellular organism control when and where particular genes are transcribed, and the resulting mRNAs translated into protein?

11.1 Gene Expression Through Time and Tissue

Knowledge of the sequence of the human genome was not necessary for geneticists to begin thinking about the control of gene expression. An excellent example was discovered half a century ago—the globin proteins that transport oxygen in the blood.

Globin Chain Switching

A hemoglobin molecule in an adult consists of four polypeptide chains, each wound into a globular conformation (**figure 11.1**). Two of the chains are 146 amino acids long, and are called "beta" (β). The other two chains are 141 amino acids long and are termed "alpha" (α). The genes for beta subunits are clustered on chromosome 11, and the alpha genes are grouped on chromosome 16. Hemoglobin provides a classic example of a change in gene expression that accompanies development. The subunits of the hemoglobin molecule change in parallel to the changes in oxygen concentration that depend upon whether oxygen arrives through the placenta or the newborn's lungs. The chemical basis for this globin chain switching is that different polypeptide subunits attract oxygen molecules to different degrees. Parts of the globin gene clusters, called locus control regions, oversee the changes in the molecule's composition and assembly.

The subunit makeup of the hemoglobin molecule differs in the embryo, fetus, and adult (**figure 11.2**). During the embryonic period, as the placenta forms, the embryo's hemoglobin consists first of two epsilon (ε) chains, which are in the beta globin group, and two zeta (ζ) chains, which are in the alpha globin group. About 4 percent of the hemoglobin in the embryo includes beta chains, a percentage that gradually grows.

As development proceeds and the embryo becomes a fetus, the epsilon and zeta chains decrease in number, as gamma (γ) and alpha chains accumulate. Hemoglobin consisting of two gamma and two alpha chains is called fetal hemoglobin. The gamma globin subunits bind very strongly to oxygen released from maternal red blood cells into the placenta, so that fetal blood carries 20 to 30 percent more oxygen than an adult's blood. As the fetus matures, beta chains gradually replace the gamma chains. At birth, however, the hemoglobin is not fully of the adult type—fetal hemoglobin (two gamma and two alpha chains) comprises from 50 to 85 percent of the blood. By four months of age, the proportion drops to 10 to 15 percent, and by four years, it is less than 1 percent. In a condition called hereditary persistence of fetal hemoglobin, gamma globin continues to be made into adulthood, with no effects on health. Activating gamma globin, the silenced fetal hemoglobin component, is used to treat disorders that result from certain mutations in the beta globin gene, discussed further in chapter 12.

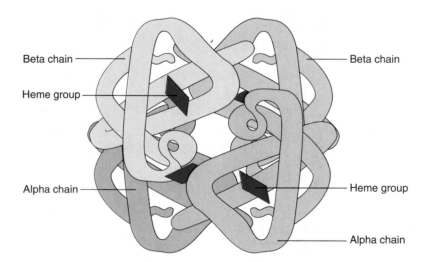

Figure 11.1 The structure of hemoglobin. A hemoglobin molecule is made up of two globular protein chains from the beta (β) globin group and two from the alpha (α) globin group, each surrounding an iron-containing chemical group called a heme.

Building Tissues and Organs

The globin chains affect one type of molecule, hemoglobin. Changing gene expression can also be observed on a larger scale. For example, blood plasma contains about 40,000 different types of proteins. Plasma is the liquid portion of blood that the red blood cells packed with hemoglobin travel through, along with white blood cells and platelets. Ten types of proteins account for 90 percent of all the plasma protein molecules, and nearly half of those are one type, albumin. This means that many thousands of types of proteins are present in vanishingly small amounts, which is why only 300 or so have been described. But change the conditions—the person develops an infection or allergic reaction—and the protein profile of the plasma can change dramatically. Behind it all is differential gene expression.

Blood is a structurally simple tissue. Imagine the complexity of a solid gland or organ, constructed from specialized cells and tissues, and that organization maintained throughout a lifetime of growth, repair, and changing external conditions. Stem cell biology is beginning to shed light on how genes are turned on and off during the development of an organ or gland. Researchers isolate individual stem cells and then see which combinations of growth factors, hormones, and other biochemicals must be added to steer development towards a particular cell type, tissue, or organ. Presumably, these manipulations mimic what happens naturally during development.

Consider the pancreas. It is a dual gland, with two types of cell clusters that have exocrine and endocrine functions (**figure 11.3**). An exocrine gland secretes into ducts, as the exocrine portion of the pancreas does with digestive enzymes. An endocrine gland secretes directly into the bloodstream, as the other portion of the pancreas does for polypeptide hormones that control nutrient utilization (**table 11.1**). The endocrine cell clusters are called pancreatic islets. As the pancreas develops in the embryo, ducts form first. Within their walls reside rare stem and progenitor cells (see figure 2.22). When a transcription factor called pdx-1 becomes activated, some of the progenitor cells divide, giving rise to daughter cells that follow an exocrine pathway, destined to produce digestive enzymes (**figure 11. 4**). Other progenitor

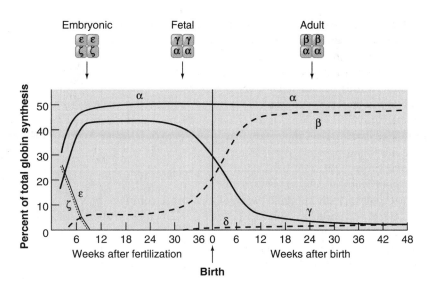

Figure 11.2 Globin chain switching. The subunit composition of human hemoglobin changes as the concentration of oxygen in the environment changes. With the switch from the placenta to the newborn's lungs to obtain oxygen, beta (β) globin begins to replace gamma (γ) globin.

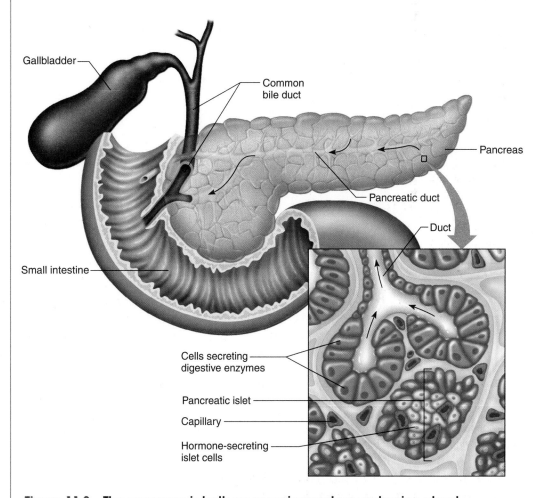

Figure 11.3 The pancreas is both an exocrine and an endocrine gland.
The expanded drawing shows the hormone-secreting pancreatic islets next to enzyme-secreting exocrine cells.

cells respond to signals to divide to yield daughters that follow the endocrine pathway. The most familiar pancreatic hormone is insulin—its absence (or the inability of cells to recognize it) causes diabetes mellitus.

Researchers can observe the specialization of pancreas cells by taking individual progenitor cells from human pancreas ducts and supplying specific growth factors at particular times. This treatment stimulates certain progenitor cells to give rise to clusters that look and function like pancreatic islets. When exposed to glucose, the cells secrete insulin! In addition, the cells, although from humans, can cure diabetes when transplanted into mice whose pancreases have been removed. The goal of this research is to provide new diabetes treatments. Perhaps one day physicians will be able to coax the body of a person with diabetes to develop its own new pancreas cells.

Proteomics

A more complete portrait of gene expression emerges through proteomics, the consideration of all proteins made in a cell, tissue, gland, organ, or entire body. **Figure 11.5** depicts a global way of tracking the proteome—comparing the relative representations of fourteen categories of proteins from conception through old age to their expression before birth. (This is accomplished using either DNA microarrays to reveal which genes are expressed in cells from different stages of prenatal development or postnatal life, or using a chemical technique called mass spectrometry to identify proteins directly.) The differences in gene expression at different times make sense. For example, transcription factors are more highly expressed in the embryo and fetus, presumably because of the extensive cell differentiation that is a hallmark of this period. During the prenatal period, enzymes are less emphasized, perhaps because the fetus receives some enzymes through the placenta. Such proteomic profiles shift with time in different tissues, and during periods of health and disease.

Another way to look at the complete proteome is by specific functions, which

Table 11.1

Pancreatic Hormones

Hormone	Function	Cell Type
Glucagon	Stimulates production of glucose	Alpha
Insulin	Stimulates cells to take up glucose	Beta
Somatostatin	Controls rate of carbohydrate absorption in blood	Delta
Pancreatic polypeptide	Controls secretion of digestive enzymes	F

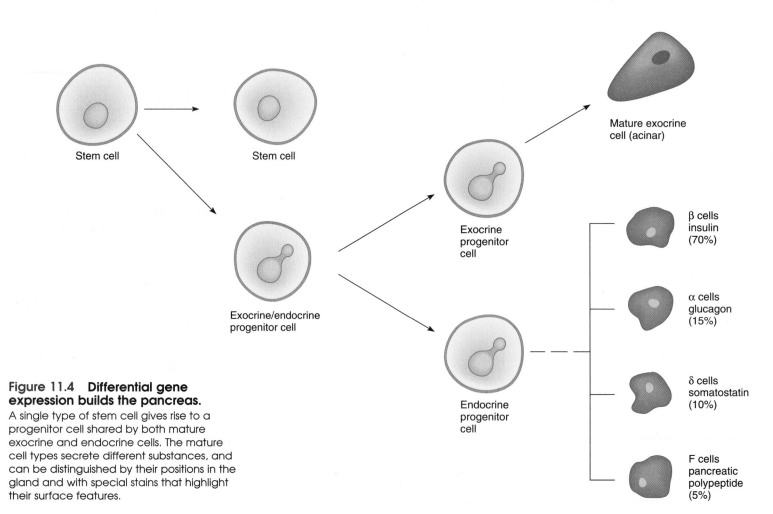

Figure 11.4 Differential gene expression builds the pancreas.

A single type of stem cell gives rise to a progenitor cell shared by both mature exocrine and endocrine cells. The mature cell types secrete different substances, and can be distinguished by their positions in the gland and with special stains that highlight their surface features.

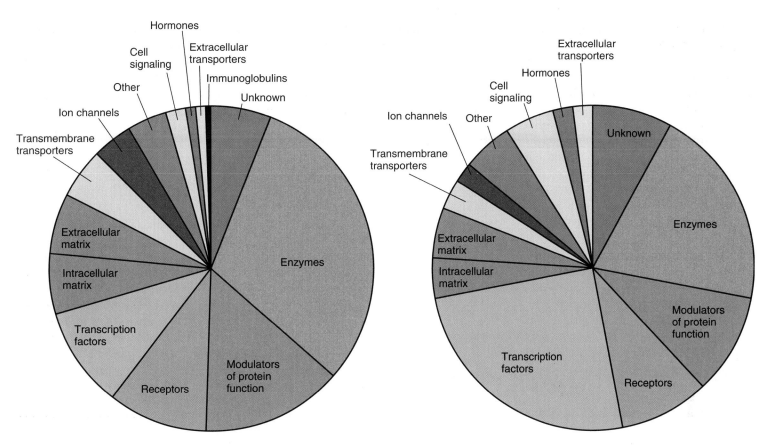

a. Distribution of health-related proteins from conception through old age

b. Distribution of health-related proteins from conception to birth

Figure 11.5 **Proteomics meets medicine.** One way to analyze the effects of genes is to categorize them by the functions of their protein products, and then to chart the relative abundance of each class at different stages of development, in sickness and in health. The pie chart in **(a)** considers 14 categories of proteins that when abnormal or missing cause disease, and their relative abundance from conception through advanced age. The pie chart in **(b)** displays the same protein categories for the prenatal period, from conception to birth. These depictions represent just one of the many new ways of looking at differential gene expression.

has led to the creation of various new "ome" words. Genes whose encoded proteins control lipid synthesis constitute the "lipidome," and those that monitor carbohydrate production and utilization form the "glycome." Genes whose products regulate the nervous system form the "neuroproteome." "Omics" can be highly specific. For example, the "kinome" consists of 518 genes that encode protein kinases, which are enzymes that add phosphate groups to other proteins. Researchers make fun of all the "omics," but the designations are helpful in sorting out the thousands of proteins a human cell can manufacture. But identifying the proteins is only a first step. The next hurdle is to determine how proteins with related functions interact.

Researchers are accumulating gene expression profiles for all sorts of cells under all sorts of conditions. Comparing gene expression profiles over time is particularly useful clinically, to chart disease progression and response to therapy. For example, 55 genes are overexpressed and 480 underexpressed in cells of a prostate cancer that has a very high likelihood of spreading. Cells from a prostate cancer that will not spread have a different gene expression profile.

Key Concepts

Gene expression changes over time and in different cell types. The subunit composition of hemoglobin changes in the embryo, fetus, and after birth.
• As a pancreas forms, progenitor cells diverge from shared stem cells and their daughters specialize.
• Proteomics tracks all of the proteins in a cell, tissue, organ, or organism under specified conditions.

11.2 Mechanisms of Gene Expression

We have already seen in a general sense how gene expression is controlled, and it is a complex, multilayered picture: Combinations of signals instruct cells to activate combinations of transcription factors, and these in turn control which genes are transcribed. The transcription factors interact, positioning DNA to facilitate its interactions with yet other proteins. We now take a closer look at two specific mechanisms of control over gene expression—how changing chromatin structure regulates DNA accessibility, and how small "interfering" RNA molecules seek and destroy selected mRNA transcripts.

The Histone Code

For many years, biologists thought that histones were simple scaffolds that wind up long DNA molecules into nucleosomes, little more than tiny spools (see figure 9.12). However, histones play a major role in exposing DNA when it is to be transcribed, and shielding it when it is to be silenced. Enzymes add or delete various small chemical groups to the histones. The resulting patterns of added chemical groups control the effect of histones on their associated protein-encoding genes.

The key to the role histones play in controlling gene expression lies in small organic molecules called acetyl groups (CH_3CO_2). At first, when acetyl groups were identified on the "tails" of certain histones, they were thought to loosen the grip between histones and genes by disrupting electrical attractions between the two. But when experiments revealed that the acetyls bind to very specific sites on certain histones, particularly to the amino acid lysine, the idea emerged that the pattern of histone binding in itself holds information, called the histone code.

For years the histone code was not much more than a controversial idea. Then, researchers at Columbia University deciphered the histone code for a particular gene—the one that encodes beta interferon, an immune system protein that combats viral infection. **Figure 11.6** shows how acetyl binding can subtly shift histone interactions in a way that eases transcription. A series of proteins moves the histone complex away from the TATA box, exposing it enough for RNA polymerase to bind and transcription to begin (see figure 10.6). First, a group of proteins called an enhanceosome attracts the enzyme (acetylase) that adds acetyl groups to specific lysines on specific histones. Then transcription factors bind, and transcription begins. Enzymes called deacetylases remove acetyl groups, which shuts off gene expression. Many researchers are now investigating whether the histone code for the beta interferon gene applies to other genes.

Methyl groups (CH_3) are also added to or taken away from histones. Recall that in genomic imprinting (see section 6.5), methyl groups silence DNA. When CH_3 binds to a specific amino acid in a specific histone type, a protein called HP1 (for heterochromatin protein) is attracted, and shuts the DNA off. (Heterochromatin is dark-staining DNA, and is discussed further in chapter 13.) This methylation spreads from the tail of one histone to the adjacent histone, propagating the gene silencing. Experiments in mice have shown that functional genes placed next to DNA covered with methylated histones are also shut off, indicating that the effect spreads along a chromosome.

The complete histone code may include binding patterns for acetyl, methyl, and perhaps also phosphate groups. Altering the chromatin by adding or removing chemical groups is termed **chromatin remodeling.** The altered state of the chromatin can be passed on when DNA replicates. This is an example of an epigenetic change, or change "outside conventional genetics." That is, these changes are heritable, but they do not directly affect the DNA sequence. How the histone code operates is not well understood. Enzymes that add or delete acetyl, methyl, and phosphate groups must be in a balance that controls which genes are expressed and which are silenced.

RNA Interference

Genetics continues to hold surprises—which makes writing a textbook difficult! Chapter 10 clearly stated that for any gene, only one strand of the DNA is transcribed. But there are exceptions. Up to 8 percent of genes may actually be transcribed from both strands, leading to a phenomenon called **RNA interference** (or RNAi) that destroys specific mRNA molecules. Transcribing both DNA strands leads to the formation of single-stranded RNAs that bind in places within themselves to generate double-stranded, hairpin-shaped structures. Through a series of interactions with proteins, these RNAs are shortened to form "small interfering RNAs," known as siRNAs, that are opened up and then find and bind their mRNA complements, tagging them for dismantling by enzymes.

The siRNAs affect gene expression in the nucleus and in the cytoplasm. In the nucleus, siRNAs help add methyls to histones, shutting off transcription at its start. Slightly smaller siRNAs in the cytoplasm bind mature mRNAs, acting after transcription ends. RNA interference is not the normal dismantling of a used mRNA, but a distinct mechanism that suppresses expression of certain genes.

The inhibiting effects of short double-stranded RNA molecules were first noted in plants, where they destroy infecting viral DNA. They were overlooked in human cells perhaps because they are so small and fleeting, and researchers focused for many years on the larger and more abundant mRNA, rRNA, and tRNA molecules.

As in other activities in the cell, several proteins and protein complexes orchestrate the steps of RNA interference (**figure 11.7**). An enzyme called dicer first cuts long double-stranded RNAs into 21- or 22-base-long pieces. Then a large protein complex called RISC (for RNA-induced silencing

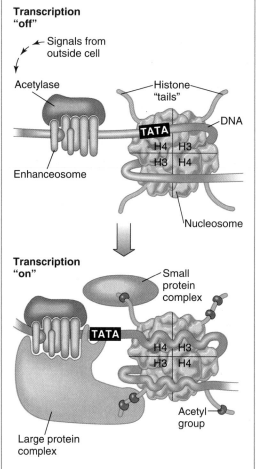

Figure 11.6 Acetylated histones allow transcription to begin.
Once acetyl groups are added to particular amino acids in the tails of certain histones, the TATA box becomes accessible to transcription factors. In this case, transcription of the beta interferon gene can begin. (H3 and H4 are histone types.)

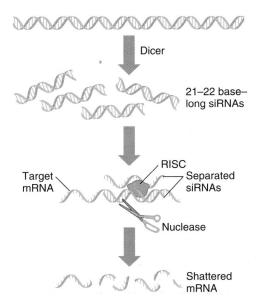

Figure 11.7 RNA interference.
Dicer cuts double-stranded portions of RNA molecules, which then associate with RNA-induced silencing complexes (RISCs). The RNAs open, revealing single strands that locate and bind specific mRNAs by complementary base pairing. Nucleases then break down the targeted mRNAs. This action controls gene expression by destroying specific transcripts.

complex) binds the pieces and unwinds them, exposing single strands. These strands then attract their complementary mRNAs, which are then chewed up by enzymes called nucleases.

Introducing siRNAs into cells is a useful research tool. An siRNA is said to "knock down" a specific mRNA, compared to other techniques, discussed in chapter 19, that "knock out" or "knock in" a function. "Knocking down" depletes the mRNA molecules representing a particular gene, whereas "knocking out" completely silences a gene and "knocking in" adds a gene. Some of the first experiments using siRNA were done on the nematode worm *Caenorhabditis elegans.* This worm is a model organism used to study development, and was one of the first to have its genome sequenced (see figure 1 in Reading 22.1). Researchers fed short double-stranded RNAs to the worms, and identified the functions of many genes by observing how each siRNA affected the animal. Experiments that used only siRNAs involved in fat metabolism identified several hundred genes that control fat deposition—suggesting new places to

look in the human genome for genes that control weight.

RNAi already has applications. In vaccine research, RNAi knocks down gene expression from the viruses that cause AIDS, polio, SARS and hepatitis C. SiRNA can knock down an enzyme required for caffeine synthesis in coffee plants, creating a better-tasting decaf. A library of siRNAs covering the entire human transcriptome—that is, all of the DNA that encodes protein—will support research and clinical applications of controlling gene expression for many years to come.

Key Concepts

Nucleosomes control gene expression through the acetylation of specific amino acids on specific histone proteins. Acetylation contorts the histone so that transcription of a nearby gene can begin. Removing the acetyl groups stops transcription. Methyl and phosphate groups control histone function, too. • In RNA interference, short double-stranded RNA molecules locate and bind to specific mRNAs, marking them for destruction, and also add methyls to DNA in the nucleus, blocking transcription.

11.3 Proteins Outnumber Genes

Cataloging protein diversity in tissue and time reveals a numerical mismatch—our 25,000 or so genes encode 200,000 or more different proteins. But this apparent paradox wasn't entirely unexpected.

The discovery of introns in 1977 first planted the idea that a number of genes could specify a larger number of proteins by mixing and matching gene parts. Research since then has revealed that many exons encode stretches of amino acids, called domains, that can be part of more than one protein. For example, the DNA that encodes a blood-clotting protein called tissue plasminogen activator (t-PA) includes sequences from genes that encode three other proteins (plasminogen, epidermal growth factor, and fibronectin)—that's four proteins from three genes. This process of combining exons is called **exon shuffling,** and it is possible because of alternate splicing patterns of mRNA molecules. **Figure 11.8** illustrates schematically how two genes can give rise to at least seven proteins. Exon shuffling is evident on a chromosomal scale. On a part of chromosome 22, for example, 245 genes yield 642 mRNA transcripts.

Introns may seem wasteful, little more than vast stretches of DNA bases that

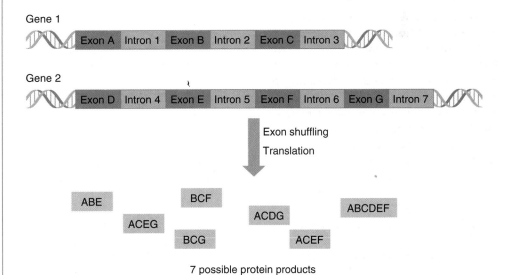

Figure 11.8 Exon shuffling expands gene number. This schematic illustration shows how two genes can encode at least seven possible distinct proteins. Considering that many genes have many more introns than this one, it's clear that exon shuffling can generate many different proteins.

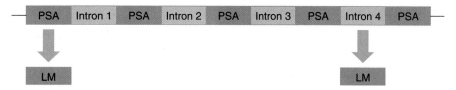

Figure 11.9 **Two genes from one.** Embedded in the PSA gene are two protein-encoded sequences—the PSA portion consists of five exons, and the PSA-LM part consists of two exons, one of which lies within an intron of PSA. (Not drawn to scale; introns are much larger than exons.)

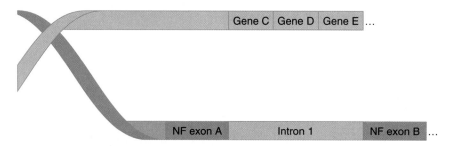

Figure 11.10 **Genes in introns.** An intron of the neurofibromin gene harbors three genes on the opposite strand.

outnumber and outsize exons. But a DNA sequence that is an intron in one context may encode protein in another. Consider prostate specific antigen (PSA), a protein found on certain cell surfaces that is overproduced in some cases of prostate cancer (**figure 11.9**). The gene for PSA has five exons and four introns, but it also encodes a second, different protein, called PSA-linked molecule (PSA-LM). Both genes have the same beginning DNA sequence, but the remainder of the PSA-LM gene is part of the fourth intron of the PSA sequence! The proteins seem to have antagonistic functions. That is, when the level of one is high, the other is low. Future blood tests to detect elevated risk of prostate cancer will likely consider levels of both proteins.

In another situation where introns may account for the overabundance of proteins compared to genes, a DNA sequence that is an intron in one gene's template strand may encode protein on the coding strand. That is, what is the template strand for one gene may be the coding strand for the other. This is the case for the gene for neurofibromin, which when mutant causes neurofibromatosis type 1 (an autosomal

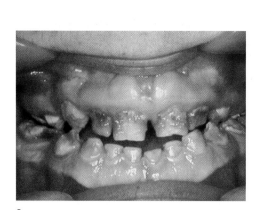

a.

Figure 11.11 **Another way to encode two genes in one.** **(a)** The misshapen, discolored, and enamel-stripped teeth of a person with dentinogenesis imperfecta were at first associated with deficiency of the protein DPP. Then researchers discovered that DSP is deficient, too, but is usually present in such small amounts that its role wasn't recognized. **(b)** Both DPP and DSP are cut from the same larger protein, but DSP is degraded faster.

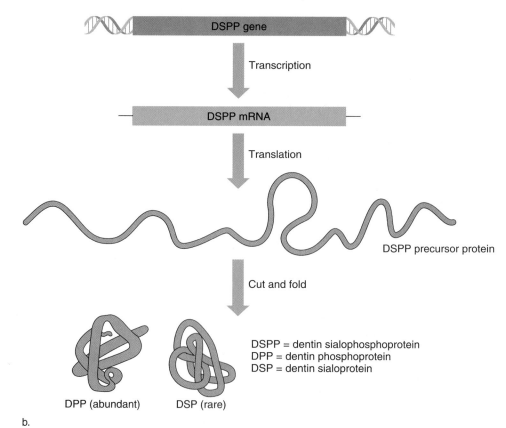

b.

DSPP = dentin sialophosphoprotein
DPP = dentin phosphoprotein
DSP = dentin sialoprotein

dominant condition that causes benign tumors beneath the skin and "café au lait" spots on the skin surface). Within an intron of the neurofibromin gene, but on the coding strand, are instructions for three other genes (**figure 11.10**). It's even possible for a single RNA to be patched together from instructions on both strands, an apparently rare occurrence called trans-splicing.

Still another way a gene can maximize its informational content is for its encoded protein to be cut to yield two products. This happens in dentinogenesis imperfecta, which causes discolored, misshapen teeth with peeling enamel (**figure 11.11**). The dentin, which is the bonelike substance beneath the enamel that forms the bulk of the tooth, is abnormal. Dentin is a complex mixture of extracellular matrix proteins. Dentin protein is 90 percent collagen, and this and most of the rest of the proteins are also found in bone. However, two proteins are unique to dentin: dentin phosphoprotein (DPP) and dentin sialoprotein (DSP). The single gene that encodes these two proteins is part of an area of chromosome 4 that seems devoted to teeth.

Researchers had associated abnormal DPP with dentinogenesis imperfecta. However, DPP, because it is much more abundant than DSP, may have overshadowed the rarer protein. Both DPP and DSP are translated from a single mRNA molecule as the precursor protein dentin sialophosphoprotein (DSPP). DPP may be much more abundant because it is longer-lived than DSP; that is, DSP degrades faster. These two proteins remain somewhat of a mystery. Often when genes with similar functions lie right next to each other on a chromosome, as these do, it is because they arose from gene duplication; the two genes are then very similar in sequence. This is not the case with the DNA sequences that encode DPP and DSP.

Key Concepts

Only a tiny proportion of the genome encodes protein, yet the number of proteins greatly outnumbers known protein-encoding genes. Exon shuffling, introns that encode protein, and single genes that encode a precursor protein later cut in two all maximize the number of proteins that DNA encodes.

11.4 The "Other" 98.5 Percent of the Human Genome

When the first generation of molecular geneticists worked out the details of transcription and translation in the 1960s, they never imagined that only 1.5 percent of the human genome encodes protein. What does the "other" 98.5 percent do? In general, this noncoding DNA falls into four categories: (1) RNAs other than mRNA (called noncoding or ncRNAs), (2) introns, (3) promoters and other control sequences, including siRNAs, and (4) repeated sequences (**table 11.2**).

Noncoding (nc) RNAs

About a third of the human genome is transcribed into RNA types other than mRNA, such as tRNA and rRNA. The rate of transcription of a cell's tRNA genes is attuned to cell specialization. The collection of proteins characteristic of a skeletal muscle cell, for example, would require different amounts of certain amino acids than the proteins of a white blood cell, and therefore different amounts of the corresponding tRNAs too.

Human tRNA genes are dispersed among the chromosomes in clusters—25 percent of them are on the sixth largest chromosome, for example. Altogether, tRNAs account for

Table 11.2

The Nonprotein Encoding Parts of the Human Genome

	Function or Characteristic
Noncoding RNA genes	
tRNA genes	Connect mRNA codon to amino acid
rRNA genes	Parts of ribosomes
Pseudogenes	DNA sequences very similar to known gene sequences that may be transcribed but are not translated
Small nucleolar RNAs	Process rRNA in nucleolus
Small nuclear RNAs	Parts of spliceosomes
Telomerase RNA	Part of ribonucleoprotein that adds bases to chromosome tips
Xist RNA	Inactivates one X chromosome in cells of females
Vault RNA	Part of "vault," a large ribonucleoprotein complex of unknown function
Introns	Parts of protein-encoding genes that are transcribed but cut out before the encoded protein is translated
Promoters and other control sequences	Guide enzymes that carry out DNA replication, transcription, or translation
Small interfering RNAs	Control transcription
Micro RNAs	Control transcription
Repeats	
Transposons	Repeats that move around the genome
Telomeres	Chromosome tips whose lengths control the cell cycle
Centromeres	Provide backdrop for proteins that form attachments for spindle fibers
Duplications of 10 to 300 kilobases	Unknown
Simple short repeats	Unknown

0.1 percent of the genome. Our 500 or so types of tRNA genes may seem like a lot, but frogs have thousands! This may reflect the fact that frog eggs are huge and contain many types of proteins.

The 243 types of rRNA genes are clustered on six chromosomes, each cluster harboring 150 to 200 copies of a 44,000-base repeat sequence. Once transcribed from these clustered genes, the rRNAs go to the nucleolus, where yet another type of ncRNA called small nucleolar RNAs (snoRNAs) cuts them into their final forms.

Hundreds of thousands of ncRNAs are neither tRNA nor rRNA, nor snoRNAs, nor the other less-abundant types described in table 11.2. Instead, they are transcribed from DNA sequences called **pseudogenes.** A pseudogene is very similar in sequence to a particular protein-encoding gene, and it may be transcribed into RNA, but it is not translated into protein. Presumably it is altered in sequence from the original gene in a way that impairs its translation—perhaps the encoded amino acids cannot fold into a functional protein. Pseudogenes may be remnants of genes past, once-functional variants that diverged from the normal sequence too greatly to encode a working protein. Pseudogenes are incredibly common in the human genome. For example, at least 324 pseudogenes shadow our tRNA genes.

Repeats

The human genome is riddled with highly repetitive sequences that appear to be gibberish, at least if we restrict the definition of genetic meaning to encoding protein. It is entirely possible that repeats represent a different type of genetic information, perhaps using a language in which meaning lies in a repeat size or number. Some types of repeats may help to hold a chromosome together.

The most abundant type of repeat is a sequence of DNA that can jump about the genome, called a transposable element, or **transposon** for short. Barbara McClintock originally identified them in corn in the 1940s, and then they were discovered in bacteria in the 1960s. Transposons comprise about 45 percent of the human genome sequence. They are repeats because they are typically present in many copies. Some transposons include parts that encode enzymes that enable them to leave one chromosomal site and integrate into another.

Transposons are classified by size, whether they are transcribed into RNA, which enzymes they use to move, and whether they resemble bacterial transposons. For example, a class of transposons called long interspersed elements (LINEs) are 6,000 bases long and are transcribed and then trimmed to 900 bases before they are "reverse transcribed" back into DNA (by an enzyme called reverse transcriptase) and re-inserted into a chromosome. In contrast, short interspersed elements (SINEs) are 100 to 500 bases long and use enzymes that are encoded in LINEs to insert.

A major class of SINEs are called Alu repeats. Each Alu repeat is about 300 bases long, and a genome may contain 300,000 to 500,000 of them. Alu repeats comprise 2 to 3 percent of the genome, and they have been increasing in number over time because they can copy themselves. Alu repeats may serve as attachment points for proteins called cohesins that bind newly replicated DNA to parental strands before anaphase, when replicated chromosomes pull apart in mitosis.

Other rarer classes of repeats include those that comprise telomeres, centromeres, and rRNA gene clusters; duplications of 10,000 to 300,000 bases (10 to 300 kilobases); copies of pseudogenes; and simple repeats of one, two, or three bases. Many repeats arise from RNAs that are reverse transcribed into DNA and are then inserted into chromosomes. In fact, the entire human genome may have duplicated once or even twice, as is discussed further in chapter 16.

Our understanding of the functions of repeats lags far behind our knowledge of the roles of the various noncoding RNA genes. Repeats may make sense in light of evolution, past and future. Pseudogenes are likely vestiges of genes that functioned in our nonhuman ancestors. Perhaps the repeats that seem to have no obvious function today will serve as raw material from which future genes may arise.

Key Concepts

The 98.5 percent of the human genome that does not specify protein encodes many types of RNA as well as introns, promoters, and other control sequences and repeats. We do not know the functions of some types of repeats.

Summary

11.1 Gene Expression Through Time and Tissue

1. Changes in gene expression occur over time at the molecular level (globin switching), at the tissue level (blood plasma), and at the organ/gland level (pancreas development).

2. Proteomics uses analytical chemistry techniques and gene expression DNA microarrays to catalog the types of proteins in particular cells, tissues, organs, or entire organisms under specified conditions.

11.2 Mechanisms of Gene Expression

3. Acetylation of certain histones enables the transcription of associated genes. Phosphorylation and methylation are also important in **chromatin remodeling.**

4. The pattern of chemical groups on histones forms an epigenetic code that spreads, can be transmitted when the cell divides, and controls gene expression.

5. **RNA interference** promotes gene silencing in the nucleus and removes certain mRNAs in the cytoplasm.

11.3 Proteins Outnumber Genes

6. Only 1.5 percent of the human genome encodes protein, yet those 25,000 or so genes specify up to 200,000 proteins.

7. Mechanisms to explain the mismatch between gene and protein diversity include **exon shuffling,** use of introns, and cutting proteins translated from a single gene.

11.4 The "Other" 98.5 Percent of the Human Genome

8. The rest of the genome includes noncoding RNAs, introns, promoters and other controls, and repeats.

Review Questions

1. Why is control of gene expression necessary?

2. What questions about DNA were raised after the genetic code was worked out in the 1960s, and then after sequencing the human genome?

3. What is the environmental signal that stimulates globin switching?

4. How does development of the pancreas illustrate differential gene expression?

5. Distinguish between a genetic and an epigenetic change.

6. How do histones control gene expression, yet genes also control histones?

7. Name two types of chemical reactions that silence transcription.

8. How is the function of siRNA in the cytoplasm similar to the function of proteasomes (see figure 10.17)?

9. In the 1960s, a gene was defined as a continuous sequence of DNA, located permanently at one place on a chromosome, that specifies a sequence of amino acids from one strand. List three ways this definition has changed.

10. Give three examples of discoveries mentioned in the chapter that changed the way we think about the genome.

11. What are the functions of each of the following proteins or protein complexes?

   a. acetylases and deacetylases

   b. dicer

   c. RISC

   d. enhanceosome

   e. locus control region

   f. pdx-1 transcription factor

12. How can one of the two dental proteins implicated in dentinogenesis imperfecta be much more abundant than the other, if they are both transcribed and translated from the same gene?

13. How can the same long stretch of amino acids be part of three different proteins?

14. State four roles of DNA other than encoding protein.

Applied Questions

1. SAGE (serial analysis of gene expression) is a technique that uses tags that correspond to many exons to detect proteins that result from alternate splicing. Gene expression DNA microarrays cannot detect splice variants. Why would it be valuable clinically to be able to identify all the proteins in which a particular exon's encoded amino acid sequence is found?

2. Invent a new "omics" to investigate genes that are functionally related in a particular way.

3. Drug companies are synthesizing compounds that inhibit the enzymes that either put acetyl groups on histones or take them off. Would you use an inhibitor of an acetylase or a deacetylase to combat a cancer caused by too little expression of a gene that normally suppresses cell division?

4. Chromosome 7 has 863 protein-encoding genes, but many more proteins. The average gene is 69,877 bases, but the average mRNA is 2,639 bases. Explain both of these observations.

5. When researchers compared the number of mRNA transcripts that correspond to a part of chromosome 19 to the number of protein-encoding genes in the region, they found 1,859 transcripts and 544 genes. State three mechanisms that could account for the discrepancy.

6. Figure 11.5 shows the distribution of types of proteins that, when abnormal or absent from a certain cell type, cause disease. Such charts have been constructed for different stages of development—prenatal, under a year, childhood, puberty to age 50, and over age 50. Explain the observation that transcription factors account for:

   • 9 percent of proteins overall (throughout development and life)

   • 25 percent of proteins before birth

   • 7 percent of proteins from birth to one year

   • 6 percent of proteins from childhood to age 50 years

   • 5 percent of proteins for those over 50 years

Web Activities

7. Many companies are offering products based on RNA interference to use in research to "knock down" gene expression. Go to one of the following websites, or find others, learn about a particular RNAi product, and suggest how it might be used. (The companies listed have all existed for many years. There are many newer ones.)

Ambion	www.ambion.com
Invitrogen	www.invitrogen.com
New England Biolabs	www.neb.com
Novagen	www.novagen.com
Qiagen	www.qiagen.com
Stratagene	www.stratagene.com

Case Studies

8. Jerrold is 38 years old. His body produces too much of the hormone estrogen and as a result, he has gynecomastia—well-developed breasts. He had a growth spurt and development of pubic hair by age 5, and then his

growth dramatically slowed so that his adult height is well below normal. He had his breasts removed, but has a very high-pitched voice and no facial hair, which are lingering signs of his excess estrogen production. Jerrold's son, Timmy, is 8 years old and has the exact same symptoms—breast enlargement and early rapid growth.

Jerrold and Timmy have an overactive gene for aromatase, an enzyme required to synthesize estrogen. Five promoters control expression of the gene in a tissue-specific manner, each promoter activated by a different combination of hormonal signals. The five promoters lead to estrogen production in skin, fat, brain, gonads (ovaries and testes) and placenta. In premenopausal women, the ovary-specific promoter is highly active, and estrogen is abundant. In men and postmenopausal women, however, only small amounts of estrogen are normally produced, in skin and fat. The father and son had a wild type aromatase gene, but high levels of estrogen in several tissues, particularly fat, skin, and blood. They do, however, have a mutation that turns around an adjacent gene so that it falls under the control of a different promoter. Suggest an explanation for their phenotype.

9. Margaret is 102 years old, and she still walks at least half a mile a day, albeit slowly. She is a trim vegetarian who has rarely been ill her entire life. Morris is an obese, balding 62-year-old man who has high blood pressure and colon cancer. How might their proteome portraits, such as the one in figure 11.5, differ? (Hint: reread Reading 3.1, The Centenarian Genome.)

Learn to apply the skills of a genetic counselor with this additional case found in the *Case Workbook in Human Genetics*:

Hypoxia-inducible factor 1

Suggested Readings

Agalioti, Theodora, et al. November 1, 2002. Deciphering the transcriptional histone acetylation code for a human gene. *Cell* 111:381–92. Is the histone code for the beta interferon gene the same as that for other genes?

Carmichael, Gordon G. April 2003. Antisense starts making more sense. *Nature Biotechnology* 21:371–72. RNAs do a lot more than encode protein; they control gene expression.

Cullen, Brayn R. July 2002. RNA interference: antiviral defense and genetic tool. *Nature Immunology* 3(7):597–99. RNA interference may have evolved to protect plants from viral infection, but today's researchers use it to knock down gene expression.

Felsenfield, Gary, and Mark Groudine. January 23, 2003. Controlling the double helix. *Nature* 421:448–53. The histone code controls expression of the genetic code.

Hannon, Gregory. July 11, 2002. RNA interference. *Nature* 418:244–51. Hannon discovered dicer, the enzyme that cuts double-stranded RNAs down to size.

Lewis, Ricki. February 24, 2003. RNA calls the shots. *The Scientist* 17(4):29–30. There are some ways RNA controls gene expression other than those mentioned in the chapter.

Lewis, Ricki, and Barry Palevitz. June 11, 2001. Genome economy. *The Scientist* 15(12):1. Some other ways RNA controls gene expression that were not mentioned in the chapter.

Mennella, Thomas. June 16, 2003. The out-of-hand omnipresent ome. *The Scientist* 17(12):52. A call for an anti-omics movement.

Ogita, Shinjiro, et al. June 19, 2003. Producing decaffeinated coffee plants. *Nature* 423:823. RNA interference already has practical applications.

Pennisi, Elizabeth. August 22, 2003. Gene counters struggle to get the right answer. *Science* 301:1040–1041. Researchers still cannot agree on the number of genes in the human genome.

Weekly updates of current news related to human genetics are available through Power Web on your Online Learning Center.

C H A P T E R

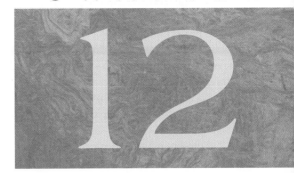

Gene Mutation

12

CHAPTER CONTENTS

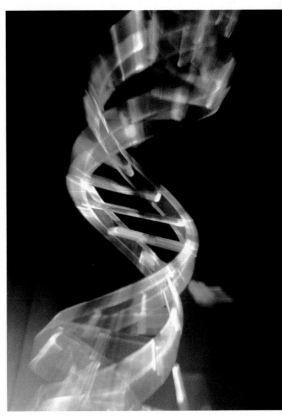

Changes in the DNA sequence can affect health or alter inherited traits.

A **mutation** is a change in a gene's nucleotide base sequence. It can occur at the molecular level, substituting one DNA base for another or adding or deleting a few bases, or at the chromosome level, the subject of chapter 13. Chromosomes can exchange parts, and genetic material can even jump from one chromosome to another. This chapter discusses mutations at the DNA level. They occur in the part of a gene that encodes a protein, in a sequence that controls transcription, in an intron, or at a site critical to intron removal and exon splicing.

The effects of mutation vary. A mutation can stop or slow production of a protein, overproduce it, or impair the protein's function—such as altering its secretion, location, or interaction with another protein. Not all mutations are harmful. For example, about 1 percent of the general population is homozygous for a recessive allele that encodes a cell surface protein called CCR5 (see figure 17.13). To enter a T cell, HIV must bind to CCR5 and to another protein. The mutation prevents CCR5 from traveling from the cytoplasm to the cell surface. HIV cannot bind and the person cannot become infected. Heterozygotes are partially protected against HIV infection—they are at considerably lower risk.

The term *mutation* refers to genotype—that is, a change at the DNA or chromosome level. The familiar term **mutant** refers to an unusual phenotype. A mutant phenotype depends upon how the alteration affects the gene's product or activity, and usually connotes an abnormal or unusual characteristic. However, it may also mean an unusual variant that is nevertheless "normal," such as a red-haired child in a class of brunettes and blondes. Detecting mutations forms the basis of the several types of genetic tests described in **table 12.1**.

In an evolutionary sense, mutation has been essential to life, because it produces individuals with variant phenotypes who are better able to survive specific environmental challenges, including illnesses. Disease-resistant gene variants that arise by mutation tend to become more common in populations over time when they exert a protective effect, because they give the people with the mutation a survival advantage. Chapter 15 further discusses the role of mutations in populations.

A mutation may be present in all the cells of an individual or just in some cells. In a **germline mutation,** the change occurs during the DNA replication that precedes *meiosis*. The resulting gamete and all the cells that descend from it after fertilization have the mutation. In contrast, in a **somatic mutation,** the change happens during DNA replication before a *mitotic* cell division. All the cells that descend from the original changed cell are altered, but they might only comprise a small part of the body. Somatic mutations are responsible for certain cancers (see Reading 18.2 and figure 18.4).

12.1 Mutations Can Alter Proteins—Three Examples

Identifying how a mutation causes symptoms has clinical applications, and also reveals the workings of biology. Following are three examples of mutant genes.

The Beta Globin Gene

The first genetic illness to be understood at the molecular level was sickle cell disease. Researchers knew in the 1940s that an inherited anemia (weakness and fatigue caused by too few red blood cells) was associated with sickle-shaped red blood cells (**figure 12.1**). In 1949, Linus Pauling discovered that hemo-

Table 12.1

Types of Genetic Tests

Type of Test	Information Provided	Example
Carrier screen	Identifies heterozygotes—people with one copy of a mutant gene	The healthy sibling of a child with CF is tested—chance of being a carrier is 2/3.
Prenatal test	Detects mutant gene in a fetus for a condition present in a family	A couple who know they are carriers of Tay-Sachs disease have a fetus tested.
Prenatal screen	Tests embryos or fetuses from a population for increased risk of a condition, not based on family history	A pregnant woman's blood is tested for elevated level of a protein indicating increased risk for neural tube defect.
Newborn screen	Populationwide testing for several treatable inborn errors of metabolism	A child identified with sickle cell disease genes at birth can prevent or delay symptoms with antibiotics.
Diagnostic test	Confirms diagnosis based on symptoms	A child with "failure to thrive" and frequent lung infections is tested for mutant alleles for CF.
Predisposition test	Detects allele(s) associated with an illness, but not absolutely diagnostic of it	A young Jewish woman with a strong family history of breast cancer has a mutant *BRCA1* allele, giving her an 85 percent lifetime risk of developing the condition.
Predictive test	Detects highly penetrant mutation with adult onset in an individual at high risk based on family history	A healthy person is tested for the *HD* allele because one of his parents has the condition.

globin from healthy people and from people with the anemia, when placed in a solution in an electrically charged field (a technique called electrophoresis), moved to different positions. Hemoglobin from the parents of people with the anemia, who were carriers, showed movement to both positions.

The difference between the two types of hemoglobin lay in beta globin. Recall from figure 11.1 that adult hemoglobin consists of two alpha polypeptide subunits and two beta subunits. Protein chemist V. M. Ingram developed a shortcut to localize the mutation in the 146-amino-acid-long protein. He cut normal and sickle hemoglobin with a protein-digesting enzyme, separated the pieces, stained them, and displayed them on filter paper. The patterns of fragments—known as peptide fingerprints—were different for the two types of hemoglobin. This meant, Ingram deduced, that the two molecules differ in amino acid sequence. Then he homed in on the difference. One piece of the molecule in the fingerprint, fragment four, occupied a different position in each of the two types of hemoglobin. Because this peptide was only 8 amino acids long,

Ingram needed to decipher only that short sequence to find the site of the mutation. It was a little like knowing which sentence on a page contains a typographical error.

Ingram identified the tiny mutation responsible for sickle cell disease: a substitution of the amino acid valine for the glutamic acid that is normally the sixth amino acid in the beta globin polypeptide chain. At the DNA level, the change was even smaller—a CTC to a CAC, corresponding to RNA codons GAG and GUG, learned after researchers deciphered the genetic code. This mutation changes the surfaces of hemoglobin molecules so that they link when in low-oxygen conditions, bending the red blood cells into rigid, fragile, sickle-shaped structures. The misshapen cells lodge in narrow blood vessels, cutting off local blood supplies and causing anemia, joint pain, and organ damage.

Sickle cell disease was the first inherited illness linked to a molecular abnormality, but it wasn't the first known condition that results from a mutation in the beta globin genes. In 1925, Thomas Cooley and Pearl Lee described severe anemia in Italian chil-

dren, and in the decade following, others described a milder version of "Cooley's anemia," also in Italian children. The disease was named thalassemia, from the Greek for "sea," in light of its high prevalence in the Mediterranean area. The two disorders turned out to be versions of the same illness. The severe form, sometimes called thalassemia major, results from a homozygous mutation in the beta globin gene. The milder form, called thalassemia minor, is associated with heterozygosity for the mutation.

Once researchers had worked out the structure of the hemoglobin molecule, and learned that different globins function in the embryonic and fetal periods, the molecular basis of thalassemia became clear. The disorder that is common in the Mediterranean area is more accurately called beta thalassemia, because the symptoms result from too few beta globin chains, which are needed to build enough hemoglobin molecules to effectively deliver oxygen to tissues. Symptoms of anemia, such as fatigue and bone pain, arise during the first year of life as the child depletes fetal hemoglobin supplies, and the "adult" beta globin genes are not transcribed and translated on schedule.

As severe beta thalassemia continues, red blood cells die because of the relative excess of alpha globin chains, and the liberated iron slowly destroys the heart, liver, and endocrine glands. People with the disorder can receive periodic blood transfusions to control the anemia, but this treatment hastens iron buildup and organ damage. Drugs called chelators that entrap the iron can extend life past early adulthood, but this treatment is very costly and is not available in developing nations.

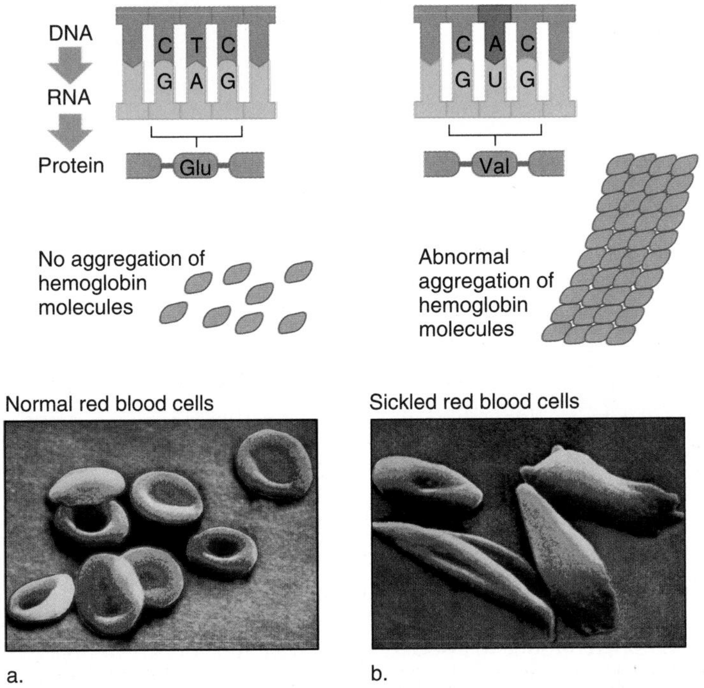

Disorders of Orderly Collagen

Much of the human body consists of the protein collagen. It accounts for more than 60 percent of the protein in bone and cartilage and provides 50 to 90 percent of the dry weight of skin, ligaments, tendons, and the dentin of teeth. Collagen is in parts of the eyes and the blood vessel linings, and it separates cell types in tissues. It is also a major component of connective tissue. Mutations in the genes that encode collagen lead to a variety of medical problems (table 12.2).

DNA → RNA → Protein

C T C / G A G — Glu

No aggregation of hemoglobin molecules

Normal red blood cells

a.

C A C / G U G — Val

Abnormal aggregation of hemoglobin molecules

Sickled red blood cells

b.

Figure 12.1 Sickle cell disease results from a single DNA base change. Hemoglobin carries oxygen throughout the body. When normal **(a)**, the globular molecules do not aggregate, enabling the cell to assume a rounded shape. In sickle cell disease **(b)**, a single DNA base change substitutes one amino acid in the protein (valine replaces glutamic acid). The result is a change in the surfaces of the molecules that causes aggregation into long, curved rods that deform the red blood cell.

Table 12.2

Collagen Disorders

Disorder	OMIM Number	Defect	Signs and Symptoms
Alport syndrome	203780	Mutation in type IV collagen interferes with tissue boundaries	Deafness and inflamed kidneys
Aortic aneurysm	100070	Missense mutation substitutes *arg* for *gly* in alpha 1 gene	Aorta bursts
Chondrodysplasia	302950	Deletion, insertion, or missense mutation replaces *gly* with bulky amino acids	Stunted growth, deformed joints
Dystrophic epidermolysis bullosa	226600	Collagen fibrils that attach epidermis to dermis break down	Skin blisters on any touch
Ehlers-Danlos syndrome	130050	Missense mutations replace *gly* with bulky amino acids; deletions or missense mutations disrupt intron/exon splicing	Stretchy, easily scarred skin, lax joints
Osteoarthritis	165720	Missense mutation substitutes *cys* for *arg* in alpha 1 gene	Painful joints
Osteogenesis imperfecta type I	166200	Inactivation of α allele reduces collagen triple helices by 50%	Easily broken bones; blue eye whites; deafness
Stickler syndrome	108300	Nonsense mutation in procollagen	Joint pain, degeneration of vitreous gel and retina

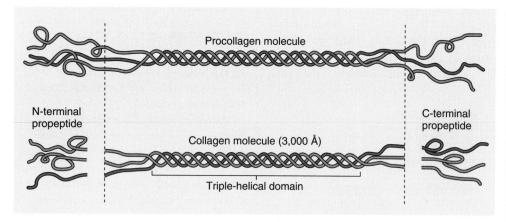

Figure 12.2 Collagen has a very precise conformation. The α1 collagen gene encodes the two blue polypeptide chains, and the α2 procollagen gene encodes the third (red) chain. The procollagen triple helix is shortened before it becomes functional, forming the fibrils and networks that comprise much of the human body.

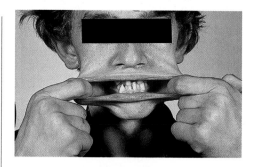

Figure 12.3 A disorder of connective tissue produces stretchy skin.
A mutation that blocks the trimming of procollagen chains to produce collagen causes the characteristic stretchy skin of Ehlers-Danlos syndrome type I. Researchers were able to find and study this gene by using a version from calves, which also inherit the condition.

This is not surprising, given collagen's diverse functions and locations.

Mutations in the collagen genes are particularly devastating because the encoded protein has an extremely precise conformation that is easily disrupted, even by slight alterations that might have little effect in proteins with other shapes (**figure 12.2**). Collagen is sculpted from a longer precursor molecule called procollagen, which consists of many repeats of a specific amino acid sequence (glycine, proline, and a modified proline). Three procollagen chains entwine. Two of the chains are identical and are encoded by one gene, and the other is encoded by a second gene. The electrical charges and interactions of these amino acids with water coil the procollagen chains into a very regular triple helix, with space in the middle only for glycine, a very small amino acid. The ragged ends of the polypeptides are snipped off by enzymes to form mature collagen. The collagen fibrils continue to associate outside the cell, building the fibrils and networks that hold the body together.

The boy in **figure 12.3** has a form of Ehlers-Danlos syndrome. A mutation prevents his procollagen chains from being cut, and collagen molecules cannot assemble. They form ribbonlike fibrils that lack the tensile strength to keep the skin from becoming too stretchy. Other collagen mutations cause missing procollagen chains, kinks in the triple helix, and defects in aggregation outside the cell.

Aortic aneurysm is a serious connective tissue disorder. Detection of the causative mutation before symptoms arise can be lifesaving. An early sign is a weakened aorta (the largest blood vessel in the body, which emerges from the heart), which can suddenly burst. A person who knows that he or she has inherited the mutant collagen gene can have frequent ultrasound exams to detect aortic weakening early enough to treat it surgically.

A Mutation That Causes Early-Onset Alzheimer Disease

The story of the discovery of the gene that causes an early-onset, autosomal dominant form of Alzheimer disease began in the 1880s, when a woman named Hannah, born in Latvia, developed progressive dementia. Hannah's condition was highly unusual; she was only in her early forties when the classic forgetfulness that heralds the disease's onset began. Apparently this form of the illness originated, in this family, in Hannah. Many of her descendants also experienced dementia—some as early as in their thirties.

In 1974, Hannah's grandson and great-grandson, both physicians, constructed an extensive pedigree tracing Alzheimer disease in their family. They circulated the pedigree among geneticists, hoping to elicit interest in identifying the family's mutation, offering their own and relatives' DNA for testing. Research teams in Mexico, the United States, and Canada began the search in 1983. By 1992, they narrowed the investigation to a portion of chromosome 14, and three years later, they pinpointed the gene. It encodes a protein called presenilin 1 that acts as a receptor anchored in the membrane of a Golgi apparatus or a vesicle (**figure 12.4**). Normally, the protein monitors the cell's storage or use of beta amyloid, the substance that accumulates in the brains of people with Alzheimer disease. Members of families that have early-onset Alzheimer disease due to mutation in this gene have elevated levels of presenilin 1 in their bloodstreams before symptoms begin. Somehow the abnormality in presenilin disrupts amyloid production, folding, or function.

So far, researchers have identified more than thirty mutations that substitute one amino acid for another in the gene for presenilin 1, impairing its function sufficiently to cause the beta amyloid buildup that eventually causes the symptoms of Alzheimer disease. Mutations in at least four other genes can cause or increase the risk of developing Alzheimer disease. **Table 12.3** offers other examples of how mutations impair health.

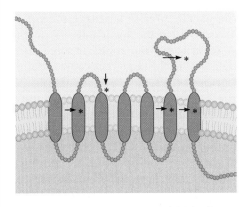

Figure 12.4 One cause of Alzheimer disease. When geneticists searched the DNA of people with very early-onset inherited Alzheimer disease, they identified a gene on chromosome 14 whose protein product, shown here, fits the well-known pattern of a receptor anchored into a membrane at seven points. This protein resides in vesicles derived from the Golgi apparatus. When abnormal, it cuts amyloid precursor proteins into abnormally-sized pieces that fuse and accumulate outside cells. Asterisks indicate sites where mutations in the gene disrupt the protein, causing symptoms.

Table 12.3

How Mutations Cause Disease

Disease	Signs and Symptoms (Phenotype)	OMIM Number	Protein	Genetic Defect (Genotype)
Cystic fibrosis	Frequent lung infection, pancreatic insufficiency	602421	Cystic fibrosis transmembrane regulator (CFTR)	Missing single amino acid or other defect alters conformation of chloride channels in certain epithelial cell plasma membranes. Water enters cells, drying out secretions.
Duchenne muscular dystrophy	Gradual loss of muscle function	310200	Dystrophin	Deletion in dystrophin gene eliminates this protein, which normally binds to inner face of muscle cell plasma membranes, maintaining cellular integrity. Cells and muscles weaken.
Familial hypercholesterolemia	High blood cholesterol, early heart disease	143890	LDL receptor	Deficient LDL receptors cause cholesterol to accumulate in blood.
Hemophilia A	Slow or absent blood clotting	306700	Factor VIII	Absent or deficient clotting factor causes hard-to-control bleeding.
Huntington disease	Uncontrollable movements, personality changes	143100	Huntingtin	Extra bases in the gene add amino acids to the protein product, which impairs certain transcription factors and proteasomes.
Marfan syndrome	Long limbs, weakened aorta, spindly fingers, sunken chest, lens dislocation	154700	Fibrillin	Too little elastic connective tissue protein in lens and aorta.
Neurofibromatosis type 1	Benign tumors of nervous tissue beneath skin	162200	Neurofibromin	Defect in protein that normally suppresses activity of a gene that causes cell division.

Multiple Mutations and Confusion

The usually precise language of science falls somewhat short when describing the consequences of mutations. In some cases, mutations in the same gene cause differing degrees of the same syndrome. This is the case for cystic fibrosis (CF). Diagnostic and prenatal tests that detect any of the more than one thousand known different mutations in the CFTR gene lead to a diagnosis of "cystic fibrosis," although patients may have different degrees or subsets of the associated symptoms. A man whose only symptom is infertility and occasional respiratory infections could have the same diagnosis as an extremely ill teenager with near-constant infections and severe malnutrition.

Mutations in the beta globin gene, in contrast, cause clinically distinct illnesses, such as sickle cell disease or beta thalassemia. These two disorders affect the same tissue, blood. More confusing are mutations in a gene called *lamin A*, which encodes a protein in the inner nuclear membrane that interacts with other proteins, producing symptoms. Mutations in *lamin A* cause the rapid-aging disorder Hutchinson-Gilford progeria syndrome (see figure 3.22 and table 3.4), and at least six other conditions, including muscular dystrophies and a heart condition.

Another source of confusion in assigning specific mutations to specific medical conditions is genetic heterogeneity—the same symptoms caused by different mutant genes. Often this situation arises when a gene is matched to a syndrome, and then exceptions are noted. This is the case for combined deficiencies of factors V and VIII, which impairs blood clotting. The disorder was initially associated with a protein called LMAN1, which is essential for secretion of both clotting factors. But large studies revealed that 30 percent of the affected individuals have a wild type *LMAN1* gene and a mutation in a different gene, *MCFD2*. The proteins the two genes encode—LMAN1 and MCFD2—act together, and are thus known as co-transporters. Both are necessary to move the clotting factors from the endoplasmic reticulum to the Golgi apparatus. Impair either, and blood does not clot normally.

Key Concepts

Mutations add, delete, or rearrange genetic material in a germline cell or somatic cell. Learning exactly how a mutation alters a protein can help explain how disease arises. In sickle cell disease, a mutation causes hemoglobin to crystallize in a low-oxygen environment, bending red blood cells into sickle shapes and impairing circulation. In beta thalassemia, beta globin is absent or scarce, causing too few complete hemoglobin molecules and buildup of free alpha globin chains and iron. • Mutations in collagen genes often disrupt the protein's precise organization. • In one form of Alzheimer disease, a mutation in a receptor protein leads to beta-amyloid buildup. • Mutations in a gene may cause either distinct illnesses or different versions of the same disease.

12.2 Causes of Mutation

A mutation can occur spontaneously or be induced by exposure to a chemical or radiation. An agent that causes mutation is called a **mutagen.**

Spontaneous Mutation

A spontaneous mutation can show up as a surprise. For example, two healthy people of normal height may have a child of extremely short stature. The child has achondroplasia (a form of dwarfism) caused by an autosomal dominant mutation. How could this happen when there are no other affected family members? If the mutation is dominant, why are the parents of normal height? The child has a genetic condition, but he did not inherit it. Instead, he originated it. His siblings have no higher risk of inheriting the condition than anyone in the general population, but each of his children will face a 50 percent chance of inheriting it. The boy with achondroplasia arose from a *de novo*, or new, mutation in his mother's oocyte or father's sperm cell. This is a spontaneous mutation—that is, it is not caused by known exposure to a mutagen. Instead, a spontaneous mutation usually originates as an error in DNA replication.

One cause of spontaneous mutation stems from the chemical tendency of free nitrogenous bases to exist in two slightly different structures, called tautomers. For extremely short times, each base is in an unstable tautomeric form. If, by chance, such an unstable base is inserted into newly forming DNA, an error will be generated and perpetuated when that strand replicates. **Figure 12.5** shows how this can happen. One of Watson and Crick's early and incorrect models of DNA structure used the rare tautomeric forms of the bases—a student suggested that they consider the more common tautomers, which eventually led to the double helix model.

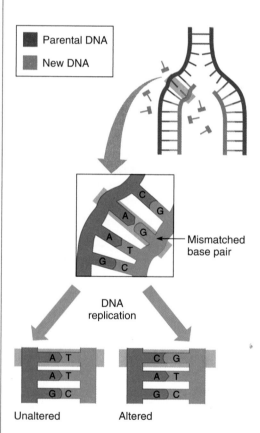

Figure 12.5 Spontaneous mutation. DNA bases are very slightly chemically unstable, and for brief moments they exist in alternate forms. If a replication fork encounters a base in its unstable form, a mismatched base pair can result. After another round of replication, one of the daughter cells has a different base pair than the one in the corresponding position in the original DNA. (This figure depicts two rounds of DNA replication.)

Spontaneous Mutation Rate

The spontaneous mutation rate varies for different genes. The dominant gene that causes neurofibromatosis type 1 (NF1), for example, has a very high mutation rate, arising in 40 to 100 of every million gametes (table 12.4). NF1 affects 1 in 3,000 births, about half in families with no prior cases. The gene's large size may contribute to its high mutability—there are more ways for its sequence to change, just as there are more opportunities for a misspelling to occur in a long sentence than in a short one.

Based on the prevalence of certain disease-causing genes, geneticists estimate that each human gene has about a 1 in 100,000 chance of mutating. Each of us probably carries a few new spontaneously mutated genes. Mitochondrial genes mutate at a higher rate than nuclear genes because they lack DNA repair mechanisms, as discussed in section 12.6.

Estimates of the spontaneous mutation rate for a particular gene are usually derived from observations of new, dominant conditions, such as the achondroplasia in the boy. This is possible because a new dominant mutation is detectable simply by observing the phenotype. In contrast, a new recessive mutation would not be obvious until two heterozygotes produced a homozygous recessive offspring with a noticeable phenotype.

The spontaneous mutation rate for autosomal genes can be estimated using the formula: number of *de novo* cases/2X, where X is the number of individuals examined. The denominator has a factor of 2 to account for the nonmutated homologous chromosome.

Spontaneous mutation rates in human genes are difficult to assess because our generation time is long—usually 20 to 30 years. In bacteria, a new generation arises every half hour or so, and mutation is therefore much more frequent. This ability to rapidly mutate can be harmful to human health when disease-causing bacteria become resistant to antibiotic drugs. Chapter 15 addresses this pressing health concern from an evolutionary viewpoint.

The genetic material of viruses also spontaneously mutates rapidly. This is why an influenza vaccine manufactured to fight one year's predominant strain may be ineffective by the next flu season. Genetic changes can alter the virus's surface to such an extent that the vaccine cannot protect. HIV poses the same challenge.

Mutational Hot Spots

Mutations may occur anywhere in a gene, but in some genes they are more likely to occur in certain regions called hot spots. Sequences that are mutational hot spots are often not random; many occur where the DNA sequence is repetitive. It is as if the molecules that guide and carry out replication become "confused" by short repeated sequences, as an editor scanning a manuscript might miss the spelling errors in the words "happpiness" and "bananana" (figure 12.6). For example, more than one-third of the many mutations that cause alkaptonuria occur at or near one or more CCC repeats, even though these repeats account for only 9 percent of the gene (see In Their Own Words, chapter 5).

The increased incidence of mutations in repeated DNA sequences has a physical basis. Within a gene, when DNA strands locally unwind to permit replication, symmetrical or repeated sequences allow base pairing to occur between bases located on the same strand, such as a stretch of ATATAT pairing with TATATA. This interferes with replication and repair enzymes, increasing the chance of an error. Mutations in the gene for clotting factor IX, which causes hemophilia B, for example, occur 10 to 100 times as often at any of 11 sites in the gene that have extensive direct repeats of CG (CGCGCG . . .).

Small additions and deletions of DNA are more likely to occur near sequences called palindromes (see figure 12.6). These

Table 12.4

Mutation Rates of Some Genes That Cause Inherited Disease

	OMIM Number	Mutations per Million Gametes	Signs and Symptoms
X-linked			
Duchenne muscular dystrophy	310200	40–105	Muscle atrophy
Hemophilia A	306700	30–60	Severe impairment of blood clotting
Hemophilia B	306900	0.5–10	Mild impairment of blood clotting
Autosomal Dominant			
Achondroplasia	100800	10	Very short stature
Aniridia	106200	2.6	Absence of iris
Huntington disease	143100	<1	Uncontrollable movements, personality changes
Marfan syndrome	154700	4–6	Long limbs, weakened blood vessels
Neurofibromatosis type 1	162200	40–100	Brown skin spots, benign tumors under skin
Osteogenesis imperfecta	166200	10	Easily broken bones
Polycystic kidney disease	600666	60–120	Benign growths in kidneys
Retinoblastoma	180200	5–12	Malignant tumor of retina

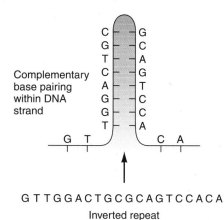

Repeat of a nucleotide   A A A A A A A A A

Direct repeat of a dinucleotide   G C G C G C G C

Direct repeat of a trinucleotide   T A C T A C T A C

Complementary base pairing within DNA strand

```
        C ─ G
        G ─ C
        T ─ A
        C ─ G
        A ─ T
        G ─ C
        G ─ C
        T   A
    G T       C A
```

G T T G G A C T G C G C A G T C C A C A

Inverted repeat

Palindrome

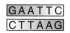

GAATTC
CTTAAG

Figure 12.6 DNA symmetry may increase the likelihood of mutation. These examples show repetitive and symmetrical DNA sequences that may "confuse" replication enzymes, causing errors.

sequences read the same, in a 5′ to 3′ direction, on complementary strands. Put another way, the sequence on one strand is the reverse of the sequence on the complementary strand. Palindromes probably increase the spontaneous mutation rate by disturbing replication.

The blood disorder alpha thalassemia illustrates the confusing effect of direct (as opposed to inverted) repeats of an entire gene. A person who does not have the disorder has four genes that specify alpha globin chains, two next to each other on each chromosome 16. Homologs with repeated genes can misalign during meiosis when the first sequence on one chromosome lies opposite the second sequence on the homolog. If crossing over occurs, a sperm or oocyte can form that has one or three of the alpha globin genes instead of the normal two (**figure 12.7**). Fertilization with a normal gamete then results in a zygote with one extra or one missing alpha globin gene.

A person with only three alpha globin genes produces enough hemoglobin, and is considered a healthy carrier. Rarely, individuals arise with only two copies of the

gene, and they are mildly anemic and tire easily. A person with a single alpha globin gene is severely anemic, and a fetus lacking alpha globin genes does not survive. Alpha thalassemia is common because carriers have an advantage—they are protected against malaria, a severe infectious illness transmitted by mosquitoes in the tropics. Chapter 16 discusses the protective effect of being heterozygous for any of several inherited disorders.

Induced Mutations

Researchers can sometimes infer a gene's normal function by observing what happens when mutation alters it. Because the spontaneous mutation rate is far too low to be a practical source of genetic variants for experiments, researchers make mutants. Geneticists have used many mutagens on a variety of experimental organisms to infer normal gene functions, yielding many collections. For example, a researcher can obtain mutant fruit flies from a facility at Indiana University, or mutant mice from the Jackson Laboratory in Bar Harbor, Maine.

Intentional Use of Mutagens

Geneticists use chemicals or radiation to induce mutation. Chemicals called alkylating agents, for example, remove a DNA base, which is replaced with any of the four bases—three of which will be a mismatch against the complementary strand. Dyes called acridines add or remove a single DNA base. Because the DNA sequence is read three bases in a row, adding or deleting a single base can destroy a gene's information, altering the amino acid sequence of the encoded protein. Several other mutagenic chemicals alter base pairs, so that an A-T replaces a G-C, or vice versa, changing a gene's DNA sequence. X rays and other forms of radiation delete a few bases or break chromosomes.

Researchers have developed several *in vitro* (in the test tube) protocols for testing the mutagenicity of a substance. The most famous of these, the Ames test, developed by Bruce Ames of the University of California, assesses how likely a substance is to harm the DNA of rapidly reproducing bacteria. One version of the test uses a strain of *Salmonella* that cannot grow when the amino acid histidine is absent from its medium. If exposure to a substance

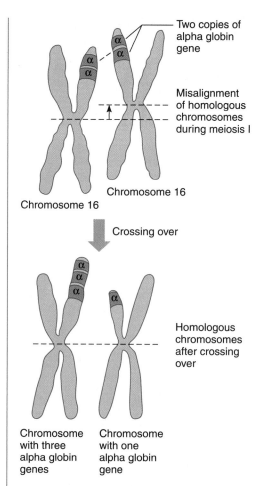

Figure 12.7 Gene duplication and deletion. The repeated nature of the alpha globin genes makes them prone to mutation by mispairing during meiosis. A person missing one alpha globin gene can develop anemia.

enables the bacteria to grow on the deficient medium, then it has undergone a mutation that allows it to do so. Another variation of the Ames test incorporates mammalian liver tissue into the medium to make the results more applicable to the response of an animal. Because many mutagens are also carcinogens (cancer-causing agents), the substances that the Ames test identifies as mutagens may also cause cancer. **Table 12.5** lists some common mutagens.

A limitation of using a mutagen is that it cannot cause a specific mutation. A technique called **site-directed mutagenesis** changes a gene in a desired way, using the polymerase chain reaction (see figure 9.16). The PCR primers include a specific base change, but are still similar enough in sequence to base pair with the gene of interest in the DNA sample. When the gene is amplified, the

Table 12.5

Commonly Encountered Mutagens

Mutagen	Source
Aflatoxin B	Fungi growing on peanuts and other foods
2-amino 5-nitrophenol	Hair dye components
2,4-diaminoanisole	"
2,5-diaminoanisole	"
2,4-diaminotoluene	"
p-phenylenediamine	"
Furylfuramide	Food additive
Nitrosamines	Pesticides, herbicides, cigarette smoke
Proflavine	Antiseptic in veterinary medicine
Sodium nitrite	Smoked meats
Tris (2,3-dibromopropyl phosphate)	Flame retardant in children's sleepwear

intentional change is replicated, just as an error in a manuscript is printed in every copy of a book. Site-directed mutagenesis is faster and more precise than waiting for nature or a mutagen to produce a useful variant. It also makes it possible to study lethal mutations that can theoretically exist, but never do because they are so drastic. Researchers can study such a lethal mutation in cell culture, or in model organisms before they cease developing.

Accidental Exposures to Mutagens

In contrast to the intentional use of mutagens in research is unintentional mutagen exposure. This occurs from contact in the workplace that occurred before the danger was known, from industrial accidents, from medical treatments such as chemotherapy and radiation, and from exposure to weapons that emit radiation.

An example of an environmental disaster that released mutagenic radiation was a steam explosion at a nuclear reactor in the former Soviet Union on April 25, 1986. Between 1:23 and 1:24 A.M., Reactor 4 at the Chernobyl Nuclear Power Station in Ukraine exploded, sending a great plume of radioactive isotopes into the air that spread for thousands of miles. The reactor had been undergoing a test, its safety systems temporarily disabled, when it overloaded and rapidly flared out of control. Twenty-eight

people died of radiation exposure in the days following the explosion.

Acute radiation poisoning is not a genetic phenomenon. Evidence of a mutagenic effect has come from the increased rate of thyroid cancer among children who were living in nearby Belarus. Rates have multiplied tenfold. The thyroid glands of young people soak up iodine, which in a radioactive form bathed the area in the first days after the explosion. Cancer rates have also risen among "liquidators," the workers who cleaned up after the disaster. Analysis of evidence of radiation exposure in their teeth is being used to assess whether cancer risk rises with degree of exposure.

Another way researchers tracked mutation rate in the wake of the Chernobyl explosion was to compare the lengths of short DNA repeats called minisatellite sequences in children born in 1994 and in their parents, who lived in the Mogilev district of Belarus at the time of the accident and have remained there. Minisatellites are the same length within all cells of an individual. A minisatellite size in a child that does not match the size of either parent indicates that a mutation occurred in a parent's gamete. Such a mutation was twice as likely to occur in exposed families than in control families living elsewhere. Mutation rates of nonrepeated DNA sequences are too low to provide useful information on the effects of radiation exposure, so investigators track minisatellites as a sensitive test of change.

Researchers learned of a new type of mutation from a young man conceived within a week of the Chernobyl accident, near the disaster site. He has extra digits, an abnormal epiglottis, and a benign growth on the hypothalamus, a group of symptoms called Pallister-Hall syndrome. On his way to a camp for "children of Chernobyl" in the summer of 2002, he stopped at the National Institutes of Health to provide a DNA sample. Researchers indeed found a mutation in the gene on chromosome 7 known to cause the syndrome—a 72-base insertion that causes a "stop" codon to form, shortening the encoded protein. The insertion matched DNA sequences known to come from the mitochondria. Apparently, the radiation damaged mitochondria in the sperm or oocyte, sending some mitochondrial DNA into the nucleus, where it inserted into the Pallister-Hall gene. Another clue to the unusual origin of this young man's condition is that it is autosomal dominant, but neither of his parents have it. Researchers are looking for other sporadic cases of autosomal dominant conditions linked to Chernobyl, to confirm whether DNA transfer from a mitochondrion to the nucleus is indeed a route to mutation.

Natural Exposure to Mutagens

The simple act of being alive exposes us to radiation that can cause mutation. Such natural environmental sources of radiation include cosmic rays, sunlight, and radioactive minerals in the earth's crust, such as radon. Contributions from medical X rays and occupational radiation hazards are comparatively minor (table 12.6). Job sites with increased radiation exposure include weapons facilities, research laboratories, health care facilities, nuclear power plants, and certain manufacturing plants. Radiation exposure is measured in units called millirems; the average annual exposure in the northern hemisphere is 360 millirems.

Most of the potentially mutagenic radiation we are exposed to is of the ionizing type, which means that it has sufficient energy to remove electrons from atoms. Unstable atoms that emit ionizing radiation both exist naturally and are made by humans. Ionizing radiation breaks the sugar-phosphate backbone of DNA.

Table 12.6

Sources of Radiation Exposure

Source	Percentage of Total
Natural (cosmic rays, sunlight, earth's crust)	81%
Medical X rays	11%
Nuclear medicine procedures	4%
Consumer products	3%
Other (nuclear fallout, occupational)	<1%

Ionizing radiation is of three major types. Alpha radiation is the least energetic and most short-lived, and the skin absorbs most of it. Uranium and radium emit alpha radiation. Beta radiation can penetrate the body farther, and emitters include tritium (an isotope of hydrogen), carbon-14, and strontium-70. Both alpha and beta rays tend not to harm health, although they can do damage if inhaled or eaten. In contrast is the third type of ionizing radiation, gamma rays. These can penetrate all the way through the body, damaging tissues as they do. Plutonium and cesium isotopes used in weapons emit gamma rays, and this form of radiation is intentionally used to kill cancer cells.

X rays are the major source of exposure to human-made radiation, and they are not a form of ionizing radiation. They have less energy and do not penetrate the body to the extent that gamma rays do.

The effects of radiation damage to DNA depend upon the functions of the mutated genes. Mutations in oncogenes or tumor suppressor genes, discussed in chapter 18, can cause cancer. Radiation damage can be widespread, too. Exposing cells to radiation and then culturing them causes a genome-wide destabilization, so that mutations may occur even after the cell has divided a few times. Cell culture studies have also identified a "bystander effect," when radiation seems to harm even cells not directly exposed. Researchers have noted which cells in an experiment received radiation, then detected chromosome breakage in cells located nearby as well as in the exposed cells. This effect is not well understood.

Chemical mutagens exist in the environment, too. Evaluating the risk that a specific chemical exposure will cause a mutation is very difficult, largely because people vary greatly in inherited suscepti-

bilities, and are exposed to many chemicals. The risk that exposure to a certain chemical will cause a mutation is often less than the natural variability in susceptibility within a population, making it nearly impossible to track the true source and mechanism of any mutational event. Human genome sequence information can be used to determine specific inherited risks for specific employees who might encounter a mutagen in the workplace. However, such testing raises ethical concerns. The Bioethics box discusses testing for sensitivity to the element beryllium.

Key Concepts

Genes have different mutation rates. Spontaneous mutations result when rare base tautomers present during replication change the sequence. Spontaneous mutations are more frequent in microorganisms and viruses because they reproduce often and lack repair. Mutations are more likely to happen when the nearby DNA is repetitive or unusually symmetrical. • Mutagens are chemicals or radiation that increase the likelihood of mutation. Researchers use mutagens to more quickly obtain mutants, which they study to reveal normal gene function. Site-directed mutagenesis uses PCR primers with intentional base mismatches to engineer and amplify specific mutations. Accidental exposure to mutagens may come on the job, from nuclear accidents, medical treatments or weapons. • Natural radiation sources include cosmic rays, sunlight, and radioactive elements in the earth's crust. Gamma rays are the most damaging form of ionizing radiation. They disrupt the sugar-phosphate backbone of DNA.

12.3 Types of Mutations

Mutations are classified by exactly how they alter DNA. **Table 12.7** summarizes the types of genetic changes described in this section using an analogy to an English sentence.

Point Mutations

A **point mutation** is a change in a single DNA base. It is a **transition** if a purine replaces a purine (A to G or G to A) or a pyrimidine replaces a pyrimidine (C to T or T to C). It is a **transversion** if a purine replaces a pyrimidine or vice versa (A or G to T or C). A point mutation can have any of several consequences—or it may have no obvious effect at all on the phenotype, acting as a silent mutation.

Missense and Nonsense Mutations

A point mutation that changes a codon that normally specifies a particular amino acid into one that codes for a different amino acid is called a **missense mutation.** If the substituted amino acid alters the protein's conformation sufficiently or occurs at a site critical to its function, signs or symptoms of disease or an observable variant of a trait may result.

The point mutation that causes sickle cell disease (see figure 12.1) is a missense mutation. The DNA sequence CTC encodes the mRNA codon GAG, which specifies glutamic acid. In sickle cell disease, the mutation changes the DNA sequence to CAC, which encodes GUG in the mRNA, which specifies valine. This mutation changes the protein's shape, which alters its function.

A point mutation that changes a codon specifying an amino acid into a "stop" codon—UAA, UAG, or UGA in mRNA—is a **nonsense mutation.** A premature stop codon shortens the protein product, which can profoundly influence the phenotype. Nonsense mutations are predictable by considering which codons can mutate to a "stop" codon.

The most common cause of factor XI deficiency, a blood clotting disorder, is a nonsense mutation that changes one GAA codon specifying glutamic acid to UAA, signifying "stop." The shortened clotting factor cannot halt the profuse bleeding that occurs

Beryllium Screening

On the surface, screening workers for a genetic variant that predisposes them to develop a possibly fatal reaction to a substance they may contact on the job seems like a good idea. But some workers say the risks outweigh uncertain benefits. The case in point: screening for chronic beryllium disease (CBD), also called berylliosis. This condition causes the person to react to the metal beryllium, used in nuclear power plants, in electronics, and in manufacturing fluorescent powders. Exposed workers include those who mine beryllium, nuclear power plant employees, and support staff such as office workers who inhale beryllium dust.

A small percentage of people exposed to beryllium dust or vapor develop an immune response that damages the lungs, producing cough, shortness of breath, fatigue, loss of appetite, and weight loss. Fevers and night sweats indicate the immune system is responding to the exposure. The steroid drug prednisone can control symptoms, but it isn't used until symptoms begin, which can be anywhere from a few months to forty years after the first exposure.

The Department of Energy and some private companies have screened more than ten thousand workers exposed to beryllium on the job using a test based on immune system response. In people who have symptoms, certain white blood cells divide in the presence of beryllium. About 45 percent of people without symptoms who test positive go on to develop the condition. A more precise and predictive genetic test will eventually replace the immune system test, but even this test is far from perfect. It detects homozygosity for a rare genetic variant that is part of the human leukocyte antigen complex, a group of genes that control immune system function. A person who tests positive on this genetic test has an

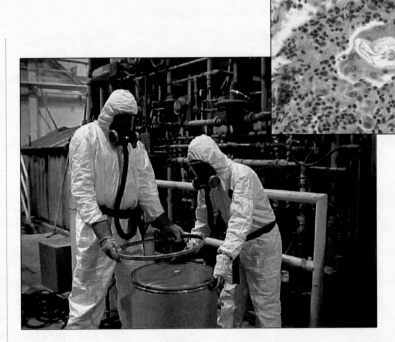

Figure 1 **Beryllium screening.** Screening for beryllium sensitivity aims to protect workers, but some people see it as an invasion of their genetic privacy. The lung tissue in the inset is granular in appearance, a sign of damage from beryllium exposure in a sensitive individual.

85 percent chance of developing CBD if exposed to beryllium (**figure 1**).

Experience so far with the immune system test suggests that screening for beryllium sensitivity using genetic tests will be controversial. So far, workers at the Department of Energy who test positive on the immune system test are not allowed to work near beryllium. Some of them resent this, preferring to decide themselves where they work. In addition, both the immune system test and genetic test are inconclusive—they detect susceptibility, meaning that some people who test positive will not develop the condition. Finally, people labeled as "sensitive" fear that their test results might have negative effects on their health insurance coverage. These issues will continue to mount as DNA tests become more powerful and precise.

The goal of CBD screening at the Department of Energy and the companies is to protect workers. Not only are sensitive individuals kept away from beryllium, but efforts have been underway for several years to minimize the dust and to make sure all beryllium workers use protective clothing and devices. Still, some people object to identifying susceptible individuals. This is yet another area where "political correctness" clashes with the reality of genetics—individuals *do* vary in their responses to many stimuli, including environmental lung irritants. To deny that is to expose certain people to potentially harmful surroundings. Genetic screening for beryllium sensitivity may set a precedent for other types of susceptibility testing that will be developed using human genome information.

---

during surgery or from injury. In the opposite situation, when a normal stop codon mutates into a codon that specifies an amino acid, the resulting protein is longer than normal, because translation proceeds through what is normally a stop codon.

Point mutations may exert profound effects by controlling how transcription proceeds. For example, in 15 percent of people who have Becker muscular dystrophy—a milder adult form of the condition—the muscle protein dystrophin is normal, but its

levels are reduced. The mutation causing the protein shortage is in the promoter for the dystrophin gene, which slows the transcription rate. Since cells then produce fewer mRNAs that encode dystrophin, the protein is scarce. Muscle function suffers. In

Table 12.7

Types of Mutations

A sentence comprised of three-letter words can provide an analogy to the effect of mutations on a gene's DNA sequence:

Normal	THE ONE BIG FLY HAD ONE RED EYE
Missense	TH**Q** ONE BIG FLY HAD ONE RED EYE
Nonsense	THE ONE BIG
Frameshift	THE ONE QBI GFL YHA DON ERE DEY
Deletion	THE ONE BIG HAD ONE RED EYE
Insertion	THE ONE BIG WET FLY HAD ONE RED EYE
Duplication	THE ONE BIG FLY FLY HAD ONE RED EYE
Expanding mutation	
generation 1	THE ONE BIG FLY HAD ONE RED EYE
generation 2	THE ONE BIG FLY FLY FLY HAD ONE RED EYE
generation 3	THE ONE BIG FLY FLY FLY FLY FLY HAD ONE RED EYE

contrast, the other 85 percent of individuals who have Becker muscular dystrophy have shortened proteins, not a deficiency of normal-length proteins.

Another way that point mutations can affect protein production is to disrupt the trimming of long precursor molecules. Such a mutation causes the type of Ehlers-Danlos syndrome that affects the boy in figure 12.3.

Splice Site Mutations

A point mutation can greatly affect a gene's product if it alters a site where introns are normally removed from the mRNA. This is called a splice site mutation. It can affect the phenotype if an intron is translated into amino acids, or an exon is skipped instead of being translated.

Retaining an intron adds bases to the protein coding portion of an mRNA. For example, in one family with severe cystic fibrosis, a missense mutation alters an intron site so that it is not removed. The encoded protein is too bulky to move to its normal position in the plasma membrane, where it should enable salt to exit the cell. As a result, chloride (a component of salt) accumulates in cells and water moves in, drying and thickening the mucus outside the cells.

A missense mutation need not alter the amino acid sequence to cause harm if it disrupts intron/exon splicing. For example, a missense mutation in the *BRCA1* gene that causes breast cancer went undetected for a long time because it does not alter the amino acid sequence. Instead, the protein is missing several amino acids. What happens is that the missense mutation creates an intron splicing site where there should not be one, and an entire exon is "skipped" when the mRNA is translated into protein, as if it were an intron. This mutation, therefore, is a deletion (missing material), but is caused by a missense mutation.

A disorder called familial dysautonomia (FD) usually results from a splice site mutation that causes exon skipping. An exon in the gene encoding an enzyme called I-kappa beta kinase-associated protein is not translated into protein because a point mutation in one of its splice sites signals the spliceosome not to translate that segment. Symptoms reflect loss of certain neurons that control sensation and involuntary responses. The In Their Own Words box in this chapter describes life for a child with FD.

A peculiarity of some disorders caused by exon-skipping mutations is that some cells seem to ignore the problem, manufacturing a normal protein from the affected

gene—after all, the amino acid sequence information is still there. Depending upon which cells function, the phenotype may be less severe than in individuals with the same disorder but with a different type of mutation in the coding portion of the gene.

Studies on various cell types from individuals with FD or who have died from the disease reveal that the cells where the exon is skipped are the cells that contribute to symptoms. That is, many cells from the brain and spinal cord are missing the exon, but cells from muscle, lung, liver, white blood cells, and various glands produce normal protein. This means there may be a way to coax nervous system cells in affected children to also produce the protein. Current clinical trials are examining the ability of several natural compounds to restore normal processing of the FD gene's information.

Deletions and Insertions Can Cause Frameshifts

In genes, the number three is very important, because triplets of DNA bases specify amino acids. Adding or deleting a number of bases that is not a multiple of three devastates a gene's function because it disrupts the gene's reading frame, which refers to the nucleotide position where the DNA begins to encode protein. Such a change that alters the reading frame is called a **frameshift mutation.** The mutation that disables the CCR5 HIV receptor is a frameshift.

A **deletion mutation** removes genetic material. A deletion that removes three or a multiple of three bases will not cause a frameshift, but can still alter the phenotype. Deletions range from a single DNA nucleotide to thousands of bases to larger pieces of chromosomes. The next chapter considers large deletions. Many common inherited disorders result from deletions. About two-thirds of people with Duchenne muscular dystrophy, for example, are missing large sections of the huge gene that encodes dystrophin. Many cases of male infertility are caused by tiny deletions in the Y chromosome.

An **insertion mutation** adds DNA and it, too, can offset a gene's reading frame. In one form of Gaucher disease, for example, an inserted single DNA base prevents production of an enzyme that

Familial Dysautonomia: Rebekah's Story

Our daughter Rebekah has familial dysautonomia. This is a rare genetic disorder that affects the functioning of the autonomic and peripheral nervous systems. Rebekah was born in 1992, but she was not diagnosed until she was almost three. Her diagnosis came as both a shock and a relief, putting her bizarre and terrifying symptoms into perspective.

Rebekah, who appeared to be healthy at birth, developed medical problems that became more serious with each passing month. Always a discontented, gassy baby, Rebekah began to decline rapidly by nine months, and within a year our lifestyle included twice monthly visits to the hospital. She suffered from frequent pneumonia, vomiting and retching, extremely high fevers, chills, rapid heartbeat, and seizures. At times, she would become covered with hot, red blotches. Other times, her hands and feet got very cold and appeared puffy and blue. Episodes of crying would precipitate breathholding, when she would turn blue and lose consciousness. As she lost ground on the growth and development charts, medical testing failed to reveal a cause for these symptoms. As we watched our baby suffer and become more ill, we wondered if we would identify the problem before she died. Our physicians, in their frustration, sometimes hinted that perhaps we were the cause. As I tried to advocate for my baby's care, more than one doctor wondered aloud if my "overbearing parenting" was the cause of my child's illness.

After more than twelve local hospitalizations and a variety of tests, we traveled to a major children's teaching hospital, hoping that a fresh team of doctors would identify Rebekah's condition. To our surprise, one doctor knew immediately that she had FD. He recognized the pattern of "dysautonomic crises"—a hallmark of FD. Two more symptoms, which we hadn't even noticed, were

diagnostic indicators. Individuals with FD do not cry tears, and they lack papillae (bumps) on the tip of the tongue. Our Eastern European, Jewish heritage was also a clue, because FD is one of a number of diseases primarily affecting this population.

To a varying degree, FD reduces sensation of pain, heat, and cold. There are problems with balance and coordination due to peripheral nerve problems, including oral motor difficulties which affect feeding, swallowing, and breathing. Most people with FD have a feeding tube, and must limit what they eat or drink by mouth due to danger of aspiration. FD causes fluctuations in blood pressure, digestive problems, and learning disabilities. Most individuals develop scoliosis, usually requiring corrective spine surgery before growth is complete. In short, FD affects every organ and system in the body.

Confronting this diagnosis was a shock, but the alternative of not knowing was even worse. Having a diagnosis has allowed us to finetune Rebekah's therapies and activities to maximize her health and well-being. With improved nutrition, excellent therapies, and wonderful teachers, Rebekah has made tremendous progress in every area. The reality of FD means we are always poised for a hospital stay, now about three times per year. Even a minor illness can set off a crisis. We have assembled a team of pediatric specialists to monitor her lungs, heart, eyes, back, and growth and development. Rebekah is a happy, good-natured child who makes friends easily and is sensitive to the needs of others. She works hard in school, and is able to keep up with her classmates when her health is good. She has learned to overcome her learning challenges, using assistive technology in school to help her with writing and organizing, areas of ongoing difficulty. This year Rebekah got a back brace to try to slow the scoliosis. As usual, she has adjusted to

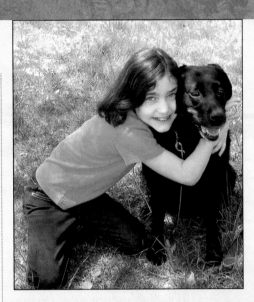

Figure 1 Rebekah with her dog, Tracy.

this new challenge with a practical, matter-of-fact attitude. When I tried to steer her to choose clothes that would deemphasize the bulk of the brace, she told me, "Mom, just relax. They're going to see it sooner or later!"

We don't know what the future holds. FD is a progressive, degenerative disease with life-threatening complications and a shortened lifespan. Any major stress, including developmental changes, surgery, a serious illness, and increased emotional stress, can exacerbate the severity. Yet, we feel hopeful for our daughter's future. With the discovery of the genetic mutations that cause FD in 2001, we know scientists are working on developing effective treatments and a cure. We are most encouraged by Rebekah herself. Her positive outlook on life, her willingness to find the good in any situation, and her ability to overcome challenges with spunk and humor inspire everyone around her. We can't predict the future, but we can say with confidence that Rebekah will be able to experience a life filled with joy and achievement. Isn't this what we all want for our children?

Lynn Lieberman

---

normally breaks down glycolipids in lysosomes. The resulting buildup of glycolipid enlarges the liver and spleen and causes easily fractured bones and neurological

impairment. Gaucher disease is common among Jewish people of eastern European descent. Although most cases arise from a missense mutation, some families have the

insertion mutation. Gaucher disease illustrates how different types of mutations in the same gene cause the same or a similar phenotype.

Another type of insertion mutation repeats part of a gene's sequence. The insertion is usually adjacent or close to the original sequence, like a typographical error repeating a word word. Two copies of a gene next to each other is called a **tandem duplication.** A form of Charcot-Marie-Tooth disease, which causes numb hands and feet, results from a one-and-a-half-million-base-long tandem duplication.

Figure 12.8 compares the effects on protein sequence of missense, nonsense, and frameshift mutations in the gene that encodes the LDL receptor, causing familial hypercholesterolemia (see figure 5.2). These three mutations exert very different effects on the protein. A missense mutation replaces one amino acid with another, bending the protein in a way that impairs its function. A nonsense mutation is much more drastic, removing a part of the protein. A frameshift mutation introduces a section of amino acids not normally found in the protein.

Pseudogenes and Transposons Revisited

Recall from chapter 11 that a pseudogene is a stretch of DNA with a sequence very similar to that of another gene. A pseudogene is not translated into protein, although it may be transcribed. The pseudogene may have descended from the original gene sequence, which was duplicated when DNA strands misaligned during meiosis. When this happens, a gene and its pseudogene end up right next to each other on the chromosome. The original gene or the copy then mutates to such an extent that it is no longer functional and becomes a pseudogene. Its duplicate lives on as the functional gene.

Although a pseudogene is not translated, its presence can interfere with the expression of the functional gene and cause a mutation. For example, some cases of Gaucher disease can result from a crossover between the working gene and its pseudogene, which has 95 percent of the same sequence located 16,000 bases away. The result is a fusion gene, which is a sequence containing part of the functional gene and part of the pseudogene. The fusion gene does not retain enough of the normal gene sequence to enable the cell to synthesize the enzyme. Gaucher disease results.

Chapter 11 also considered transposons, or "jumping genes." Transposons can alter

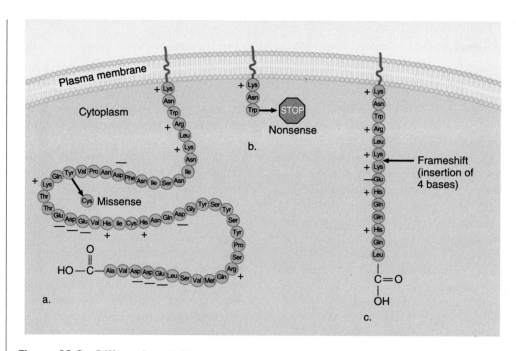

Figure 12.8   Different mutations in a gene can cause the same disorder.
In familial hypercholesterolemia, several types of mutations may disrupt the portion of the LDL receptor normally anchored in the cytoplasm. LDL receptor **(a)** bears a missense mutation—a substitution of a cysteine for a tyrosine. The receptor is bent enough to impair its function, causing disease. The short LDL receptor in **(b)** results from a nonsense mutation, in which a stop codon replaces a tryptophan codon. In **(c)**, a 4-base insertion alters the reading frame, so that a sequence of amino acids not normally in this protein forms until a stop codon occurs.

gene function in several ways. They can disrupt the site they jump from, shut off transcription of the gene they jump into, or alter the reading frame of their destination if they are not a multiple of three bases. For example, a boy with X-linked hemophilia A had a transposon in his factor VIII gene—a sequence that was also in his carrier mother's genome, but on her chromosome 22. Apparently, in the oocyte, the transposon jumped into the factor VIII gene on the X chromosome, causing the boy's hemophilia.

Expanding Repeats Lead to Protein Misfolding

Until 1992, myotonic dystrophy was a very puzzling disorder because it worsened and began at an earlier age as it passed from one generation to the next. This phenomenon is called "anticipation," and for many years it was thought to be psychological. A grandfather might experience only mild weakness in his forearms, and cataracts. In the next generation, a daughter might have more noticeable arm and leg weakness, and a characteristic flat facial expression. By the third generation, children who inherit the genes

experience severe muscle impairment—worse if the affected parent was the mother.

With the ability to sequence genes, researchers found that myotonic dystrophy indeed worsens with each generation because the gene expands! The gene for the disorder, on chromosome 19, has an area rich in repeats of the DNA triplet CTG. A person who does not have myotonic dystrophy usually has from 5 to 37 copies of the repeat, whereas a person with the disorder has from 50 to thousands of copies (**figure 12.9**). Myotonic dystrophy is an example of an **expanding triplet repeat** disorder.

So far, expanding triplet repeats have been discovered in more than fifteen human inherited disorders. Usually, a repeat number of fewer than 40 copies is stably transmitted to the next generation and doesn't produce symptoms. Larger repeats are unstable, increasing in number with each generation and causing symptoms that are more severe and begin sooner. Reading 12.1 describes the first triplet repeat disorder to be discovered, fragile X syndrome.

The mechanism behind the triplet repeat disorders lies in the DNA sequence. The base composition of the repeated triplets

Fragile X Syndrome—The First of the Triplet Repeat Disorders

In the 1940s, geneticists hypothesized that a gene on the X chromosome confers mental retardation, because more affected individuals are male. It wasn't until 1969, though, that a clue emerged to the genetic basis of X-linked mental retardation. Two retarded brothers and their mother had an unusual X chromosome. The tips at one chromosome end dangled, separated from the rest of each chromatid by a thin thread (**figure 1**). When grown under specific culture conditions (lacking folic acid), this part of the X chromosome was very prone to breaking—hence, the name fragile X syndrome. Although fragile X syndrome was first detected at the chromosomal level, it turned out that the cause is a mutation at the DNA level—but of a type never seen before.

Fragile X syndrome is second only to Down syndrome in genetic or chromosomal causes of mental retardation. Worldwide, it affects 1 in 2,000 males, accounting for 4 to 8 percent of all males with mental retardation. One in 4,000 females is affected. They usually have milder cases because of the presence of a second, normal X chromosome.

Youngsters with fragile X syndrome do not appear atypical, but by young adulthood, certain similarities become apparent. The fragile X patient has a very long, narrow face. The ears protrude, the jaw is long, and the testicles are very large. Mental impairment and behavioral problems vary, and relate to difficulty in handling environmental stimuli. They include mental retardation, learning disabilities, repetitive speech, hyperactivity, shyness, social anxiety, a short attention span, language delays, and temper outbursts.

Fragile X syndrome is inherited in an unusual pattern. Because the fragile chrom-

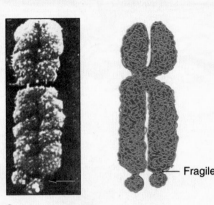

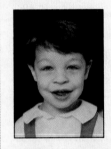 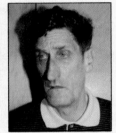

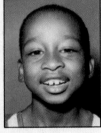 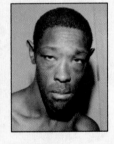

Figure 1   Fragile X syndrome.
A fragile site on the tip of the long arm of the X chromosome **(a)** is associated with mental retardation and a characteristic long face that becomes pronounced with age **(b)**.

osome is the X, the associated syndrome should be transmitted as any X-linked trait is, from carrier mother to affected son. However, penetrance is quite low. One-fifth of males who inherit the chromosomal abnormality have no symptoms. However, because they pass on the affected chromosome to all their daughters—half of whom have some degree of mental impairment—they are called "transmitting males." A transmitting male's grandchildren may inherit the condition.

Researchers in the 1980s were on the right track when they proposed two states of the X chromosome region responsible for fragile X signs and symptoms—a premutation form that does not cause symptoms but does transmit the condition, and a full mutation form that usually causes mental impairment. Still, it took a molecular-level look in 1991 to begin to clarify the inheritance pattern of fragile X syndrome.

In unaffected individuals, the fragile X area contains 6 to 50 repeats of the DNA sequence CGG, as part of a gene called the fragile X mental retardation gene (*FMR1*). In people who have the fragile chromosome and show its effects, this region is greatly expanded to 200 to 2,000 CGG repeats. Transmitting males, as well as females with mild symptoms, often have a premutation consisting of an intermediate number of repeats—50 to 200 copies.

The *FMR1* gene encodes fragile X mental retardation protein (FMRP). This protein, when abnormal, binds to and disables several different mRNA molecules whose encoded proteins are crucial for brain neuron function. The fact that a mutation in *FMR1* ultimately affects several proteins explains the several signs and symptoms of fragile X syndrome.

implicated in the expansion diseases, unlike others, bond to each other in ways that bend the DNA strand into shapes, such as hairpins. These shapes then interfere with replication, which causes the expansion. Once translated, the extra-long proteins shut down

cells in various ways—binding to parts of transcription factors that have stretches of amino acid repeats similar to or matching the expanded repeat; blocking proteasomes and thereby enabling misfolded proteins to persist; and directly triggering apoptosis.

Triplet repeat proteins may also enter the nucleus when their wild type versions would function in the cytoplasm, or vice versa.

The triplet repeat disorders are described as causing a "dominant toxic gain of function." This means that they cause something novel to happen, rather than removing a function, such as is often associated with recessive enzyme deficiencies. The idea of a gain of function arose from the observation that deletions of these genes do not cause symptoms. **Table 12.8** describes several triplet repeat disorders. Particularly common are the "polyglutamine diseases" that have repeats of the mRNA codon CAG, which encodes the amino acid glutamine.

For some triplet repeat disorders, the mutation thwarts gene expression before a protein is even manufactured. In myotonic dystrophy type I—the gene variant on chromosome 19 in which triplet repeats were discovered—the expansion occurs in the initial untranslated region of the gene, resulting in a huge mRNA. When genetic testing became available for myotonic dystrophy, researchers discovered a second form of the illness. Myotonic dystrophy type II is caused by an expanding quadruple repeat of (CCTG)n in a gene on chromosome 3. Affected individuals have more than 100 copies of the repeat, compared to the normal fewer than 10 copies. When researchers realized that this second repeat mutation was also in a non-protein-encoding part of the gene—an intron—a mechanism of disease became apparent: the mRNA is simply too big to get out of the nucleus. In myotonic dystrophy type I, the excess material is tacked onto the front end of the gene; in type II, it appears in an intron that is not excised.

A lesson learned from the expanding triplet and now quadruple repeat disorders is that a DNA sequence is more than just one language that can be translated into another. Whether a sequence is random—CGT CGT ATG CAT CAG, for example—or highly repetitive—such as CAG CAG CAG

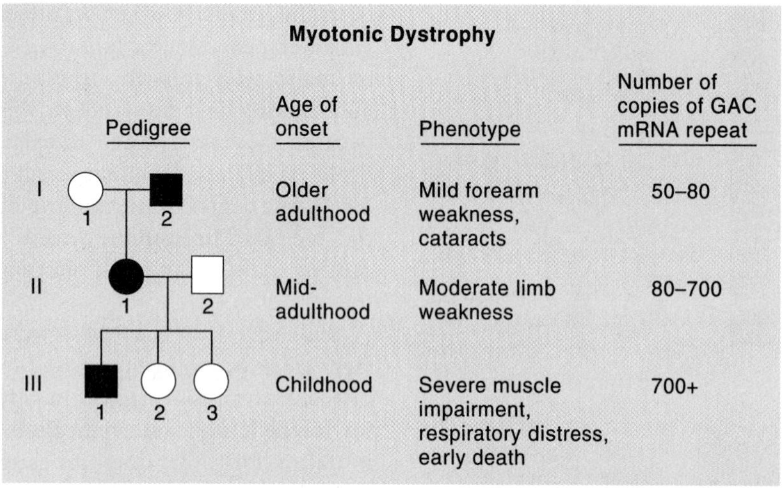

Figure 12.9 Expanding genes explain anticipation. In some disorders, symptoms that worsen from one generation to the next—a phenomenon termed *anticipation*—have a physical basis: the gene is expanding as the number of repeats grows.

Table 12.8

Triplet Repeat Disorders

Disease	OMIM Number	mRNA Repeat	Normal Number of Copies	Disease Number of Copies	Symptoms
Fragile X syndrome	309550	CGG or CCG	6–50	200–2,000	Mental retardation, large testicles, long face
Friedreich ataxia	229300	GAA	6–29	200–900	Loss of coordination and certain reflexes, spine curvature, knee and ankle jerks
Haw River syndrome	140340	CAG	7–25	49–75	Loss of coordination, uncontrollable movements, dementia
Huntington disease	143100	CAG	10–34	40–121	Personality changes, uncontrollable movements
Jacobsen syndrome	147791	CGG	11	100–1,000	Poor growth, abnormal face, slow movement
Myotonic dystrophy type I	160900	CTG	5–37	80–1,000	Progressive muscle weakness; heart, brain, and hormone abnormalities
Myotonic dystrophy type II	602668	CCTG	<10	>100	Progressive muscle weakness; heart, brain, and hormone abnormalities
Spinal and bulbar muscular atrophy	313200	CAG	14–32	40–55	Muscle weakness and wasting in adulthood
Spinocerebellar ataxia (5 types)	271245	CAG	4–44	40–130	Loss of coordination

CAG on and on—can affect transcription, translation, or the ways that proteins interact. Several lines of evidence indicate that DNA may harbor more meaning than the simple specification of amino acid sequences:

- Synthetic DNAs with random sequences migrate differently in electrical fields than do synthetic DNAs of the same length with repeated sequences.

- Transcription factors interact differently with random and repeated sequences.

- Repeats of CTG and CGG make the double helix more flexible.

- DNA with many CTG repeats winds more tightly about histone proteins to form nucleosomes than other DNA sequences do, affecting the accessibility of genes for transcription.

- DNA with many repeats can fold into a variety of structures as it is being replicated or transcribed. These include loops, triple and quadruple helices, and "slipped-strand" formations where the same repeats on homologs misalign, increasing the chance of mutation.

Key Concepts

A point mutation alters a single DNA base and can occur in any part of a gene. In a transversion, a purine replaces a pyrimidine, or vice versa; in a transition, a purine replaces a purine or a pyrimidine replaces a pyrimidine. A missense mutation replaces one amino acid with another. A nonsense mutation alters an amino-acid-coding codon into a "stop" codon, shortening the protein. A stop codon that changes to an amino-acid-coding codon lengthens the protein. Mutations in intron/exon splice sites, promoters, or other control regions also affect gene function. • Inserting or deleting bases can cause a frameshift mutation. Tandem duplications repeat a section of a gene. Pseudogenes are nonfunctional sequences very similar to nearby functional genes. Transposons can move, insert into genes, and cause illness. • Expanded repeats disturb brain function, with several effects that arise from protein misfolding. The degree of repetition in a DNA region may affect its structure and function.

12.4 The Importance of a Mutation's Position in the Gene

The degree to which a mutation alters the phenotype depends to a great extent upon where in the gene the change occurs, and how the mutation affects the conformation, activity, or expression of an encoded protein. A mutation that replaces an amino acid with a very similar one would probably not affect the phenotype greatly, because it wouldn't substantially change the conformation of the protein. Even substituting a very different amino acid would not have much effect if the change is in part of the protein not crucial to its function. Yet sickle cell disease and the disorders of collagen illustrate that even a small change in a gene can drastically alter the encoded protein's function. The effects of specific mutations are well-studied in the hemoglobin molecule. They are less understood, but still fascinating, in the gene that encodes prion protein.

Globin Variants

Because the globin gene mutations were the first to be analyzed in humans, and because some variants are easily detected using electrophoresis, hundreds of globin gene mutations have been known for years. Mutations in these genes can cause anemia with or without sickling, or cause cyanosis (a blue pallor due to poor oxygen binding), or, rarely, boost the molecule's affinity for oxygen. Some globin gene variants exert no effect on the phenotype at all, and are thus considered "clinically silent." Oddly, hemoglobin S and hemoglobin C each change the sixth amino acid in the beta globin polypeptide, but in different ways. Homozygotes for hemoglobin S have sickle cell disease, yet homozygotes for hemoglobin C are healthy. Both types of homozygotes are resistant to malaria because the unusual hemoglobin alters the shapes and surfaces of red blood cells in ways that keep out the parasite that causes the illness. (The hemoglobin/malaria link is discussed further in chapter 15.) **Table 12.9** lists some hemoglobin variants with differing effects, along with the nature of the mutations that define them.

An interesting consequence of certain mutations in either the alpha or beta globin chains is hemoglobin M. Normally, the iron in hemoglobin is in the ferrous form, which means that it has two positive charges. In hemoglobin M, the mutation stabilizes the ferric form, which has three positive charges and cannot bind oxygen. Fortunately, an

Table 12.9

Globin Mutations

Associated Phenotype	Name	Mutation
Clinically silent	Hb Wayne	Single-base deletion in alpha gene causes frameshift, changing amino acids 139–141 and adding amino acids
	Hb Grady	Nine extra bases add three amino acids between amino acids 118 and 119 of alpha chain
Oxygen binding	Hb Chesapeake	Change from arginine to leucine at amino acid 92 of beta chain
	Hb McKees Rock	Change from tyrosine to STOP codon at amino acid 145 in beta chain
Anemia	Hb Constant Spring	Change from STOP codon to glutamine elongates alpha chain
	Hb S	Change from glutamic acid to valine at amino acid 6 in beta chain causes sickling
	Hb Leiden	Amino acid 6 deleted from beta chain
Protection against malaria	Hb C	Change from glutamic acid to lysine at amino acid 6 in beta chain causes sickling

enzyme converts the abnormal ferric iron to the normal ferrous form, so that the only symptom is usually cyanosis. The condition has been known for more than two hundred years in a small town in Japan. Many people there have "blackmouth" because of the cyanosis caused by the faulty hemoglobin. It is autosomal dominant.

Even more noticeable than people with blackmouth are the "blue people of Troublesome Creek." Seven generations ago, a French orphan who settled in this area of Kentucky brought in a recessive gene that causes a form of methemoglobinemia. He was missing an enzyme (cytochrome b5 reductase) that normally converts a type of hemoglobin with poor oxygen affinity, called methemoglobin, back into normal hemoglobin by causing it to gain an electron. This man chose a wife who, unfortunately, carried the same disease. After extensive inbreeding in the isolated community, a large pedigree of "blue people" of both sexes arose. The excess oxygen-poor hemoglobin causes a dark blue complexion. Carriers may have frighteningly bluish lips and fingernails at birth, though this usually improves. This form of methemoglobinemia is also seen in the Navajo and Eskimos. A second form of methemoglobinemia results from absence of a protein that must be present for cytochrome B5 reductase to function. This is another example of genetic heterogeneity, because the same phenotype—blueness—results from mutations in different genes. Treatment is simple: a tablet of methylene blue, a commonly used dye, paradoxically adds the electron back to methemoglobin, converting it to normal hemoglobin.

Inherited Susceptibility to Prion Disorders

For the prion protein gene, as with the globin genes, certain mutations exert drastic effects, while others don't. Recall from chapter 10 that a prion is a protein with an unknown function that assumes both stable conformations and infectious conformations that convert other prion proteins, spreading brain destruction. A prion disease can be inherited, such as fatal familial insomnia, or acquired, such as developing variant Creutzfeldt-Jakob disease from eating beef from a cow that had bovine spongiform encephalopathy. The prion protein has at least eight distinct conformations. The normal form of the protein has a central core made up of helices. In a disease-causing form, the helices open into a sheet (see figure 10.19). Precise genetic changes make all the difference in the plasticity of the prion protein—and in the health of the person.

The nature of the amino acid at position 129 in the prion protein is key to developing the disease. In people who inherit these disorders, amino acid 129 is either valine in all copies of the protein (genotype VV) or methionine in all copies (genotype MM). These people are homozygous for this small part of the gene. Most people, however, are heterozygous, with valine in some prion proteins and methionine in others (genotype VM). Perhaps having two different amino acids at this position enables the proteins to assemble and to carry out their normal functions, without damaging the brain. Further studies on the gene revealed that a mutation at a different site raises the risk of brain disease even higher. Comparing the prion proteins of healthy individuals to those who inherited a prion disorder showed that normally prion protein folds so that amino acid 129 is near amino acid 178, which is aspartic acid. People who inherit prion diseases are homozygous for the gene at position 129, and have another mutation that changes amino acid 178 to asparagine. Interestingly, people with two valines at position 129 develop fatal familial insomnia, whereas those with two methionines develop a form of Creutzfeldt-Jakob syndrome. Other genes affect susceptibility to prion disorders, too.

Key Concepts

Whether a mutation alters the phenotype, and how it does so, depends upon where in the protein the change occurs. Mutations in globin genes are well-studied and diverse; they may cause anemia or cyanosis, or they may be silent. Hemoglobin M affects the ability of the iron in the molecule to bind oxygen. • Mutations in two parts of the prion protein gene predispose an individual to developing a prion disorder.

12.5 Factors That Lessen the Effects of Mutation

Mutation is a natural consequence of DNA's ability to change. It has been and continues to be essential for evolution because it generates new variants, some of which may resist environmental change and enable a population or even a species to survive. However, many factors minimize the deleterious effects of mutations on phenotypes.

Synonymous codons render many alterations in the third codon position "silent." For example, a change from RNA codon CAA to CAG does not alter the designated amino acid, glutamine, so a protein whose gene contains the change would not be altered. The genetic code has other nuances that protect against drastically altered proteins. Mutations in the second codon position sometimes replace one amino acid with another that has a similar conformation. Often, this does not disrupt the protein's form too drastically. For example, a GCC mutated to GGC replaces alanine with equally small glycine.

A **conditional mutation** affects the phenotype only under certain conditions. This can be protective if an individual avoids the exposures that trigger symptoms. Consider a common variant of the X-linked gene that encodes glucose 6-phosphate dehydrogenase (G6PD), an enzyme that immature red blood cells use to extract energy from glucose. One hundred million people worldwide have G6PD deficiency, which can cause life-threatening hemolytic anemia, but only under rather unusual conditions—eating fava beans, inhaling pollen in Baghdad, or taking a certain antimalarial drug.

In the fifth century B.C., the Greek mathematician Pythagoras wouldn't allow his followers to consume fava beans—he had discovered that it would make some of them ill. During the second World War, several soldiers taking the antimalarial drug primaquine developed hemolytic anemia. A study began shortly after the war to investigate the effects of the drug on volunteers at the Stateville Penitentiary in Joliet, Illinois. Researchers soon identified abnormal G6PD in people who developed anemia when they took the drug.

What do fava beans, antimalarial drugs, and dozens of other triggering substances have in common? They "stress" red blood cells by exposing them to oxidants, chemicals that strip electrons from other compounds. Without the enzyme, the stress bursts the red blood cells.

Another example of a disorder caused by a conditional mutation is trichothiodystrophy. Symptoms of brittle hair and nails and scaly skin arise in some patients only during periods of fever that persist long enough for hair, nail, and skin changes to become noticeable. Heat destabilizes an enzyme that functions in base excision repair, discussed in the next section.

12.6   DNA Repair

Any manufacturing facility tests a product in several ways to see whether it has been assembled correctly. Mistakes in production are rectified before the item goes on the market—at least, most of the time. The same is true for a cell's manufacture of DNA.

DNA replication is incredibly accurate—only about 1 in 100 million bases is incorrectly incorporated. DNA polymerase as well as repair enzymes oversee the fidelity of replication.

All eukaryotes can repair their nuclear DNA, although some species do so more efficiently than others. Mitochondrial DNA cannot repair itself, which accounts for its higher mutation rate. The master at DNA repair is a large, reddish microbe that *The Guinness Book of World Records* named "the world's toughest bacterium." *Deinococcus radiodurans* was discovered in a can of spoiled ground meat at the Oregon Agricultural Experiment Station in Corvallis in 1956, where it had withstood the radiation used to sterilize the food. It tolerates 1,000 times the radiation level that a person can, and it can even live amidst the intense radiation of a nuclear reactor. The bacterium realigns its radiation-shattered pieces of genetic material and enzymes bring in new nucleotides and stitch together the pieces.

The discovery of DNA repair systems began with observations in the late 1940s that when fungi were exposed to ultraviolet radiation, those cultures nearest a window grew best. The researchers who noted these effects were not investigating DNA repair, but using UV light in other experiments. Therefore, DNA repair was known before the structure of DNA. In fact, James Watson worked on DNA repair as a graduate student. The DNA-damaging effect of ultraviolet radiation, and the ability of light to correct it, was soon observed in a variety of organisms.

Types of DNA Repair

Since its beginning, the Earth has been periodically bathed in ultraviolet radiation. Volcanoes, comets, meteorites, and supernovas all depleted ozone in the atmosphere, which allowed ultraviolet wavelengths of light to reach organisms. The shorter wavelengths—UVA—are not dangerous, but the longer UVB wavelengths damage DNA by forming an extra covalent bond between adjacent (same-strand) pyrimidines, particularly thymines (**figure 12.10**). The linked thymines are called thymine dimers. Their extra bonds kink the double helix sufficiently to disrupt replication and lead to possible insertion of a noncomplementary base. For example, an A might be inserted opposite a G or C, instead of opposite a T. Thymine dimers also disrupt transcription.

Early in the evolution of life, organisms that could handle UV damage had a survival advantage. Enzymes enabled them to do this, and thus DNA repair came to persist. In many modern species, three types of DNA repair mechanisms peruse the genetic material for mismatched base pairs. In the first type of DNA repair, enzymes called photolyases absorb energy from visible light and use it to detect and bind to pyrimidine dimers, then break the extra bonds. This type of repair, called photoreactivation, is what enables ultraviolet-damaged fungi to recover when exposed to sunlight. Humans do not have this repair mechanism.

In the early 1960s, researchers discovered a second type of DNA self-mending,

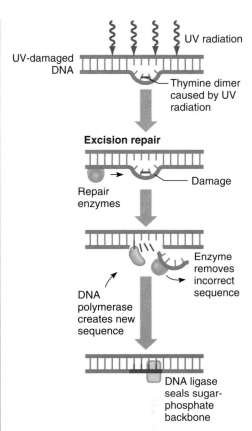

Figure 12.10   Excision repair.
Human DNA damaged by UV light is repaired by excision repair, which removes and replaces the pyrimidine dimer and a few surrounding bases.

called **excision repair,** in mutant *E. coli* that were unable to repair ultraviolet-induced DNA damage. The enzymes that carry out excision repair cut the bond between the DNA sugar and base and snip out—or excise—the pyrimidine dimer and surrounding bases (see figure 12.10). Then, a DNA polymerase fills in the correct nucleotides, using the exposed template as a guide. DNA polymerase also detects and corrects mismatched bases in newly replicated DNA.

Humans have two types of excision repair. **Nucleotide excision repair** replaces up to 30 nucleotides and removes errors that result from several types of insults, including exposure to chemical carcinogens, UVB in sunlight, and oxidative damage. Thirty different proteins carry out nucleotide excision repair, functioning together as a structure called a repairosome. The second type of excision repair, **base excision repair,** replaces one to five nucleotides at a time, but specifically corrects errors that result from oxidative damage. Oxygen free radicals are highly reactive forms of oxygen that arise during chemical reactions such as those of metabolism and transcription. Free radicals damage DNA. Genes that are very actively transcribed face greater oxidative damage from free radicals; base excision repair targets this type of damage.

A third mechanism of DNA repair is called **mismatch repair.** Enzymes "proofread" newly replicated DNA for small loops that emerge from the double helix. The enzymes excise the mismatched base so that it can be replaced (**figure 12.11**). These loops indicate an area where the two strands are not precisely aligned, as they should be if complementary base pairing is occurring at every point. Such slippage and mismatching tend to occur in chromosome regions where very short DNA sequences repeat. These sequences, called microsatellites, are scattered throughout the genome. Like minisatellites, microsatellite lengths can vary from person to person, but within an individual, they are usually all the same length. Excision and mismatch repair differ in the cause of the error—ultraviolet-induced pyrimidine dimers versus replication errors—and in the types of enzymes involved.

The three forms of DNA repair in human cells relieve the strain on thymine dimers or replace incorrectly inserted bases. Another form of repair can heal a broken sugar-phosphate backbone in both strands, which can result from exposure to ionizing radiation or oxidative damage. This insult breaks a chromosome, an event which is associated with cancer. At least two types of multiprotein complexes reseal the backbone, either by rejoining the broken ends or recombining with DNA on the unaffected homolog.

In yet another variation on DNA repair called damage tolerance, a "wrong" DNA base is left in place, but replication and transcription proceed. "Sloppy" DNA polymerases, with looser adherence to the base-pairing rules, read past the error, randomly inserting any other base, although it could adversely affect the encoded protein. It is a little like retaining a misspelled wrod in a sentence—usually the meaning remains clear. **Table 12.10** summarizes DNA repair mechanisms.

DNA Repair Disorders

The ability to repair DNA is crucial to health. Mutations in any of the genes whose protein products take part in DNA repair can cause problems. A particular repair disorder may be genetically heterogeneic because it can be caused by mutations in any of several genes that participate in the same repair mechanism. That is, different single-gene defects can cause the same symptoms.

At the crux of the decision as to whether a cell whose DNA has been damaged can be repaired is a protein called p53. Signal transduction activates the p53 protein, stabilizing it and causing it to aggregate into complexes consisting of four proteins. These quartets bind to the DNA by recognizing four palindromic repeats that indicate genes that slow the cell cycle. The cycle must slow so that repair can take place. If the damage is too severe to be repaired, the p53 protein quartets instead increase the rate of transcription of genes that promote apoptosis. At the same time, p53 increases transcription of yet another protein that regulates the synthesis of the p53 protein, so that it can shut off its own production.

DNA repair disorders fail to fix chromosome breakage caused by other factors, such as radiation. Mutations in repair genes therefore greatly increase susceptibility to certain types of cancer following exposure to ionizing radiation or chemicals that affect cell division. These conditions develop because errors in the DNA sequence accumulate and are perpetuated to a much greater extent than they are in people with functioning repair systems. **Table 12.11** lists several disorders that result from faulty DNA replication or repair. We conclude this chapter with a closer look at a few of them.

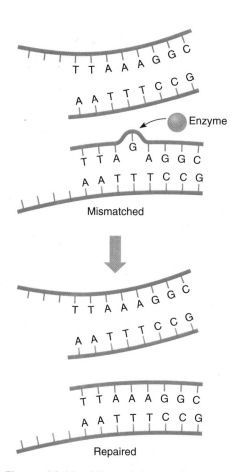

Figure 12.11 Mismatch repair.
In this form of DNA repair, enzymes detect loops and bulges in newly replicated DNA that indicate mispairing. The enzymes correct the error. Highly repeated sequences are more prone to this type of error.

Table 12.10	
DNA Repair	

Mechanism	Events
Nucleotide excision repair	Repairosome cuts 30-base segments out that include environmentally damaged DNA (due to ultraviolet radiation or oxidative damage)
Base excision repair	Enzymes remove 1 to 5 bases missed by nucleotide excision repair, countering oxidative damage
Mismatch repair	Enzymes remove individual mismatched bases incorrectly inserted during replication
Double-stranded breaks	Enzymes join ends of broken sugar-phosphate backbone, or recombine damaged sections using homolog
Damage tolerance	"Sloppy" DNA polymerase bypasses mismatched base

Table 12.11

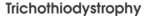

Some DNA Replication and Repair Disorders

Disorder	OMIM Number	Frequency	Defect
Ataxia telangiectasis	208900	1/40,000	Deficiency in kinase that controls the cell cycle
Bloom syndrome	278700	100 cases since 1950	DNA ligase is inactive or heat sensitive, slowing replication
Fanconi anemia	227650	As high as 1/22,000 in some populations	Deficient excision repair
Hereditary nonpolyposis colon cancer	120435	1/200	Deficient mismatch repair
Werner syndrome	277700	3/1,000,000	Deficient helicase
Xeroderma pigmentosum	278700	1/250,000	Deficient excision repair
Trichothiodystrophy	601675	Fewer than 100 cases	Deficient excision repair

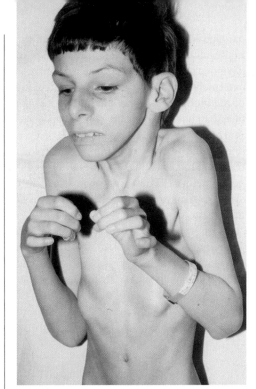

a.

Trichothiodystrophy

At least five different genes can cause tri-chothiodystrophy. At its worst, this condition causes dwarfism, mental retardation, and failure to develop, in addition to the scaly hair with low sulfur content that gives the illness its name. Although the child may appear to be normal for a year or two, growth soon slows dramatically, signs of premature aging begin, and life ends early. Hearing and vision may fail. Interestingly, the condition does not increase the risk of cancer. Symptoms reflect accumulating oxidative damage. Individuals have faulty nucleotide excision repair, base excision repair, or both (**figure 12.12a**).

Inherited Colon Cancer

Hereditary nonpolyposis colon cancer (HNPCC) was linked to a DNA repair defect when researchers discovered that these cancer cells exhibit different-length microsatellites within an individual. Because mismatch repair normally keeps a person's microsatellites all the same length, researchers hypothesized that people with this type of colon cancer might be experiencing a breakdown in this form of DNA repair. The causative gene is located on chromosome 2 and is remarkably similar to a corresponding mismatch repair gene in *E. coli*. HNPCC is a common repair disorder, affecting 1 in 200 people.

Xeroderma Pigmentosum (XP)

A child with XP lives, intentionally, indoors in artificial light, because even the briefest exposure to sunlight causes painful blisters. Failing to cover up and use sunblock can result in skin cancer (figure 12.12b). More than half of all children with XP develop the cancer before they reach their teens. People with XP have a 10,000-fold increased risk of developing skin cancer compared to others.

XP is autosomal recessive. It can reflect malfunction of excision repair or deficient "sloppy" DNA polymerase, both of which allow thymine dimers to stay and block replication. It is extremely rare—only about 250 people in the world are known to have it. A family living in upstate New York runs a special summer camp for children with XP, where they turn night into day, as they have done for their own affected daughter Katie. Activities take place at night, or in special areas where the windows are covered and light comes from low-ultraviolet incandescent lightbulbs.

Ataxia Telangiectasis (AT)

This multisymptom disorder is the result of a defect in a kinase that functions as a cell cycle checkpoint (see figure 2.17). Cells proceed through the cell cycle without pausing just after replication to inspect the new DNA and to repair any mispaired bases. Some cells die through apoptosis if the

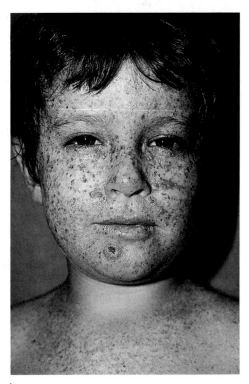

b.

Figure 12.12 DNA repair disorders.
(a) Trichothiodystrophy (a form called Cockayne syndrome) causes a child to appear aged. Excision repair fails. **(b)** The marks on this child's face are a result of sun exposure. He is highly sensitive because he has inherited xeroderma pigmentosum (XP), also an impairment of excision repair. The large lesion on his chin is a skin cancer.

damage is too great to repair. Because of the malfunctioning cell cycle, individuals who have this autosomal recessive disorder have extremely high rates of cancers, particularly of the blood. Additional symptoms include poor balance and coordination (ataxia), red marks on the face (telangiectasia), delayed sexual maturation, and high risk of contracting lung infections and developing diabetes mellitus. These symptoms probably arise from disruption of other functions of the kinase.

AT is rare, but heterozygotes are not. They make up from 0.5 to 1.4 percent of various populations. Carriers may have mild radiation sensitivity, which causes a two- to sixfold increase in cancer risk over the general population. Some physicians advise people who know they are AT carriers to avoid or limit medical X rays, because for them even low exposure may cause cancer.

DNA's changeability, so vital for evolution of a species, comes at the cost of occasional harm to individuals. The DNA repair systems are, like many genetic functions, more complex than researchers originally envisioned. The human genome sequence will probably reveal several dozen DNA repair genes, which will perhaps be studied as a "repairome."

We continue looking at mutation in chapter 13, at the chromosomal level.

Key Concepts

Many genes encode enzymes that search for and correct errors in replicating DNA. A common cause of noncomplementary base insertion is an ultraviolet radiation-induced pyrimidine dimer. Photoreactivation or excision repair can unlink pyrimidine dimers. Mismatch repair corrects noncomplementary base pairs that form in newly replicated DNA. Repair also seals broken sugar-phosphate backbones. DNA damage tolerance allows replication to proceed past a mismatched base. • Abnormal repair genes cause disorders that are usually associated with chromosome breaks and predisposition to cancer.

Summary

12.1 Mutations Can Alter Proteins—Three Examples

1. A **mutation** is a change in a gene's nucleotide base sequence that is rare and can cause a **mutant** phenotype.

2. A **germline mutation** originates in meiosis and affects all cells of an individual. A **somatic mutation** originates in mitosis and affects a subset of cells.

3. A mutation causes illness by disrupting the function or amount of a protein. In sickle cell disease, beta globin is misshapen; in beta thalassemia, it is absent or reduced. Mutations readily disrupt the highly symmetrical gene encoding collagen. One form of Alzheimer disease is caused by mutation in a receptor protein. Whether different mutations in a gene cause the same or distinct illnesses varies.

12.2 Causes of Mutation

4. A spontaneous mutation arises due to chemical phenomena or to an error in DNA replication. Spontaneous mutation rate is characteristic of a gene and is more likely to occur in repeated or symmetrical DNA sequences.

5. **Mutagens** are chemicals or forms of radiation that can induce mutation by deleting, substituting, or adding bases. An organism may be exposed to a mutagen intentionally, accidentally, or naturally.

12.3 Types of Mutations

6. A **point mutation** alters a single DNA base. It may be a **transition** (purine to purine or pyrimidine to pyrimidine) or a **transversion** (purine to pyrimidine or vice versa). A **missense mutation** substitutes one amino acid for another, while a **nonsense mutation** substitutes a "stop" codon for a codon that specifies an amino acid, shortening the protein product. Point mutations in splice sites can lead to many extra or missing amino acids.

7. Adding or deleting genetic material may upset the reading frame or otherwise alter protein function.

8. A **pseudogene** results when a duplicate of a gene mutates. It may disrupt chromosome pairing, causing mutation.

9. **Transposons** may disrupt the functions of genes they jump into.

10. Expanding triplet repeat mutations add stretches of the same amino acid to a protein, usually one that functions in the brain. They expand because they attract each other, which affects replication. This type of mutation may add a function, often leading to a neurodegenerative disease when the number of repeats exceeds a threshold level.

12.4 The Importance of a Mutation's Position in the Gene

11. Several types of mutations can affect a gene.

12. Mutations in the globin genes may affect the ability of the blood to transport oxygen, or have no effect.

13. Susceptibility to prion disorders requires one to inherit two mutations that affect different parts of the protein that interact as the amino acid chain folds.

12.5 Factors That Lessen the Effects of Mutation

14. Synonymous codons limit the effects of mutation. Changes in the second codon position often substitute a similarly shaped amino acid, so the protein's function may not be impaired.

15. **Conditional mutations** are expressed only in response to certain environmental triggers.

12.6 DNA Repair

16. DNA polymerase proofreads DNA, but repair enzymes correct errors in other ways.

17. Photoreactivation repair uses light energy to split pyrimidine dimers that kink the DNA.

18. In **excision repair,** pyrimidine dimers are removed and the area is filled in correctly. **Nucleotide excision repair** replaces up to 30 nucleotides from various sources of mutation. **Base excision repair** fixes up to five bases that paired incorrectly due to oxidative damage.

19. **Mismatch repair** proofreads newly replicated DNA for loops that indicate noncomplementary base pairing.

20. DNA repair also fixes the sugar-phosphate backbone. Damage tolerance enables replication to continue beyond a mismatch.

21. Mutations in repair genes lead to chromosome breakage and increased cancer risk.

Review Questions

1. Distinguish between a germline and a somatic mutation. Which is likely to be more severe? Which can be transmitted to offspring?

2. Why is the collagen gene prone to mutation?

3. How can a spontaneous mutation arise?

4. What is the physical basis of a mutational hot spot?

5. What are three different types of mutations that cause Gaucher disease?

6. Cite three ways in which the genetic code protects against the effects of mutation.

7. List four ways that DNA can mutate without affecting the phenotype.

8. What is a conditional mutation?

9. List two types of mutations that can alter the reading frame.

10. Why can a mutation that retains an intron's sequence and a triplet repeat mutation have a similar effect on a gene's encoded protein?

11. Cite two ways a jumping gene can disrupt gene function.

12. List two reasons it takes many years to detect induction of recessive mutations in a human population.

13. What is a physical, molecular explanation for anticipation, the worsening of an inherited illness over successive generations?

14. Compare and contrast how short repeats within a gene, long triplet repeats within a gene, and repeated genes can cause disease.

15. What criteria should be used to determine whether mutations in a gene are likely to cause different disorders or differing degrees of the same disorder?

16. How do excision and mismatch repair differ?

Applied Questions

1. A condition called "congenital insensitivity to pain with anhidrosis" causes loss of the ability to feel pain, inability to sweat, fever, mental retardation, and self-mutilation. The genetic cause is a mutation that replaces a glycine (*gly*) with an arginine (*arg*). List every type of mutation that might cause this change.

2. Retinitis pigmentosa causes night blindness and loss of peripheral vision before age 20. A form of X-linked retinitis pigmentosa is caused by a frameshift mutation that deletes 199 amino acids. How can a simple mutation have such a drastic effect?

3. One form of Ehlers-Danlos syndrome (not the "stretchy skin" type described in the chapter) can be caused by a mutation that changes a C to a T. This change results in the formation of a "stop" codon and premature termination of procollagen. Consult the genetic code table and suggest how this can happen.

4. Townes-Brocks syndrome causes several unrelated problems, including extra thumbs, a closed anus, hearing loss, and malformed ears. The causative mutation occurs in a transcription factor. How can a mutation in one gene cause such varied symptoms?

5. Susceptibility to developing prion diseases entails a mutation from aspartic acid (*asp*) to asparagine (*asn*). Which nucleotide base changes make this happen?

6. Two teenage boys meet at a clinic set up to treat muscular dystrophy. The boy who is more severely affected has a two-base insertion at the start of his dystrophin gene. The other boy has the same two-base insertion but also has a third base inserted a few bases away. Explain why the second boy's illness is milder.

7. About 10 percent of cases of amyotrophic lateral sclerosis (also known as ALS and Lou Gehrig disease) are inherited. This disorder causes loss of neurological function over a five-year period. Two missense mutations cause ALS. One alters the amino acid asparagine (*asn*) to lysine (*lys*). The other changes an isoleucine (*ile*) to a threonine (*thr*). List the codons involved and describe how single-base mutations alter the amino acids they specify.

8. In one family, Tay-Sachs disease stems from a four-base insertion, which changes an amino-acid-encoding codon into a "stop" codon. What type of mutation is this?

9. Epidermolytic hyperkeratosis is an autosomal dominant condition that produces scaly skin. It can be caused by a missense mutation that substitutes a histidine (*his*) amino acid for an arginine (*arg*). Write the mRNA codons that could account for this change.

10. Fanconi anemia is an autosomal recessive condition that causes bone marrow abnormalities and an increased risk of certain cancers. It is caused by a transversion mutation that substitutes a valine (*val*) for an aspartic acid (*asp*) in the amino acid sequence. Which mRNA codons are involved?

11. Aniridia is an autosomal dominant eye condition in which the iris is absent. In one family, an 11-base insertion in the gene causes a very short protein to form. What kind of mutation must the insertion cause?

12. A biotechnology company has encapsulated DNA repair enzymes in fatty bubbles called liposomes. Why would this be a valuable addition to a suntanning lotion?

Web Activities

13. Children with Hutchinson-Gilford progeria syndrome age extremely rapidly. In 2003, researchers identified the gene that encodes lamin A as the cause of the disorder. In 18 of 20 children whose DNA was sequenced, a single base change alters a C to a T, but this mutation removes 50 amino acids from the encoded protein. In all 20 children, the parents do not have the mutation.

    a. Is the mutation in the 18 children *de novo* or induced? What is the evidence for this distinction?

    b. How can a change in a single base remove 50 amino acids?

    c. Using OMIM, list and describe six other disorders caused by mutation in the lamin A gene.

Case Studies

14. Jan and Marcia meet at a clinic for college students who have cystic fibrosis. They are both studying genetics, and they become interested in learning about the particular mutations in their families. Jan's mutation results in exon skipping. Marcia's mutation is a nonsense mutation. Which young woman probably has more severe symptoms? Cite a reason for your answer.

15. Marshall and Angela have skin cancer resulting from xeroderma pigmentosum. They meet at an event for teenagers with cancer. However, their mutations affect different genes. They decide to marry but not to have children because they believe that each child would have a 25 percent chance of inheriting XP because it is autosomal recessive. Are they correct? Why or why not?

Learn to apply the skills of a genetic counselor with additional cases found in the *Case Workbook in Human Genetics:*

 Bloom syndrome

 DNA repair

 Gyrate atrophy

 Open-angle glaucoma

 Otospondylomegaepiphyseal dysplasia

 Tay-Sachs disease

 von Willebrand disease

Suggested Readings

Darnell, Jennifer C., et al. November 16, 2001. Fragile X mental retardation protein targets G quartet mRNAs important for neuronal function. *Cell* 107:489–99. Fragile X syndrome results from a cascade of disrupted protein function.

Friedberg, Errol C. January 23, 2003. DNA damage and repair *Nature* 421:436–40. Cells mend damaged DNA in several ways.

Green, P. M., et al. December 1999. Mutation rates in humans. 1. Overall and sex-specific rates obtained from a population study of hemophilia B. *The American Journal of Human Genetics* 65:1572. The mutation rate for the gene that, when mutant, causes hemophilia B is two to eight mutations per million gametes.

Hunter, Philip. September 8, 2003. Protein folding: theory meets disease. *The Scientist,* 17(17):24–25. The list of diseases caused by improper protein folding is growing.

Ingram, V. M. 1957. Gene mutations in human hemoglobin: The chemical difference between normal and sickle cell hemoglobin. *Nature* vol. 180. The classic paper explaining the molecular basis for sickle cell disease.

Lewis, Ricki. May 19, 2003. Huntington disease pathology unfolds. *The Scientist* 17(10):32–33. HD was one of the first triplet repeat disorders discovered.

Mirkin, Sergei M., and Ekaterina V. Smirnova. May 2002. Positioned to expand. *Nature Genetics* 31:5–6. Certain DNA repeats expand because they bond with themselves.

Tapscott, Stephen J., and Charles A. Thornton. August 3, 2001. Reconstructing myotonic dystrophy. *Science* 293:864–67. Triplet and even quadruplet repeats can have devastating effects on gene expression, even if they are not in exons.

Turner, Clesson, et al. February 2003. Human genetics disease caused by *de novo* mitochondrial-nuclear DNA transfer. *Human Genetics* 112(3):303–9. Did radiation from the Chernobyl disaster fling DNA into the nucleus, causing disease?

Withgott, Jay. July–August 2001. Evolving under UV. *Natural History.* DNA repair systems evolved to help organisms cope with environmental UV exposure.

Weekly updates of current news related to human genetics are available through Power Web on your Online Learning Center.

VISIT YOUR ONLINE LEARNING CENTER

Visit your online learning center for additional resources and tools to help you master this chapter. See us at

www.mhhe.com/lewisgenetics6.

Chromosomes

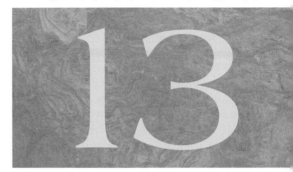

CHAPTER CONTENTS

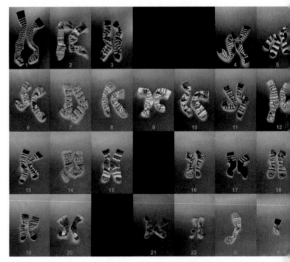

Different styles of socks can be arranged in a pattern similar to that used to show paired chromosomes.

Genetic health is largely a matter of balance—inheriting the "correct" number of genes, usually on the "correct" number of chromosomes (46, for humans). Too much or too little genetic material, particularly among the autosomes, can cause syndromes (groups of signs and symptoms). A person with Down syndrome, for example, usually has an extra chromosome 21 and, therefore, extra copies of all the genes on that chromosome. The extra genes cause mental retardation and various medical problems, but, as **figure 13.1** illustrates, people with Down syndrome can lead full and productive lives.

Abnormal numbers of genes or chromosomes are a form of mutation. Mutations range from the single-base changes described in chapter 12, to missing or extra pieces of chromosomes or entire chromosomes, to entire extra sets of chromosomes. A mutation is considered a chromosomal aberration if it is large enough to see with a light microscope using stains and/or fluorescent tags to highlight missing, extra, or moved material. The mutations described in chapter 12 and this chapter represent a continuum—they differ in scale and in our ability to detect them.

In general, excess genetic material has milder effects on health than a deficit. Still, most chromosomal abnormalities are so harmful that prenatal development ceases in the embryo. As a result, only a few—0.65 percent—of all newborns have chromosomal abnormalities that produce symptoms. An additional 0.20 percent have chromosomal rearrangements; their chromosome parts have flipped or been swapped, but they do not produce symptoms unless they disrupt genes that are crucial to health.

Cytogenetics is the subdiscipline within genetics that links chromosome variations to specific traits, including illnesses. Data from the human genome project are adding to our cytogenetics knowledge by identifying which genes contribute which symptoms to chromosome-related syndromes, and by comparing the gene contents of the chromosomes. For example, for decades geneticists did not understand why the most frequently seen extra autosomes in newborns are chromosomes 13, 18, and 21.

The human genome sequence revealed that these chromosomes have the lowest gene densities—that is, they carry considerably fewer protein-encoding genes than the other autosomes, compared to their total amount of DNA. Therefore, extra copies of these chromosomes are tolerated well enough for some individuals with them to survive to be born.

This chapter explores several ways that chromosome structure can deviate from normal and the consequences of these variations.

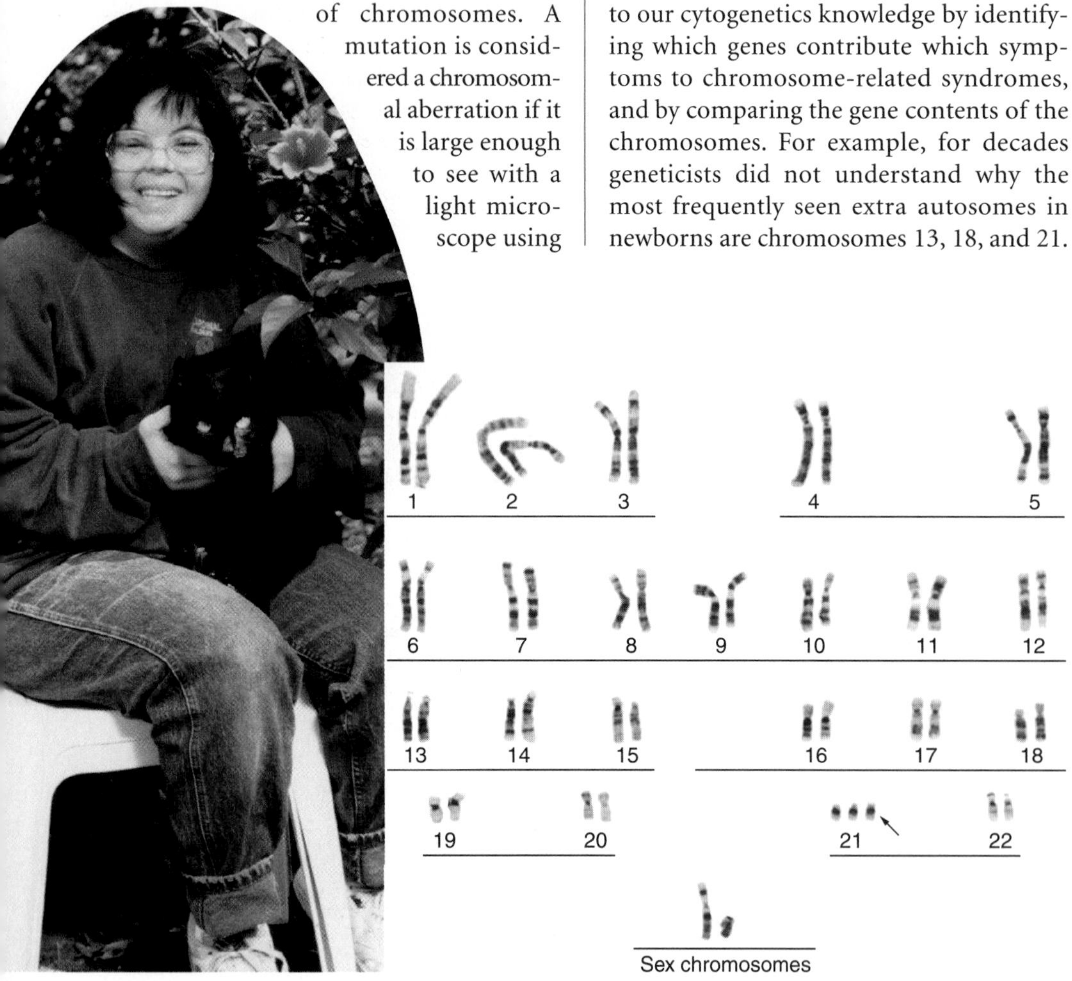

13.1 Portrait of a Chromosome

A chromosome is a structure that consists primarily of DNA and proteins that is duplicated and transmitted, via mitosis or meiosis, to the next cell generation. Cytogeneticists have long described and distinguished chromosome types by size and shape, and used stains and dyes to contrast dark **heterochromatin,** which is mostly repetitive DNA sequences, with lighter **euchromatin,** which harbors more protein-encoding genes (**figure 13.2**). Human genome sequence information is continually augmenting these earlier depictions.

Telomeres and Centromeres Are Essential

A chromosome must include structures that enable it to replicate and remain intact—everything else is essentially informational cargo (the protein-encoding genes) and DNA sequences that impart stability to the overall structure. The absolutely essential parts of a chromosome, in terms of navigating cell division, are:

- telomeres

- origin of replication sites, where replication forks begin to form

- the centromere

Recall from figure 2.18 that **telomeres** are chromosome tips, each consisting of many repeats of the sequence TTAGGG that are whittled down with each mitotic cell division.

The **centromere** is the largest constriction of a chromosome, and is the place where spindle fibers attach. A chromosome without a centromere is no longer a

| 1 | 2 | 3 | | 4 | 5 |

| 6 | 7 | 8 | 9 | 10 | 11 | 12 |

| 13 | 14 | 15 | | 16 | 17 | 18 |

| 19 | 20 | | 21 | 22 |

Sex chromosomes

a.   b.

Figure 13.1 Trisomy 21 Down syndrome. (a) Wendy Weisz enjoys studying art at Cuyahoga Community College. **(b)** A karyotype (chromosome chart) for trisomy 21 Down syndrome shows the extra chromosome 21.

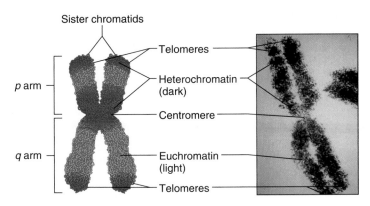

Sister chromatids

Telomeres

Heterochromatin (dark)

p arm

Centromere

q arm

Euchromatin (light)

Telomeres

Figure 13.2 Portrait of a chromosome. Tightly wound, highly repetitive heterochromatin forms the centromere (the largest constriction) and the telomeres (the tips). Elsewhere, lighter-staining euchromatin includes protein-encoding genes. The centromere divides this chromosome into a short arm (*p*) and a long arm (*q*).

chromosome—it vanishes from the cell as soon as division begins, because it cannot attach to the spindle.

In humans, many of the hundreds of thousands of DNA bases that form the centromere are repeats of a 171-base DNA sequence called an **alpha satellite.** (In this usage, *satellite* refers to the fate of these sequences when chromosomal DNA is shattered and different pieces settle in a density gradient. Because this part of the chromosome settles out at a density separate from the rest of the chromosome, it is called a satellite, just as the moon is a lump derived from the Earth.) The size and number of repeats in alpha satellites are similar in many species even if the sequence differs, suggesting that they have a structural role in maintaining chromosomes rather than encoding protein.

Centromeres also include **centromere-associated proteins.** Some of these are synthesized only when mitosis is imminent, forming a structure called a **kinetochore** that emanates from the centromere and contacts the spindle fibers. The kinetochore appears at prophase and vanishes during telophase.

Centromeres are replicated toward the end of S phase. A protein that may control this process is called centromere protein A, or CENP-A. Molecules of CENP-A remain associated with centromeres as chromosomes are replicated, covering about half a million DNA base pairs. When the replicated (sister) chromatids separate at anaphase, each member of the pair retains some CENP-A. The protein is therefore passed to the next cell generation, but it is *not* DNA. The amino acid sequence of CENP-A is nearly identical in diverse species. Researchers hypothesize that

CENP-A and other centromere-associated proteins are the critical parts of centromeres, rather than the alpha satellite DNA sequences. Evidence comes from DNA sequences that function as "neocentromeres." These are sequences, found throughout the genome in noncentromeric regions, that can function as centromeres if moved, even if they lack alpha satellites.

Centromeres lie within vast stretches of heterochromatin. The arms of the chromosome lie outward from the centromere. Gradually, the terrain of the DNA includes more protein-encoding sequences as distance from the centromere increases. Here, gene density varies greatly among the chromosome types. Chromosome 21 is a gene "desert," harboring a million-base stretch with no protein-encoding genes at all. Chromosome 22, in contrast, is a gene "jungle." These two tiniest chromosomes are at opposite ends of the gene-density spectrum. They are remarkably similar in size, but chromosome 22 contains 545 genes to chromosome 21's 225. **Table 13.1** compares some basic characteristics of the first five autosomes sequenced, and **figure 13.3** shows disorders associated with just one chromosome. Reading 13.1 describes the technique of creating chromosomes.

The chromosome parts between protein-rich areas and the telomeres are termed **subtelomeres (figure 13.4).** These areas extend from 8,000 to 300,000 bases inward toward the centromere from the telomeres.

Table 13.1

Five Autosomes

Chromosome	Size in Megabases (millions of bases)	% of Genome	Genes of Interest
5	194.00	6	Acute myelogenous leukemia Basal cell carcinoma Colorectal cancer Dwarfism Salt resistant hypertension
16	98.00	3	Adult polycystic kidney disease Breast cancer Crohn disease Prostate cancer
19	60.00	2	Atherosclerosis Type I diabetes mellitus DNA repair
21	33.55	1	Alzheimer disease Amyotropic lateral sclerosis Bipolar disorder susceptibility Homocystinuria Usher syndrome
22	33.46	1	Cat eye syndrome Chronic myelogenous leukemia DiGeorge syndrome Schizophrenia susceptibility

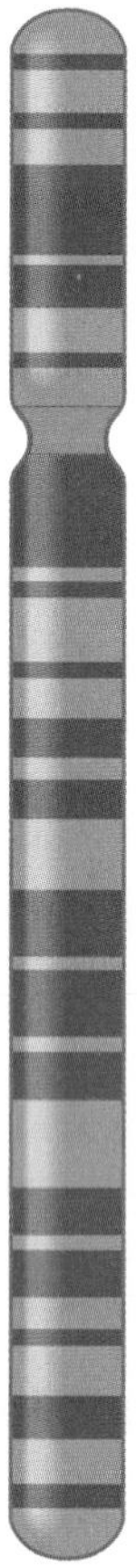

Chromosome 12
143 million bases
Dentatorubro-pallidoluysian atrophy
Emphysema
Alzheimer disease, susceptibility to
Inflammatory bowel disease
Leukemia, acute lymphoblastic
Hypertension, essential, susceptibility to
Leukemia factor, myeloid
Spastic paraplegia, autosomal dominant
Taste receptors
Glycogen storage disease, type 0
Hypertension with brachydactyly
Alzheimer disease, familial
Retinoblastoma-binding protein
Ichthyosis bullosa of Siemens
Telangiectasia, hereditary hemorrhagic
Leukemia: myeloid, lymphoid, or mixed-lineage
Allgrove syndrome
Diabetes insipidus, nephrogenic, dominant and recessive
Human papillomavirus type 18 integration site
Epidermolytic hyperkeratosis
Keratoderma, palmoplantar, nonepidermolytic
Cyclic ichthyosis with epidermolytic hyperkeratosis
White sponge nevus
Pachyonychia congenita
Fundus albipuctatus
Glioma
Myxoid liposarcoma
Stickler syndrome, type I
SED congenita
Kniest dysplasia
Glycogen storage disease
Rickets, pseudovitamin D deficiency
Interferon, immune deficiency
Cornea plana congenita, recessive
Growth retardation with deafness and mental retardation
Spinal muscular atrophy, congenital nonprogressive
Cardiomyopathy, hypertrophic
Brachydactyly, type C
Noonan syndrome
Cardiofaciocutaneous syndrome
Tyrosinemia, type III
Lymphoma, B-cell non-Hodgkin, high-grade
Holt-Oram syndrome
Alcohol intolerance, acute
Tumor rejection antigen
Human immunodeficiency virus-1 expression
Amyloidosis, renal

Figure 13.3 Anatomy of a chromosome. The centromere is indicated in red, and the bands represent classic staining patterns. When proteins associate with the DNA and the chromosome condenses, the centromere often appears as a constriction. Updated chromosome maps are available at www.ornl.gov/hgmis/posters/chromosome.

Telomere
Centromere
Subtelomere
ACACACTTTCGCGAATAAT...TTAAGGTTAGGGTTAGGGTAAGGG...TTAGGGTTAGGG...
(Short repeats)
(6-base repeats similar to telomeres)
(Telomere)

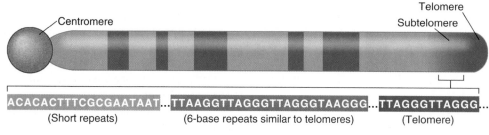

Figure 13.4 Subtelomeres. The repetitive sequence of a telomere gradually diversifies toward the centromere. A subtelomere consists of from 8,000 to 300,000 bases from the telomere inward on a chromosome arm. In this and other figures, the centromere is depicted as a buttonlike structure to more easily distinguish it. The centromere is composed of DNA, however, just like the rest of the chromosome.

Subtelomeres include some protein-encoding genes and therefore bridge the gene-rich regions and the telomere repeats. The transition is gradual. Areas of 50 to 250 bases, right next to the telomeres, consist of 6-base repeats, many of them very similar to TTAGGG. Then, moving inward from the 6-base zone are many shorter repeats, each present in a few copies. Their function isn't known. Finally the sequence diversifies and protein-encoding genes appear.

When researchers compared subtelomeres to known gene sequences, they found more than 500 matches. About half of these identified genes are members of multigene families (groups of genes of very similar sequence next to each other) that include pseudogenes. These multigene families may reflect recent evolution: Apes and chimps have only one or two genes for many of the gene families in humans. Such gene organization is one explanation for why our genome sequence is so very similar to that of our primate cousins—but we are clearly different animals. Our genomes differ more in gene copy number and chromosomal organization than in base sequence similarity. Chapter 16 compares primate genomes in greater detail.

Karyotypes Are Chromosome Charts

Even in this age of genomics, the standard chromosome chart, or **karyotype,** remains a major clinical genetic tool. A karyotype displays chromosomes by size and by physical landmarks that appear during mitotic metaphase, when DNA coils especially tightly.

The 24 human chromosome types are numbered from largest to smallest—1 to 22—although chromosome 21 is actually the smallest. The other two chromosomes are the X and the Y. Early attempts to size-order chromosomes resulted in generalized groupings because many of the chromosomes are of similar size.

Centromere position is one distinguishing feature of chromosomes. A chromosome is **metacentric** if the centromere divides it into two arms of approximately equal length. It is **submetacentric** if the centromere establishes one long arm and one short arm, and **acrocentric** if it pinches off only a small amount of material toward one end (**figure 13.5**). Some species have

HACs—Human Artificial Chromosomes

What are the minimal building blocks necessary to form a chromosome? Cytogeneticists knew from work on other species that a chromosome consists of three basic parts:

1. Telomeres

2. Origins of replication, estimated to occur every 50 to 350 kilobases (thousands of bases) in human chromosomes

3. Centromeres

All of these elements enable the entire unit to replicate during cell division and the original and replicated DNA double helices to be distributed into two cells from one.

The 24 types of human chromosomes range in size from 50 to 250 megabases (millions of bases). Researchers considered two ways to construct a chromosome—pare down an existing chromosome to see how small it can get and still hold together, or build a new chromosome from DNA pieces.

To trim an existing chromosome, researchers swapped in a piece of DNA that included telomere sequences. New telomeres formed at the insertion site, like periods added to the middle of a sentence, prematurely ending it. This technique formed chromosomes as small as 3.5 megabases—but researchers couldn't get them out of cells for further study.

Huntington Willard and his colleagues at Case Western Reserve University tried the building-up approach. They sent separately

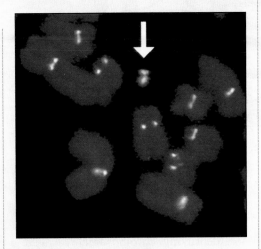

Figure 1 **Human artificial chromosomes.** Researchers introduced telomere sequences, centromere sequences, and other DNA pieces into cells in culture. The pieces aligned and assembled into human artificial chromosomes.

(John Harrington, Huntington Willard, et al. 1997. *Nature Genetics* 4:345–55.)

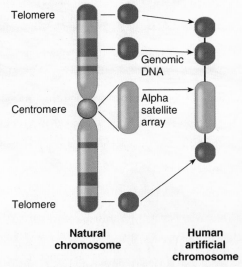

Figure 2 **Creating a human artificial chromosome.** Human artificial chromosomes (HACs) are formed by combining isolated telomeres, centromeric DNA from alpha satellite arrays, and genomic DNA derived from natural chromosomes.

(Modified from Willard, 1998. *Curr Opin Genet Dev* 8:219–25.)

into cultured cells telomere DNA alpha satellites and random pieces of DNA from the human genome containing origin-of-replication sites (**figures 1 and 2**). In the cells, some of the pieces assembled in a correct orientation to form structures 6 to 10 megabases long. These "human artificial chromosomes"—HACS—withstand repeated rounds of cell division. They have the integrity of a natural chromosome.

Other researchers have whittled down combinations of telomeres, neocentromeres, and other sequences to 0.7 to 1.8 megabases. Neocentromeres consist of centromere DNA sequences minus the alpha satellite repeats. The human genome contains several dozen of them, scattered among the chromosomes.

Constructing ever-smaller artificial chromosomes is revealing what a chromosome is—an autonomous nucleic acid/protein partnership that can replicate. More practically, artificial chromosomes may one day ferry healing genes to cells where gene activity is missing or abnormal.

---

telocentric chromosomes that have only one arm, but humans do not. The long arm of a chromosome is designated q, and the short arm p (p stands for "petite").

Five human chromosomes (13, 14, 15, 21, and 22) are distinguished further by bloblike ends, called satellites, that extend from a thinner, stalklike bridge from the rest of the chromosome. (This use of the word *satellite* differs from the usage of the term in centromeric repeats.) The stalklike regions are areas that do not bind stains well. The stalks

carry many repeats of genes coding for ribosomal RNA and ribosomal proteins, areas called nucleolar organizing regions. They coalesce to form the nucleolus, a structure in the nucleus where ribosomal building blocks are produced and assembled.

Karyotypes are useful at several levels. When a baby is born with the distinctive facial features of Down syndrome, a karyotype confirms the clinical diagnosis. Within families, karyotypes are used to identify relatives with a particular chrom-

osomal aberration that can affect health. For example, in one family, several adult members died from a rare form of kidney cancer. Because the cancer was so unusual, researchers karyotyped the affected individuals and found that they all had an exchange called a **translocation** between chromosome 3 and 8. When karyotypes showed that two young family members had the translocation, physicians examined and monitored their kidneys, detecting cancer very early and treating it successfully.

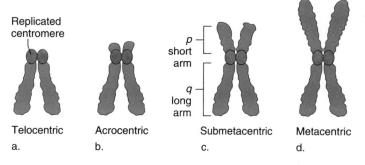

Figure 13.5 Centromere position is used to distinguish chromosomes. (a) A telocentric chromosome has the centromere at one end. Humans do not have any telocentric chromosomes. (b) An acrocentric chromosome has the centromere near an end. (c) A submetacentric chromosome's centromere creates a long arm (*q*) and a short arm (*p*). (d) A metacentric chromosome's centromere creates equal-sized arms.

Karyotypes of individuals from different populations can reveal the effects of environmental toxins, if abnormalities appear only in a group exposed to a particular contaminant. Because chemicals and radiation that can cause cancer and birth defects often break chromosomes into fragments or rings, detecting this genetic damage can alert physicians to the possibility that certain cancers may appear in the population.

Karyotypes compared between species can clarify evolutionary relationships. The more recent the divergence of two species from a common ancestor, the more closely related we presume they are, and the more alike their chromosome banding patterns should be. Our closest relative, according to karyotypes, is the pygmy chimpanzee (bonobo). The human karyotype is also remarkably similar to that of the domestic cat (see figure 16.12), and somewhat less similar to those of mice, pigs, and cows. It is least like the karyotype of the aardvark, indicating that this is a primitive placental mammal.

Key Concepts

A chromosome minimally includes telomeres, origins of replication, and centromeres, which enable the entire structure to replicate. A centromere consists of alpha satellite repeats and associated proteins, some of which form the kinetochore, to which spindle fibers attach. Centromere protein A enables the centromere to replicate. Subtelomeres contain telomerelike repeats and protein-encoding multigene families.
• Chromosomes are distinguishable by size, centromere location, satellites, and staining. Karyotypes are size-order charts of chromosomes.

13.2 Visualizing Chromosomes

Extra or missing chromosomes are easily detected by counting a number other than 46. Identifying chromosome rearrangements, such as an inverted sequence or an exchange of parts between two chromosomes, requires a way to distinguish among the chromosomes. A combination of stains and DNA probes applied to chromosomes allows this. A **DNA probe** is a labeled piece of DNA that binds to its complementary sequence on a particular chromosome.

Obtaining Cells for Chromosome Study

Any cell other than a mature red blood cell (which lacks a nucleus) can be used to examine chromosomes, but some cells are easier to obtain and culture than others. For adults, white blood cells separated from a blood sample or skinlike cells collected from the inside of the cheek are usually used for a chromosome test. A person might require such a test if he or she has a family history of a chromosomal abnormality or seeks medical help because of infertility.

For blood-borne cancers (leukemias and lymphomas), cytogeneticists examine chromosomes from bone marrow cells, which give rise to blood cells. DNA microarray tests are replacing karyotypes in matching cancers to the most effective chemotherapies. Figure 18.2 shows how such microarrays distinguished a newly-recognized form of leukemia, revealing why patients showed poor response to standard treatment—they were being treated for a different disease. The distinctions were detectable by gene

expression pattern, but not by symptoms or the appearance of the affected cells.

Chromosome tests are most commonly performed on cells from fetuses. Couples who receive a prenatal diagnosis of a chromosome abnormality can arrange for treatment of the newborn, if possible; learn more about the condition and contact support groups and plan care; or terminate the pregnancy. These choices are highly individual and personal and are best made after a genetic counselor or physician provides information on the medical condition and treatment options.

Amniocentesis

The first fetal karyotype was constructed in 1966 by a technique called **amniocentesis.** A doctor removes a small sample of fetal cells and fluids from the uterus with a needle passed through the woman's abdominal wall (**figure 13.6a**). The cells are cultured for a week to 10 days, and typically 20 cells are karyotyped. DNA probes can detect chromosomes in a day or two. The sampled amniotic fluid is also examined for deficient, excess, or abnormal biochemicals that could indicate certain inborn errors of metabolism. Amniocentesis takes just a few minutes and causes a feeling of pressure. Ultrasound is used to follow the needle's movement, and is also used to visualize particular fetal parts, such as the profile in **Figure 13.7.**

Amniocentesis can detect approximately 800 of the more than 5,000 known chromosomal and biochemical problems. Additional tests for single-gene disorders must be requested. The most common chromosomal abnormality detected is an extra chromosome, called a **trisomy.** Amniocentesis is usually performed between 14 and 16 weeks gestation, when the fetus isn't yet very large but amniotic fluid is plentiful, but can be carried out anytime after this point.

Doctors recommend amniocentesis if the risk that the fetus has a detectable condition exceeds the risk that the procedure will cause a miscarriage, which is about 1 in 350 (**table 13.2**). The most common candidate for the test is a pregnant woman over age 35. This "advanced maternal age" is statistically associated with increased risk that the fetus will have an extra or missing chromosome. Amniocentesis is also warranted if a couple has had several spontaneous abor-

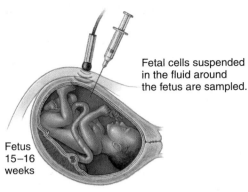

Fetal cells suspended in the fluid around the fetus are sampled.

Fetus 15–16 weeks

a. Amniocentesis

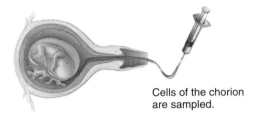

Cells of the chorion are sampled.

b. Chorionic villi sampling

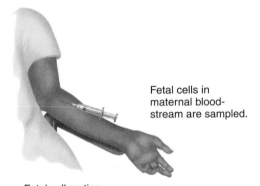

Fetal cells in maternal blood-stream are sampled.

c. Fetal cell sorting

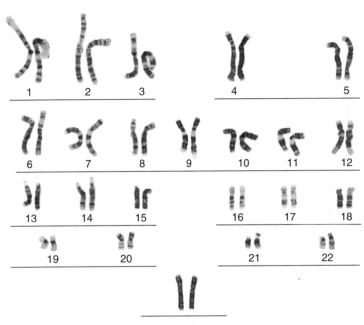

1	2	3	4	5
6	7	8	9	10	11	12
13	14	15	16	17	18
19	20	21	22	

Sex chromosomes

d. Fetal karyotype (normal female)

Figure 13.6 Three ways of checking a fetus's chromosomes.
(a) Amniocentesis draws out amniotic fluid, harvesting fetal cells shed into the fluid. **(b)** Chorionic villus sampling removes cells that would otherwise develop into the placenta. Since these cells came from the fertilized ovum, they should have the same chromosomal constitution as the fetus. **(c)** Improved techniques for identifying and extracting specific cells allow researchers to detect fetal cells in a sample of blood from the woman. **(d)** For all three techniques, the harvested cells are allowed to reach metaphase, when chromosomes are most visible, and then broken open on a slide. The chromosomes are stained or their DNA probed, then arranged into a karyotype.

tions or children with birth defects or a known chromosome abnormality.

Another reason to seek amniocentesis is if a blood test on the pregnant woman reveals low levels of a fetal liver protein called alpha fetoprotein (AFP) and high levels of human chorionic gonadotropin (hCG). These signs may indicate a fetus with a small liver, which may reflect a condition caused by an extra chromosome, such as Down syndrome. Such **maternal serum marker tests** may assess a third or fourth biochemical, too (estriol or inhibin). Yet another maternal serum marker, pregnancy-associated plasma protein A (PAPP), is detectable only during the first trimester.

Maternal serum marker tests are useful for pregnant women younger than 35 who would not routinely undergo age-related amniocentesis. Doctors use maternal serum

marker tests to screen their patients to identify those who may require genetic counseling and perhaps further, more invasive testing. For example, one four-marker test measures AFP, hCG, estriol, and inhibin during the second trimester. Considering maternal age along with the four markers reveals risk of trisomy 18 and trisomy 21. A risk of greater than 1 in 270 is typically sufficient for a physician to suggest a more definitive test, such as amniocentesis. About 7 percent of pregnant women tested are above this risk level, but only one in six of them actually carries a fetus with trisomy 21 Down syndrome. The AFP, hCG, and estriol values can also reflect elevated risk of trisomy 18. About 0.3 percent of all women tested are found to carry a fetus at high risk of having trisomy 18, and one in 15 of these fetuses is actually affected. Both of these conditions

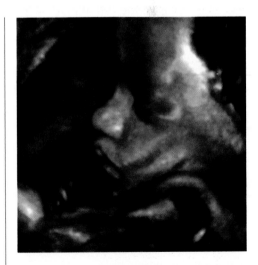

Figure 13.7 Ultrasound. In an ultrasound exam, sound waves are bounced off the embryo or fetus, and the pattern of deflected sound waves is converted into a "three-dimensional" image.

Table 13.2

Amniocentesis or Chorionic Villus Sampling (CVS)?

Procedure	Time (weeks)	Cell Source	Route	Added Risk of Miscarriage
CVS	10–12	Chorionic villi	Vagina	0.8%
Amniocentesis	14–16	Skin, bladder, digestive system cells in amniotic fluid	Needle in abdomen	0.3%

are discussed later in the chapter. In addition to the high number of false positives (high risk on the screen but normal fetus), maternal serum markers also have false negatives (low risk on the screen but an affected fetus). The four-marker test detects only 80 percent of trisomy 18 cases. This lack of precision is why maternal serum marker tests are considered screens rather than diagnostic tests.

Chorionic Villus Sampling

During the 10th through 12th week of pregnancy, **chorionic villus sampling** (CVS) obtains cells from the chorionic villi, the structures that develop into the placenta (figure 13.6b). A karyotype is prepared directly from the collected cells, rather than first culturing them, as in amniocentesis. Results are ready in days.

Because chorionic villus cells descend from the fertilized ovum, their chromosomes should be identical to those of the embryo and fetus. Occasionally, a chromosomal aberration occurs only in an embryo, or only in chorionic villi. This results in a situation called chromosomal mosaicism—that is, the karyotype of a villus cell differs from that of an embryo cell. Chromosomal mosaicism has great clinical consequences. If CVS indicates an aberration in villus cells that is not also in the fetus, then a couple may elect to terminate the pregnancy based on misleading information—that is, the fetus is actually chromosomally normal, although CVS indicates otherwise. In the opposite situation, the results of the CVS may be normal, but the fetus has abnormal chromosomes.

CVS is slightly less accurate than amniocentesis, and in about 1 in 1,000 to 3,000 procedures, it halts development of the feet and/or hands, a condition termed trans-verse limb defects. Also, CVS does not sample amniotic fluid, so tests for inborn errors of metabolism are not possible.

Couples expecting a child are sometimes asked to choose between amniocentesis and CVS. The advantage of CVS is earlier results, but the disadvantage is a greater risk of spontaneous abortion. Although CVS is slightly more invasive and dangerous to the fetus, its greater risk reflects the fact that CVS is done earlier in pregnancy. Since most spontaneous abortions occur early in pregnancy, more will follow CVS than amniocentesis. The spontaneous abortion rate after the 12th week of pregnancy is about 5 percent, and the additional risk that CVS poses is 0.8 percent. In contrast, the spontaneous abortion rate after the 14th week is 3.2 percent, and amniocentesis adds 0.3 percent to the risk.

Fetal Cell Sorting

Fetal cell sorting, a newer technique that separates fetal cells from the woman's bloodstream, is safer than amniocentesis and CVS but is still experimental (figure 13.6c) in the United States. The technique traces its roots to 1957, when a pregnant woman died when cells from a very early embryo lodged in a major blood vessel in her lung, blocking blood flow. The fetal cells were detectable because they were from a male, and contained the telltale Y chromosome. This meant that fetal cells could enter a woman's circulation. By studying the blood of other pregnant women, researchers found that fetal cells enter the maternal circulation in up to 70 percent of pregnancies. Cells from female embryos, however, cannot be distinguished from the cells of the pregnant woman on the basis of sex chromosome analysis. But fetal cells from either sex can be distinguished from maternal cells using a device called a fluorescence-activated cell sorter. It separates fetal cells from maternal blood by identifying surface characteristics that differ from those on the woman's cells. The fetal cells are then karyotyped (figure 13.6d) and fetal DNA extracted and amplified for specific gene tests. Free fetal DNA can also be isolated from maternal blood.

Rarely, other techniques are used to sample specific fetal tissues, such as blood, skin, liver, or muscle. These biopsy procedures are usually done by using ultrasound to guide a hollow needle through the woman's abdominal wall to reach the fetus. Such an invasive test is performed if the family has a disease affecting the particular tissue, and a DNA-based test is not available.

Instead of examining chromosomes, ultrasound can be used to identify physical features that are part of chromosomal syndromes. For example, ultrasound scans can enable a physician to detect increased fluid at the back of the neck (called nuchal translucency) and absent or underdeveloped nasal bones, both characteristic of Down syndrome and part of its initial description in 1866. In one study, 75 percent of fetuses with Down syndrome had these characteristics, compared to 0.5 percent of fetuses who did not have Down syndrome. Ultrasound scanning is less precise, but safer than obtaining chromosomes with amniocentesis or CVS. Ultrasound scans and maternal serum marker tests are sometimes combined. Particularly valuable, because it can be done in the first trimester, is nuchal translucency plus detection of two serum markers, which can identify 90 percent of trisomy 21 Down syndrome cases.

Preparing Cells for Chromosome Observation

Cytogeneticists have tried to describe and display human chromosomes since the late nineteenth century (**figure 13.8** and the Technology Timeline). Then, the prevailing view held that humans had an XO sex determination system, with females having an extra chromosome (XX). Estimates of the human chromosome number ranged from 30 to 80. In 1923, Theophilus Painter published sketches of human chromosomes

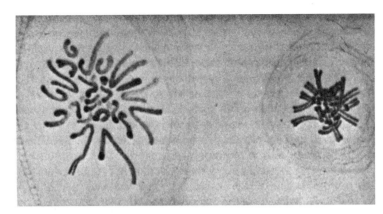

Figure 13.8 Viewing chromosomes. **(a)** The earliest drawings of chromosomes, by German biologist Walter Flemming, date from 1882. His depiction captures the random distribution of chromosomes as they splash down on a slide. **(b)** A micrograph of actual chromosomes, before a computer program arranges them into size-ordered pairs, echoes the old sketches. **(c)** A karyotype was once constructed with scissors and tape. Several websites enable you to create a karyotype the old-fashioned way. It isn't easy!

a.

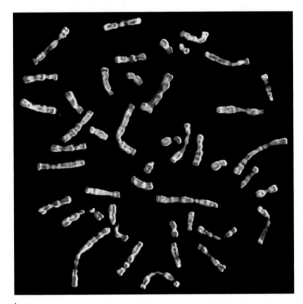

b.

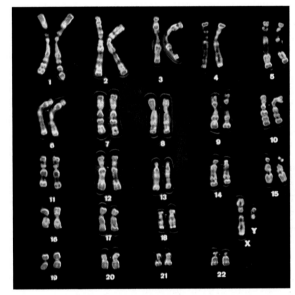

c.

from three patients at a Texas state mental hospital. The patients had been castrated in an attempt to control their abusive behavior, and Painter was able to examine the tissue. He could not at first tell whether the cells had 46 or 48 chromosomes, but finally decided that he saw 48. Painter later showed that both sexes have the same chromosome number.

The difficulty in distinguishing between 46 or 48 chromosomes was physical—it is challenging to prepare a cell in which chromosomes do not overlap. To easily count the chromosomes, scientists had to find a way to capture them when they are most condensed—during cell division— and also spread them apart. Since the 1950s, cytogeneticists have used colchicine, an extract of the chrysanthemum plant, to arrest cells during division.

Technology Timeline

1923	Theophilus Painter's chromosome sketches are published; human chromosome number thought to be 48
1951	Method to detangle chromosomes discovered by accident
1953	Albert Levan and Joe-Hin Tjio develop "squash and stain" technique for chromosome preparation
1956	Using tissue culture cells, Levan, Tjio, and Biesele determine chromosome number to be 46
1956	J. L. Hamerton and C. E. Ford identify 23 chromosomes in human gametes
1959	First chromosome abnormalities identified
1960	Phytohemagglutinin added to chromosome preparation protocol to separate and stimulate division in white blood cells
1970s	Several chromosome stains implemented to improve resolution of karyotypes
1970s	FISH developed
1990s	Spectral karyotyping combines FISH probes to distinguish each chromosome

Swelling, Squashing, and Untangling

How to untangle the spaghettilike mass of chromosomes was solved by accident in 1951. A technician mistakenly washed white blood cells being prepared for chromosome analysis in a salt solution that was less concentrated than the interiors of the cells. Water rushed into the cells, swelling them and separating the chromosomes.

Two years later, cell biologists Albert Levan and Joe-Hin Tjio found that when they drew cell-rich fluid into a pipette and dropped it onto a microscope slide prepared with stain, the cells burst open and freed the mass of chromosomes. Adding a glass coverslip spread the chromosomes enough that they could be counted. Another researcher, a former student of Painter, John Biesele, suggested that Levan and Tjio use cells from tissue culture, and by 1956, they finally agreed that 46 chromosomes are in a diploid human cell. In the same year, J. L. Hamerton and C. E. Ford identified 23 chromosomes in human gametes. In 1960 came another advance in visualizing chromosomes—use of a kidney bean extract called phytohemagglutinin to stimulate white blood cells to divide.

Until recently, a karyotype was constructed using a microscope to locate a cell in which the chromosomes were not touching, photographing the cell, developing a print, cutting out the individual chromosomes, and arranging them into a size-ordered chart. A computerized approach has largely replaced the cut-and-paste method. The device scans ruptured cells in a drop of stain and selects one in which the chromosomes are the most visible and well-spread. Then image analysis software recognizes the band patterns of each stained chromosome pair, sorts the structures into a size-ordered chart, and prints the karyotype—in minutes. If the software recognizes an abnormal band pattern, a database pulls out identical or similar karyotypes from other patients, providing clinical information on the anomaly. Genome sequence information is also scanned. However, the expert eyes of a skilled technician are still needed to detect subtle abnormalities in chromosome structure.

Staining

In the earliest karyotypes, dyes stained the chromosomes a uniform color. Chromosomes were grouped into size classes, designated A through G, in decreasing size order. In 1959, scientists described the first chromosomal abnormalities—Down syndrome (an extra chromosome 21), **Turner syndrome** (also called XO syndrome, a female with only one X chromosome), and **Klinefelter syndrome** (also called XXY syndrome, a male with an extra X chromosome). Before this, women with Turner syndrome were thought to be genetic males because they lack Barr bodies (see figure 6.12), while men with Klinefelter syndrome were thought to be genetic females because their cells have Barr bodies. Visualizing and distinguishing the sex chromosomes revealed the causes of these conditions.

The first stains applied to chromosomes could highlight large deletions and duplications, but usually researchers only vaguely understood the nature of a chromosomal syndrome. In 1967, a mentally retarded child with material missing from chromosome 4 would have been diagnosed as having a "B-group chromosome" disorder. Today, geneticists can identify the exact genes that are missing.

Describing smaller-scale chromosomal aberrations required better ways to distinguish among the chromosomes. In the 1970s, Swedish scientists developed more specific chromosome stains that create banding patterns unique to each chromosome. Stains are specific for AT-rich or GC-rich stretches of DNA, or for heterochromatin, which stains darkly at the centromere and telomeres.

The ability to detect missing, extra, inverted, or misplaced bands allowed researchers to link many more syndromes with specific chromosome aberrations. In the late 1970s, Jorge Yunis at the University of Minnesota improved chromosome staining further by developing a way to synchronize white blood cells in culture, arresting them in early mitosis. His approach of high-resolution chromosome banding revealed many more bands. Today, **fluorescence *in situ* hybridization,** or FISH, improves banding further by highlighting individual genes.

FISHing

One drawback of conventional chromosome stains is that they are not specific to particular chromosomes. Rather, they generate different banding patterns among the 24 human chromosome types. FISH uses DNA probes complementary to specific DNA sequences, and if those sequences are unique to a particular chromosome, the technique can identify it. FISH probes are attached to molecules that fluoresce when illuminated, producing a flash of color precisely where the probe binds to a chromosome in a patient's sample.

FISH is based on a technique, developed in 1970, called *in situ* hybridization, which originally used radioactive rather than fluorescent labels. *In situ* hybridization took weeks to work, because it relied on exposing photographic film to reveal bound DNA probes. The danger of working with radioactivity, and the crudeness of the results, prompted researchers to seek alternative ways to detect DNA probes.

FISH is used to identify specific chromosomes and to "paint" entire karyotypes, providing a different color for each chromosome. Many laboratories that perform amniocentesis or chorionic villus sampling use FISH probes specific to chromosomes 13, 18, 21, and the sex chromosomes to quickly identify the most common chromosome abnormalities. **Figure 13.9** shows FISH revealing the extra chromosome 21 in cells from a fetus with trisomy 21 Down syndrome. In an application of FISH called spectral karyotyping, each chromosome is probed with several different fluorescent molecules. A computer integrates the images and creates a false color for each chromosome (see figure 13.8*b*).

A new approach to prenatal chromosome analysis called quantitative PCR amplifies certain repeated sequences on chromosomes 13, 18, 21, X, and Y. The technique distinguishes paternally derived from maternally derived repeats on each homolog for these five chromosomes. An abnormal ratio of maternal to paternal repeats indicates a numerical problem, such as two copies of one parent's chrom-

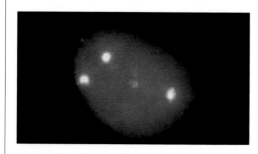

Figure 13.9 FISHing for genes and chromosomes. FISH shows three fluorescent dots that correspond to three copies of chromosome 21.

osome 21. Combined with the one chromosome 21 from the other parent, this situation would produce a fertilized ovum with three copies of chromosome 21, which causes Down syndrome. Quantitative PCR is less accurate than culturing cells or performing FISH, but it gives results in only hours, which can greatly reduce parental anxiety.

Chromosomal Shorthand

Geneticists abbreviate the pertinent information in a karyotype. They list chromosome number first, then sex chromosome constitution, then abnormal autosomes. Symbols describe the type of aberration, such as a deletion or translocation. Numbers are listed that correspond to specific bands. A normal male is 46,XY; a normal female is 46,XX. Geneticists use this notation to describe gene locations. For example, the β-globin subunit of hemoglobin is located at 11p15.5. **Table 13.3** gives some examples of chromosomal shorthand.

Chromosome information is displayed in an **ideogram,** which is a graphical representation of a karyotype (**figure 13.10**). Bands appear as stripes, and they are divided into numbered regions and subregions. Specific gene loci known from mapping data are listed on the righthand side with information from the human genome sequence. Ideograms are becoming so crowded with notations indicating specific genes that they may soon become obsolete.

Key Concepts

Karyotypes are charts that display chromosomes in size order. Chromosomes can be obtained from any cell that has a nucleus and can be cultured. Fetal karyotypes are constructed from cells obtained by amniocentesis, chorionic villus sampling, or fetal cell sorting from maternal blood. Ultrasound can detect physical signs of chromosome abnormalities. • To detect a chromosome abnormality, cytogeneticists obtain cells; display, stain, and probe chromosomes with fluorescent molecules; and then arrange them in a karyotype. Chromosomal shorthand summarizes the number of chromosomes, sex chromosome constitution, and type of aberration. Ideograms are maps of the distinguishing features of individual chromosomes.

Table 13.3

Chromosomal Shorthand

Abbreviation	What It Means
46,XY	Normal male
46,XX	Normal female
45,X	Turner syndrome (female)
47,XXY	Klinefelter syndrome (male)
47,XYY	Jacobs syndrome (male)
46,XY del (7q)	A male missing part of the long arm of chromosome 7
47,XX,+21	A female with trisomy 21 Down syndrome
46,XY t (7;9)(p21.1; q34.1)	A male with a translocation between the short arm of chromosome 7 at band 21.1 and the long arm of chromosome 9 at band 34.1

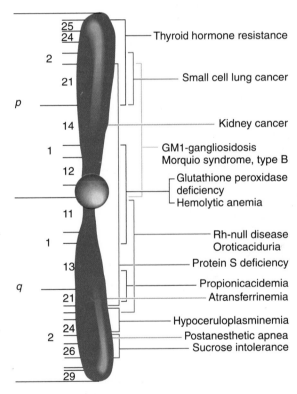

Figure 13.10 Ideogram. An ideogram is a schematic chromosome map. It indicates chromosome arm (p or q), major regions delineated by banding patterns, and the loci of known genes. This is a partial map of human chromosome 3.

13.3 Abnormal Chromosome Number

A human karyotype is abnormal if the number of chromosomes is not 46, or if individual chromosomes have extra, missing, or rearranged genetic material. **Table 13.4** summarizes the types of chromosome abnormalities in the order in which they are discussed.

Abnormal chromosomes account for at least 50 percent of spontaneous abortions. Yet only 0.5 to 0.7 percent of newborns have abnormal chromosomes. Therefore, most embryos and fetuses with abnormal chromosomes stop developing before birth.

Polyploidy

The most drastic upset in chromosome number is an entire extra set. A cell with extra sets of chromosomes is **polyploid.** An individual whose cells have three copies of each chromosome is a triploid (designated 3N, for three sets of chromosomes). Two-thirds of all triploids result from fertilization of an oocyte by two sperm. The other cases arise from formation of a diploid gamete, as when a normal haploid sperm fertilizes a diploid oocyte. Triploids account for 17 percent of spontaneous abortions (**figure 13.11**). Very rarely, an infant survives for a few days, with defects in nearly all organs.

Polyploids are very common among flowering plants, including roses, cotton, barley, and wheat. Individual cells in a human body may be polyploid. The liver, for example, has some tetraploid (4N) and even octaploid (8N) cells.

Aneuploidy

Cells missing a single chromosome or having an extra one are **aneuploid,** which means "not good set." Rarely, aneuploids can have more than one missing or extra chromosome, indicating defective meiosis in a parent. A normal chromosome number is **euploid,** which means "good set."

Most autosomal aneuploids (with a missing or extra non-sex chromosome) are spontaneously aborted. Those that survive have specific syndromes, with symptoms depending upon which chromosomes are missing or extra. Mental retardation is common in an individual who survives with aneuploidy, because development of the brain is so complex and of such long duration that nearly any chromosome-scale disruption involves genes whose protein products affect the brain. Sex chromosome aneuploidy usually produces milder symptoms.

Most children born with the wrong number of chromosomes have an extra chromosome (a **trisomy**) rather than a missing chromosome (a **monosomy**). Most monosomies are so severe that an affected embryo ceases developing. Trisomies and monosomies are named according to the chromosome involved, and the associated syndrome has traditionally been named for the investigator who first described it. Today, cytogenetic terminology is used

Table 13.4	
Chromosome Abnormalities	
Type of Abnormality	**Definition**
Polyploidy	Extra chromosome sets
Aneuploidy	An extra or missing chromosome
Monosomy	One chromosome absent
Trisomy	One chromosome extra
Deletion	Part of a chromosome missing
Duplication	Part of a chromosome present twice
Translocation	Two chromosomes join long arms or exchange parts
Inversion	Segment of chromosome reversed
Isochromosome	A chromosome with identical arms
Ring chromosome	A chromosome that forms a ring due to deletions in telomeres, which cause ends to adhere

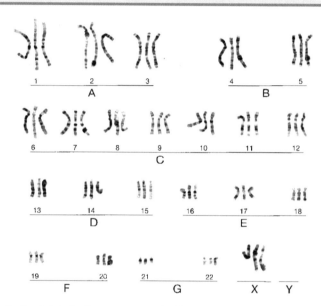

Figure 13.11 **Polyploids in humans are lethal.** Individuals with three copies of each chromosome (triploids) account for 17 percent of all spontaneous abortions and 3 percent of stillbirths and newborn deaths.

because it is more precise. For example, Down syndrome can result from an extra chromosome 21 (a trisomy) or a translocation. The distinction is important in genetic counseling. Translocation Down syndrome, although accounting for only 4 percent of cases, has a much higher recurrence risk within a family than the trisomy 21 form, a point we will return to later in the chapter.

The meiotic error that causes aneuploidy is called **nondisjunction.** Recall that in normal meiosis, homologs separate, and each of the resulting gametes receives only one member of each chromosome pair. In nondisjunction, a chromosome pair fails to

separate at anaphase of either the first or second meiotic division. This produces a sperm or oocyte that has two copies of a particular chromosome, or none, rather than the normal one copy (**figure 13.12**). When such a gamete fuses with its mate at fertilization, the zygote has either 45 or 47 chromosomes, instead of the normal 46. Different trisomies tend to be caused by nondisjunction in the male or female, at meiosis I or II.

A cell can have a missing or extra chromosome in 49 ways—an extra or missing copy of each of the 22 autosomes, plus the five abnormal types of sex chromosome combinations—Y, X, XXX, XXY, and XYY.

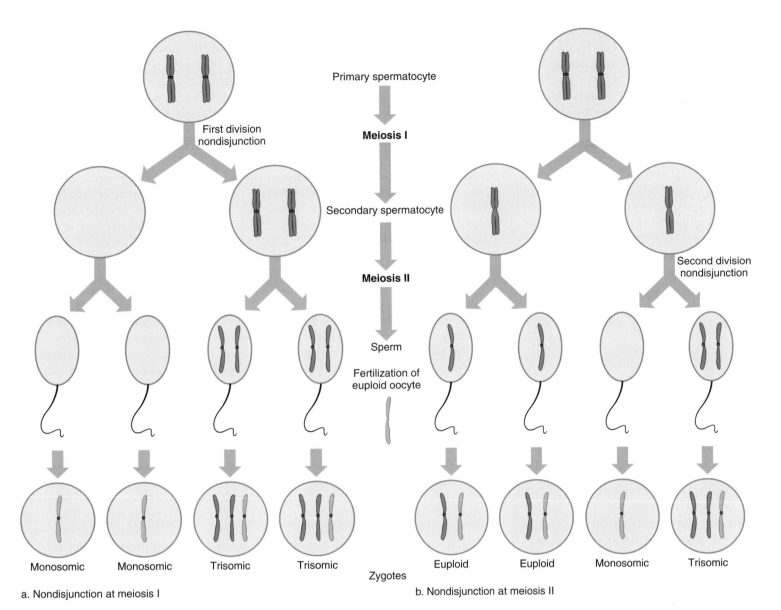

Figure 13.12 **Extra and missing chromosomes—aneuploidy.** Unequal division of chromosome pairs can occur at either the first or second meiotic division. **(a)** A single pair of chromosomes is unevenly partitioned into the two cells arising from meiosis I in a male. The result: two sperm cells have two copies of the chromosome, and two sperm cells have no copies. When a sperm cell with two copies of the chromosome fertilizes a normal oocyte, the zygote is trisomic; when a sperm cell lacking the chromosome fertilizes a normal oocyte, the zygote is monosomic. **(b)** This nondisjunction occurs at meiosis II. Because the two products of the first division are unaffected, two of the mature sperm are normal and two are aneuploid. Oocytes can undergo nondisjunction as well, leading to zygotes with extra or missing chromosomes when normal sperm cells fertilize them.

(Sometimes individuals have four or even five sex chromosomes.) However, only nine types of aneuploids are known in newborns. Others are seen in spontaneous abortions or fertilized ova intended for *in vitro* fertilization.

Most of the 50 percent of spontaneous abortions that result from extra or missing chromosomes are 45,X individuals (missing an X chromosome), triploids, or trisomy 16. About 9 percent of spontaneous abortions are trisomy 13, 18, or 21. Although

these are the most common autosomal aneuploids seen in newborns, they are still rare, affecting only 0.1 percent of all children. Put another way, more than 95 percent of newborns with abnormal chromosome numbers have an extra 13, 18, or 21, or an extra or missing X or Y chromosome.

Types of chromosome abnormalities seem to differ between the sexes. Abnormal oocytes mostly have extra or missing chromosomes, whereas abnormal sperm more often have structural variants, such as

inversions or translocations, discussed later in the chapter.

Aneuploidy and polyploidy also arise during mitosis, producing groups of somatic cells with the extra or missing chromosome. An individual with two chromosomally distinct cell populations is a mosaic. If only a few cells are altered, health may not be affected. However, a mitotic abnormality that occurs early in development, so that many cells descend from the unusual one, can affect health. A chromosomal mosaic for a trisomy may have a mild version of the associated condition. This is usually the case for the 1 to 2 percent of people with Down syndrome who are mosaic. For example, a person may have the extra chromosome that causes Down syndrome in 5 of 20 sampled fetal cells. This individual would not be as severely mentally impaired as a person who has the extra chromosome in every cell. The phenotype depends upon which cells have the extra chromosome. A fetus with affected cells in the brain would later show a greater mental impairment than a fetus with the affected cells mostly in the skin. Unfortunately, prenatal testing cannot reveal which cells are affected.

Autosomal Aneuploids

Most autosomal aneuploids are very rarely seen in live births, due to the lethality of a large imbalance of genetic material. Following are descriptions of the most common autosomal aneuploids among liveborns, summarized in **table 13.5**.

Trisomy 21 Down Syndrome The most common autosomal aneuploid among liveborns is trisomy 21. The characteristic extra folds in the eyelids, called epicanthal folds, and flat face of a person with trisomy 21 prompted Sir John Langdon Haydon Down to term the condition *mongoloid* when he described it in 1866. As the medical superintendent of a facility for the profoundly mentally retarded, Down noted that about 10 percent of his patients resembled people of Mongolian heritage. The resemblance is superficial and meaningless. Males and females of all ethnic groups can have Down syndrome.

Down syndrome may have been recognized as early as 1515 in the Flemish painting "The Adoration of the Christ Child." An angel next to Mary has the characteristic facial features and short fingers of the condition.

Researchers suspected a link between Down syndrome and an abnormal chromosome number as long ago as 1932. In 1958, improved chromosome visualization techniques revealed 47 chromosomes in cells of a person with trisomy 21 Down syndrome. By 1959, researchers had implicated chromosome 21. In 1960, they discovered Down syndrome caused by a translocation between chromosome 21 and another chromosome, and in 1961, researchers identified mosaic Down syndrome. The affected girl had physical signs of the condition, but normal intelligence.

A person with Down syndrome is usually short and has straight, sparse hair and a tongue protruding through thick lips. The hands have an abnormal pattern of creases, the joints are loose, and poor reflexes and muscle tone give a "floppy" appearance. Developmental milestones (such as sitting, standing, and walking) come slowly, and toilet training may take several years. Intelligence varies greatly. Parents of a child with Down syndrome can help their child reach maximal potential by providing a stimulating environment.

Many people with Down syndrome have physical problems, including heart and kidney defects, and hearing and vision loss. A suppressed immune system can make influenza deadly. Digestive system blockages are common and require surgical correction. A child with Down syndrome is 15 times more likely to develop leukemia than a child who does not have the syndrome, but this is only a 1 percent risk. Many of the medical problems associated with Down syndrome are treatable, so that more than 70 percent of affected individuals live beyond age 30. In 1910, life expectancy was only nine years.

Persons with Down syndrome who pass age 40 often develop the black fibers and tangles of amyloid protein in their brains characteristic of Alzheimer disease, although they usually do not become severely demented. The chance of a person with trisomy 21 developing Alzheimer disease is 25 percent, compared to 6 percent for the general population. A gene on chromosome 21 causes one inherited form of Alzheimer disease. Perhaps the extra copy of the gene in trisomy 21 has a similar effect to a mutation in the gene that causes Alzheimer disease. In a person with Down syndrome, Alzheimer disease seems like an acceleration in the forgetfulness that can accompany aging.

Before the human genome sequence became available, researchers studied people who have a third copy of only part of chromosome 21 to identify specific genes that could cause symptoms. That region has been narrowed down to about 2.5 million bases, but the responsible area may not be just one stretch of genes—that is, the genes that exert effects when present in an extra copy may be distributed over this area. **Table 13.6** lists some of the genes known to contribute to trisomy 21 Down syndrome symptoms.

The likelihood of giving birth to a child with Down syndrome increases dramatically with the age of the mother. The overall frequency of trisomy 21 Down syndrome is 1 in about 800 births. For women under 30, the chances are 1 in 952. But at age 35, the risk is 1 in 378, and at age 40, 1 in 106. By age 45, risk jumps to 1 in 30, and by age 48, it is 1 in 14. However, 80 percent of children with trisomy 21 are born to women under age 35. This is because younger women are more likely to become pregnant and less likely to undergo amniocentesis. About 90 percent of trisomy 21 conceptions are due to nondisjunction during meiosis I in the female. The 10 percent of cases due to the male result from nondisjunction during meiosis I or II.

The chance that trisomy 21 will recur in a family, based on empirical data (how often it actually does recur in families), is 1 percent. Genetic counselors consider this figure, along with maternal age, to present a worst-case scenario.

The age factor in Down syndrome may reflect the fact that meiosis in the female ends after conception. The older a woman is, the longer her oocytes have been arrested

Table 13.5		

Comparing and Contrasting Trisomies 13, 18, and 21

Type of Trisomy	Incidence at Birth	Percent of Conceptions That Survive 1 Year After Birth
13 (Patau)	1/12,500–1/21,700	<5%
18 (Edward)	1/6,000–1/10,000	<5%
21 (Down)	1/800–1/826	85%

Table 13.6

Genes Associated with Trisomy 21 Down Syndrome

Gene	OMIM Number	Associated Symptoms
Amyloid precursor protein (APP)	104760	Protein deposits in brain
Chromatin assembly factor I (CAF1A)	601245	Impaired DNA synthesis
Collagen type VI (COL6A1)	120220	Heart defects
Crystallin (CRYA1)	123580	Cataracts
Cystathione beta synthase (CBS)	236200	Impaired metabolism and DNA repair
Interferon receptor 1 (IFNAR)	107450	Impaired immunity
Kinase 1 (DYRK1A)	600855	Mental retardation
Oncogene ETS2 (ETS2)	164740	Skeletal abnormalities, cancer
Phosphoribosylglycinamide formyltransferase (GART)	138440	Impaired DNA synthesis and repair
Superoxide dismutase (SOD1)	147450	Premature aging

on the brink of completing meiosis. During this time, the oocytes may have been exposed to toxins, viruses, and radiation. A variation on this idea suggests that females have a pool of aneuploid oocytes resulting from nondisjunction, which for an unknown reason do not mature. As a woman ages, selectively releasing normal oocytes each month, the abnormal ones remain, much as black jellybeans accumulate as people preferentially eat the colored ones.

The association between maternal age and Down syndrome has been recognized since the nineteenth century, when physicians noticed that affected babies were often the youngest children in large families. The condition was thought to be caused by syphilis, tuberculosis, thyroid malfunction, alcoholism, or emotional trauma. In 1909, a study of 350 affected infants revealed an overrepresentation of older mothers, prompting some researchers to attribute the link to "maternal reproductive exhaustion." In 1930, another study found that the increased risk of Down syndrome correlated to maternal age, and not to the number of children in the family.

Trisomy 18—Edward Syndrome

Trisomies 18 and 13 were described in the same research report in 1960. Only 1 in 6,000 to 10,000 newborns has trisomy 18, but as table 13.5 indicates, most affected individuals do not survive to be born. The severe symptoms of trisomy 18 explain why few affected fetuses survive and also make the syndrome relatively easy to diagnose prenatally using ultrasound—yet the symptoms are presumably milder than those associated with most aneuploids, which are spontaneously aborted. Affected children have great physical and mental disabilities, with developmental skills stalled at the six-month level. Major abnormalities include heart defects, a displaced liver, growth retardation, and oddly clenched fists. Milder signs and symptoms include overlapping placement of fingers (**figure 13.13**), a narrow and flat skull, abnormally shaped and low-set ears, a small mouth and face, unusual or absent fingerprints, short large toes with fused second and third toes, and "rocker-bottom" feet. Most cases of trisomy 18 are traced to nondisjunction in meiosis II of the oocyte.

Trisomy 13—Patau Syndrome

Trisomy 13 is very rare, but, as is the case with trisomy 18, the number of newborns with the anomaly reflects only a small percentage of affected conceptions. Trisomy 13 has a different set of signs and symptoms than trisomy 18. Most striking, although rare, is a fusion of the developing eyes, so that a fetus has one large eyelike structure in the center of the face. More common is a small or absent eye. Major abnormalities affect the heart, kidneys, brain, face, and limbs. The nose is often malformed, and cleft lip and/or palate is present in a small head. Extra fingers and toes may occur. Appearance of a facial cleft and extra digits on an ultrasound exam are considered sufficient evidence to pursue chromosome analysis of the fetus to detect or rule out trisomy 13.

Ultrasound examination of an affected newborn often reveals more extensive anomalies, such as an extra spleen, abnormal liver, rotated intestines, and an abnormal pancreas. A few individuals have survived until adulthood, but they do not progress developmentally beyond the six-month level.

Sex Chromosome Aneuploids

People with sex chromosome aneuploidy have extra or missing sex chromosomes. **Table 13.7** indicates how these aneuploids can arise. Note that some conditions can result from nondisjunction in meiosis in the male or female.

Turner Syndrome (45,X)

In 1938, at a medical conference, a U.S. endocrinologist named Henry Turner described seven young women, aged 15 to 23, who were sexually undeveloped, short, had folds of skin on the back of their necks, and had malformed elbows. (Eight years earlier, an English physician named Ullrich had described the

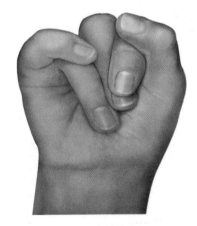

Figure 13.13 Trisomy 18 (Edward syndrome). An infant with trisomy 18 clenches its fist in a characteristic manner, with fingers overlapping.

Table 13.7

How Nondisjunction Leads to Sex Chromosome Aneuploids

Situation	Oocyte	Sperm	Consequence
Normal	X	Y	46,XY normal male
	X	X	46,XX normal female
Female nondisjunction	XX	Y	47,XXY Klinefelter syndrome
	XX	X	47,XXX triplo-X
		Y	45,Y nonviable
		X	45,X Turner syndrome
Male nondisjunction (meiosis I)	X		45,X Turner syndrome
	X	XY	47,XXY Klinefelter syndrome
Male nondisjunction (meiosis II)	X	XX	47,XXX triplo-X
	X	YY	47,XYY Jacobs syndrome
	X		45,X Turner syndrome

syndrome in young girls, so it is called Ullrich syndrome in the U.K.) Alerted to what would become known as Turner syndrome in the United States, other physicians soon began identifying such patients in their practices. Physicians assumed that a hormonal insufficiency caused the symptoms. They were right, but there was more to the story—a chromosomal imbalance caused the hormone deficit.

In 1954, at a London hospital, P. E. Polani discovered that cells from Turner patients lacked a Barr body, the dark spot that indicates a second X chromosome (see figure 6.12). Might lack of a sex chromosome cause the symptoms, particularly failure to mature sexually? By 1959, karyotyping confirmed the absence of an X chromosome in cells of Turner syndrome patients. Later, researchers learned that only 50 percent of people with Turner syndrome are XO. The rest have partial deletions or are mosaics, with only some cells affected.

Like the autosomal aneuploids, Turner syndrome is found more frequently among spontaneously aborted fetuses than among newborns—99 percent of affected fetuses die before birth. The syndrome affects 1 in 2,000 female births. However, people with the condition usually do not know they have a chromosome abnormality until they lag behind their classmates in sexual development. Two X chromosomes are necessary for normal sexual development in females.

In childhood, signs of Turner syndrome include wide-set nipples, slight webbing at the back of the neck, short stature, coarse facial features, and a low hairline at the back of the head. About half of people with Turner syndrome have impaired hearing and frequent ear infections due to a small defect in the shape of the cochlea, the coiled part of the inner ear. They cannot hear certain frequencies of sound. At sexual maturity, sparse body hair develops, but the girls do not ovulate or menstruate, and they have underdeveloped breasts. The uterus is very small, but the vagina and cervix are normal. However, in the ovaries, oocytes speed through development, depleting the supply during infancy. Intelligence is normal, and these women can lead fairly normal lives if they receive hormone supplements. Using growth hormone adds up to three inches or so of height. Although women with Turner syndrome are infertile, individuals who are mosaics may have children.

Women with Turner syndrome who do become pregnant are at high risk of carrying a fetus with an abnormal number of chromosomes. In one study of 138 pregnancies, 82 produced infants, and 23 of them had birth defects, 10 of these with abnormal chromosomes. *In vitro* fertilization (IVF), discussed in chapter 21, can be used to select oocytes that have a normal chromosome number. Interestingly, Turner syndrome is the only aneuploid condition that seems unrelated to the age of the mother.

For many years, it was thought that Turner syndrome had no effects in adulthood, but this was largely because most studies of common adult disorders did not consider chromosome status. Researchers in Edinburgh have been tracking the health of 156 women with Turner syndrome for more than 25 years as part of an abnormal karyotype registry. Having Turner syndrome apparently does affect lifespan. For example, 68 percent of the 156 participants reached age 60, compared to 88 percent of the general British population. Adults with Turner syndrome are more likely to develop certain disorders than the general population (**figure 13.14**).

The many signs and symptoms of Turner syndrome result from the loss of specific genes. For example, loss of a gonadal dysgenesis gene accounts for the ovarian failure, whereas absence of a homeobox gene, which is a transcription factor, causes short stature. Another gene causes the unusual hearing defect that is part of the syndrome.

Extra X Chromosomes   About 1 in every 1,000 females has an extra X chromosome in each of her cells, a condition called triplo-X. The only symptoms seem to be taller stature and menstrual irregularities. Although triplo-X females are rarely mentally retarded, they tend to be less intelligent than their siblings. The lack of symptoms associated with having extra X chromosomes reflects the protective effect of X inactivation—all but one of the X chromosomes is inactivated.

About 1 in 1,000 males has an extra X chromosome, which causes Klinefelter syndrome (XXY). Physicians first described the signs and symptoms in 1942, and geneticists identified the underlying chromosomal anomaly in 1959. Men severely affected with Klinefelter syndrome are underdeveloped sexually, with rudimentary testes and prostate glands and sparse pubic and facial hair. They have very long arms and legs, large hands and feet, and may develop breast tissue. Klinefelter syndrome is the most common genetic or chromosomal cause of male infertility, accounting for 4 to 6 percent of infertile men.

Testosterone injections during adolescence can limit limb lengthening and prompt development of secondary sexual characteristics. Boys and men with Klinefelter syndrome may be slow to learn, but they are usually

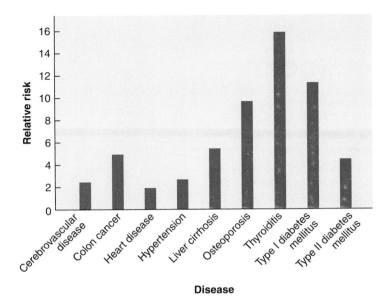

Figure 13.14 Turner syndrome in adulthood. For many years, geneticists thought Turner syndrome did not affect individuals in middle adulthood, because such women did not report problems. But it turned out that nobody asked! Women with Turner syndrome do not look different, so until recently, there were no data on their higher risk of developing certain conditions. (Chapter 1 discusses relative risk.)

not mentally retarded unless they have more than two X chromosomes, which happens rarely.

Many textbooks include photographs of very extreme cases of Klinefelter syndrome, which may give the erroneous impression that the syndrome is always severe. Actually, many men who have the condition discover it only when they have an infertility problem. Some affected men probably never learn that they have Klinefelter syndrome. The photograph of the young man who wrote "A Personal Look at Klinefelter Syndrome" on page 256 shows that affected individuals can look like anyone else.

Some men with Klinefelter syndrome have fathered children, using IVF and intracytoplasmic sperm injection (ICSI), also discussed in chapter 21. Using these methods, doctors can identify and select sperm that contain only one sex chromosome and use them to fertilize oocytes. Sperm from men with Klinefelter syndrome are more likely to have extra chromosomes—usually X or Y, but also autosomes—compared to sperm from men who do not have Klinefelter syndrome.

XYY Syndrome

One male in 1,000 has an extra Y chromosome. Awareness of this condition arose in 1961, when a tall, healthy, middle-aged man, known for his boisterous behavior, underwent a routine chromosome check after fathering a child with Down syndrome. The man had an extra Y chromosome. A few other cases were detected over the next several years.

In 1965, researcher Patricia Jacobs published results of a survey among 197 inmates at Carstairs, a high-security prison in Scotland. Of 12 men with unusual chromosomes, seven had an extra Y. Might their violent or aggressive behavior be linked to their extra Y chromosome? Jacobs's findings were repeated in studies in English and Swedish mental institutions. Soon after, *Newsweek* magazine ran a cover story on "congenital criminals." In 1968, defense attorneys in France and Australia pleaded their violent clients' cases on the basis of an inherited flaw, the extra Y of what became known as Jacobs syndrome. Meanwhile, the National Institute of Mental Health, in Bethesda, Maryland, held a conference on the condition, lending legitimacy to the hypothesis that an extra Y predisposes to violent behavior.

In the early 1970s, newborn screens began in hospital nurseries in England, Canada, Denmark, and Boston. Social workers and psychologists visited XYY children and offered "anticipatory guidance" to the parents on how to deal with their toddling future criminals. By 1974, geneticists and others halted the program, pointing out that singling out these boys on the basis of a few statistical studies was inviting self-fulfilling prophecy.

Today, we know that 96 percent of XYY males are apparently normal. The only symptoms attributable to the extra chromosome may be great height, acne, and perhaps speech and reading problems. An explanation for the continued prevalence of XYY among mental-penal institution populations may be more psychological than biological. Large body size may lead teachers, employers, parents, and others to expect more of these people, and a few of them may deal with this stress with aggression.

Jacobs syndrome can arise from nondisjunction in the male, producing a sperm with two Y chromosomes that fertilizes an X-bearing oocyte. Geneticists have never observed a sex chromosome constitution of one Y and no X. Since the Y chromosome carries little genetic material, and the gene-packed X chromosome would not be present, the absence of so many genes makes development beyond a few cell divisions in a YO embryo impossible.

Key Concepts

Polyploids have extra sets of chromosomes and do not survive for long. Aneuploids have extra or missing chromosomes. Nondisjunction during meiosis causes aneuploidy. Trisomics are more likely to survive than monosomics, and sex chromosome aneuploidy is less severe than autosomal aneuploidy. • Mitotic nondisjunction produces chromosomal mosaics. Down syndrome (trisomy 21) is the most common autosomal aneuploid, followed by trisomies 18 and 13. Sex chromosome aneuploids include people with Turner syndrome (XO), triplo-X, Klinefelter syndrome (XXY), and XYY syndrome.

13.4 Abnormal Chromosome Structure

Structural chromosomal defects include missing, extra, or inverted genetic material within a chromosome or combined or exchanged parts of nonhomologs (translocations) (**figure 13.15**).

A Personal Look at Klinefelter Syndrome

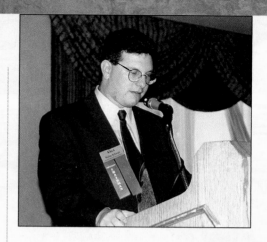

I was diagnosed with Klinefelter syndrome (KS) at age 25, in February 1996. Being diagnosed has been . . . a big sigh of relief after a life of frustrations. Throughout my early childhood, teens, and even somewhat now, I was very shy, reserved, and had trouble making friends. I would fly into rages for no apparent reason. My parents knew when I was very young that there was something about me that wasn't right.

I saw many psychologists, psychiatrists, therapists, and doctors, and their only diagnosis was "learning disabilities." In the seventh grade, I was told by a psychologist that I was stupid and lazy, and I would never amount to anything. After barely graduating high school, I started out at a local community college. I received an associate degree in business administration, and never once sought special help. I transferred to a small liberal arts college to finish up my bachelor of science degree, and spent an extra year to complete a second degree. Then I started a job as a software engineer for an Internet-based company. I have been using computers for 20 years and have learned everything I needed to know on my own.

To find out my KS diagnosis, I had gone to my general physician for a physical. He noticed that my testes were smaller than they should be and sent me for blood work. The karyotype showed Klinefelter syndrome, 47,XXY. After seeing the symptoms of KS and what effects they might have, I found it described me perfectly. But, after getting over the initial shock and dealing with the denial, depression, and anger, I decided that there could be things much worse in life. I decided to take a positive approach.

There are several types of treatments for KS. I give myself a testosterone injection in the thigh once every two weeks. My learning and thought processes have become stronger, and I am much more outgoing and have become more of a leader. Granted, not all of this is due to the increased testosterone level, some of it is from a new confidence level and from maturing.

I feel that parents who are finding out prior to the birth of their son [that he will have Klinefelter syndrome] or parents of affected infants or young children are very lucky. There is so much they can do to help their child have a great life. I have had most all of the symptoms at some time in my life, and I've gotten through and done well.

Stefan Schwarz

(Stefan Schwarz runs a Boston-area support group for KS.)

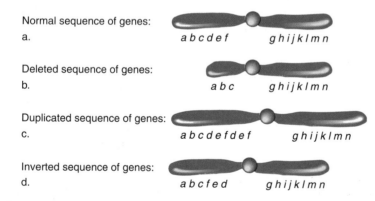

Figure 13.15 Chromosome abnormalities. If a hypothetical normal gene sequence appears as shown in **(a)**, then **(b)** represents a deletion, **(c)** a duplication, and **(d)** an inversion.

Deletions and Duplications

A **deletion** is missing genetic material. Deletions range greatly in size, with the larger ones tending to have greater effects because they remove more genes. Consider cri-du-chat syndrome (French for "cat's cry"), caused by deletion of part of the short arm of chromosome 5 (also called 5p⁻ syndrome). Affected children have a high-pitched cry similar to the mewing of a cat, have pinched facial features, and are mentally retarded and developmentally delayed. The chromosome region responsible for the catlike cry is distinct from the region that causes mental retardation and developmental delay. The cri-du-chat deletion also removes the gene for telomerase reverse transcriptase, which normally keeps telomeres long in cells that divide often. The gene's absence may contribute to the shortened lifespan of affected individuals.

A cytogeneticist can determine by examining a detailed karyotype whether a child will have only the catlike cry and perhaps poor weight gain, or will have all of the signs and symptoms, which include low birth weight, poor muscle tone, a small head, and impaired language skills. In Their Own Words on page 257 describes a child who had 5p⁻ syndrome.

A **duplication** is a region of a chromosome where genes are repeated. Duplications, like deletions, are more likely to cause symptoms if they are extensive. For example, duplications of chromosome 15 do not produce a phenotype unless they repeat several

Ashley's Message of Hope

What is it like to have a child born with cri-du-chat syndrome? How does this affect the family and its future? What kinds of assistance can the medical community offer the family?

The birth of any child raises many questions. Will she have my eyes, her dad's smile? What will she want to be when she grows up? But the biggest question for every parent is "Will she be healthy?" If complications occur during birth or if the child is born with a genetic disorder, the questions become more profound and immediate. "How did this happen?" "Where do we go from here?" "Will this happen again?"

Our daughter, Ashley Elizabeth Naylor [figure 1], was born August 12, 1988. We had a lot of mixed emotions the day of her birth, but mainly we felt fear and despair. The doctors suspected complications, which led to a cesarean section, but the exact problem was not known. Two weeks after her birth, chromosome analysis revealed cri-du-chat (cat cry) syndrome, also known as 5p$^-$ syndrome because part of the short arm of one copy of chromosome 5 is missing. The prognosis was uncertain. This is a rare disorder, we were told, and little could be offered to help our daughter. The doctors used the words "profoundly retarded," which cut like a knife through our hearts and our hopes. It wasn't until a few years later that we realized how little the medical community actually knew about cri-du-chat syndrome and especially about our little girl!

Ashley defied all the standard medical labels, as well as her doctors' expectations. Her spirit and determination enabled her to walk with the aid of a walker and express herself using sign language and a communication device. With early intervention and education at United Services for the Handicapped, Ashley found the resources and additional encouragement she needed to succeed. In return, Ashley freely offered one of her best-loved and sought-after gifts—her hugs. Her bright eyes and glowing smile captured the hearts of everyone she met.

In May of 1994, Ashley's small body could no longer support the spirit that inspired so many. She passed away after a long battle with pneumonia. Her physical presence is gone, but her message remains: hope.

If you are a parent faced with similar profound questions after the birth of your child, do not assume one doctor has all the answers. Search for doctors who respect your child enough to talk to her, not just about her. Above all, find an agency or a school that can help you give your child a chance to succeed. Early education for your child and support for yourself are crucial.

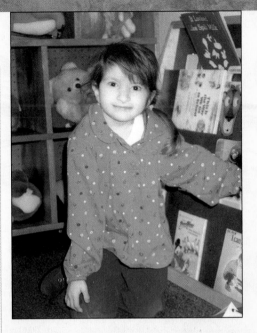

Figure 1 Ashley Naylor brought great joy to her family and community during her short life.
Courtesy of Kathy Naylor.

If you are a student in a health field, become as knowledgeable as possible and stay current with the latest research, but most importantly, be sensitive to those who seek your help. Each word you speak is taken to heart. Information is important, but hope can make all the difference in a family's future.

Kathy Naylor

---

genes. **Figure 13.16** shows three duplicated chromosome 15s, with increasing amounts of material repeated. Many people have the first two types of duplications and have no symptoms. However, several unrelated individuals with the third, larger duplication have seizures and mental retardation. A duplication elsewhere on chromosome 15 is associated with panic attacks and other anxiety disorders.

FISH can detect tiny deletions and duplications that are smaller than the bands of conventional chromosome staining. Small duplications are generally not dangerous, but some "microdeletions" are associated with a number of syndromes. Certain microdele-tions in the Y chromosome, for example, cause male infertility. Deletions and duplications can arise from chromosome rearrangements, which include translocations, inversions, and ring chromosomes.

Translocations

In a translocation, different (nonhomologous) chromosomes exchange or combine parts. Exposure to certain viruses, drugs, and radiation can cause translocations, but often they arise for no apparent reason.

There are two major types of translocations. In a **Robertsonian translocation,** the short arms of two different acrocentric chromosomes break, leaving sticky ends that cause the two long arms to join, forming a single, large chromosome with two long arms. The tiny short arms are lost, but their DNA sequences are repeated elsewhere in the genome, so their absence in a person with a Robertsonian translocation does not cause symptoms. The person with the large, translocated chromosome, called a **translocation carrier,** has 45 chromosomes, but may not have symptoms if no crucial genes have been deleted or damaged. Even so, he or she may produce unbalanced gametes—sperm or oocytes with too many or too few genes. This can lead to spontaneous abortion or birth defects.

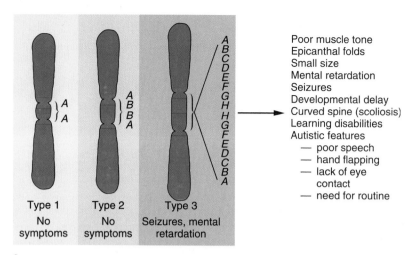

Type 1
No
symptoms

Type 2
No
symptoms

Type 3
Seizures, mental
retardation

A B C D E F G H H G F E D C B A

Poor muscle tone
Epicanthal folds
Small size
Mental retardation
Seizures
Developmental delay
Curved spine (scoliosis)
Learning disabilities
Autistic features
— poor speech
— hand flapping
— lack of eye
contact
— need for routine

a.

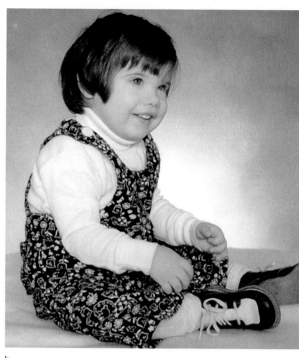

b.

Figure 13.16 **A duplication.** A study of duplications of parts of chromosome 15 revealed that small duplications do not affect the phenotype, but larger ones may. **(a)** The letters indicate specific DNA sequences, which serve as markers to compare chromosome regions. Note that the duplication is also inverted. **(b)** This child, who has "inv dup (15) syndrome," appears normal but has minor facial anomalies characteristic of the condition.

In 1 in 20 cases of Down syndrome, a parent has a Robertsonian translocation between chromosome 21 and another, usually chromosome 14. The individual with the translocation produces some gametes that lack either of the involved chromosomes and some gametes that have extra material from one of the translocated chromosomes (**figure 13.17**). In such a case, each fertilized ovum has a 1 in 2 chance of ending in spontaneous abortion, and a 1 in 6 chance of developing into an individual with Down syndrome. The risk of having a child with Down syndrome is theoretically 1 in 3, because the spontaneous abortions are not births. However, because some Down syndrome fetuses spontaneously abort, the actual risk of a couple in this situation having a child with Down syndrome is about 15 percent. The other two outcomes—a fetus with normal chromosomes or a translocation carrier like the parent—have normal phenotypes. Either a male or a female can be a translocation carrier, and the condition is not related to age. The second most common type of Robertsonian translocation occurs between chromosomes 13 and 14, causing symptoms of Patau syndrome because of an excess of chromosome 13 material.

Because Robertsonian translocations are among the more common chromosomal aberrations, an intriguing theory has arisen—they could one day lead to a human karyotype of 44 instead of 46 chromosomes, and perhaps even two types of people! Individuals who have one Robertsonian translocation have 45 chromosomes, and therefore may make gametes missing a chromosome, which impairs fertility. A person who has two different Robertsonian translocations would have 44 chromosomes, but the normal amount of genetic material. Two such people could have children together, the male producing sperm and the female producing oocytes with 22 chromosomes each. Robertsonian translocations affect one in 1,000 individuals. The chance of two people with different single translocations passing both to shared offspring is about 1 in 4 million—unlikely, yet possible.

In a **reciprocal translocation,** two different chromosomes exchange parts (**figure 13.18**). FISH can be used to highlight the involved chromosomes. If the chromosome exchange does not break any genes, then a person who has both translocated chromosomes is healthy and is also a translocation carrier. He or she has the normal amount of genetic material, but it is rearranged.

A reciprocal translocation carrier can have symptoms if one of the two breakpoints lies in a gene, disrupting its function. **Figure 13.19** shows a father and

son who have a reciprocal translocation between chromosomes 2 and 20 that causes Alagille syndrome. Apparently the exchange disrupts a gene on chromosome 20 that causes the condition, because families with the syndrome have deletions in this region of the chromosome. Alagille syndrome produces a characteristic face, absence of bile ducts in the liver, abnormalities of the eyes and ribs, heart defects, and severe itching. The symptoms are so variable that some people do not know they have it. The father in figure 13.19 did not realize he had the syndrome until he had a child with a more severe case. Sometimes, a *de novo* translocation arises in a gamete that leads to a new individual with a disorder, as opposed to inheriting a translocated chromosome from a parent.

A translocation carrier produces some unbalanced gametes—sperm or oocytes that have deletions or duplications of some of the genes in the translocated chromosomes. The resulting phenotype depends upon the particular genes that the chromosomal rearrangement disrupts and whether they are extra or missing.

Information from the human genome sequence and from other chromosomal abnormalities can explain how some translocations affect health. For example, a child was born with a reciprocal transloca-

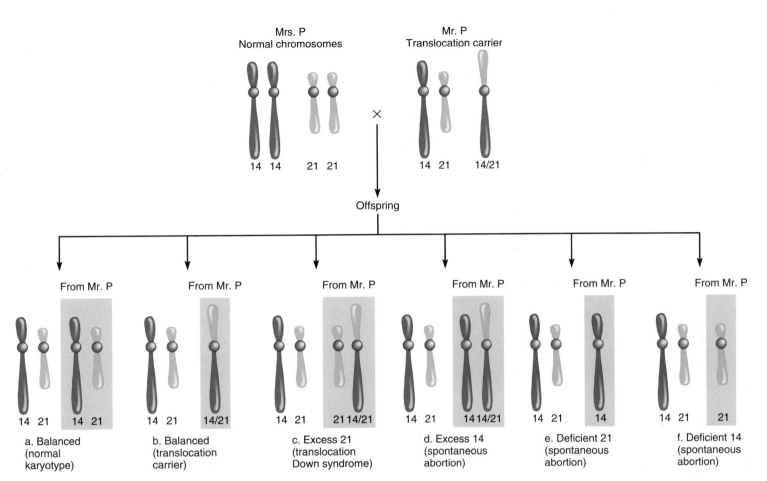

Figure 13.17 A Robertsonian translocation. Mr. P. has only 45 chromosomes because the long arm of one chromosome 14 has joined the long arm of one chromosome 21. He has no symptoms. Mr. P. makes six types of sperm cells, and they determine the fate of offspring. **(a)** A sperm with one normal chromosome 14 and one normal 21 yields a normal child. **(b)** A sperm carrying the translocated chromosome produces a child who is a translocation carrier, like Mr. P. **(c)** If a sperm contains Mr. P.'s normal 21 and his translocated chromosome, the child receives too much chromosome 21 material and has Down syndrome. **(d)** A sperm containing the translocated chromosome and a normal 14 leads to excess chromosomal 14 material, which is lethal in the embryo or fetus. If a sperm lacks either chromosome 21 **(e)** or 14 **(f)**, it leads to monosomies, which are lethal prenatally. (Chromosome arm lengths are not precisely accurate.)

tion between chromosomes 12 and 22. The distinctive symptoms of language delay, mild mental retardation, loose joints, minor facial anomalies, and a narrow, long head matched those of another chromosome problem, called 22q13.3 deletion syndrome. That condition is caused by absence of a gene (called *ProSAP2*) that forms scaffolds for neurons in the cerebral cortex and cerebellum. Apparently, the translocation cuts this gene, abolishing its function just as a deletion does. As a result, these parts of the brain malfunction.

A genetic counselor becomes alerted to the possibility of a translocation if a family has had multiple birth defects and spontaneous abortions. People with translocations have been very valuable to medical genetics

research. Studies to identify disease-causing genes often began with people whose translocations pointed the way toward a gene of interest.

Inversions

An inverted sequence of chromosome bands indicates that part of the chromosome has flipped around. Empirical studies show that 5 to 10 percent of inversions cause health problems, probably because they disrupt important genes. Sometimes inversions are detected in fetal chromosomes, but physicians do not know whether symptoms will be associated with the problem. The parents can have their chromosomes checked. If one of them has the inversion and is healthy,

then the child will most likely not have symptoms related to the inversion. If neither parent has the inversion, then the anomaly arose in a gamete, and effects may depend on which genes are involved.

Like a translocation carrier, an adult can be heterozygous for an inversion and be healthy, but have reproductive problems. One woman had an inversion in the long arm of chromosome 15 and had two spontaneous abortions, two stillbirths, and two children with multiple problems who died within days of birth. She did eventually give birth to a healthy child. How did the inversion cause these problems?

Inversions with such devastating effects can be traced to meiosis, when a crossover occurs between the inverted chromosome

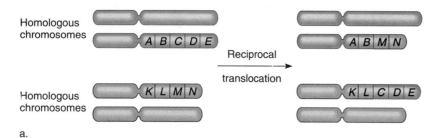

Homologous chromosomes

Homologous chromosomes

Reciprocal translocation

a.

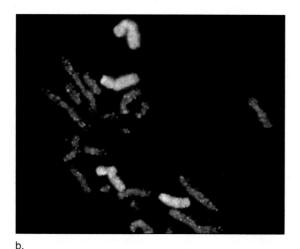

b.

Figure 13.18 A reciprocal translocation. In a reciprocal translocation, two nonhomologous chromosomes exchange parts. In **(a)**, genes *C, D,* and *E* on the blue chromosome exchange positions with genes *M* and *N* on the red chromosome. Part **(b)** highlights a reciprocal translocation using FISH. The pink chromosome with the dab of blue, and the blue chromosome with a small section of pink, are the translocated chromosomes.

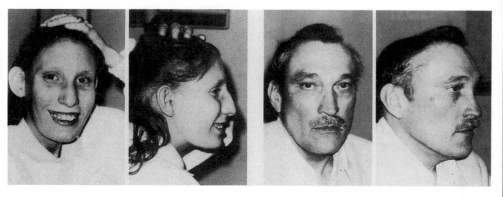

Figure 13.19 A translocation syndrome. In one family with Alagille syndrome, a reciprocal translocation occurs between chromosomes 2 and 20. Distinctive facial features are part of the condition.

segment and the noninverted homolog. To allow the genes to align, the inverted chromosome forms a loop. When crossovers occur within the loop, some areas are duplicated and some deleted in the resulting recombinant chromosomes. In inversions, the abnormal chromosomes result from the chromatids that crossed over.

Two types of inversions are distinguished by the position of the centromere relative to

the inverted section. A **paracentric inversion** does not include the centromere (**figure 13.20**). A single crossover within the inverted segment gives rise to two very abnormal chromosomes. The other two chromosomes are normal. One abnormal chromosome retains both centromeres and is **dicentric.** When the cell divides, the two centromeres are pulled to opposite sides of the cell, and the chromosome breaks, leav-

ing pieces with extra or missing segments. The second type of abnormal chromosome resulting from a crossover within an inversion loop is a small piece that lacks a centromere, called an acentric fragment. When the cell divides, the fragment is lost.

A **pericentric inversion** includes the centromere within the loop. A crossover in it produces two chromosomes that have duplications and deletions, but one centromere each (**figure 13.21**).

Isochromosomes and Ring Chromosomes

Another meiotic error that leads to unbalanced genetic material is the formation of an **isochromosome,** which is a chromosome that has identical arms. This occurs when, during division, the centromeres part in the wrong plane (**figure 13.22**). Isochromosomes are known for chromosomes 12 and 21 and for the long arms of the X and the Y. Some women with Turner syndrome do not have the more common monosomy XO, but an isochromosome in which the long arm of the X chromosome is duplicated but the short arm is absent.

Chromosomes shaped like rings form in 1 out of 25,000 conceptions. Ring chromosomes may arise when telomeres are lost, leaving sticky ends that adhere. Exposure to radiation can form rings. They can involve any chromosome, and may occur in addition to a full diploid chromosome set, or account for 1 of the 46 chromosomes.

Ring chromosomes can produce symptoms when they add genetic material. For example, a small ring chromosome of DNA from chromosome 22 causes cat eye syndrome. Affected children have vertical pupils, are mentally retarded, have heart and urinary tract anomalies, and have skin growing over the anus. They have 47 chromosomes—the normal two chromosome 22s and a ring. A syndrome resulting from one normal chromosome and one other homolog that is a ring is marked by mental delay, poor coordination, muscle weakness, and speech problems. The severity reflects the amount of DNA missing from the ring chromosome.

A study from Japan examined fifteen women who have a ring X chromosome in some cells, in addition to the other two complete X chromosomes. Nine of the women

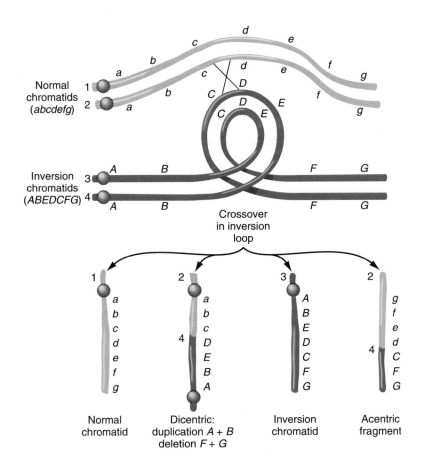

Figure 13.20 Paracentric inversion.
A crossover between a chromosome with a paracentric inversion and its normal homolog, when in the region of the inversion, produces one normal chromatid, one inverted chromatid, one with two centromeres (dicentric), and one with no centromere (an acentric fragment). The letters *a* through *g* denote genes. (These chromosomes are depicted as less condensed than those in other figures to ease following the crossovers.)

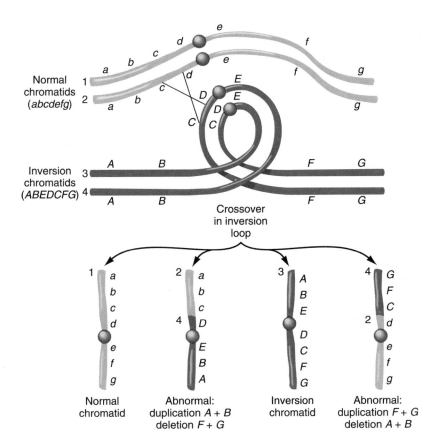

Figure 13.21 Pericentric inversion.
A pericentric inversion in one chromosome leads to two chromatids with duplications and deletions, one normal chromatid, and one inverted chromatid that arises if a crossover occurs.

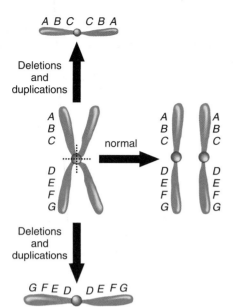

A B C   C B A

Deletions and duplications

A B C   normal   A B C   A B C
D E F G   D E F G   D E F G

Deletions and duplications

G F E D   D E F G

Figure 13.22 Isochromosomes have identical arms. They form when chromatids divide along the wrong plane (in this depiction, horizontally rather than vertically).

Table 13.8

Causes of Chromosomal Aberrations

	Causes
Numerical Abnormalities	
Polyploidy	Error in cell division (meiosis or mitosis) in which not all chromatid pairs separate in anaphase Multiple fertilization
Aneuploidy	Nondisjunction (in meiosis or mitosis) leading to lost or extra chromosomes
Structural Abnormalities	
Deletions and duplications	Translocation Crossover between a chromosome that has a pericentric inversion and its noninverted homolog
Translocation	Exchange between nonhomologous chromosomes
Inversion	Breakage and reunion of fragment in same chromosome, but with wrong orientation
Dicentric and acentric	Crossover between a chromosome with a paracentric inversion and its noninverted homolog
Ring chromosome	A chromosome loses telomeres and the ends fuse, forming a circle

were mentally retarded, and in all of them, the ring X chromosome did not include the *XIST* site. Recall from chapter 6 that *XIST* normally shuts off all but one X chromosome. In these nine women, too much expressed X chromosome material caused the mental retardation. In the other six women, the ring chromosome clearly included *XIST,* and so presumably was silenced.

In a very unusual case, identical twin girls each inherited two ring chromosomes. FISH analysis revealed that about two-thirds of the examined cells from both girls had one ring derived from chromosome 1 and one from chromosome 16. The remainder of the cells had either one ring or neither. Double rings had only been reported once previously—and never for twins. The twins' extra genetic material caused them many medical woes. The girls were hospitalized as newborns for several months for a variety of problems, and at 2 years of age, each still required supplemental oxygen, was developmentally delayed, had an undersized head, and was small. The girls' symptoms and distinctive faces led physicians to call in cytogeneticists. They identified the ring chromosomes and deduced that the twins arose from a single fertilized egg that developed the rings at the 2- or 4-

cell stage, then split to yield two individuals that have the rings in most of their cells. In other cases, ring chromosomes detected on routine amniocentesis present a challenging problem in genetic counseling, because rings usually do not affect health—often, they consist of highly repeated DNA sequences that do not encode proteins.

Table 13.8 summarizes the causes of different types of chromosomal aberrations.

Key Concepts

Chromosome rearrangements can cause deletions and duplications. In a Robertsonian translocation, the long arms of two different acrocentric chromosomes join to form one large chromosome. In a reciprocal translocation, two chromosomes exchange parts. If a translocation leads to a deletion or duplication, or disrupts a gene, symptoms may result. Gene duplications and deletions can occur in isochromosomes and ring chromosomes, and when crossovers involve inversions. An isochromosome has two identical arms, thereby introducing duplications and deletions, and ring chromosomes can add genetic material.

13.5 Uniparental Disomy—Two Genetic Contributions from One Parent

If nondisjunction occurs in both of the gametes that join to become a fertilized ovum, a pair of homologs (or parts of them) can come solely from one parent, rather than one from each parent, as Mendel's law of segregation predicts. For example, if a sperm lacking a chromosome 14 fertilizes an ovum with two copies of that chromosome, it produces an individual with the normal 46 chromosomes, but one homologous pair that comes only from the female. This very rare situation of inheriting two chromosomes or two segments of chromosomes from one parent is called **uniparental disomy** (UPD). It means "two bodies from one parent," with "bodies" referring to chromosomes. The alternative state—normal segregation of chromosome pairs—is termed biparental inheritance. UPD can also arise from a trisomic embryo in which some cells lose the extra chromosome, restoring diploidy, but leaving two chromosomes from one parent.

Because UPD requires the simultaneous occurrence of two very rare events—either nondisjunction of the same chromosome in gametes that join, or trisomy followed by chromosome loss—it is exceedingly rare. In addition, many cases are probably never seen, because bringing together identical homologs inherited from one parent could give the fertilized ovum a homozygous set of lethal alleles. Development would halt. Other cases of UPD may go undetected if they cause known recessive conditions and both parents are assumed to be carriers, when actually only one parent contributed to the offspring's illness. This was how UPD was discovered.

In 1988, Arthur Beaudet of the Baylor College of Medicine saw a very unusual patient with cystic fibrosis. Beaudet was comparing CF alleles in the patient to those in her parents, and he found that only the mother was a carrier—the father had two normal alleles. Didn't both parents have to be carriers for a child to inherit this autosomal recessive disorder? Beaudet did further testing and constructed haplotypes for each parent's chromosome 7, which includes the CF gene. He found that the daughter had two copies from her mother, and none from her father (**figure 13.23**). How did this happen?

Apparently, in the patient's mother, nondisjunction of chromosome 7 in meiosis II led to formation of an oocyte bearing two identical copies of the chromosome, instead of the usual one. A sperm that had also undergone nondisjunction and lacked a chromosome 7 then fertilized the abnormal oocyte. The mother's extra genetic material compensated for the father's deficit, and an offspring developed. Unfortunately, she inherited a double dose of the mother's chromosome that carried the mutant CF allele. In effect, inheriting two of the same chromosome from one parent shatters the protection that

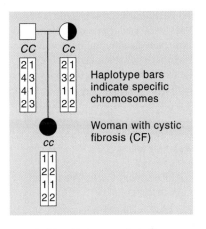

Figure 13.23 Uniparental disomy.
Uniparental disomy doubles part of one parent's genetic contribution. According to the law of segregation, a child with cystic fibrosis (CF) cannot be born to a person who is homozygous dominant for the wild type allele. But it can happen. In this family, the woman with CF inherited two copies of her mother's chromosome 7, and neither of her father's. Unfortunately, it was the chromosome with the disease-causing allele that she inherited in a double dose.

combining genetic material from two individuals offers, a protection that is the defining characteristic of sexual reproduction.

UPD may also cause disease if it removes the contribution of the important parent for an imprinted gene. Recall from chapter 6 that an imprinted gene is expressed if it comes from one parent, but silenced if it comes from the other (see figure 6.15). If UPD removes the parental genetic material that must be present for a critical gene to be expressed, a mutant phenotype results. The classic example is the 20 to 30 percent of Prader-Willi syndrome and Angelman syndrome cases caused by UPD (see figure

6.16). These disorders arise from mutations in different genes that are closely linked in a region of the long arm of chromosome 15, where imprinting occurs. They both cause mental retardation and a variety of other symptoms, but are quite distinct.

In 1989, researchers found that some children with Prader-Willi syndrome have two parts of the long arm of chromosome 15 from their mothers. The disease results because the father's Prader-Willi gene must be expressed for the child to avoid the associated illness. For Angelman syndrome, the situation is reversed. Children have a double dose of their father's DNA in the same chromosomal region implicated in Prader-Willi syndrome, with no maternal contribution. The mother's gene must be present for health.

People usually learn their chromosomal makeup only when something goes wrong—when they have a family history of reproductive problems, exposure to a toxin, cancer, or symptoms of a known chromosomal disorder. While researchers analyze the human genome sequence, chromosome studies will continue to be part of medical care—beginning before birth.

Key Concepts

Uniparental disomy (UPD) results when two chromosomes or chromosome parts are inherited from the same parent. It can arise from a trisomy and subsequent chromosome loss, or from two nondisjunction events. Uniparental disomy can cause disease if it creates a homozygous recessive condition, or if it disrupts imprinting.

Summary

13.1 Portrait of a Chromosome

1. Mutation can occur at the chromosomal level. **Cytogenetics** is the study of chromosome aberrations and their effects on phenotypes.

2. **Heterochromatin** stains darkly and harbors many DNA repeats. **Euchromatin** is light staining and contains many protein-encoding genes.

3. A chromosome consists of DNA and proteins. Essential parts are the

telomeres, centromeres, and origin of replication sites.

4. Centromeres include **alpha satellites** and **centromere-associated proteins,** some of which form **kinetochores** that contact spindle fibers. CENP-A is a protein that may control centromere duplication.

5. **Subtelomeres** have telomerelike repeats that gradually disappear, as some protein-encoding genes occur. Chromosomes vary in gene density.

6. Chromosomes are distinguishable by size, centromere position, satellites, DNA probes to specific sequences, and staining patterns.

7. A **karyotype** is a size-ordered chromosome chart. A **metacentric** chromosome has two fairly equal arms. A **submetacentric** chromosome has a large arm designated q and a short arm designated p. An **acrocentric** chromosome's centromere is near a tip, so that it has one long arm and one very short arm.

13.2 Visualizing Chromosomes

8. Chromosomes can be obtained from any cell that has a nucleus. Prenatal diagnostic techniques that obtain fetal chromosomes include **amniocentesis, chorionic villus sampling,** and **fetal cell sorting.**

9. Hand-cut karyotypes and stains to view chromosomes are giving way to computerized karyotyping and chromosome-specific **fluorescence *in situ* hybridization (FISH). Ideograms** are diagrams that display chromosome bands, FISH data, and gene loci.

10. Chromosomal shorthand indicates chromosome number, sex chromosome constitution, and the nature of the specific chromosomal abnormality.

13.3 Abnormal Chromosome Number

11. A **euploid** somatic human cell has 22 pairs of autosomes and one pair of sex chromosomes.

12. **Polyploid** cells have extra chromosome sets.

13. **Aneuploids** have extra or missing chromosomes. **Trisomies** (an extra chromosome) are less harmful than **monosomies** (lack of a chromosome), and

sex chromosome aneuploidy is less severe than autosomal aneuploidy. **Nondisjunction** is uneven distribution of chromosomes in meiosis. It causes aneuploidy. Most autosomal aneuploids cease developing as embryos. The most common at birth are trisomies 21, 13, and 18, because these chromosomes are gene-poor. Sex chromosome anomalies (XXY; 45, X; XXX; XYY) are less severe.

13.4 Abnormal Chromosome Structure

14. Deletions and/or duplications can result from crossing over after pairing errors occur in synapsis. Crossing over in an inversion heterozygote can also generate deletions and duplications.

15. In a **Robertsonian translocation,** the short arms of two acrocentric chromosomes break, leaving sticky ends on the long arms that join to form an unusual, large chromosome.

16. In a **reciprocal translocation,** two nonhomologous chromosomes exchange parts. In both types of translocation, a **translocation carrier** may have an associated phenotype if the translocation disrupts a vital gene. A translocation carrier also produces a predictable percentage of

unbalanced gametes, which can lead to birth defects and spontaneous abortions.

17. A heterozygote for an **inversion** may have reproductive problems if a crossover occurs between the inverted region and the noninverted homolog, generating deletions and duplications. A **paracentric inversion** does not include the centromere; a **pericentric inversion** does.

18. **Isochromosomes** repeat one chromosome arm but delete the other. They form when the centromere divides in the wrong plane during meiosis. Ring chromosomes form when telomeres are removed, leaving sticky ends that then adhere.

13.5 Uniparental Disomy—Two Genetic Contributions from One Parent

19. In **uniparental disomy,** a chromosome, or a part of one, doubly represents one parent. It can result from nondisjunction in both gametes, or from a trisomic cell that loses a chromosome.

20. Uniparental disomy causes symptoms if it creates a homozygous recessive state associated with an illness, or if it affects an imprinted gene.

Review Questions

1. What are the essential components of a chromosome? of a centromere?

2. How does the DNA sequence change with distance from the telomere?

3. How are centromeres and telomeres alike?

4. What happens during meiosis to produce each of the following?
   a. an aneuploid
   b. a polyploid
   c. the increased risk of trisomy 21 Down syndrome in the offspring of a woman over age 40 at the time of conception
   d. recurrent spontaneous abortions to a couple in which the man has a pericentric inversion
   e. several children with Down syndrome in a family where one parent is a translocation carrier

5. A human liver has patches of cells that are octaploid—that is, they have eight sets of chromosomes. Explain how this might arise.

6. Describe an individual with each of the following chromosome constitutions. Mention the person's sex and possible phenotype.
   a. 47,XXX
   b. 45,X
   c. 47,XX, trisomy 21

7. Which chromosomal anomaly might you expect to find more frequently among the members of the National Basketball Association than in the general population? Cite a reason for your answer.

8. List three examples illustrating the idea that the amount of genetic material involved in a chromosomal aberration affects the severity of the associated phenotype.

9. List three types of chromosomal aberrations that can cause duplications and/or deletions, and explain how they do so.

10. Why would having the same inversion on both members of a homologous chromosome pair *not* lead to unbalanced

gametes, as having the inversion on only one chromosome would?

11. Define or describe the following technologies:
   a. high-resolution chromosome banding
   b. FISH
   c. amniocentesis
   d. chorionic villus sampling
   e. fetal cell sorting
   f. maternal serum markers
   g. quantitative PCR
   h. human artificial chromosomes

12. What is the evidence that trisomies 13 and 18 are lethal primarily before birth? Why are they more common than trisomies 5 or 16?

13. How many chromosomes would a person have who has Klinefelter syndrome and also trisomy 21?

14. Explain why a female cannot have Klinefelter syndrome and a male cannot have Turner syndrome.

15. List three causes of Turner syndrome.

Applied Questions

1. The following is part of a chart used to provide genetic counseling on maternal age effect on fetal chromosomes. Answer questions a–e based on this chart.

Maternal Age	Trisomy 21 Risk	Risk for Any Aneuploid
20	1/1,667	1/526
24	1/1,250	1/476
28	1/1,053	1/435
30	1/952	1/385
32	1/769	1/322
35	1/378	1/192
36	1/289	1/156
37	1/224	1/127
38	1/173	1/102
40	1/106	1/66
45	1/30	1/21
48	1/14	1/10

a. If the risk that amniocentesis will cause spontaneous abortion is 1 in 250 at a particular obstetrical practice, at what age should patients in this practice undergo the test?

b. The Willoughbys have a son who has trisomy 21 Down syndrome. The mother, Suzanne, is 24 years old and pregnant. The Martinis do not have any relatives who have Down syndrome or any other chromosomal condition. Karen Martini is pregnant, and is 32 years old. Who has the lower risk of having a child with Down syndrome, Suzanne Willoughby or Karen Martini?

c. Why are the risks in the righthand column higher than those in the middle column?

d. Sam and Alice Dekalb receive genetic counseling because of "advanced maternal age"—Alice is 40 years old. When amniocentesis reveals trisomy 13, the couple is shocked, explaining that they thought the risk of a chromosomal problem was less than 1 percent. How have they misinterpreted the statistics?

e. A 40-year-old woman wants to have children, but would like to postpone becoming pregnant until she is 45. How much will her risk of conceiving a child with trisomy 21 increase in that time?

2. Amniocentesis indicates that a fetus has the chromosomal constitution 46, XX,del(5)(p15). What does this mean? What might the child's phenotype be?

3. What type of test would you use to determine whether a triploid infant resulted from a diploid oocyte fertilized by a haploid sperm, or from two sperm fertilizing one oocyte?

4. For an exercise in a college genetics laboratory course, a healthy student constructs a karyotype from a cell in a drop of her blood. She finds only one chromosome 3 and one chromosome 21, plus two unusual chromosomes that do not seem to have matching partners.

   a. What type of chromosomal abnormality does she have?

   b. Why doesn't she have any symptoms?

   c. Would you expect any of her relatives to have any particular medical problems? If so, which medical conditions?

5. A fetus ceases developing in the uterus. Several of its cells are karyotyped. Approximately 75 percent of the cells are diploid, and 25 percent are tetraploid (containing four copies of each chromosome). What do you think happened? When in development did it probably occur?

6. Distinguish among Down syndrome caused by aneuploidy, mosaicism, and translocation.

7. A couple has a son diagnosed with Klinefelter syndrome. Explain how the son's chromosome constitution could have arisen from either parent.

8. DiGeorge syndrome causes abnormal parathyroid glands, disrupting blood calcium levels; heart defects; and an underdeveloped thymus gland, impairing development of the immune system. About 85 percent of patients have a microdeletion of a particular area of chromosome 22. In one family, a girl, her mother, and a maternal aunt have very mild cases of DiGeorge syndrome, and they also all have a reciprocal translocation involving chromosomes 22 and 2.

   a. How can a microdeletion and a translocation cause the same set of symptoms?

   b. Why were the cases of people with the translocation less severe than those of people with the microdeletion?

   c. What other problems might arise in the family with the translocation?

9. Refer to this list of all of the human chromosomes, the number of protein-encoding genes on each, and the number of bases to answer these questions:

Chromosome	Number of Genes	Number of Bases
Chromosome 1	2,968	279 million bases
Chromosome 2	2,288	251 million bases
Chromosome 3	2,032	221 million bases
Chromosome 4	1,297	197 million bases
Chromosome 5	1,643	198 million bases
Chromosome 6	1,963	176 million bases
Chromosome 7	1,443	163 million bases
Chromosome 8	1,127	148 million bases
Chromosome 9	1,299	140 million bases
Chromosome 10	1,440	143 million bases
Chromosome 11	2,093	148 million bases
Chromosome 12	1,652	142 million bases
Chromosome 13	748	118 million bases
Chromosome 14	1,098	107 million bases
Chromosome 15	1,122	100 million bases
Chromosome 16	1,098	104 million bases
Chromosome 17	1,576	88 million bases
Chromosome 18	766	86 million bases
Chromosome 19	1,454	72 million bases
Chromosome 20	927	66 million bases
Chromosome 21	303	45 million bases
Chromosome 22	288	48 million bases
Chromosome X	1,184	163 million bases
Chromosome Y	231	51 million bases

   a. Which two chromosomes are out of order, and why?

   b. Which chromosome has the greatest proportion of its DNA sequence that encodes protein?

   c. Which chromosome has the greatest proportion of noncoding sequence?

   d. How much larger is the largest chromosome compared to the smallest?

Web Activities

10. Go to http://gslc.genetics.utah.edu/units/disorders/karyotype/karyotype.cfm, the Genetic Science Learning Center at the Eccles Institute of Human Genetics at the University of Utah. Follow the instructions to create a karyotype.

11. Go to the Human Genome Landmarks poster at www.ornl.gov/hgmis/posters/chromosome, the source of figure 13.3. Select a chromosome, and use Online Mendelian Inheritance in Man (OMIM) to describe four traits or disorders associated with it. Or, consult www.ornl.gov/hgmis/launchpad for information on four genes carried on a specific chromosome.

Case Studies

12. The medical literature includes 18 cases of children with a syndrome consisting of poor growth before birth, developmental delay, premature puberty, loose joints, a large head, short stature, and small hands. In a different syndrome, children have a small chest, ears, and facial features as well as rib and finger defects. Children with the first condition have both copies of the entire long arm of chromosome 14 from their mothers, whereas children with the second condition inherit the same chromosome part from their fathers.

   a. What type of chromosomal aberration is responsible for these two disorders?

   b. Describe how each of the conditions might arise.

   c. Describe how these conditions might result from a deletion mutation.

13. Two sets of parents who have children with Down syndrome meet at a clinic. The Phelps know that their son has trisomy 21. The Watkins have two affected children, and Mrs. Watkins has had two spontaneous abortions. Why should the Watkins be more concerned about future reproductive problems than the Phelps? How are the offspring of the two families different, even though they have the same symptoms?

Learn to apply the skills of a genetic counselor with additional cases found in the *Case Workbook in Human Genetics.*

DiGeorge syndrome
Down syndrome
Tetrasomy 12p
Turner syndrome
Williams syndrome

Suggested Readings

Dobson, Roger. January 18, 2003. Painting is earliest example of portrayal of Down syndrome. *The British Medical Journal* 326:126. An artist's depiction of people with Down syndrome, from 1515, suggests that they were not regarded as different from other people.

Lewis, Ricki. June 12, 2000. Chromosome 21 reveals sparse gene content. *The Scientist* 14(12):1. When it comes to chromosomes, size doesn't matter—gene content and density do.

Lewis, Ricki. October 15, 2001. Mapping subtelomeres. *The Scientist* 15(20):12. The regions next to telomeres are more than just buffers.

Lewis, Ricki. November 25, 2002. Toward 2N–44. *The Scientist* 16(23):8. Could Robertsonian translocations one day divide our species?

Lewis, Ricki. July 28, 2003. Y envy. *The Scientist* 17(15):64. A lighthearted look at the Y chromosome.

Lewis, Ricki. October 20, 2003. Genetic testing timeline. *The Scientist* 17(20):23. Depictions of the chromosomes that bear genes for four familiar diseases.

Mennuti, Michael T. and Deborah A. Driscoll. October 9, 2003. Screening for Down's syndrome—too many choices? *The New England Journal of Medicine* 349(15):1471–72. Maternal serum screening is not as informative as amniocentesis or CVS, but it is safer.

Ranke, Michael R., and Paul Saenger. July 28, 2001. Turner's syndrome. *The Lancet* 358:309–14. Having an XO chromosome constitution raises the risk of some more common disorders.

Willard, Huntington F. May 8, 2001. Neocentromeres and human artificial chromosomes: An unnatural act. *Proceedings of the National Academy of Sciences* 98:5374–76. The human genome harbors several dozen potential centromeric sequences.

Weekly updates of current news related to human genetics are available through Power Web on your Online Learning Center.

VISIT YOUR ONLINE LEARNING CENTER

Visit your online learning center for additional resources and tools to help you master this chapter. See us at

www.mhhe.com/lewisgenetics6.

CHAPTER

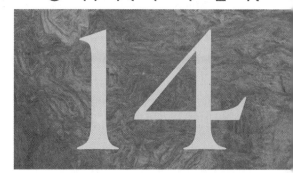

When Allele Frequencies Stay Constant

14

CHAPTER CONTENTS

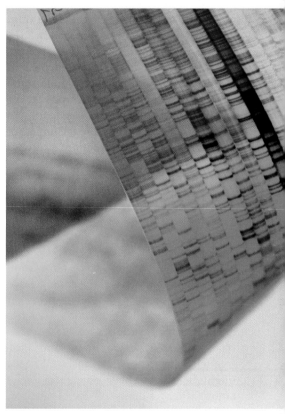

Rows of bands reveal identities, courtesy of DNA profiling techniques.

So far, we've considered the gene as a "character" that transmits traits, and as a biochemical blueprint for building a specific protein. Genes can also be considered at the population level.

A **population** is any group of members of the same species in a given geographical area. Human populations might include the students in a class, a stadium full of people, or the residents of a community, state, or nation. **Population genetics** is a branch of genetics that considers all the alleles in a population, which constitute the **gene pool.** The "pool" in gene pool refers to a collection of gametes. An offspring can be considered as a sample of two gametes taken from the pool. Alleles can move between populations when individuals migrate and mate. This movement, termed **gene flow,** underlies evolution. At the population level, genetics reflects history, anthropology, human behavior, and sociology, enabling us to trace our beginnings and to understand our diversity. This chapter introduces the major principle of population genetics, and the next two chapters explore the impact of population genetics on evolution.

14.1 The Importance of Knowing Allele Frequencies

Thinking about genes at the population level begins by considering frequencies—that is, how often a particular gene variant occurs in a particular population. Such frequencies can be calculated for alleles, genotypes, or phenotypes. For example, an allele frequency for the cystic fibrosis (CF) gene might be the number of $\Delta F508$ alleles among the residents of San Francisco. $\Delta F508$ is the most common allele that, when homozygous, causes the disorder. The allele frequency derives from the two $\Delta F508$ alleles in each person with CF, plus those carried in heterozygotes, as a proportion of all alleles for that gene in the gene pool. The genotype frequencies are the proportions of heterozygotes and the two types of homozygotes in the population. Finally, a phenotypic frequency is simply the percentage of people in the population who have CF (or who do not). With multiple alleles for a single gene, the situation becomes more complex.

Phenotypic frequencies are determined empirically—that is, by observing how common a condition or trait is in a population. These figures have value in genetic counseling in estimating the risk that a particular inherited disorder will occur in an individual when there is no family history of the illness. **Table 14.1** shows disease incidence for phenylketonuria (PKU), an inborn error of metabolism that causes mental retardation unless the person follows a special low-protein diet from birth. Note how the frequency differs in different populations.

On a broader level, shifting allele frequencies in populations reflect the small steps of genetic change, called **microevolution,** that collectively constitute evolution. Allele frequencies can change when any of the following conditions are met:

1. Individuals of one genotype are more likely to produce offspring with each other than with those of other genotypes (*nonrandom mating*).

2. Individuals *migrate* between populations.

3. Reproductively isolated small groups form within or separate from a larger population (*genetic drift*).

4. *Mutation* introduces new alleles into a population.

5. People with a particular genotype are more likely to be able to produce viable, fertile offspring under a specific environmental condition than individuals with other genotypes (*natural selection*).

Table 14.1
Frequency of PKU in Various Populations

Population	Frequency of PKU
Chinese	1/16,000
Irish, Scottish, Yemenite Jews	1/5,000
Japanese	1/119,000
Swedes	1/30,000
Turks	1/2,600
United States Caucasians	1/10,000

Because these conditions are operating more often than not, genetic equilibrium—when allele frequencies are *not* changing—is rare. Thus, microevolution is not only possible, but also nearly unavoidable. Chapter 15 considers these factors in this order, in depth.

When enough microevolutionary changes accumulate to keep two fertile organisms of opposite sex from successfully producing fertile offspring together, **macroevolution,** or the formation of a new species, has occurred. In contrast, this chapter discusses the interesting, but unusual, situation in which allele frequencies stay constant, a condition called **Hardy-Weinberg equilibrium.**

Key Concepts

Population genetics is the study of allele frequencies in groups of organisms of the same species in the same geographic area. The genes in a population comprise its gene pool. Microevolution reflects changes in allele frequencies in populations. It is not occurring if allele frequencies stay constant from generation to generation (called Hardy-Weinberg equilibrium). This happens only if mating is random and the population is large, with no migration, genetic drift, mutation, or natural selection.

14.2 When Allele Frequencies Stay Constant

Gregor Mendel worked with phenotypes, and inferred the genotypes, in crosses of individual plants. Population genetics also looks at phenotypes and genotypes, but among large numbers of individuals. Here, allele frequencies reveal the underlying rules. Considering the alleles in a population—the gene pool—is more precise than assessing phenotypes, because the same phenotype can result from different genotypes. (Recall Mendel's *TT* and *Tt* tall plants.)

Hardy-Weinberg Equilibrium

In 1908, a Cambridge University mathematician named Godfrey Harold Hardy (1877–1947) and Wilhelm Weinberg

(1862–1937), a German physician interested in genetics, independently used algebra to explain how allele frequencies can be used to predict phenotypic and genotypic frequencies in populations of diploid, sexually reproducing organisms.

Hardy unintentionally cofounded the field of population genetics with a simple letter published in the journal *Science*—he did not consider his idea to be worthy of the more prestigious British journal *Nature*. The letter began with a curious mix of modesty and condescension:

I am reluctant to intrude in a discussion concerning matters of which I have no expert knowledge, and I should have expected the very simple point which I wish to make to have been familiar to biologists.

Hardy continued to explain how mathematically inept biologists had deduced from Mendel's work that dominant traits would increase in populations, while recessive traits would become rarer. This seems to make sense, but is actually untrue, because recessive alleles are introduced by mutation or migration and maintained in heterozygotes. Hardy and Weinberg disproved the assumption that dominant traits increase while recessive traits decrease using the language of algebra.

The expression of population genetics in algebraic terms begins with the simple equation

$$p + q = 1.0$$

where p represents all dominant alleles for a gene, and q represents all recessive alleles. The expression "$p + q = 1.0$" simply means that all the dominant alleles and all the recessive alleles comprise all the alleles for that gene in a population.

Next, Hardy and Weinberg described the possible genotypes for a gene with two alleles using the binomial expansion

$$p^2 + 2pq + q^2 = 1.0$$

In this equation, p^2 represents homozygous dominant individuals, q^2 represents homozygous recessive individuals, and $2pq$ represents heterozygotes (**table 14.2**). The letter p designates the frequency of a dominant allele, and q is the frequency of a recessive allele. **Figure 14.1** shows how the binomial expansion is derived from allele frequencies. Note

Table 14.2

The Hardy-Weinberg Equation

Algebraic Expression	What It Means
$p + q = 1.0$ (allele frequencies)	All dominant alleles plus all recessive alleles add up to all alleles for a particular gene in a population.
$p^2 + 2pq + q^2 = 1.0$ (genotype frequencies)	For a particular gene with 2 alleles, all homozygous dominant individuals (p^2) plus all heterozygotes ($2pq$) plus all homozygous recessives (q^2) add up to all of the individuals in the population.

that the derivation is conceptually the same as tracing alleles in a monohybrid cross.

The binomial expansion used to describe genes in populations became known as the Hardy-Weinberg equation. It can reveal the allele frequency changes that underlie evolution. If the proportion of genotypes remains the same from generation to generation, as the equation indicates, then that gene is not evolving (changing). This situation, Hardy-Weinberg equilibrium, is an idealized state. It is possible only if the population is large, if its members mate at random, and if no migration, genetic drift, mutation, or natural selection takes place.

Hardy-Weinberg equilibrium is rare for protein-encoding genes that affect the phenotype, because an organism's appearance and health affect its ability to reproduce. That is, genes that affect the phenotype are subject to natural selection—allele combinations that harm the individual are weeded out of the population. However, Hardy-Weinberg equilibrium is seen in repeats and other DNA sequences that do not affect the phenotype, and therefore are not subject to natural selection.

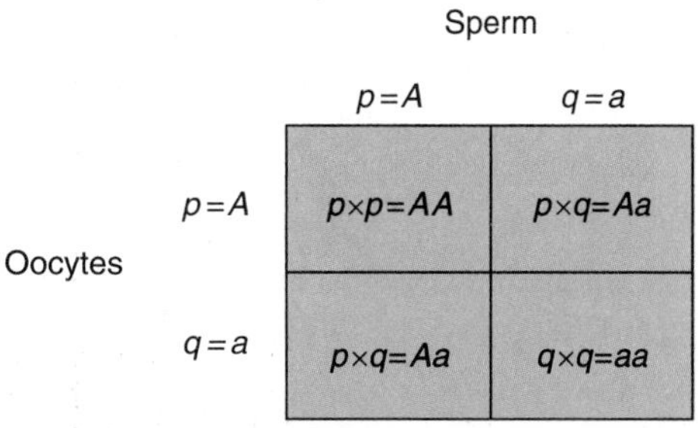

Figure 14.1 Source of the Hardy-Weinberg equation. A variation on a Punnett square reveals how random mating in a population in which gene A has two alleles—A and a—generates genotypes aa, AA, and Aa, in the relationship $p^2 + 2pq + q^2$.

Solving a Problem: The Hardy-Weinberg Equation

We can follow the frequency of two alleles of a particular gene from one generation to the next to understand Hardy-Weinberg equilibrium. Mendel's laws underlie such population genetics calculations.

Consider an autosomal recessive trait: a middle finger shorter than the second and fourth fingers. If we know the frequencies of the dominant and recessive alleles, then we can calculate the frequencies of the genotypes and phenotypes and trace the trait through the next generation. The dominant allele D confers normal-length fingers; the recessive allele d confers a short middle finger (**figure 14.2**). We can figure out the frequencies of the dominant and recessive alleles by observing the frequency of homozygous recessives, because this phenotype reflects only one genotype. If 9 out of 100 individuals in a population have short fingers—genotype dd—the frequency is 9/100 or 0.09. Since dd equals q^2, then q equals 0.3. Since $p + q = 1.0$, knowing that q is 0.3 means that p is 0.7.

Next, calculate the proportions of the three genotypes that arise when gametes combine at random:

homozygous dominant $= DD$
$= 0.7 \times 0.7 = 0.49$
$= 49$ percent of individuals in generation 1
homozygous recessive $= dd$
$= 0.3 \times 0.3 = 0.09$
$= 9$ percent of individuals in generation 1
heterozygous $= Dd + dD$
$= 2pq = (0.3)(0.7) + (0.3)(0.7) = 0.42$
$= 42$ percent of individuals in generation 1

The proportion of homozygous individuals is calculated simply by multiplying the allele frequency for the recessive or dominant allele by itself. The heterozygous calculation is $2pq$ because there are two ways of combining a D with a d gamete—a D sperm with a d egg, and a d sperm with a D egg.

In this population, 9 percent of the individuals have a short middle finger. Now jump ahead a few generations, and assume that people choose mates irrespective of finger length. This means that each genotype of a female (DD, Dd, or dd) is equally likely to mate with each of the three types of males (DD, Dd, or dd), and vice versa. **Table 14.3** multiplies the genotype frequencies for each possible mating, which leads to offspring in the familiar proportions of 49 percent DD, 42 percent Dd, and 9 percent dd. This gene, therefore, is in Hardy-Weinberg equilibrium—the allele and genotype frequencies do not change from one generation to the next.

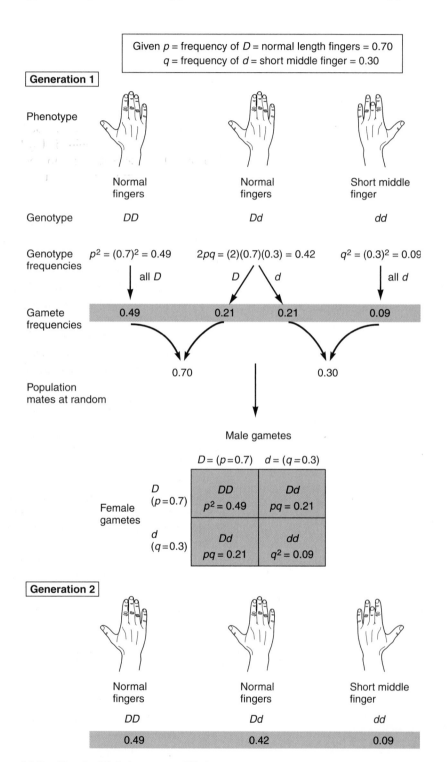

Figure 14.2 Hardy-Weinberg equilibrium. In Hardy-Weinberg equilibrium, allele frequencies remain constant from one generation to the next.

Key Concepts

For any two alleles of a gene in a population, the proportion of homozygous dominants equals the square of the frequency of the dominant allele (p^2), and the proportion of homozygous recessives equals the square of the frequency of the recessive allele (q^2). The proportion of heterozygotes equals $2pq$. If we know the genotype proportions in a population, we can calculate allele frequencies. The frequency of the recessive allele equals the proportion of homozygous recessives plus one-half that of carriers, and the frequency of the dominant allele equals the proportion of homozygous dominants plus that of one-half the carriers. In Hardy-Weinberg equilibrium, allele frequencies do not change from one generation to the next.

14.3 Practical Applications of Hardy-Weinberg Equilibrium

The Hardy-Weinberg equation is applied to population statistics on genetic disease incidence to derive carrier risks. To determine allele frequencies for autosomal recessively inherited characteristics, we need to know the frequency of one genotype in the population. This is typically the homozygous recessive class, for the same reason that this group is used to do a test cross when tracing inheritance of a single trait—its phenotype indicates its genotype.

The known incidence of an autosomal recessive disorder can be used to help calculate the risk that a particular person is a heterozygote. Returning to the example of CF, the incidence of the disease, and therefore also of carriers, may vary greatly in different populations (**table 14.4**). **Figure 14.3** provides another example of an illness common in one population, but exceedingly rare elsewhere.

Table 14.3

Hardy-Weinberg Equilibrium—When Allele Frequencies Stay Constant

Possible Matings			Frequency of Offspring Genotypes		
Male	Female	Proportion in Population	DD	Dd	dd
0.49 DD	0.49 DD	0.2401 (DD × DD)	0.2401		
0.49 DD	0.42 Dd	0.2058 (DD × Dd)	0.1029	0.1029	
0.49 DD	0.09 dd	0.0441 (DD × dd)		0.0441	
0.42 Dd	0.49 DD	0.2058 (Dd × DD)	0.1029	0.1029	
0.42 Dd	0.42 Dd	0.1764 (Dd × Dd)	0.0441	0.0882	0.0441
0.42 Dd	0.09 dd	0.0378 (Dd × dd)		0.0189	0.0189
0.09 dd	0.49 DD	0.0441 (dd × DD)		0.0441	
0.09 dd	0.42 Dd	0.0378 (dd × Dd)		0.0189	0.0189
0.09 dd	0.09 dd	0.0081 (dd × dd)			0.0081
		Resulting offspring frequencies:	0.49	0.42	0.09
			DD	Dd	dd

Table 14.4

Carrier Frequency for Cystic Fibrosis

Population Group	Carrier Frequency
African Americans	1 in 66
Asian Americans	1 in 150
Caucasians of European descent	1 in 23
Hispanic Americans	1 in 46

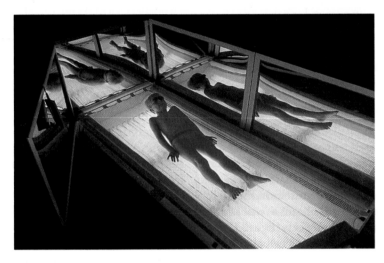

Figure 14.3 Disease incidence varies in populations.   Of the 60 cases of Crigler-Najjar syndrome known worldwide, many are in the Mennonite and Amish community of Lancaster County, Pennsylvania. This enzyme deficiency causes the buildup of a substance called bilirubin, producing severe jaundice (yellowing of the skin and eyes). If untreated, the syndrome rapidly results in fatal brain damage. Fortunately, exposure to ultraviolet light breaks down excess bilirubin, but children must sleep unclothed under the lights every night. The Mennonite and Amish populations have many other autosomal recessive illnesses that are extremely rare elsewhere, because these people descended from a few founding families and marry among themselves.

Cystic fibrosis affects 1 in 2,000 Caucasian newborns. Therefore, the homozygous recessive frequency—*cc* if *c* represents the disease-causing allele—is 1/2,000, or 0.0005 in this population. This equals q^2. The square root of q^2 is about 0.022, which equals the frequency of the *c* allele. If *q* equals 0.022, then *p*, or $1 - q$, equals 0.978. Carrier frequency is equal to $2pq$, which equals (2)(0.978)(0.022), or 0.043—about 1 in 23.

If there is no cystic fibrosis in a family, a person's risk of having an affected child, derived from population statistics, is relatively low. Consider a Caucasian couple with no family history of cystic fibrosis asking a genetic counselor to calculate the risk that they could conceive a child with this illness. The genetic counselor tells them that the chance of *each* potential parent being a carrier is about 4.3 percent, or 1 in 23. But this is only part of the picture. The chance that *both* of these people are carriers is 1/23 multiplied by 1/23—or 1 in 529—because the probability that two independent events will occur equals the product of the probability that each event will happen alone. However, if they *are* both carriers, each of their children would face a 1 in 4 chance of inheriting the illness, based on Mendel's first law of gene segregation. Therefore, the risk that two unrelated Caucasian individuals with no family history of cystic fibrosis will have an affected child is $1/4 \times 1/23 \times 1/23$, or 1 in 2,116. This couple has learned their chance of producing an affected child from disease incidence statistics.

For X-linked traits, different predictions of allele frequencies apply to males and females. For a female, who can be homozygous recessive, homozygous dominant, or a heterozygote, the standard Hardy-Weinberg equation of $p^2 + 2pq + q^2$ applies, as it usually would to an autosomal recessive trait. However, in males, the allele frequency is the phenotypic frequency, because a male who inherits an X-linked recessive allele exhibits it in his phenotype.

The incidence of X-linked hemophilia (X^hY), for example, is 1 in 10,000 male births. Therefore, *q* (the frequency of the *h* allele) equals 0.0001. Using the formula $p + q = 1$, the frequency of the wild type allele is 0.9999. The incidence of carriers (X^hX^H), who are all female, equals $2pq$, or (2)(0.0001)(0.9999), which equals 0.00019; this is 0.0002, or 0.02 percent, which equals about 1 in 5,000. The incidence of a female having hemophilia (X^hX^h) is q^2, or $(0.0001)^2$, or about 1 in 100 million.

In the real world of medical genetics, neat allele frequencies such as 0.6 and 0.4, or 0.7 and 0.3, are unusual. Mendelian disorders are usually very rare, and the *q* component of the Hardy-Weinberg equation contributes little. Because this means that

DNA Profiling Relies on Molecular Genetics and Population Genetics

DNA profiling has rapidly become a standard and powerful tool used in forensic investigations, agriculture, paternity testing, and historical investigations. Section 1.5 discussed several interesting examples. But until 1986, DNA profiling was unheard of outside of scientific circles. A dramatic rape case changed that.

Tommie Lee Andrews became the first person in the United States to be convicted of a crime on the basis of DNA evidence. Andrews picked his victims months before he attacked and watched them so that he knew exactly when they would be home alone. On a balmy Sunday night in May 1986, Andrews awaited Nancy Hodge, a young computer operator at Disney World, at her home in Orlando, Florida. The burly man surprised her when she was in the bathroom removing her contact lenses. He covered her face, then raped and brutalized her repeatedly.

Andrews was very careful not to leave fingerprints, threads, hairs, or any other indication that he had ever been in Hodge's home. But he had not counted on the new technology of DNA profiling. Thanks to a clear-thinking crime victim and scientifically informed lawyers, Andrews was soon at the center of a trial—not only his trial, but one that would judge the technology that helped to convict him.

After the attack, Hodge went to the hospital, where she provided a vaginal secretion sample containing the rapist's sperm cells. Two district attorneys who had read about DNA profiling sent some of the sperm to a biotechnology company that extracted DNA and cut it with restriction enzymes. The sperm's DNA pieces were then mixed with labeled DNA probes that bound to complementary sequences.

The same procedure of extracting, cutting, and probing the DNA was done on white blood cells from Nancy Hodge and Tommie Lee Andrews, who had been apprehended and held as a suspect in several assaults. When the radioactive DNA pieces from each sample, which were the sequences where the probes had bound, were separated and displayed according to size, the resulting pattern of bands—the DNA profile—matched exactly for the sperm sample and Andrews's blood, differing from Nancy Hodge's DNA (**figure 1**).

Because Tommie Lee Andrews is black, his allele frequencies were compared to those for a representative African American population. At his first trial in November 1987, the judge, perhaps fearful that too much technical information would overwhelm the jury, did not allow the prosecution to cite population-based statistics. Without the appropriate allele frequencies, DNA profiling was reduced to a comparison of smeary lines on test papers to see whether the patterns of DNA pieces in the forensic sperm sample looked like those for Andrews's white blood cells. The probabilities determined from population-based statistics indicated that the possibility that Tommie Lee Andrews's DNA would match the evidence by chance was 1 in 10 billion. But the prosecution could not mention this.

After a mistrial was declared, the prosecution cited the precedent of using population statistics to derive databases on standard blood types. So when Andrews stood trial just three months later for the rape of a different woman, the judge permitted population analysis, and Andrews was convicted. Today, in jail, he keeps a copy of the *Discover* magazine article (written by this author) that describes his role in the first case tried using DNA profiling.

The sizes of the DNA pieces in the type of DNA profile used in the Andrews case vary from person to person because of differences in DNA sequence in the regions surrounding the probed genes. The discriminating power of the technology stems from the fact that there are many more ways for the 3 billion bases of the human genome to vary than there are people. However, this theoretical variation is tempered by the fact that certain gene combinations are more prevalent in some populations because of marriage, travel, and other social customs. That is, within ethnic groups, some people may be more alike genetically, and distinguishing among them might be more difficult. In one case, for example, DNA profiling could not reveal whether a man or his father had committed a rape.

Today, many DNA profiles analyze short, tandem repeats, or STRs, which are 4 or 5 bases long. STRs are analyzed using the polymerase chain reaction (PCR). Recall from chapter 9 that PCR uses primer sequences that flank a gene of interest and replication enzymes to rapidly mass produce a sequence. The more repeats, the longer the PCR product. PCR works well on degraded DNA and requires only a few cells—conditions common for biological evidence from crime scenes.

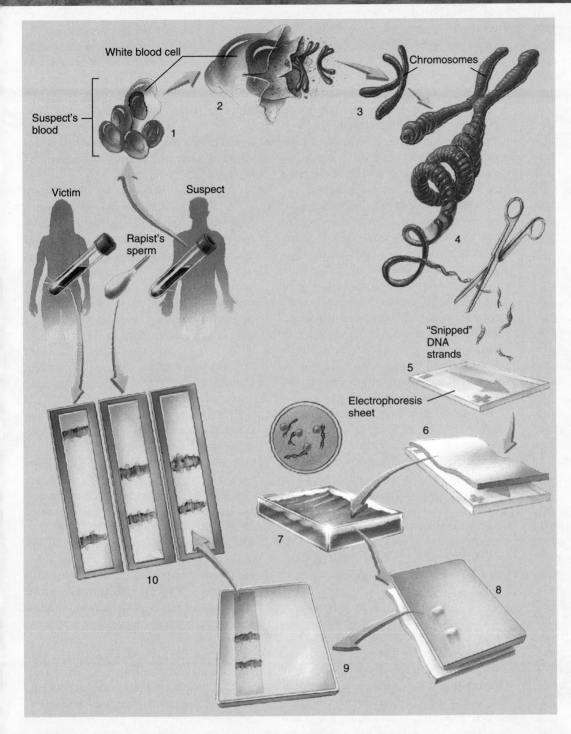

Figure 1 DNA profiling. A blood sample (1) is collected from the suspect. White blood cells are separated and burst open (2), releasing DNA (3). Restriction enzymes snip the strands into fragments (4), and electrophoresis aligns them by size in a groove on a sheet of gel (5). The resulting pattern of DNA fragments is transferred to a nylon sheet (6). It is then exposed to radioactively tagged probes (7) that home in on the DNA areas used to establish identity. When the nylon sheet is placed against a piece of X-ray film (8) and processed, black bands appear where the probes stuck (9). This pattern of bands constitutes a DNA profile (10). This profile may then be compared to the victim's DNA pattern, the rapist's DNA obtained from sperm cells, and other biological evidence. Originally, DNA profiling used radioactively tagged probes, but today fluorescent labels are often used.

Labels within figure: White blood cell; Chromosomes; Suspect's blood; Victim; Suspect; Rapist's sperm; "Snipped" DNA strands; Electrophoresis sheet; 1; 2; 3; 4; 5; 6; 7; 8; 9; 10

The Hardy-Weinberg equation and the product rule are used to derive the statistics that back up a DNA profile shown in **figure 14.7**. First, the DNA profile pattern indicates whether an individual is a homozygote or a heterozygote for each repeat, because a homozygote only has one band representing that gene. Genotype frequencies are then calculated using parts of the Hardy-Weinberg equation; that is, p^2 and q^2 denote the two homozygotes for a two-allele gene, and $2pq$ represents the heterozygote. The genotype frequencies are multiplied using the product rule, and the result is the probability that this particular combination of DNA sequences would occur in the population. Logic then enters the equation. If an allele combination is very rare in the population the suspect comes from, and if it is found both in the suspect's DNA and in crime scene evidence, the suspect's guilt appears to be highly likely.

The accuracy and meaning of a DNA profile depend upon the population that is the source for the allele frequencies used. If populations are too broadly defined, then allele frequencies are typically quite low, leading to very large estimates of the likelihood that a suspect matches evidence based on chance alone. In one oft-quoted trial, the prosecutor concluded, "The chance of the DNA fingerprint of the cells in the evidence matching blood of the defendant by chance is 1 in 738 trillion." The numbers themselves were not at fault, but some population geneticists questioned the validity of the databases. Did they really reflect the gene pool compositions of actual human populations? By 1991, half a dozen judges had rejected DNA evidence because population geneticists had testified that the databases do not correspond directly to true allele frequencies because they greatly oversimplify human population structure. Therefore, the odds that crime scene DNA matched suspect DNA were not as reliable as originally suggested.

The first DNA profiling databases that were consulted neatly shoehorned many different groups into just three—Caucasian, black, or Hispanic—designations not necessarily biologically meaningful. People from Poland, Greece, or Sweden would all be considered white, and a dark-skinned person from Jamaica and one from Somalia would be lumped together as blacks. Perhaps the most incongruous of all were the Hispanics.

Cubans and Puerto Ricans are part African, whereas people from Mexico and Guatemala have mostly Native American gene variants. Spanish and Argentinians have neither black African nor Native American genetic backgrounds. Yet these diverse peoples were considered a single population! Other groups were left out, such as Native Americans and Asians. Ultimately, analysis of these three databases revealed significantly more homozygous recessives for certain polymorphic genes than the Hardy-Weinberg equation would predict, confirming what many had suspected—allele frequencies were not in equilibrium.

Giving meaning to the allele frequencies necessary to interpret DNA profiles requires more restrictive ethnic databases. A frequency of 1 in 1,000 for a particular allele in all whites may actually be much higher or lower in, for example, only Italians, because they (and many others) tend to marry among themselves. On the other hand, narrowly defined ethnic databases may be insufficient to interpret DNA profiles from people of mixed heritages, such as someone whose mother was Scottish/French and whose father was Greek/German.

We may need to develop mathematical models to account for real population structures. Perhaps the first step will be to understand the forces that generate genetic substructures within more broadly defined populations, which means taking into account history and human nature. Chapter 15 explores these factors.

DNA Profiling to Identify World Trade Center Victims

During the second half of September, 2001, Myriad Genetics Inc., a biotechnology company in Salt Lake City that normally provides breast cancer tests, was flooded with a very different type of medical sample—frozen DNA from people who had presumably perished in the terrorist attack on the World Trade Center on the 11th. The laboratory also received cheek brush scrapings from relatives of the missing, amassed at DNA collection centers set up throughout New York City in the days after the disaster, and tissue from the victims' toothbrushes, razors, and hairbrushes. The workers used the polymerase chain reaction to determine the numbers of copies of four-base short tandem repeats at 13 loca-

tions in the genome. They also determined the sex chromosome constitution. The probability that any two individuals have the same 13 markers by chance is 1 in 250 trillion; if the STR pattern of a sample from the crime scene matched a sample from a victim's toothbrush, identification was fairly certain. Myriad sent its results to the New York State Forensic Laboratory, where investigators matched family members to victims. Meticulous records were kept so that when an individual was identified more than once, the bad news wasn't delivered to the family again.

The most difficult part of the massive DNA profiling effort was right at the beginning—obtaining victim samples, because most of the bodies were incinerated. Myriad performed STR analysis on whatever pieces of soft tissue were found. Sadly, their job ended within a few weeks, but the DNA analysis continued. Bone bits, which can persist despite the ongoing fire at the site, were sent to a laboratory in Virginia where DNA was extracted. The DNA was then sent to Celera Genomics Corp. in Rockville, Maryland, where DNA profiling was done on mitochondrial DNA, which can yield information from tissue too degraded for the more accurate STR typing. (The armed forces handled DNA profiling of the victims at the Pentagon.) At the time, STR analysis required pieces of DNA 200 to 400 bases long. By September 11, 2003, STR and mitochondrial DNA analysis had identified slightly more than half of the 2,800 victims, who were represented by about 20,000 pieces of evidence, some of it just bits of tissue. The slow pace led to improvement in technique; STR analysis became possible on much smaller pieces of DNA. A biotechnology company also developed a way to identify remains using SNPs.

DNA profiling provides much more reliable information on identity than traditional forensic techniques such as dental patterns, scars, and fingerprints, and clues such as jewelry, wallets, and rolls of film found with the victim. Consider the case of Jose Guadalupe and Christopher Santora, two of the fifteen firefighters lost from one engine company on September 11, 2001. Rescue workers brought a body found beside a fire truck next to the destroyed towers to the Medical Examiner's office on September 13th. Other firefighters identified the remains as belonging to Guadalupe based on where the body had

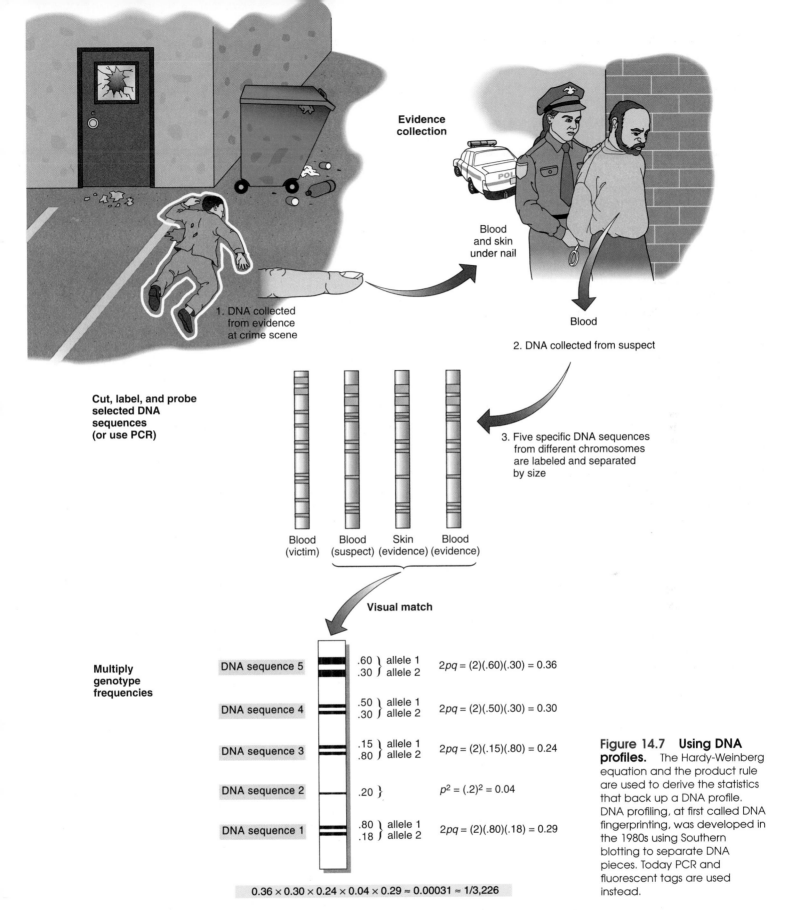

Evidence collection

Blood and skin under nail

Blood

1. DNA collected from evidence at crime scene

2. DNA collected from suspect

Cut, label, and probe selected DNA sequences (or use PCR)

3. Five specific DNA sequences from different chromosomes are labeled and separated by size

Blood (victim) · Blood (suspect) · Skin (evidence) · Blood (evidence)

Visual match

Multiply genotype frequencies

DNA sequence 5 — .60 } allele 1, .30 } allele 2 — $2pq = (2)(.60)(.30) = 0.36$

DNA sequence 4 — .50 } allele 1, .30 } allele 2 — $2pq = (2)(.50)(.30) = 0.30$

DNA sequence 3 — .15 } allele 1, .80 } allele 2 — $2pq = (2)(.15)(.80) = 0.24$

DNA sequence 2 — .20 } — $p^2 = (.2)^2 = 0.04$

DNA sequence 1 — .80 } allele 1, .18 } allele 2 — $2pq = (2)(.80)(.18) = 0.29$

$0.36 \times 0.30 \times 0.24 \times 0.04 \times 0.29 \approx 0.00031 \approx 1/3,226$

Figure 14.7 Using DNA profiles. The Hardy-Weinberg equation and the product rule are used to derive the statistics that back up a DNA profile. DNA profiling, at first called DNA fingerprinting, was developed in the 1980s using Southern blotting to separate DNA pieces. Today PCR and fluorescent tags are used instead.

Conclusion: The probability that another person in the suspect's population group has the same pattern of these alleles is approximately 1 in 3,226.

been found, because he had been the chauffeur of the fire truck. The body also had a gold chain that the men recognized, and X rays revealed a birth defect in the neck bone that he was known to have had. Guadalupe was buried on October 1—but it wasn't Guadalupe who was buried. It turned out that Christopher Santora had the same necklace and the same neck condition! A DNA sample taken from the buried man's remains and from Santora's relatives matched.

The scale of the DNA profiling task that followed the September 11, 2001 attack was unprecedented, and particularly difficult because there was no list of victims, as there is in the case of a plane crash. It was very distressing for the technicians and researchers whose jobs suddenly shifted from detecting breast cancer and sequencing genomes to helping identify human remains. Said J. Craig Venter, president of Celera Genomics when the samples from the World Trade Center began to arrive, "I never, ever thought we would have to do DNA forensics at this level, and for this reason."

Key Concepts

DNA profiles are based on SNPs or differences in the sizes of highly repeated DNA sequences among individuals, based on the idea that the human genome sequence can vary in more ways than there are people. • Population statistics are applied to determine the probability that the same pattern would occur by chance in two individuals. A limitation of the method is that databases may not adequately represent real human populations. Developing narrower ethnic databases and considering historical and social factors may make population statistics more realistic. • DNA profiling of nuclear and mitochondrial DNA was performed on evidence from the September 11 terrorist attacks.

Summary

1. A **population** is a group of interbreeding members of the same species in a particular area. Their genes constitute the **gene pool.**

14.1 The Importance of Knowing Allele Frequencies

2. **Population genetics** considers allele, genotype, and phenotype frequencies to reveal whether **microevolution** is occurring. Phenotypic frequencies can be determined empirically, then used in algebraic expressions to derive other frequencies.

3. Allele frequencies change if migration, nonrandom mating, genetic drift, mutations, or natural selection operate. In **Hardy-Weinberg equilibrium,** allele frequencies are not changing.

14.2 When Allele Frequencies Stay Constant

4. Hardy and Weinberg proposed an algebraic equation to explain the constancy of allele frequencies. This would show why dominant traits do not increase and recessive traits do not decrease in populations. The Hardy-Weinberg equation is a binomial expansion used to represent genotypes in a population.

5. Hardy-Weinberg equilibrium is demonstrated by following gamete frequencies as they recombine in the next generation. In Hardy-Weinberg equilibrium, these genotypes remain constant from generation to generation if evolution is not occurring. When the equation $p^2 + 2pq + q^2$ represents a gene with one dominant and one recessive allele, p^2 corresponds to the frequency of homozygous dominant individuals; $2pq$ stands for heterozygotes; and q^2 represents the frequency of the homozygous recessive class. The frequency of the dominant allele is p, and of the recessive allele, q.

14.3 Practical Applications of Hardy-Weinberg Equilibrium

6. If we know either p or q, we can calculate genotype frequencies, such as carrier risks. Often such information comes from knowing the q^2 class, which corresponds to the frequency of homozygous recessive individuals in a population.

7. For X-linked recessive traits, the mutant allele frequency for males equals the trait frequency. For very rare disorders or traits, the value of p approaches 1, so the carrier frequency ($2pq$) is approximately twice the frequency of the rare trait (q).

14.4 DNA Profiling—A Practical Test of Hardy-Weinberg Assumptions

8. A highly variable gene variant or DNA sequence present in more than 1 percent of the population is a **polymorphism.**

9. **Restriction enzymes** or PCR are used to isolate polymorphic repeats, and polyacrylamide gel electrophoresis is used to separate and display labeled DNA fragments by size. The fragment pattern is the DNA profile.

10. To interpret DNA profiles, allele frequencies are derived from population data, and genotype frequencies are calculated and then multiplied. The result estimates the likelihood that two individuals from a given population share the same genotype for all of the DNA sequences examined.

11. DNA profiling will become a more powerful tool when we can more specifically define and analyze human populations.

12. DNA profiling based on short tandem repeats, SNPs, and mitochondrial DNA was used to identify victims of the World Trade Center disaster on September 11, 2001.

Review Questions

1. "We like him, he seems to have a terrific gene pool," say the parents upon meeting their daughter's latest boyfriend. Why doesn't their statement make sense?

2. What is *not* happening in a population in Hardy-Weinberg equilibrium?

3. Why is knowing the incidence of a homozygous recessive condition in a population important in deriving allele frequencies?

4. Two couples want to know their risk of conceiving a child with cystic fibrosis. In one couple, neither partner has a family history of the disease; in the other, one partner knows he is a carrier. How do their risks differ?

5. Why are short DNA repeats more likely to be in Hardy-Weinberg equilibrium than protein-encoding genes?

6. Why are specific databases necessary to interpret DNA fingerprints?

7. How is the Hardy-Weinberg equation used to predict the recurrence of X-linked recessive traits?

Applied Questions

1. Glutaric aciduria type I causes progressive paralysis and brain damage. It is very common in the Amish of Lancaster County, Pennsylvania—0.25 percent of newborns have the disorder. Calculate the percentage of newborns that are carriers for this condition, and the percentage that do not have the disease-causing allele.

2. Torsion dystonia is a movement disorder that affects 1 in 1,000 Jewish people of eastern European descent (Ashkenazim). What is the carrier frequency in this population?

3. Factor IX deficiency is a clotting disorder affecting 1 in 190 Ashkenazim living in Israel. It affects 1 in 1,000,000 Japanese, Korean, Chinese, German, Italian, African American, English, Indian, and Arab people.

   a. What is the frequency of the mutant allele in the Israeli population?

   b. What is the frequency of the normal allele in this population?

   c. Calculate the proportion of carriers in the Israeli population.

   d. Why might the disease incidence be very high in the Israeli population but very low in others?

4. The Finnish population has a 1 percent carrier frequency for a seizure disorder called myoclonus epilepsy. Two people who have no relatives with the illness ask a genetic counselor to calculate the risk that they will conceive an affected child, based on their belonging to this population group. What is the risk?

5. Maple syrup urine disease (MSUD) is an autosomal recessive inborn error of metabolism that causes mental and physical retardation, difficulty feeding, and a sweet odor to urine. In Costa Rica, 1 in 8,000 newborns inherits the condition. Calculate the carrier frequency of MSUD in this population.

6. The amyloidoses are a group of inborn errors of metabolism in which sticky protein builds up in certain organs. Amyloidosis, caused by a mutation in the gene encoding a blood protein called transthyretin, affects the heart and/or nervous system. It is autosomal recessive. In a population of 177 healthy African Americans, four proved, by blood testing, to have one mutant allele of the transthyretin gene. What is the carrier frequency in this population?

7. Ability to taste phenylthiocarbamide (PTC) is mostly determined by the *T* gene. *TT* individuals taste a strong, bitter taste; *Tt* people experience a slightly bitter taste; *tt* individuals taste nothing.

   A fifth-grade class of 20 students tastes PTC that has been applied to small pieces of paper, rating the experience as "very yucky" (*TT*), "I can taste it" (*Tt*), and "I can't taste it" (*tt*). For homework, the students test their parents, with these results:

   Of 6 *TT* students, 4 have 2 *TT* parents; one has one parent who is *TT* and one parent who is *Tt*. The sixth *TT* student has one parent who is *Tt* and one who is *tt*.

   Of 4 students who are *Tt*, 2 have 2 parents who are *Tt*, and 2 have one parent who is *TT* and one parent who is *tt*.

   Of the 10 students who can't taste PTC, 4 have 2 parents who also are *tt*, but 4 students have one parent who is *Tt* and one who is *tt*. The remaining 2 students have 2 *Tt* parents.

   Calculate the frequencies of the *T* and *t* alleles in the two generations. Is Hardy-Weinberg equilibrium maintained, or is this gene evolving?

Web Activities

8. On December 5, 1984, Theresa Fusco was raped and strangled near a roller-skating rink on Long Island, New York. Two similar crimes had occurred in previous months. Three young men were charged with the crime and then convicted, all the while proclaiming their innocence, maintaining that their confessions had been coerced and witnesses had lied. At their trial in 1990, defense lawyers requested DNA profiling, but the judge ruled that the technology was too unproven to use. In 2003, the case was reopened. Stored semen was taken from the "rape kit" and subjected to DNA testing, and the three men were exonerated. They had not killed Theresa Fusco after all—but they had spent more than a decade in prison.

   a. Why, specifically, might the judge have refused to consider DNA testing in 1990?

   b. List the types of cells that could have been used to settle this case.

   c. What information on the three suspects would be needed to interpret DNA patterns?

   d. Do you think it is fair to decide whether or not a science-based forensic test or tool be used based on how well a judge, jury, lawyers, or the public—who may have little or no training in genetics—understands how it works?

   e. In 1992, lawyers Barry Scheck and Peter Neufeld, of the Cardozo School of Law in New York City, founded the nonprofit Innocence Project, a legal clinic to reopen cases where DNA profiling could have made a difference in the verdict. They have vindicated more than 140 individuals. Consult the website (http://www.innocenceproject.org), click on "Case Profiles," and select a case, describing how the DNA evidence exonerated a prisoner.

Case Studies

9. An extra row of eyelashes is an autosomal recessive trait that occurs in 900 of the 10,000 residents of an island in the south Pacific. Greta knows that she is a heterozygote for this gene, because her eyelashes are normal, but she has an affected parent. She wants to have children with a homozygous dominant man, so that the trait will not affect her offspring. What is the probability that a person with normal eyelashes in this population is a homozygote for this gene?

10. In a true crime that took place in Israel, a man knocked a woman unconscious with a cement block and then raped her. He was careful not to leave any hairs at the crime scene. But he left behind eyeglasses with unusual frames, and an optician helped police locate him. The man also left a half-eaten lollipop at the scene. DNA from blood taken from the suspect matched DNA from cheek-lining cells collected from the base of the telltale lollipop. Forensic scientists obtained the DNA profile shown here by looking at four genes and considering their allele frequencies in the man's ethnic group in Israel.

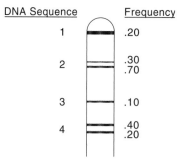

DNA Sequence	Frequency
1	.20
2	.30 / .70
3	.10
4	.40 / .20

a. Which of the tested genes has two alleles? How do you know this?

b. What is the possibility that the suspect's DNA matches that of the lollipop rapist by chance? (Do the calculation.)

c. The man's population group is highly inbred—many people have children with relatives. How does this information affect the accuracy or reliability of the DNA profile?

d. If a fifth gene was added to the analysis and the lollipop rapist was found to have just one allele of this gene that has a frequency of 0.45 in his population, how would it affect the probability that the man is guilty?

(P.S.—He was so frightened by the DNA analysis that he confessed!)

Learn to apply the skills of a genetic counselor with this additional case found in the *Case Workbook in Human Genetics:*

The Ice Maiden

Suggested Readings

Altman, Lawrence K. September 25, 2001. Now, doctors must identify the dead. *The New York Times,* F1. It isn't doctors, but genetic researchers, who did the DNA profiling of World Trade Center victims.

Crow, James F. February 15, 2001. The beanbag lives on. *Nature* 409:771. A very clear explanation of Hardy-Weinberg equilibrium.

Gootman, Elissa. June 11, 2003. DNA evidence frees three men in 1984 murder of L. I. girl. *The New York Times,* F1. Add another three people to the list of those exonerated by DNA evidence.

Grady, Denise. June 29, 1999. At gene therapy's frontier, the Amish build a clinic. *The New York Times.* The gene that causes Crigler-Najjar syndrome is far from Hardy-Weinberg equilibrium.

Hand, Larry. October 14, 2002. SNP technology focuses on terror victims' IDs. *The Scientist* 16(20):20. Single-base differences made it possible to identify some Sept. 11 victims.

Hoffert, Stephen P. May 11, 1998. Taking the clinic to the patients gave researcher sense of purpose. *The Scientist* 12:1. The Amish and Mennonites of Lancaster County, Pennsylvania, have high frequencies of alleles that are extremely rare elsewhere.

Kleinfeld, N. R. November 28, 2001. Error puts body of one firefighter in a grave of a firehouse colleague. *The New York Times,* F1. DNA profiling adds precision to forensics.

Lewis, Ricki. June 1988. Witness for the prosecution. *Discover* vol. 9. The story of one of the first DNA profiling cases.

Oransky, Ivan. September 9, 2003. DNA identification of Sept. 11 victims continues. *The Scientist* daily news. www.the-scientist.com. Two years after the terrorist attacks against the U.S., DNA profiling had identified remains of 54 percent of the victims.

Weekly updates of current news related to human genetics are available through Power Web on your Online Learning Center.

CHAPTER

15

Changing Allele Frequencies

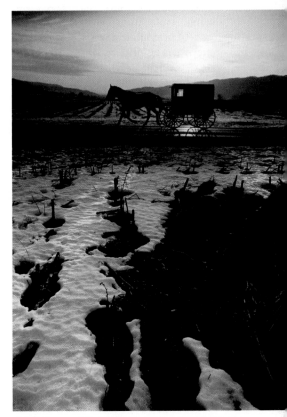

Certain genetic disorders are much more
common in Amish communities than elsewhere because of an initial founder effect,
followed by restriction of marriage to others
within the group.

Historically, we seem to have gone out of our way to see that the very specific conditions necessary for Hardy-Weinberg equilibrium—unchanging allele frequencies from generation to generation—do not occur, at least for some genes. Wars and persecution kill certain populations. Economic and political systems enable some groups to have more children than others. Religious restrictions and personal preferences guide our choices of mates. We travel extensively, shuttling our genes in and out of populations. Natural disasters and new infectious diseases reduce populations to a few individuals, who then rebuild their numbers, but at the expense of genetic diversity. Add to all this the forces of mutation and the reshuffling of genes that occurs in each generation, and it is clear that a gene pool is a very fluid entity. These ever-present and interacting forces of nonrandom or selective mating, migration, genetic drift, mutation, and natural selection work to differing degrees to shape populations. This chapter addresses the factors that shake up gene pools.

15.1   Nonrandom Mating

In the theoretical state of Hardy-Weinberg equilibrium, individuals of all genotypes are presumed equally likely to mate and to choose partners at random. But in reality, we give great thought to selecting mates—it is hardly a random process. We choose partners based on physical appearance, ethnic background, intelligence, and shared interests. Surveys show that we marry people similar to ourselves about 80 percent of the time. Worldwide, about one-third of all marriages occur between people who were born fewer than ten miles apart! Such nonrandom mating is a major factor in changing allele frequencies in human populations.

Another form of nonrandom mating on a population level occurs when certain individuals contribute disproportionately to the next generation. This is common in agriculture when an animal or plant with valuable characteristics is bred extensively. For example, semen from one prize bull may be used to artificially inseminate thousands of cows. Such an extreme situation can arise in a human population when a man fathers many children. A striking mutation can reveal such behavior. In the Cape population of South Africa, for example, a Chinese immigrant known as Arnold had a very rare dominant genetic disease that causes one's teeth to fall out before age 20. Arnold had seven wives. Of his 356 living descendants, 70 have the dental disorder. The frequency of this allele in the Cape population is exceptionally high, thanks to Arnold. Similarly, Y chromosome analysis reveals that Genghis Khan, a Mongolian warrior who lived from 1162 to 1227, was so attentive to his many wives that today, 1 in every 200 males living between Afghanistan and northeast China shares his Y—that's 16 million men (**figure 15.1**)!

The high frequency of people with autosomal recessive albinism among Arizona's Hopi Indians also reflects nonrandom mating. Albinism is uncommon in the general U.S. population, but it affects 1 in 200 Hopi Indians. The reason for the trait's prevalence is cultural—men with albinism often stay back and help the women, rather than risk severe sunburn in the fields with the other men. They contribute more children to the population because they have more contact with the women.

The events of history reflect nonrandom mating patterns. When a group of people is subservient to another, genes tend to "flow" from one group to the other as the males of the ruling class have children with females of the underclass. Historical records and chromosome DNA sequences reveal this directional gene flow phenomenon.

Despite our partner preferences, many traits do mix randomly in the next generation. This may be because we are unaware of these characteristics or they are not considered in choosing a partner. In populations where AIDS is extremely rare or nonexistent, for example, the two mutations that render a person resistant to HIV infection are in Hardy-Weinberg equilibrium. This would change, over time, if HIV arrives, because the people with these mutations would become more likely to survive to produce offspring—some of whom would perpetuate the protective mutation. Natural selection would intervene, ultimately altering allele frequencies. Interestingly, one of the mutations that removes the receptor for HIV on human cells also blocks infection by the bacterium that causes plague. Seven centuries ago, in Europe, the "Black Death" plague epidemic led to increase of the protective allele in the population. Today it makes 3 million people in the U.S. and the United Kingdom resistant to HIV infection.

Many blood types are in Hardy-Weinberg equilibrium because we do not select life partners on the basis of blood type. Yet sometimes the opposite occurs. People with mutations in the same gene meet when their families participate in a program for people with the resulting inherited condition, such as summer camps for children with cystic fibrosis. More than two-thirds of the relatives visiting such a camp are likely to be carriers for CF, compared to the 1 in 23 or fewer in large population groups. In the reverse situation, an organization called Dor Yeshorim offers carrier tests for more than a dozen diseases more common among Ashkenazi (Eastern European descended) Jews. In certain religious Jewish communities, young people are encouraged to take these tests before they begin dating. The results are stored in a database with a numerical identifier rather than a name. When two people contemplate marriage, they can find out if they are carriers for the same disorder. If so, they may elect not to have children or not to marry. Dor Yeshorim has tested more than 100,000 young people, and is partly responsible for the falling incidence of Tay-Sachs disease among Ashkenazi Jews—today it is lower than for other population groups.

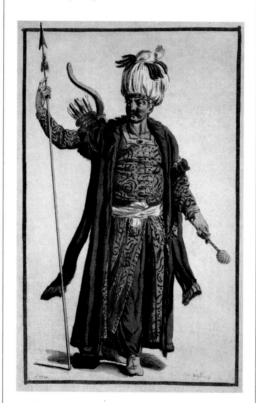

Figure 15.1   A prevalent Y.
Genghis Khan left his mark, in the form of his Y chromosome, on many men.

A population that practices consanguinity has very nonrandom mating. Recall from chapter 4 that a consanguineous relationship is one in which "blood" relatives have children together. On the family level, this practice increases the likelihood that harmful recessive alleles from shared ancestors will be passed to the same offspring, causing disease. The birth defect rate in offspring is 2.5 times the normal rate of about 3 percent. On a population level, consanguinity decreases genetic diversity. The proportion of homozygotes rises as that of heterozygotes falls.

Some populations encourage marriage between cousins, resulting in an increase in the incidence of certain recessive disorders. In certain parts of the middle east, Africa, and India, from 20 to 50 percent of all marriages are between cousins, or uncles and nieces. The tools of molecular genetics can reveal these relationships. Researchers traced DNA sequences on the Y chromosome and in mitochondria among residents of an ancient, geographically isolated "micropopulation" on the island of Sardinia, near Italy. They consulted archival records dating from the village's founding by 200 settlers around 1000 A.D. to determine familial relationships. Between 1640 and 1870, population size doubled, reaching 1,200 by 1990. Fifty percent of the present population descends from just two paternal and four maternal lines, and 86 percent have the same X chromosome. Researchers are analyzing medical conditions that are especially prevalent in this population, which include hypertension and a kidney disorder.

Worldwide, about 960 million married couples are related, and know of their relationship. Also contributing to nonrandom mating is endogamy, which is marriage within a community. In this case, spouses may be distantly related and unaware of the connection.

Key Concepts

People choose mates for many reasons, and they do not contribute the same numbers of children to the next generation. This changes allele frequencies in populations. Traits lacking obvious phenotypes may be in Hardy-Weinberg equilibrium. Consanguinity and endogamy in populations increase the proportion of homozygotes at the expense of heterozygotes.

15.2 Migration

Large cities, with their pockets of ethnicity, defy Hardy-Weinberg equilibrium by their very existence. Waves of immigrants formed the population of New York City, for example. The original Dutch settlers of the 1600s had different alleles than those in today's metropolis, which include alleles from the English, Irish, Slavics, Africans, Hispanics, Italians, Asians, and others.

Historical Clues

We can trace the genetic effects of migration by correlating allele frequencies in present-day populations to events in history, or by tracking how allele frequencies change from one geographical region to another, and then inferring in which directions ancient peoples traveled. **Figure 15.2** depicts the great changes in frequency of the allele that causes galactokinase deficiency in several European populations. This autosomal recessive disorder causes cataracts (clouding of the lens) in infants. It is very common among a population of 800,000 gypsies, called the Vlax Roma, who live in Bulgaria. It affects 1 in 1,600 to 2,500 people among them, and 5 percent of the people are carriers. But among all gypsies in Bulgaria as a whole, the incidence drops to 1 in 52,000. As the map in figure 15.2 shows, the disease becomes rarer to the west. This pattern may have arisen when people with the allele settled in Bulgaria, with only a few individuals or families moving westward.

Allele frequencies reflect who rules whom. The frequency of ABO blood types in certain parts of the world today mirrors past Arab rule. The distribution of ABO blood types is very similar in northern Africa, the Near East, and southern Spain. These are precisely the regions where Arabs ruled until 1492. The uneven distribution of allele frequencies can also reveal when and where nomadic peoples stopped for awhile. For example, in the eighteenth century, European caucasians called trekboers migrated to the Cape area of South Africa. The men stayed and had children with the native women of the Nama tribe. The mixed society remained fairly isolated, leading to the distinctive allele frequencies found in the present-day people of color of the area.

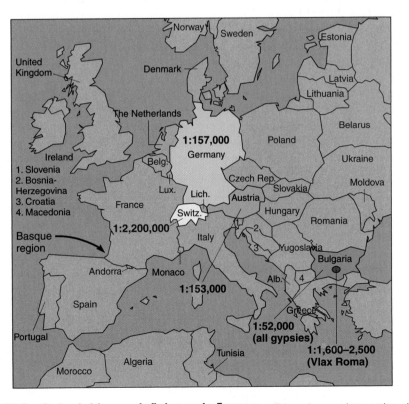

Figure 15.2 Galactokinase deficiency in Europe. This autosomal recessive disorder that causes blindness varies in prevalence across Europe. It is most common among the Vlax Roma gypsies in Bulgaria. The condition becomes much rarer to the west, as indicated by the shading from dark to light green.

Genetic analyses can corroborate migration patterns in the historical records. This is the case for Creutzfeldt-Jakob disease (CJD). Recall from chapters 10 and 11 that this prion disorder can be caused by a mutation in the prion protein gene on chromosome 20. It is rare, but more than 70 percent of affected families worldwide share the same mutation, suggesting a common origin. Researchers examined the implicated section of the chromosome in 62 affected families from 11 populations, looking at a haplotype that included repeated DNA sequences and a SNP. They identified the same haplotype in families from certain groups in Libya, Tunisia, Italy, Chile, and Spain—the exact populations that were expelled from Spain in the Middle Ages. These groups apparently took the CJD gene with them, where it persists today, causing the rare inherited form of this disease.

Geographical and Linguistic Clues

Sometimes allele frequencies change from one neighboring population to another in a gradient termed a **cline.** Changing allele frequencies usually reflect migration patterns, as immigrants introduced alleles and emigrants removed them. Clines may be gradual, reflecting unencumbered migration paths, but barriers often cause more abrupt changes in allele frequencies. Geographical formations such as mountains and bodies of water may block migration, maintaining population differences in allele frequencies. Language differences may isolate alleles, as people who cannot communicate verbally tend not to have children together.

Allele frequencies up and down the lush strip of fertile land that hugs the Nile River illustrate the concept of clines. In one study, researchers analyzed specific DNA sequences in the mitochondrial DNA of 224 people who live on either side of the Nile, an area settled for fifteen thousand years. The researchers found a gradual change in mitochondrial DNA sequences. The farther apart two individuals live along the Nile, the less alike their mitochondrial DNA. This is consistent with evidence from mummies and historical records that the area once consisted of a series of kingdoms separated by wars and language differences. If the area had been one

large interacting settlement, then the DNA sequences would have been more mixed. Instead, the researchers suggest, the Nile may have served as a "genetic corridor" between Egypt and sub-Saharan Africa.

Another pattern of changing allele frequencies reflects the human dependence on communication. In one study, population geneticists correlated twenty blood types to geographically defined regions of Italy and to areas where a single dialect is spoken. They chose Italy because it is rich in family history records and linguistic variants. Six of the blood types varied more consistently with linguistically defined subregions of the country than with geographical regions. Perhaps differences in language prevent people from socializing, sequestering alleles within groups that speak the same dialect because these people marry each other.

15.3 Genetic Drift

When a small group of individuals separate from a larger population, or reproduces only among themselves within a larger population, allele frequencies may change as a result of chance sampling from the whole. This change in allele frequency that occurs when a small group separates from the larger whole is termed **genetic drift.** It can be compared to reaching into a bag of jellybeans and, by chance, grabbing only green and yellow ones. The allele frequency changes that occur with genetic drift are random and therefore unpredictable, just as reaching into the jellybean bag a second time might yield mostly black and orange candies.

Genetic drift occurs when the population size plummets, due either to migration, to a natural disaster that isolates small pockets of a population, or to the consequences of human behavior. In a common sociological scenario, members of a small community choose to reproduce

only among themselves, which keeps genetic variants within their ethnic group. Pittsburgh, Pennsylvania, for example, is made up of many distinct neighborhoods whose residents are more similar to each other genetically than they are to others in the city. New York City, too, is more a hodgepodge of groups with distinct ethnic flavors, rather than a "melting pot" of mixed heritage.

Some groups of people become isolated in several ways—geographically, linguistically, and by choice of partners. Such populations often have a high incidence of several otherwise rare inherited conditions. Consider the native residents of the Basque country in the western part of the Pyrenees Mountains between France and Spain. They still speak remnants of Euskera, a language that the first European settlers who arrived during the late Paleolithic period brought over 10,000 years ago. The Basques have unusual frequencies of certain ABO and Rh blood types, rare mitochondrial DNA sequences and cell surface antigen patterns, and a high incidence of a mild form of muscular dystrophy. We return to them at the end of the chapter.

The Founder Effect

A common type of genetic drift in human populations is the **founder effect,** when small groups of people leave their homes to found new settlements. The new colony may have different allele frequencies than the original population.

Founder populations amplify certain alleles while maintaining great stretches of uniformity in other DNA sequences. This shows up in increased disease frequencies. Among a population of 18,000 who live in northeastern Finland, for example, the lifetime risk of developing schizophrenia is 3.2 percent, nearly triple the national average. This group traces its ancestry to forty families who settled in the region at the end of the seventeenth century. The population has been easy to study because the Finnish church has records of births, deaths, marriages, and moves, and hospital records are available. **Table 15.1** lists some other founder populations.

A powerful founder effect appears in the French Canadian population of Quebec. They lack diversity in disease-causing mutations, which reflects a long history of isolation. Consider breast cancer caused by the *BRCA1* gene. More than 500 alleles are known worldwide, yet only four are seen among French Canadians. Several inborn errors of metabolism are also more common in this group than in others. The French Canadians have what one researcher calls "optimum characteristics for gene discovery." These include many generations since founding (14), a small number of founders (about 2,500), a high rate of population expansion (74 percent increase per generation), a large present-day population (about 6 million), and minimal marriage outside the group.

The French-Canadian population exemplifies genetic drift because the people have remained mostly among themselves, within a larger population. The French founded Quebec City in 1608. Until 1660, the population grew as immigrants arrived from France, and then began to increase from births. More than 10,000 French had arrived by the time the British took over in 1759, but many of them had headed westward, taking their genes with them. Meanwhile, in Quebec, religious, language, and other cultural differences kept the French and English gene pools largely separate. The French Canadian population of Quebec grew from 2,000 to 4,000 founding genotypes to about 6 million individuals today.

The cultural and physical isolation in Canada created an unusual situation—a founder effect within a founder effect. In the nineteenth century, when agricultural lands opened up about 150 miles north of Quebec, some families migrated north. Their descendants, who remained in the remote area, form an incredibly genetically homogeneous subpopulation of founders split off from the original set of founders.

A classic example of a founder effect within a larger population is the Dunker community of Germantown, Pennsylvania. Excellent historical records combined with distinctive or measurable traits enabled geneticists to clearly track genetic drift from the larger surrounding population. The Dunkers came from Germany between 1719 and 1729, but they have lived among others since that time. Still, the frequencies of some genotypes are different among the Dunkers than among their non-Dunker neighbors, and they are also different from the frequencies seen among people living in their native

Table 15.1

Founder Populations

Population	Number of Founders	Number of Generations	Population Size Today
Costa Rica	4,000	12	2,500,000
Finland	500	80–100	5,000,000
Hutterites	80	14	36,000
Japan	1,000	80–100	120,000,000
Iceland	25,000	40	300,000
Newfoundland	25,000	16	500,000
Quebec	2,500	12–16	6,000,000
Sardinia	500	400	1,660,000

Table 15.2

Genetic Drift and the Dunkers

Blood Type	Population		
	U.S.	Dunker	European
ABO System			
A	40%	60.0%	45%
B, AB	15%	5.0%	15%
Rh⁻	15%	11.0%	15%
MN System			
M	30%	44.5%	30%
MN	50%	42.0%	50%
N	20%	13.5%	20%

German village. The Dunkers have a different distribution of blood types (**table 15.2**) and much higher incidence of attached earlobes, hyperextensible thumbs, hairs in the middle of their fingers, and left-handedness compared to the other two groups.

Founder effects can be studied at the phenotypic and genotypic levels. Phenotypically, a founder effect is indicated when a community of people, known from local history to have descended from a few founders, have their own collection of inherited traits and illnesses that are rare elsewhere in the world. This is striking among the Old Order Amish and Mennonites of Lancaster County, Pennsylvania. Often, worried parents would bring their ill children to medical facilities in Philadelphia, and over the years,

researchers realized that these people are subject to an array of extremely rare conditions (**table 15.3** and **figure 15.3**). For example, Victor McKusick, of *Online Mendelian Inheritance in Man* fame, discovered and described cartilage-hair hypoplasia. In 1965, six Amish children died at a Philadelphia hospital from chickenpox. Part of their inherited syndrome was impaired immunity, and the children could not recover from this usually mild illness. Until McKusick made the connection, other symptoms—including dwarfism, sparse hair, and anemia—were not recognized as part of a syndrome. Today, as many geneticists study inherited diseases common among the Amish and Mennonites, treatments are becoming available, from special diets to counter

Table 15.3

Inherited Conditions Common Among the Amish and Mennonites of Lancaster County, Pennsylvania

Illness	Symptoms
Ataxia telangiectasia	Increased sensitivity to radiation, loss of balance and coordination, red marks on face, delayed sexual maturation, lung infections, diabetes, high risk of cancer
Bipolar affective disorder	Mood swings (manic depression)
Cartilage-hair hypoplasia (metaphyseal chondrodysplasia, McKusick type)	Dwarfism, sparse hair, anemia, poor immunity
Crigler-Najjar syndrome	Bilirubin buildup, jaundice, brain damage
Ellis-van Creveld syndrome	Dwarfism, short fingers, underdeveloped nails, polydactyly, hair "blaze" pattern, heart disease, fused bones, teeth at birth
Glutaric aciduria type I	Paralysis, brain damage
Homocystinuria	Damaged blood vessels, stroke, heart attack
Limb-girdle muscular dystrophy	Progressive muscle weakness in limbs
Maple syrup urine disease	Sweet-smelling urine, sleepiness, vomiting, mental retardation
Metachromatic leukodystrophy	Rigid muscles, convulsions, mental deterioration
Morquio syndrome	Clouded corneas, abnormal skeleton and aortic valve

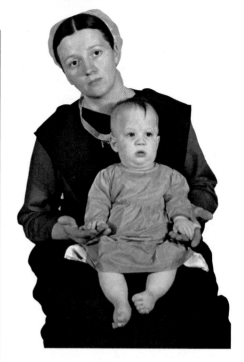

Figure 15.3   Ellis-van Creveld syndrome. This Amish child has inherited Ellis-van Creveld syndrome. He has short-limbed dwarfism, extra fingers, heart disease, fused wrist bones, and had teeth at birth. The condition is autosomal recessive, and the mutant allele occurs in 7 percent of the people of this community, reflecting consanguinity. Homozygous recessive individuals have the severe dwarfism, but heterozygotes have the milder condition Weyers acrodental dysostosis. These were thought to be different disorders until the gene was discovered in early 2000.

inborn errors of metabolism, to the "bili lights" that treat children with Crigler-Najjar syndrome (see figure 14.3), to gene therapy.

In addition to historical records, raw numbers provide evidence of a founder effect when allele frequencies in the smaller population are compared to those in the general population. The incidence of certain diseases in Lancaster County is astounding. Maple syrup urine disease, for example, affects 1 in 225,000 newborns in the United States, but 1 in 400 newborns among the Lancaster families! Similarly, a doctor new to the community and involved in a gene therapy project was startled when he took a walk at night, and noted house after house where an eerie blue glow emanated from a window. Inside each house, a child with Crigler-Najjar syndrome was being treated with bili lights. In another example, D. Holmes Morton, a research fellow at Children's Hospital in Philadelphia, discovered in 1989 that several young children from Lancaster County with cerebral palsy presumably caused by oxygen deprivation at birth actually had an inborn error of metabolism called glutaric aciduria type I. Morton went from farm to farm, tracking cases

against genealogical records, and found that *every family* that could trace its roots back to the founders had members who had the disease! Today, 0.5 percent of newborns in this population have the condition.

A mutation that is the same in all affected individuals in a population is strong evidence of a founder effect. The Bulgarian gypsies who have galactokinase deficiency, for example, all have a mutation that is extremely rare elsewhere. Similarly, an isolated group of Jewish people who settled in the Belmonte area of Portugal after being driven from Spain in the late 1400s has its own form of retinitis pigmentosa, which causes blindness. Their gene maps to a different chromosome than the genes that cause other forms of the illness.

Very often a disease-associated allele is identical in DNA sequence among people in the same population, and so is the DNA surrounding the gene. This pattern indicates that a portion of a chromosome has been passed among the members of the population from its founders. For this reason, many studies that trace founder effects examine haplotypes, which indicate very tightly linked genes that reflect linkage disequilibrium.

When historical or genealogical records are particularly well kept, founder effects can sometimes be traced to the very beginning. This is the case for the Afrikaner population of South Africa. The 2.5 million Afrikaners descended from a small group of Dutch, French, and German immigrants who had huge families, often with as many as ten children. In the nineteenth century, some Afrikaners migrated northeast to the Transvaal Province, where they lived in isolation until the Boer War in 1902 resulted in the introduction of better transportation.

Today, 30,000 Afrikaners have porphyria variegata, an autosomal dominant deficiency of one of the enzymes required to manufacture heme, the iron-containing part of hemoglobin. Symptoms include nervous attacks, abdominal pain, very fragile and sun-sensitive skin, and a severe reaction to a particular barbiturate anesthetic. All affected people descended from one couple who came from the Netherlands in 1688! Today's allele frequency in South Africa is far higher than that in the Netherlands because the founding couple had many children—who, in turn, had large families, passing on and amplifying the dominant gene.

In a similar extreme example of a founder effect, all of the cases of polydactyly (extra digits) among the Old Order Amish in Lancaster stem from one founder (see figure 15.3). Today, thanks to large families and restricted marriages, the number of cases of polydactyly among the Amish exceeds the total number in the rest of the world!

Founder effects are also evident in more common illnesses, where different populations may have different mutations in the same gene. This is the case for *BRCA1* breast cancer. The disease is most prevalent among Ashkenazi Jewish people. Nearly all affected individuals in this population have the same deletion mutation. In contrast, *BRCA1* breast cancer is quite rare in blacks, but it has affected families from the Ivory Coast in Africa, the Bahamas, and the southeastern United States. These families all share a 10-base deletion mutation in the *BRCA1* gene, probably inherited from West Africans who were ancestors of all three modern groups. Slaves brought the disease to the United States and the Bahamas between 1619 and 1808, but some of their relatives who stayed in Africa have perpetuated the gene variant there as well.

Population Bottlenecks

A **population bottleneck** occurs when many members of a group die, and only a few are left, by chance, to replenish the numbers. A bottleneck is genetically significant because the new population has only those alleles present in the small group that survived the catastrophe. An allele in the small remnant population might become more common in the replenished population than it was in the original larger group. Therefore, the new population has a much more restricted gene pool than the larger ancestral population, with some variants amplified.

Population bottlenecks sometimes occur when people (or other animals) colonize islands. An extreme example is seen among the Pingelapese people of the eastern Caroline islands in Micronesia. Between 4 and 10 percent are born with "Pingelapese blindness," an autosomal recessive combination of colorblindness, nearsightedness, and cataracts. It is also called achromatopsia. Nearly 30 percent of the Pingelapese are carriers. Elsewhere, only 1 in 20,000 to 50,000 people inherits the condition. The prevalence of the blindness among the Pingelapese has been traced to a typhoon that decimated the population in 1780. Only 9 males and 10 females survived, and they founded the present-day population. This severe population bottleneck, combined with geographic and cultural isolation, increased the frequency of the blindness gene as the population recovered its numbers.

Figure 15.4 illustrates schematically the dwindling genetic diversity that results from a population bottleneck, shown against a backdrop of a cheetah. Today's cheetahs live in just two isolated populations of a few thousand animals in South and East Africa. Their numbers once exceeded 10,000. The South African cheetahs are so alike genetically that even unrelated animals can accept skin grafts from each other. Researchers attribute the cheetahs' genetic uniformity to two bottlenecks—one that occurred at the end of the most recent ice age, when habitats were altered, and another following mass slaughter by humans in the nineteenth century. However, the good health of the animals today indicates that the genes that have survived enable the cheetahs to thrive in their environment.

Human-wrought disasters that kill many people can also cause population bottlenecks—perhaps even more severely, because aggression is typically directed at particular groups, while a typhoon indiscriminately kills anyone in its path. The Chmielnicki massacre is an example of one of the many attacks aimed against the Ashkenazi Jewish people. Overall, these acts have left a legacy of several inherited diseases that are at least ten times more common among Jewish people than in other populations (**table 15.4**).

The Chmielnicki massacre began in 1648, when a Ukrainian named Bogdan Chmielnicki led a massacre against the Polish people, including peasants, nobility, and the Jewish people, in retaliation for a Polish nobleman's seizure of his possessions. By 1654, Russians, Tartars, Swedes, and others joined the Ukrainians in wave after wave of violence against the Polish people. Thousands perished, with only a few thousand Jewish people remaining.

The Jewish people have survived many massacres, and therefore many population bottlenecks; after the Chmielnicki massacre, like the others, their numbers grew again. From 1800 to 1939, the Jewish population in Eastern Europe swelled to several million. Yet massacres continued. Jewish people also tended to have children only with each other.

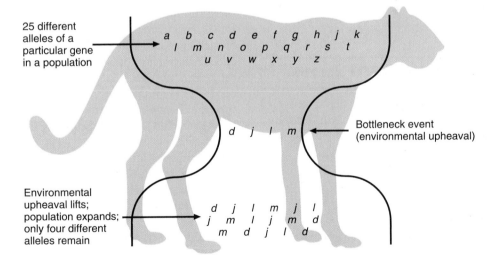

Figure 15.4 Population bottlenecks. A population bottleneck occurs when the size of a genetically diverse population drastically falls, remains at this level for a time, and then expands again. The new population loses some genetic diversity if alleles are lost in the bottleneck event. Cheetahs are difficult to breed in zoos because sperm quality is poor and many newborns die—both due to lack of genetic diversity.

Table 15.4

Autosomal Recessive Genetic Diseases Prevalent Among Ashkenazi Jewish Populations

Condition	Symptoms	Carrier Frequency
Bloom syndrome	Sun sensitivity, short stature, poor immunity, impaired fertility, increased cancer risk	1/110
Breast cancer	Malignant breast tumor caused by mutant *BRCA1* or *BRCA2* genes	3/100
Canavan disease	Brain degeneration, seizures, developmental delay, death by 18 months of age	1/40
Familial dysautonomia	No tears, cold hands and feet, skin blotching, drooling, difficulty swallowing, excess sweating	1/32
Gaucher disease	Enlarged liver and spleen, bone degeneration, nervous system impairment	1/12
Niemann-Pick disease type A	Lipid accumulation in cells, particularly in the brain; mental and physical retardation, death by age three	1/90
Tay-Sachs disease	Brain degeneration causing developmental retardation, paralysis, blindness, death by age four	1/26
Fanconi anemia type C	Deficiencies of all blood cell types, poor growth, increased cancer risk	1/89

Both of these factors—nonrandom mating and population bottlenecks—changed allele frequencies and contributed to the high incidence of certain inherited diseases seen among the Ashkenazim today. Several genetic testing companies offer "Jewish genetic disease" panels that are not meant to discriminate or stereotype, but are based on a genetic fact of life—some illnesses are more common in certain populations.

Key Concepts

Genetic drift occurs when a subset of a population contains different allele frequencies than the larger population because it is a small sample. • The founder effect occurs when a few individuals leave a community to start a new settlement. The resulting population may, by chance, either lack some alleles present in the original population or have high frequencies of others. • In a population bottleneck, many members of a population die, and only a few individuals contribute genetically to the next generation.

15.4 Mutation

A major and continual source of genetic variation is mutation—when one allele changes into another. (Chapters 12 and 13 discussed mutation.) Genetic variability also arises from crossing over and independent assortment during meiosis, but these events recombine existing traits rather than introduce new ones. If a DNA base change occurs in a part of a gene that encodes a portion of a protein necessary for its function, then an altered trait may result. If the mutation occurs in a gamete, then the change can pass to future generations and affect an allele's frequency in the population.

Natural selection eliminates deleterious alleles that are expressed in the phenotype and affect an individual's ability to reproduce. Yet these alleles are maintained in heterozygotes, where they do not exert a noticeable effect, and are reintroduced by new mutation. Therefore, all populations have some alleles that would be harmful if homozygous. The collection of such deleterious alleles in a population is called its **genetic load.**

Overall, the contribution that mutation makes to counter Hardy-Weinberg equilibrium is quite small compared to the influence of migration and nonrandom mating. The spontaneous mutation rate is only about 30 bases per haploid genome in each gamete. Each of us probably has only 5 to 10 recessive lethal alleles. Fortunately, most mutations do not alter the phenotype due to the degeneracy of the genetic code and changes that do not alter protein function. Some mutations actually increase the chance of survival, such as the *CCR5* mutation that blocks infection by HIV and the bacterium that causes plague (see figure 17.13).

Key Concepts

Mutation alters gene frequencies by introducing new alleles. Heterozygotes and mutations maintain the frequencies of deleterious alleles in populations, even if homozygotes die.

15.5 Natural Selection

Environmental change can alter allele frequencies when individuals with certain phenotypes are more likely to survive and reproduce than others. This differential survival based on phenotype, and therefore genotype, is called **natural selection.** It may be negative—removal of alleles—or positive—retention of alleles. For example, gene variants that confer the ability to taste bitter substances tend to be more prevalent where the environment includes toxin-containing plants that people might eat. Since toxins often taste bitter, those with more sensitive palates would be more likely to taste, and spit out, poisons—and live to transmit those genes.

The appearance or reemergence of infectious diseases can reveal the effect of natural selection on allele frequencies. If such an illness kills before reproductive age or impairs fertility, its spread will ultimately remove from the population gene variants that make an individual susceptible to infection. It will be interesting to track changes in allele frequencies in years to come that result from populationwide exposure to the virus that causes the apparently new severe acute respiratory syndrome (SARS) if it spreads. **Table 15.5** lists the changes that have accompanied the spread of West Nile virus infection.

Table 15.5

Evolution of an Emerging Infectious Disease: West Nile Virus (WNV)

Year	Event
1937	"Old World" WNV infects but does not kill birds in Uganda.
early 1990s	Virus mutates and spreads more rapidly among birds.
1996	WNV variant identified in Romania in humans.
1998	Dead goose in Israel has new variant of WNV.
1999	"New World" WNV sickens several New York City residents, possibly through an Israeli goose.
2000	WNV spreads rapidly throughout the U.S., killing thousands of birds and horses. Humans infected.
2002	New World WNV is genetically different from 1999 strain. Human case count in U.S.: 4,156 sick, 284 fatalities.

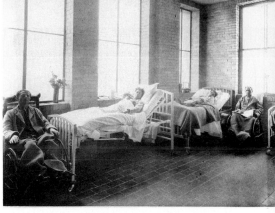

a.

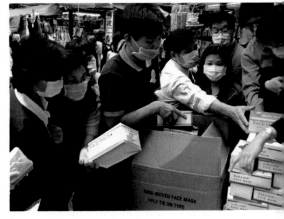

b.

Figure 15.5 Infectious diseases involve allele frequency changes in the pathogen and the host. (a) Early in the twentieth century, tuberculosis was controlled by isolating infected people in sanitaria. TB has returned, due to complacency and ease of infection among immunosuppressed individuals.
(b) Severe acute respiratory syndrome (SARS) was first noted in China in late 2002, and the responsible virus identified and its genome sequenced in record time. But initial population studies were confined to those with obvious infections. Perhaps individuals elsewhere who developed fevers and coughs in 2003 also had the illness, but were simply not tested.

Tuberculosis Ups and Downs—and Ups

The spread of tuberculosis (TB) in the Plains Indians of the Qu'Appelle Valley Reservation in Saskatchewan, Canada, strikingly illustrates natural selection. When TB first appeared there in the mid-1880s, it struck swiftly and lethally, infecting many organs. Ten percent of the population died. But by 1921, TB tended to affect only the lungs, and only 7 percent of the population died annually from it. By 1950, mortality was down to 0.2 percent.

Outbreaks of TB ran similar courses in other human populations. The disease appeared in crowded settlements where the bacteria easily spread from person to person in exhaled droplets. In the 1700s, TB raged through the cities of Europe. Immigrants brought it to the United States in the early 1800s, where it also swept the cities. Many people thought TB was hereditary until German bacteriologist Robert Koch identified the causative bacterium in 1882.

As in the Plains Indians, TB incidence and virulence fell dramatically in the cities of the industrialized world in the first half of the twentieth century—before antibiotic drugs were discovered. What tamed tuberculosis?

Natural selection, operating on both the bacterial and human populations, lessened the virulence of the infection. Some people inherited resistance and passed this beneficial trait on. At the same time, the most virulent bacteria killed their hosts so quickly that the victims had no time to spread the infection. As the deadliest bacteria were selected out of the population (negative selection), and as people who inherited resistance mutations contributed disproportionately to the next generation (positive selection), TB gradually evolved from a severe, acute, systemic infection to a rare chronic lung infection. This was true until the late 1980s.

A series of recent unrelated events has created conditions just right for the resurgence of TB, but in a form resistant to many of the eleven drugs used to treat it. Some health officials trace the return of tuberculosis to complacency; researchers turned to other projects when funding became scarce for this seemingly controlled disease. Patients became complacent, too. When antibiotics eased symptoms in two to three months, patients felt cured and stopped taking the drugs, even though they unknowingly continued to spread live bacteria for up to 18 months. The *Mycobacterium tuberculosis* bacteria had time to mutate, and mutant strains to flourish, eventually evolving the drug resistances that make the newest cases so difficult to treat (Reading 15.1). Tuberculosis treatment in the 1950s was actually more effective; patients were isolated for a year or longer in rest homes called sanitaria and were not released until the bacteria were gone (**figure 15.5**).

Today, 1 in 7 new tuberculosis cases is resistant to several drugs, and 5 percent of these patients die. People living in crowded, unsanitary conditions with poor health care are especially susceptible to drug-resistant TB. Another reservoir of new TB infection is persons infected with HIV. Tuberculosis develops so quickly in people with suppressed immunity that it can kill before physicians have determined which drugs to use—physicians have died of the infection while treating patients. The resurgence of TB should remind us never to underestimate the fact that evolution operates in all organisms—and does so unpredictably.

Antibiotic Resistance—Stemming a Biological Arms Race

The sudden appearance of an infectious disease often reflects evolution. Natural selection may favor persistence of a particular pathogen under certain environmental conditions, or a bacterium or virus may be brought to a new part of the world where host populations have not evolved resistance. Infectious diseases that were once prevalent are resurging, including diphtheria, tuberculosis, dengue, cholera, and yellow fever (**figure 1**). Infections spreading to new places include West Nile virus, SARS, and monkeypox.

Mutation also plays a role in the appearance or resurgence of an infectious disease. Bacteria and viruses can mutate in a way that enables them to produce a new toxin, infect a new species, or exist in novel places. Changes in weather patterns caused by global warming may be responsible for some recent shifts in infectious disease patterns. Unfortunately, we cannot do much to prevent mutation—it is a consequence of DNA replication. We can, however, intervene at the level of natural selection, countering environmental changes that favor pathogens.

The current crisis of antibiotic-resistant infectious bacteria illustrates the interplay

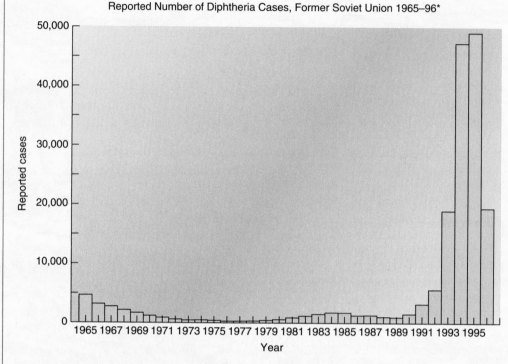

Reported Number of Diphtheria Cases, Former Soviet Union 1965–96*

Figure 1   Diphtheria—an old foe returns.   In the former Soviet Union, incomplete vaccination of the population caused the reemergence of a toxic strain of diphtheria. Crowded conditions and forced migrations helped spread the infection. Diphtheria causes a white coating of the throat, along with a fever and cough; it may also affect the skin, heart, kidneys, and nervous tissue.

*Source: CDC, Emerging Infectious Disease, vol. 4, no. 4, October–December, 1998.

Evolving HIV

Because the RNA or DNA of viruses replicates often and is not repaired, viral mutations accumulate rapidly. Like bacteria, the viruses in a human body form a population, including naturally occurring genetic variants. In HIV infection, natural selection controls the diversity of HIV genetic variants within a human body as the disease progresses. The human immune system and drugs to slow the infection become the environmental factors that select (favor) resistant viral variants.

HIV infection can be divided into three stages, both from the human and the viral perspective (**figure 15.6**). A person infected with HIV may experience an initial acute phase, with symptoms of fever, night sweats, rash, and swollen glands. In a second period, lasting from 2 to 15 years, health usually returns. In a third stage, immunity collapses, the virus replicates explosively, and opportunistic infections and cancer eventually cause death.

The HIV population changes and expands throughout the course of infection, even when the patient seems to maintain the same condition for long periods of time. New mutants continuously arise, and they alter such traits as speed of replication and the patterns of molecules on the viral surface.

In the first stage of HIV infection, as the person battles acute symptoms, viral variants that replicate swiftly predominate. In the second stage, the immune system starts to fight back and symptoms abate, as viral replication slows and many viruses are destroyed. Now natural selection acts—those viral variants that persist reproduce and mutate, giving rise to a diverse viral population. Ironically, drugs used to treat AIDS may further select against the weakest HIV variants. Gradually, the HIV population overtakes the immune system cells, but years may pass before immunity begins to noticeably decline.

The third stage, full-blown AIDS, occurs when the virus overwhelms the immune

of mutation and natural selection in the spread of infectious disease. Bacteria in a human body constitute a population of organisms that includes different genetic variants. Some bacterial strains inherit the ability to survive in the presence of a particular antibiotic drug. When the bacteria infect a person, the immune system responds, causing such symptoms as inflammation and fever. The person goes to the doctor, and a course of antibiotics seems to help; but a month later, symptoms return. What has happened?

The drug probably killed most of the bacteria, but a few survived because they have a fortuitous (for them) mutation that enables them to withstand the antibiotic assault. Over a few weeks, as sensitive bacteria die, those few mutants reproduce, taking over the niche the antibiotic-sensitive bacteria vacated. Soon, the person has enough antibiotic-resistant bacteria to feel ill again. The next step is to try a drug that works differently—and hope that the bacteria haven't mutated around that one, too. Antibiotic resistance is, in a sense, a biological arms race.

Antibiotic drugs do not cause mutations in bacteria; they select for preexisting resistant variants. (This doesn't happen in viruses because viruses are not cells, and antibiotics have no effect on them.) Bacteria with drug-resistance mutations circumvent antibiotic actions in several ways. Penicillin kills bacteria by tearing apart their cell walls. Resistant microbes produce enzyme variants that dismantle penicillin, or have altered cell walls that the drug cannot bind. Erythromycin, streptomycin, tetracycline, and gentamicin kill bacteria by attacking their ribosomes, which are different from ribosomes in a human. Drug-resistant bacteria have altered ribosomes that the drugs cannot bind.

Bacteria acquire antibiotic resistance in several ways. Their DNA may spontaneously mutate—this is how drug-resistant tuberculosis arose. They may receive a resistance gene from another bacterium in a process called transformation—this is how the sexually transmitted disease gonorrhea gained resistance to penicillin. Bacteria can acquire resistance to several drugs at once by taking up a small circle of DNA, called a plasmid, from another bacterium. Not only can plasmids transmit multiple drug resistances, but they flit freely from one species of bacteria to another.

Practical steps to halt the growing threat of antibiotic-resistant bacteria include:

- Limiting antibiotic use to bacterial infections diagnosed by a physician.

- Taking the full schedule of doses so that the infection does not return in a drug-resistant form.

- Developing new antibiotic drugs. Many models for new pharmaceuticals come from natural products. Therefore, preserving natural habitats can help to preserve potential sources of new anti-infective agents.

- Improving public health measures. These include having health care workers wash their hands frequently and thoroughly, rapidly identifying and isolating patients with drug-resistant infections, improving sewage systems and water purity, and using clean needles.

system. Now, with the selective pressure off, viral diversity again diminishes, and the fastest-replicating variants predominate. HIV wins. The entire scenario of HIV infection reflects the value of genetic diversity—to enable the survival of a population or species in the face of an environmental threat. When that threat—an immune attack or drugs—diminishes, one genotype may come to prevail.

Knowing that HIV diversifies early in the course of infection has yielded clinical benefits. Patients now take combinations of drugs that act in different ways to squelch several viral variants simultaneously, slowing the course of the infection.

Balanced Polymorphism

If natural selection eliminates individuals with detrimental phenotypes from a population, then how do harmful mutant alleles remain in a gene pool? Harmful recessive alleles are replaced in two ways: by new mutation, and by persistence in heterozygotes.

Sometimes, a recessive condition remains particularly prevalent because the heterozygote enjoys some unrelated health advantage, such as being resistant to an infectious disease or able to survive an environmental threat. This "heterozygous advantage" that maintains a recessive, dis-

ease-causing allele in a population is called **balanced polymorphism.** Recall that *polymorphism* means variant; the effect is *balanced* because the protective effect of the noninherited condition counters the negative effect of the deleterious allele, maintaining its frequency in the population. (Balanced polymorphism is a type of balancing selection, which more generally refers to maintaining heterozygotes in a population.)

Sickle Cell Disease and Malaria

Recall that sickle cell disease is an autosomal recessive disorder that causes anemia,

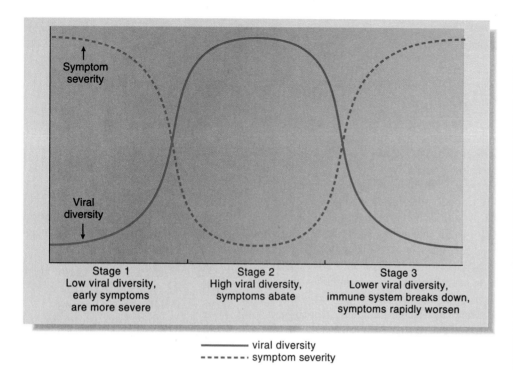

viral diversity
- - - - - symptom severity

Figure 15.6 Natural selection of HIV Natural selection controls the genetic diversity of an HIV population in a person's body. Before the immune system gathers strength, and after it breaks down, HIV diversity is low. A rapidly reproducing viral strain predominates, although new mutations continually arise. During the 2- to 15-year latency period, viral variants that can evade the immune system gradually accumulate.

joint pain, a swollen spleen, and frequent, severe infections (see figure 2.1c). It is the classic example of balanced polymorphism: carriers are resistant to malaria, or develop very mild cases. Malaria is an infection by the parasite *Plasmodium falciparum* that causes debilitating cycles of chills and fever. The parasite spends the first stage of its life cycle in the salivary glands of the mosquito *Anopheles gambiae.* When an infected mosquito bites a human, malaria parasites enter red blood cells, which transport them to the liver. The red blood cells burst, releasing parasites throughout the body.

In people with sickle cell disease, many of the red blood cells burst prematurely, which expels the parasites before they can cause rampant infection. The blood of a person with sickle cell disease is also thicker than normal, which may hamper the parasite's ability to infect. A sickle cell disease carrier's blood is abnormal enough to be inhospitable to the malaria parasite.

A clue to the protective effect of sickle cell disease heterozygosity came from striking differences in the incidence of the

two diseases in different parts of the world (**figure 15.7**). In the United States, 8 percent of African Americans are sickle cell carriers, whereas in parts of Africa, up to 45 to 50 percent are carriers. In 1949, British geneticist Anthony Allison found that the frequency of sickle cell carriers in tropical Africa was higher in regions where malaria rages all year long. Blood tests from children hospitalized with malaria showed that nearly all were homozygous for the wild type sickle cell allele. The few sickle cell carriers among them had the mildest cases of malaria. Was malaria enabling the sickle cell allele to persist by felling people who did not inherit it? The fact that sickle cell disease is rarer where malaria is rare supports the idea that sickle cell heterozygosity protects against the infection.

The sickle cell allele may have been brought to Africa by people migrating from Southern Arabia and India, or it may have arisen directly by mutation in East Africa. However it happened, people who inherited one copy of the sickle cell allele

survived or never contracted malaria. These carriers had more children and passed the protective allele to approximately half of them. Gradually, the frequency of the sickle cell allele in East Africa rose from 0.1 percent to 45 percent in 35 generations. Carriers paid the price for this genetic protection, however, whenever two of them produced a child with sickle cell disease.

Glucose-6-Phosphate Dehydrogenase Deficiency and Malaria

Recall from chapter 12 that G6PD deficiency is an X-linked recessive enzyme deficiency that causes life-threatening hemolytic anemia under specific conditions, such as eating fava beans or taking certain drugs. Among African children with severe malaria, heterozygous females ($X^G X^g$) and affected (hemizygous) males ($X^g Y$) for G6PD deficiency are underrepresented. This suggests that carrying or inheriting G6PD deficiency protects against malaria. Cell culture studies confirm that the parasite enters the red blood cells of carriers or affected males but cannot reproduce sufficiently to cause infection.

The fact that G6PD deficiency is X-linked introduces a possibility not seen with sickle cell disease, which is an autosomal recessive disorder. Because in G6PD deficiency heterozygotes and hemizygotes (males with the disease) have an advantage, the mutant allele should eventually predominate in a malaria-exposed population as homozygotes and hemizygotes for the normal allele die of malaria. However, this doesn't happen—there are still males hemizygous and females homozygous for the normal allele. The reason again relates to natural selection.

Table 15.6 shows how natural selection acts in two directions on the two types of hemizygous males—selecting for the mutant allele because it protects against malarial infection, yet also selecting for the normal allele because it protects against an enzyme deficiency. This is the "balance" of balanced polymorphism.

Studies of different G6PD mutations in different populations confirm that the

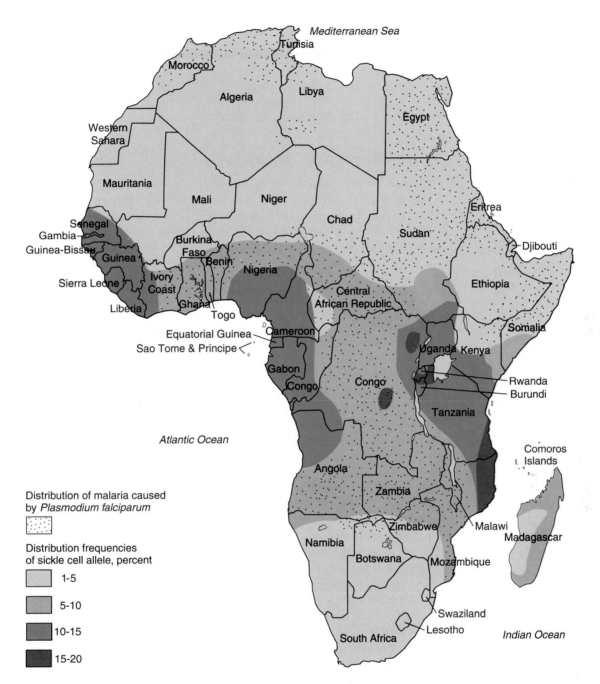

Figure 15.7 Balanced polymorphism. Comparing the distribution of people with malaria and people with sickle cell disease in Africa reveals balanced polymorphism. Carriers for sickle cell disease are resistant to malaria because changes in the blood caused by the sickle cell allele are not severe enough to impair health, but do inhibit the malaria parasite.

Table 15.6

G6PD Deficiency Protects Against Malaria

Genotypic Class	Enzyme Deficiency	Malaria Susceptibility
Normal male X^GY	no	yes
G6PD male X^gY	yes	no
Heterozygous female X^GX^g	no	no
Homozygous female X^GX^G	no	yes
Homozygous female X^gX^g	yes	no

beginning of a mutation's prevalence coincides with the onset of agriculture. These protective mutations are only seen where agriculture and malaria coexist— that is, the mutations do not accumulate where farming exists but not malaria. One researcher wrote that G6PD and malaria offer "a striking example of the signature of selection on the human genome."

PKU and Fungal Infection

Being a heterozygote for the autosomal recessive condition phenylketonuria (PKU) may protect a fetus from fungal infection. In PKU, a missing enzyme causes the amino acid phenylalanine to build up, which devastates the nervous system unless the individual avoids eating the amino acid. Carriers have elevated phenylalanine levels—not sufficient to cause symptoms, but high enough to lower the risk of miscarriage by inactivating a fungal poison, ochratoxin A.

Historical evidence links PKU heterozygosity to protection against a fungal toxin. PKU is most common in Ireland and western Scotland, and many affected families living elsewhere trace their roots to this part of the world. PKU spread eastward in Europe when the Vikings brought wives and slaves back from the Celtic lands. In the moist environment of Ireland and Scotland, the fungi that produce ochratoxin A— *Aspergillis* and *Penicillium*—grow on grains. During the famines that have plagued these nations, starving people ate moldy grain. If PKU carriers were more likely to have children than noncarriers because of the protective effects of the PKU gene, over time, the disease-causing allele would have increased prevalence in this population.

Prion Disease and Cannibalism

Being a heterozygote for the prion protein gene may protect against the disorders of protein folding called transmissible spongiform encephalopathies (see figures 10.18 and 10.19, Reading 10.1, and section 12.4). The best studied such illness is kuru, which caused brain degeneration among the Foré people in Papua, New Guinea until the Australian government halted the practice of ritual cannibalism in the mid-1950s. A recent investigation of the prion protein gene among 30 elderly Foré women who had participated in many of the brain-eating feasts revealed more heterozygotes than would exist if the gene were in Hardy-Weinberg equilibrium. That is, the excess suggests natural selection at work. Specifically, of the 30 women, 23 are heterozygotes; 15 would have been expected if selection was not acting on this gene, based on Hardy-Weinberg equilibrium observed among 140 Foré who had not participated in the ritual. In the heterozygotes, some of the normal prion proteins have a valine at amino acid position 129, and some a methionine. The presence of two amino acids, encoded one on each homolog in a heterozygote, apparently prevents the infectious misfolding that occurs to the prion protein when a person encounters an abnormal prion protein—as happens in cannibalism. (All of the people in the United Kingdom who have developed variant CJD, the human form of "mad cow disease," have only methionine at position 129.)

The overrepresentation of heterozygotes among the Foré survivors led to the hypothesis that balancing selection has favored this genotype in the population, and that canni-

balism may have been the driving force. That is, homozygotes who were cannibals died of a prion disorder before reproducing, leaving the resistant heterozygotes to slowly accumulate in the population. John Collinge, at the Medical Research Council in London, who has proposed this idea, took it one controversial step farther— attributing the finding that heterozygote frequency for this gene varies greatly in different populations to past cannibalism in some of those populations.

This new genetic view of cannibalism supports anthropological evidence that eating human flesh has occurred in many times and places in human prehistory and history. Evidence of cannibalism is found in Neanderthal caves in France and Croatia, in the American Southwest, and even in the records of the famous Donner Party forced to engage in the practice when stranded in the Sierra Nevada during the winter of 1846–47. Evidence of cannibalism is human bones damaged in ways similar to the bones of animals prepared for consumption, such as scratch marks to remove muscle and signs of breaking and crushing to obtain marrow. Biochemical evidence for past cannibalism includes human myoglobin, found only in human muscle, in fossilized human excrement.

Cystic Fibrosis and Diarrheal Disease

Balanced polymorphism may explain why cystic fibrosis is so common—the cellular defect that underlies CF protects against diarrheal illnesses such as cholera and typhus.

Diarrheal disease epidemics have left their mark on many human populations. Severe diarrhea rapidly dehydrates the body and leads to shock, kidney and heart failure, and death in days. In cholera, bacteria produce a toxin that opens chloride channels in cells of the small intestine. As salt (NaCl) leaves the intestinal cells, water rushes out, producing diarrhea. Cholera opens chloride channels, releasing chloride (in salt) and water. The CFTR protein does just the opposite, closing chloride channels and trapping salt and water in cells, which dries out mucus and other secretions. A person with CF is very unlikely to contract cholera, because the toxin cannot open the chloride channels in the small intestine cells.

CF carriers enjoy the mixed blessing of balanced polymorphism. They do not have enough abnormal chloride channels to cause the labored breathing and clogged pancreas of cystic fibrosis, but they do have enough of a defect to prevent the cholera toxin from taking hold. During the devastating cholera epidemics that have occurred throughout history, individuals carrying mutant CF alleles had a selective advantage, and they disproportionately transmitted those alleles to future generations.

However, because CF arose in western Europe and cholera originated in Africa, an initial increase in CF heterozygosity may have been a response to a different diarrheal infection—typhoid fever. The causative bacterium, *Salmonella typhi*, rather than producing a toxin, enters cells lining the small intestine—but only if functional CFTR channels are present (see figure 2.1*b*). The cells of people with severe CF manufacture CFTR proteins that never reach the cell surface, and therefore no bacteria get in. Cells of CF carriers admit some bacteria.

Diabetes Mellitus and Surviving Famine

Type II (non-insulin-dependent) diabetes mellitus (NIDDM) is a gradual failure of cells to respond to insulin and take up glucose from the bloodstream. It is a complex trait—a first-degree relative has a tenfold increased risk of developing the condition. Studies on many populations indicate that a person can inherit a susceptibility to develop NIDDM that becomes reality only if the diet is unhealthy or lifestyle sedentary, such as Arizona's Pima Indians (see figure 7.15).

The "thrifty genotype" hypothesis suggests that NIDDM is common today because the gene or genes that predispose to it might once have been beneficial, a variation on the balanced polymorphism theme. The reasoning is that NIDDM prevents the breakdown of fat and alters the body's ability to store glucose. In times past, extra fat stores and altered glucose metabolism enabled people to survive famine. Today, these abilities cause weight gain and diabetes.

P-Glycoprotein and Resistance to AIDS Drugs

Selection is a response to environmental change. When an environment changes, a trait that has been selected for may no longer be advantageous. This is the case for a gene, *MDR1,* that encodes the protein portion of a glycoprotein (called P-glycoprotein) that dots the surfaces of intestinal lining cells and T lymphocytes. An allele that causes overexpression of the gene became prevalent in some populations because the encoded protein enables cells to pump out poisons such as naturally occurring toxins in plants. But in the different circumstance of intentionally taking a poison—such as a drug to combat cancer—these pumps lose their value. A population-based study reveals that variants in this gene may explain why drugs to fight HIV infection are less effective in Africans than in other groups.

Researchers identified a polymorphism in an exon of the *MDR1* gene that correlates with overexpression, creating an allele called *C.* Another allele that leads to very few P-glycoproteins is called *T.* The resulting genotypes and phenotypes are therefore:

TT (very few P-glycoproteins)

TC (intermediate number of P-glycoproteins)

CC (many P-glycoproteins)

Researchers genotyped 172 individuals from West Africa, 41 African Americans, 537 Caucasians, and 50 Japanese, all healthy. The results were startling **(figure 15.8).** The *CC* genotype is clearly overrepresented among West Africans (83%) and African Americans (61%), compared to Caucasians (26%) and Japanese (34%). The finding makes sense in terms of natural selection—the *CC* genotype confers resistance to many bacteria and viruses that cause gastroenteritis, a major killer of children in Africa. But the same genotype ejects chemotherapeutic drugs, AIDS drugs, and antirejection transplant drugs.

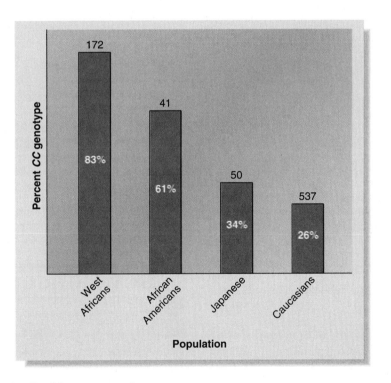

Figure 15.8 Resistance genotypes. An advantageous trait can turn disadvantageous when the environment changes. The *C/C* genotype of the *MDR1* gene enables a person's cells to pump out poisons. The genotype became prevalent in populations with African ancestry, possibly because it protected against viral and bacterial infections of the gastrointestinal tract in the African environment. Today, the same genotype may hamper the efficacy of AIDS drugs.

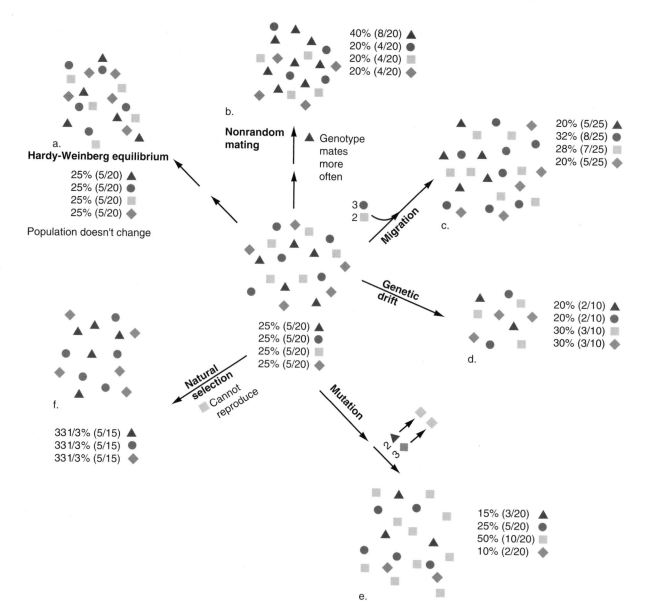

Figure 15.9 **Forces that change allele frequencies.** Several factors alter allele frequencies and thereby contribute to microevolution. The different-colored shapes represent individuals with distinctive genotypes. **(a)** In Hardy-Weinberg equilibrium, allele frequencies stay constant. **(b)** Nonrandom mating increases some allele frequencies and decreases others because individuals with certain genotypes mate more often than others. **(c)** Migration removes alleles from or adds alleles to populations. **(d)** Genetic drift samples a portion of a population, altering allele frequencies. **(e)** Mutation changes some alleles into others. **(f)** Natural selection operates when environmental conditions lower the probability that individuals of certain genotypes will reproduce.

Using this information, physicians will be able to identify people with the *CC* genotype, and perhaps give them higher doses of certain drugs.

The forces of nonrandom mating, migration, genetic drift, mutation, and natural selection interact in complex ways. **Figure 15.9** reviews and summarizes the forces that alter allele frequencies and therefore impact evolution. Reading 15.2 looks at intentional shrinking of gene pools—the "artificial selection" used to breed cats and dogs.

Key Concepts

Because of natural selection, different alleles are more likely to confer a survival advantage in different environments. Cycles of infectious disease prevalence and virulence often reflect natural selection.
• Balanced polymorphism is a type of natural selection in which a particular disease-causing allele is maintained or increases in a population because heterozygotes resist a certain infectious illness or environmental condition.

15.6   Gene Genealogy

Identifying different mutations in a gene is useful in charting the evolution and spread of genetic variants. An assumption in deciphering gene origins is that the more prevalent an allele is, the more ancient it is, because it has had more time to spread and accumulate in a population. Correlating allele frequencies with historical, archeological, and linguistic evidence provides fascinating peeks at the evolution of modern peoples.

Dogs and Cats: Products of Artificial Selection

The pampered poodle may win in the show ring, but it is a poor specimen in terms of genetics and evolution. Human notions of attractiveness in pets can lead to breeds that might never have evolved naturally. Behind carefully bred traits lurk small gene pools and extensive inbreeding—all of which spell disaster to the health of many highly prized and highly priced show animals. Purebred dogs suffer from more than 300 types of inherited disorders!

The sad eyes of the basset hound make him a favorite in advertisements, but his runny eyes can hurt. Short legs make him prone to arthritis, his long abdomen causes back injuries, and his floppy ears often hide infection. The eyeballs of the Pekingese protrude so much that a mild bump can pop them out of their sockets. The tiny jaws and massive teeth of bulldogs cause dental and breathing problems, as well as sinusitis, bad colds, and "dog breath." Larger breeds, such as the Saint Bernard, have bone problems and short life spans.

The modern dog closest to what canines were like before people controlled their breeding is the dingo, the wild dog of Australia. It was introduced from southeast Asia in a tiny founder population, about 5,000 years ago.

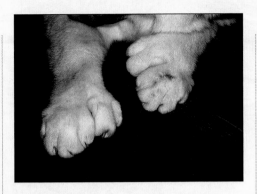

Figure 1 Multitoed cats are common in New England but rare elsewhere.

We artificially select natural oddities in cats, too. One of every 10 New England cats has six or seven toes on each paw, thanks to a multitoed ancestor in colonial Boston (**figure 1**). Elsewhere, these cats are rare. The sizes of the blotched tabby populations in New England, Canada, Australia, and New Zealand correlate with the time that has passed since cat-loving Britons colonized each region. The Vikings brought the orange tabby to the islands off the coast of Scotland, rural Iceland, and the Isle of Man, where these feline favorites flourished.

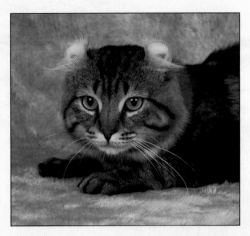

Figure 2 An American curl cat.

The American curl cat's origin traces back to a stray female who wandered into the home of a cat-loving family in Lakewood, California, in 1981 and passed her unusual, curled-up ears to future generations (**figure 2**). The cause—a dominant gene that leads to formation of extra cartilage lining the outer ear. Cat breeders hope that the gene does not have other less lovable effects. Cats with floppy ears, for example, tend to have large feet, stubbed tails, and lazy natures.

PKU Revisited

The diversity of PKU mutations suggests that the disease has arisen more than once. Mutations common to many groups of people probably represent more ancient mutational events, which perhaps occurred before many groups spread into disparate populations. This was the case for CJD among groups that left Spain in the Middle Ages, mentioned earlier in the chapter. In contrast, mutations found only in a small geographical region, or perhaps in a single family, are more likely to be of recent origin. They have had less time to spread. For example, Turks, Norwegians, French Canadians, and Yemenite Jews have their own PKU alleles. Analysis of the frequencies of PKU mutations in different populations, plus logic, can reveal the roles that genetic drift, mutation, and balanced polymorphism have played in maintaining the mutation.

A high mutation rate cannot be the sole reason for the continued prevalence of PKU because some countries, such as Denmark, continue to have only one or two mutations. If the gene were unstable, so that it mutated frequently, all populations would have several different types of PKU mutations. This is not the case.

In some isolated populations, such as French Canadians and Yemenite Jews, migration and the founder effect have maintained certain PKU alleles. Consider the history of PKU among Yemenite Jews.

In most populations, point mutations in the phenylalanine hydroxylase (*PAH*) gene cause PKU. Virtually all of the Yemenite Jews in Israel who have PKU instead have a 6,700-base deletion in the third exon of the *PAH* gene. An eclectic group of researchers—including geneticists, cell biologists, Jewish history scholars, and pediatricians—traced the spread of this PKU mutation from North Africa to Israel.

The researchers tested for the telltale deletion in the grandparents of the 22 modern Yemenite Jewish families with PKU in Israel. By asking questions and consulting court and religious records, which this close-knit community kept meticulously, the team found that all clues pointed to

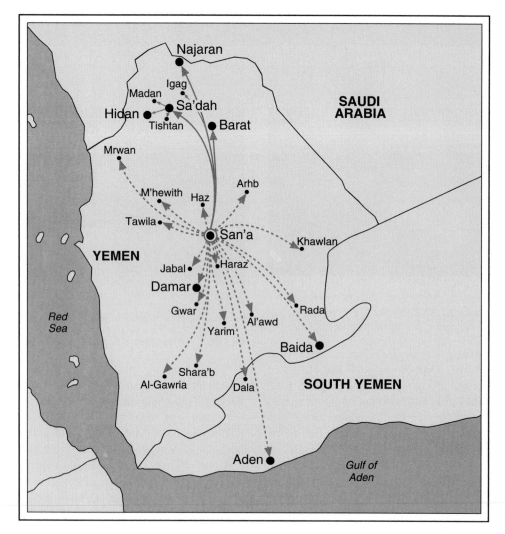

Figure 15.10 **The origin of PKU.** The exon 3 deletion in Israeli Yemenite Jews probably arose in San'a, Yemen, in the mid–18th century. The allele spread northward as families moved from San'a in 1809 (solid arrows) and subsequently spread to other regions (broken arrows).
Source: Data from Smadar Avigad, et al., A single origin of phenylketonuria in Yemenite Jews, *Nature* 344:170, March 8, 1990.

San'a, the capital of Yemen. The earliest records identify two families with PKU in San'a, and indicate that the mutation originated in one person before 1800. By 1809, religious persecution and hard economic times led nine families carrying the mutation to migrate north and settle in three towns (**figure 15.10**). Four of the families then moved farther northward, into four more towns. Twenty more families spread from San'a to inhabit 17 other towns. All of this migration took place from 1762 through the mid-1900s, and eventually led to Israel.

A more recent example of the effect history and politics can have on gene frequency is the influx of families with PKU into northwest Germany after the second world war, when Germans from the east moved westward. Future shifts in allele frequencies may parallel the breakdown of the former Soviet Union.

CF Revisited

Tracing allele distributions in modern populations known to have very ancient roots offers clues to how early genetic disorders plagued humankind. For example, the CF allele $\Delta F508$ is very prevalent among northern Europeans, but not as common in the south (**figure 15.11**). This distribution might mean that early farmers migrating from the Middle East to Europe in the Neolithic period, up until about 10,000 years ago, brought the allele to Europe. At this time, people were just beginning to give up a hunter-gatherer lifestyle for semipermanent settlements, exhibiting the first activities of agriculture.

The origin, or at least the existence, of $\Delta F508$ may go farther back, to the Paleolithic age more than 10,000 years ago. People then were hunter-gatherers who occasionally lived in caves and tents. They used tools of chipped stone, followed a lunar calendar, and created magnificent cave art.

Geneticists were led back to the Paleolithic by an intriguing group of people, the Basques. Researchers studied 45 families from the Basque country (in the mountains between France and Spain) with cystic fibrosis and identified affected children with four pure Basque grandparents by their distinctive double surnames. For 87 percent of the pure Basque CF patients, $\Delta F508$ was the causative mutation—a frequency higher than for most European populations, indicating a more ancient origin. Families of "mixed Basque" background, whose Basque ancestors interbred with French or Spanish neighbors, showed $\Delta F508$ only 58.3 percent of the time. Among the nearby Spanish population, the frequency of $\Delta F508$ is 50 percent. Today's remaining Basque people, then, may carry a pocket of cystic fibrosis mutations that arose long ago.

Key Concepts

Mutational analysis in various populations indicates that PKU originated more than once, and that genetic drift, balanced polymorphism, and perhaps mutation have affected its prevalence. Studies of allele prevalence place the origin of cystic fibrosis farther back in history than once thought.

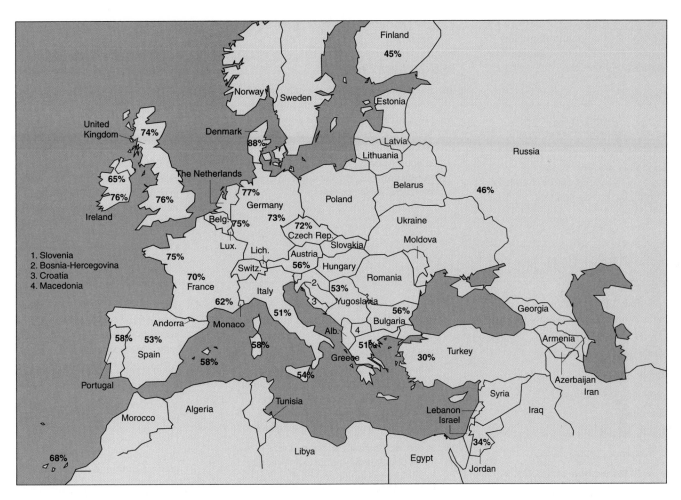

Figure 15.11 CF allele frequencies vary. The most common allele causing cystic fibrosis, ∆F508, occurs with vastly different frequencies in different populations. This map indicates the percentage of CF alleles that are ∆F508 in these nations.
Source: European Working Group on Cystic Fibrosis Genetics, Gradient of distribution in Europe of the major CF mutation and of its associated haplotype, *Human Genetics* 85:436–45, 1990.

Summary

15.1 Nonrandom Mating

1. Hardy-Weinberg equilibrium assumes that all individuals mate with the same frequency and choose mates without regard to phenotype. This rarely, if ever, happens in real human populations. We choose mates based on certain characteristics, and some individuals have many more children than others.

2. DNA sequences that do not cause a phenotype important in mate selection or reproduction may be in Hardy-Weinberg equilibrium.

3. Consanguinity increases the proportion of homozygotes in a population, which may lead to increased incidence of recessive illnesses or traits.

15.2 Migration

4. **Clines** are changes in allele frequencies from one geographic area to another.

5. Clines may reflect geographical barriers or linguistic differences and may be either abrupt or gradual.

6. Human migration patterns through history explain many cline boundaries. Forces behind migration include escape from persecution and a nomadic lifestyle.

15.3 Genetic Drift

7. **Genetic drift** occurs when a small population separates from a larger one, and its members breed only among themselves, perpetuating allele frequencies that are not characteristic of the ancestral population.

8. Genetic drift is random and may occur within a larger group or apart from it.

9. A **founder effect** is a type of genetic drift that occurs when a few individuals found a settlement and their alleles form a new gene pool, amplifying their alleles and eliminating others.

10. A **population bottleneck** is a narrowing of genetic diversity that occurs after many members of a population die and the few survivors rebuild the gene pool.

15.4 Mutation

11. Mutation continually introduces new alleles into populations. It occurs as a consequence of DNA replication errors.

12. Mutation does not have as great an influence on disrupting Hardy-Weinberg equilibrium as the other factors.

13. The **genetic load** is the collection of deleterious alleles in a population.

15.5 Natural Selection

14. Environmental conditions influence allele frequencies via **natural selection,** as the rise and fall of infectious disease indicates. Alleles that do not enable an individual to reproduce in a particular environment are selected against and diminish in the population, unless conditions change. Beneficial alleles are retained.

15. In **balanced polymorphism,** the frequencies of some deleterious alleles are maintained when heterozygotes have a reproductive advantage under certain conditions, such as resisting an infection.

15.6 Gene Genealogy

16. Frequencies of different mutations in different populations provide information on the natural history of alleles and on the relative importance of nonrandom mating, genetic drift, and natural selection in deviations from Hardy-Weinberg equilibrium.

Review Questions

1. Give examples of how each of the following can alter gene frequencies from Hardy-Weinberg equilibrium:
   a. nonrandom mating
   b. migration
   c. a population bottleneck
   d. mutation

2. Explain the influence of natural selection on
   a. the virulence of tuberculosis.
   b. bacterial resistance to antibiotics.
   c. the changing degree of genetic diversity in an HIV population during infection.
   d. the prevalence of cystic fibrosis.

3. Why is increasing homozygosity in a population detrimental?

4. Explain how misuse of antibiotics can add to the problem of antibiotic-resistant bacteria.

5. Why might a mutant allele that causes an inherited illness when homozygous persist in a population?

6. Give an example of an inherited disease allele that protects against an infectious illness.

7. Porphyria variegata, which resulted from a founder mutation in the Afrikaner population, is inherited as an autosomal dominant with incomplete penetrance. How can this mode of inheritance complicate analysis of the condition?

8. A disease-causing allele that is very rare in most populations is unusually prevalent in a particular population. What type of information might enable you to determine whether the prevalence reflects a founder effect, balanced polymorphism, or a population bottleneck?

9. Provide two examples of how molecular evidence confirms the presence of genetic uniformity.

10. Explain how table 15.2 indicates that genetic drift has occurred among the Dunkers.

11. Would a carrier test to detect the common cystic fibrosis allele ΔF508 be more accurate in France or Finland? Cite a reason for your answer.

12. What type of molecular evidence indicates a founder effect?

13. How does a founder effect differ from a population bottleneck?

14. Describe two scenarios in human populations, one of which accounts for a gradual cline, and one for an abrupt cline.

15. How do genetic drift, nonrandom mating, and natural selection interact?

16. Define:
   a. founder effect
   b. linkage disequilibrium
   c. balanced polymorphism
   d. genetic load

17. How does a knowledge of history, sociology, and anthropology help geneticists to interpret allele frequency data?

Applied Questions

1. About half of the Melanesian people of Papua, New Guinea are resistant to malaria and have shortened glycophorin C proteins, found on the surfaces of red blood cells. These people are homozygous recessive for a deletion in part of the gene. One way the malaria parasite enters red blood cells is through glycophorin C. Normally, the protein anchors the plasma membrane to the cytoskeleton. However, because other proteins do this, too, no symptoms arise from being homozygous recessive for the glycophorin C deletion mutation. Is this an example of balanced polymorphism? Give a reason for your answer.

2. Though some suggest that the ability to taste bitter substances is advantageous in avoiding poisoning, others argue that people who find many foods taste bitter might not eat the vegetables that contain chemicals that protect against cancer. Devise an experiment, perhaps based on population data, to test either hypothesis—that the ability to taste bitter substances is either protective or harmful.

3. Many people think that evolution is the transformation of one species into another, such as chimpanzees to humans, and is "just a theory," to quote a former president. State the genetic definition of microevolution, and give three examples, either from the chapter or from the news, that show evolution is going on right now.

4. The high prevalence of Tay-Sachs disease among the Ashkenazim was once attributed to natural selection—in particular, to a case of balanced polymorphism in which being a carrier protects against respiratory infections. This hypothesis arose from the observation that survivors of the Warsaw ghetto, where Jews were massacred during World War II, did not succumb to tuberculosis and other respiratory illnesses as frequently as other people did. A recent study, however, concluded that the high incidence of Tay-Sachs disease is due to genetic drift, not balanced polymorphism. The evidence is that a dozen other genetic diseases are about equally prevalent in the Ashkenazim. How does this evidence argue against balanced polymorphism?

5. Use the information in chapters 14 and 15 to explain why

   a. porphyria variegata is more prevalent among Afrikaners than other South African populations.

   b. many people among the Cape population in South Africa lose their teeth before age 20.

   c. cystic fibrosis and sickle cell disease remain common Mendelian illnesses.

   d. the Pima Indians have an extremely high incidence of non-insulin-dependent diabetes mellitus.

   e. the Amish in Lancaster County and certain Pakistani groups have a high incidence of genetic diseases that are very rare elsewhere.

   f. the frequency of the allele that causes galactokinase deficiency varies across Europe.

   g. a haplotype associated with Creutzfeldt-Jakob disease is the same in populations from Spain, Chile, Libya, Italy, and Tunisia.

   h. mitochondrial DNA sequences vary gradually in populations along the Nile River valley.

   i. disease-causing *BRCA1* alleles are different in Jewish people of eastern European descent and African Americans.

6. Which principles discussed in this chapter do the following science fiction film plots illustrate?

   a. In *When Worlds Collide,* the Earth is about to be destroyed. One hundred people are selected to colonize a new planet.

   b. In *The Time Machine,* set in the distant future on Earth, one group of people is forced to live on the planet's surface while another group is forced to live in caves. Over many years, they come to look and behave differently. The Morlocks that live below ground have dark skin, dark hair, and are very aggressive, whereas the Eloi that live aboveground are blond, fair-skinned, and meek.

   c. In *Children of the Damned,* all of the women in a small town are suddenly made pregnant by genetically identical beings from another planet.

   d. In *The War of the Worlds,* Martians cannot survive on Earth because they are vulnerable to infection by terrestrial microbes.

7. Treatment for PKU has been so successful that, over the past 30 years, many people who would otherwise have been profoundly mentally retarded have led normal lives and become parents. How has this treatment altered Hardy-Weinberg equilibrium for the mutant alleles that cause PKU?

8. Ashkenazim, French Canadians, and people who live in southwestern Louisiana all have a much higher incidence of Tay-Sachs disease than other populations, yet each of these groups has a different mutation. How is this possible?

9. Syndrome X consists of obesity, type II diabetes, hypertension, and heart disease. Researchers surveyed and sampled blood from nearly all of the 2,188 residents of the Pacific Island of Kosrae, and found that 1,709 of them are part of the same pedigree. The incidence of all of the symptoms of syndrome X is much higher in this population than for other populations. Suggest a reason for this finding, and indicate why it would be difficult to study these particular traits, even in an isolated population.

10. A single allele enables a person to manufacture lactase, the enzyme that digests the milk sugar lactose. People who lack this allele suffer the stomach cramps of lactose intolerance. Most people in societies where everyone drinks a great deal of milk, including northern Europeans and nomadic tribes of Africa and the Middle East, produce the enzyme. Which of the following factors has probably most influenced the frequency of the allele that enables one to digest lactose—migration, mutation, nonrandom mating, or natural selection?

11. People with familial Mediterranean fever have an unusually low incidence of asthma. What force may help maintain this disorder in populations?

12. By which mechanisms discussed in this chapter do the following situations alter Hardy-Weinberg equilibrium?

   a. Ovalocytosis is a rare genetic abnormality that is not only symptomless, but seems to be beneficial. A protein that anchors the red blood cell plasma membrane to the cytoplasm is abnormal, making the membrane unusually rigid. As a result, the parasites that cause malaria cannot enter the red blood cells of individuals with ovalocytosis.

   b. In the mid-1700s, a multitoed male cat from England crossed the sea and settled in Boston, where he left behind quite a legacy of kittens—about half of whom also had six, seven, eight, or even nine digits on their paws. Today, in Boston and nearby regions, multitoed cats are far more common than in other parts of the United States.

   c. Many slaves in the United States arrived in groups from Nigeria, which is an area in Africa with many ethnic subgroups. They landed at a few sites and settled on widely dispersed plantations. Once emancipated, former slaves in the South were free to travel and disperse.

Web Activities

13. Go to http://www.cdc.gov/ncidod/eid/. This is the journal *Emerging Infectious Diseases,* from the U.S. Centers for Disease Control and Prevention. Using this resource, describe an infectious disease that is evolving, and cite the evidence for this.

Case Studies

14. The human population of India is divided into many castes, and the people follow strict rules governing who can marry whom. Researchers from the University of Utah compared several genes among 265 Indians of different castes and 750 people from Africa, Europe, and Asia. The study found that the genes of higher Indian castes most closely resembled those of Europeans, and that the genes of the lowest castes most closely resembled those of Asians. In addition, the study found that maternally inherited genes (mitochondrial DNA) more closely resembled Asian versions of those genes, but paternally inherited genes (on the Y chromosome) more closely resembled European DNA sequences. Construct an historical scenario to account for these observations.

Learn to apply the skills of a genetic counselor with these additional cases found in the *Case Workbook in Human Genetics:*

Type III 3-methyl glutaconic aciduria

Ulnar-mammary syndrome

Suggested Readings

Dayton, Leigh. October 24, 2003. On the trail of the first dingo. *Science* 302:555–56. A founder effect introduced the dingo to Australia, where it reverted to wild ways.

Holden, Constance. February 21, 2003. Mongolian big daddy. *Science* 299:1179. Ghengis Khan left his Y in many modern men.

Lewis, Ricki. June 2, 2003. The bitter truth about PTC tasting. *The Scientist* 17(11):32. Opposite forces are pulling on the prevalence of bitter taste alleles.

Lewis, Ricki. January 7, 2002. SNPs as windows on evolution. *The Scientist* 16(1):16–18. SNP patterns reveal natural selection in action.

Lewis, Ricki, April 16, 2001. Founder populations fuel gene discovery. *The Scientist* 15(8):8. Founder populations enable geneticists to zero in on disease-causing genes.

Lewis, Ricki. April 17, 2000. West Nile Virus—Part II? *The Scientist* 14(8):1. Viruses evolve rapidly because they cannot repair their DNA.

Marshall, Eliot. October 24, 2003. Preventing toxicity with a gene test. *Science* 302:588–90. Different populations have different percentages of people with alleles that render certain drugs toxic.

McKusick, Victor A. March 2000. Ellis-van Creveld syndrome and the Amish. *Nature Genetics* 24:203. McKusick did some of the first genetic studies on the Amish.

May, Robert. August 1995. The rise and fall and rise of tuberculosis. *Nature Medicine,* vol. 1. Natural selection has molded the virulence of this reemerging infection.

Pennisi, Elizabeth. April 11, 2003. Cannibalism and prion disease may have been rampant in ancient humans. *Science* 300:227–28. Heterozygosity for the prion protein gene persists in times of dining on fellow humans.

Risch, Neil, et al. April 2003. Geographic distribution of disease mutations in the Ashkenazi Jewish population supports genetic drift over selection. *American Journal of Human Genetics* 72:812–22. Because all of the "Jewish genetic diseases" have similar allele frequencies, their clustering in this population more likely reflects genetic drift than natural selection.

Sachs, Oliver. 1998. *The Island of the Colorblind.* New York: Random House Vintage Books. The story of Pingelapese blindness.

Schaeffeler, Elke, et al. April 4, 2001. Frequency of C3435T polymorphism of *MDR1* gene in African people. *The Lancet* 358:383–84. A polymorphism that once protected against infection today blocks AIDS drugs.

Tishkoff, Sarah A., et al. July 20, 2001. Haplotype diversity and linkage disequilibrium at human *G6PD:* Recent origin of alleles that confer malarial resistance. *Science* 293:455–62. Rise of the protective *G6PD* allele parallels rise of malaria.

White, Tim D. 2003. Once were cannibals. *Scientific American* Special Edition 13(2):88–93. Evidence for cannibalism lies in bones with telltale marks of intentional damage.

Weekly updates of current news related to human genetics are available through Power Web on your Online Learning Center.

CHAPTER

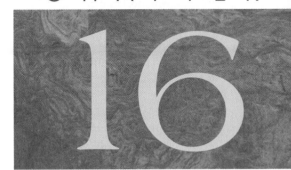

Human Origins and Evolution

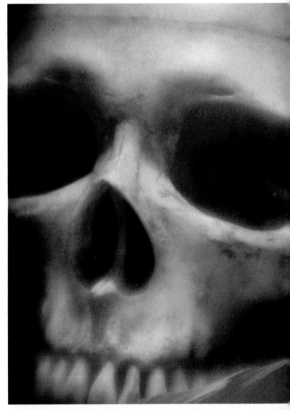

Comparing skulls among modern humans, our modern primate cousins, and fossilized hominids can reveal much about our forebears and our evolution.

Imagine being asked to build a story from the following elements:

1. A pumpkin that turns into a coach

2. A prince who hosts a ball

3. A poor but beautiful young woman with dainty feet who has two mean and ugly stepsisters with large feet

Chances are that unless you're familiar with the fairytale "Cinderella," you wouldn't come up with that exact story. In fact, ten people given the same pieces of information might construct ten very different tales.

So it is with the sparse evidence we have of our own beginnings—pieces of a puzzle in time, some out of sequence, many missing. Traditionally, paleontologists (scientists who study evidence of ancient life) have consulted the record in the earth's rocks—fossils—to glimpse the ancestors of *Homo sapiens,* our own species. Researchers assign approximate ages to fossils by observing which rock layers the fossils are located in and by extrapolating the passage of time from the ratios of certain radioactive chemicals in surrounding rock.

Fossils aren't the only way to peek into species' origins and relationships. Modern organisms also provide intriguing clues to the past, in their DNA. In this chapter, we explore human origins, genetic and genomic evidence for evolution, and how we attempt to alter the evolution of our own species and others.

16.1 Human Origins

A species includes individual organisms that are alike enough that they can successfully produce healthy offspring. *Homo sapiens* ("the wise human") probably first appeared during the Pleistocene epoch, about 200,000 years ago. Our ancestry reaches farther back, to about 60 million years ago when rodent-like insect eaters flourished. These first primates gave rise to many new species. Their ability to grasp and to perceive depth provided the flexibility and coordination necessary to dominate the treetops.

About 30 to 40 million years ago, a monkeylike animal the size of a cat, *Aegyptopithecus,* lived in the lush tropical forests of Africa. Although the animal probably spent most of its time in the trees, fossilized remains of limb bones indicate it could run on the ground, too. Fossils of different individuals found together indicate that they were social animals. *Aegyptopithecus* had fangs it might have used for defense. The large canine teeth seen only in males suggest that males may have provided food for their smaller female mates. *Propliopithecus* was a monkey-like contemporary of *Aegyptopithecus.* Both animals are possible ancestors of gibbons, apes, and humans.

From 22 to 32 million years ago, Africa was home to the first **hominoids,** animals ancestral to apes and humans only. One such resident of southwestern and central Europe was called *Dryopithecus,* meaning "oak ape," because its fossilized bones were found with oak leaves (**figure 16.1**). The way the bones fit together suggests that this animal lived in the trees but could swing and walk farther than *Aegyptopithecus.*

More abundant fossils represent the middle-Miocene apes of 11 to 16 million years ago. These apes were about the size of a human seven-year-old and had small brains and pointy snouts. (*Miocene* refers to the geologic time period).

Apelike animals similar to *Dryopithecus* and the mid-Miocene apes flourished in Europe, Asia, and the Middle East during the same period. Because of the large primate population in the forest, selective pressure to venture onto the grasslands in search of food and habitat space must have been intense. Many primate species probably vanished as the protective forests shrank. Of all

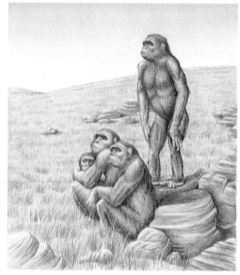

a. *Dryopithecus*

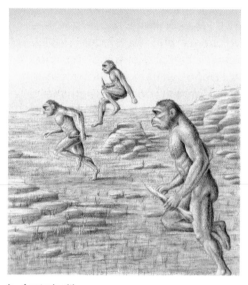

b. *Australopithecus*

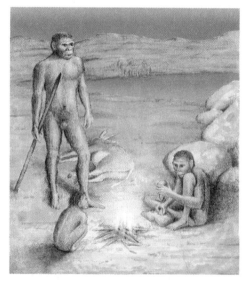

c. *Homo erectus*

Figure 16.1 Human forerunners.

(a) The "oak ape" *Dryopithecus,* who lived from 22 to 32 million years ago, was more dextrous than his predecessors. **(b)** Several species of *Australopithecus* lived from 2 to slightly more than 4 million years ago. These hominids walked upright on the plains. **(c)** *Homo erectus* made tools out of bone and stone, used fire, and dwelled communally in caves from 1.6 million years ago to possibly as recently as 35,000 years ago.

of the abundant middle-Miocene apes, one survived to give rise to humans and African apes. Eventually, animals ancestral to humans only, called **hominids,** arose and eventually thrived. (Some researchers use *hominim* instead of *hominid.*)

Hominoid and hominid fossils from 4 to 19 million years ago are scarce. This was the time when the stooped ape gradually became the upright ape-human. A seven-million-year-old fossilized skull and teeth found in northern Chad is from *Sahelanthropus tchadensis,* which may have been the most recent ancestor we share with chimps.

The Australopithecines—and Others?

Four million years ago, human forebears diversified as bipedalism—the ability to walk upright—opened up vast new habitats on the plains. Several species of a hominid called *Australopithecus* lived at this time, from 2 to 4 million years ago, probably following a hunter-gatherer lifestyle. **Figure 16.2** depicts the probable relationships among some known australopithecines, members of the genus *Homo,* and our closest modern primate relatives.

Australopithecines had flat skull bases, as do all modern primates except humans. They stood about 1.2 to 1.5 meters (four to five feet) tall and had brains about the size of a gorilla's, with humanlike teeth. The angle of preserved pelvic bones, plus the discovery of *Australopithecus* fossils with those of grazing animals, indicate that this ape-human had left the forest.

The most ancient species of australopithecine known, *Australopithecus anamensis,* lived about 4.1 million years ago. It led to *A. afarensis,* represented by a famous fossilized partial skeleton named "Lucy" discovered in 1974. She lived about 3.6 million years ago in the grasses along a lake in the Afar region of Ethiopia (**figure 16.3**). Her skull was shaped more like a human's than an ape's, with a less prominent face and larger brain than her predecessors had. The condition of her skeleton indicated that she died, with arthritis, at about the age of 20.

Much of what we know about the australopithecines comes from two parallel paths of footprints, preserved in volcanic ash in the Laetoli area of Tanzania. Archaeologist Mary Leakey and her team discovered them by accident in 1976. The 89-foot-long trail of footprints, left about 3.6 million years ago, was probably made by a large and small individual walking close together, and a third following in the steps of the larger animal in front. The shape of the prints indicates that their feet and gait were remarkably like ours.

A partial skull discovered near a lake in northern Kenya in 2001 may have belonged to a hominid that was an australopithecine or a contemporary. The animal's tentative name is *Kenyanthropus platyops,* for "flat-faced man of Kenya." It lived between 3.2 and 3.5 million years ago in grasslands bordering woods, with many other mammals. *K. platyops* had a novel combination of traits that included small earholes similar to those of chimpanzees and *Australopithecus anamensis.* It had the small brain and flat nose of *A. afarensis,* but not the prominent teeth and protruding face of Lucy. The huge flat face with elongated cheekbones is what compelled the paleontologists who discovered *K. platyops*—Meave and Louise Leakey—to place it in its own genus, calling the australopithecines a "garbage can" genus because they include so many types of fossils. *Kenyanthropus platyops* and the australopithecines may have coexisted, because their different facial structures suggest that they ate different things, enabling them to have shared habitats without competing for food.

Another type of australopithecine, *Australopithecus africanus,* lived about 2.8 million years ago, according to scant fossil evidence, and therefore lived closer in time to members of genus *Homo* than Lucy or *Kenyanthropus platyops* did. However, because this hominid lived far from the site of the earliest known *Homo* fossils, paleontologists hypothesized that there must have been some other ape-human "missing link" that lived, intermediate in time and place, between the known australopithecines and the earliest members of *Homo.* Paleontologists may have found a missing link in 1999, with the discovery of evidence of three individuals from a species named *Australopithecus garhi.* Trying to understand how this human forebear lived is a little like piecing together the Cinderella story. Researchers found:

1. Remains of an antelope that had been butchered. It was dismembered, and the ends of the long bones had been cleanly cut with tools, the marrow

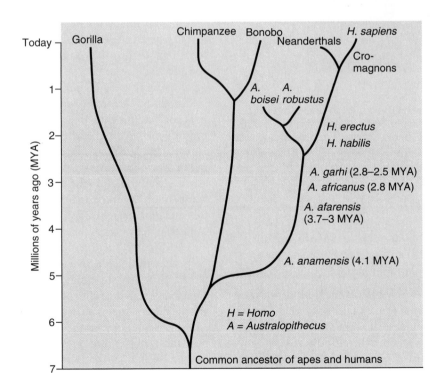

Figure 16.2 Evolutionary tree. An evolutionary tree diagram indicates the relationships among primates, past and present.

Several dating techniques place its existence at about 2.5 million years ago. The fossils were found in a desert in eastern Ethiopia, near later *Homo* fossils. The limb lengths and cranial capacity suggest a transitional form. In addition, *A. garhi* hunted.

Homo

Like the Cinderella story, the tale of how *Australopithecus* became or was replaced by *Homo* is built on sparse clues. Some australopithecines were "dead ends," dying off or leading to the Neanderthals, a branch of the *Homo* family tree that eventually vanished. Clues suggest that by 2.3 million years ago, *Australopithecus* coexisted with *Homo habilis*—a more humanlike cave dweller who cared intensively for its young. *Habilis* means handy, and this primate was the first to use tools for tasks more challenging than stripping meat from bones. *H. habilis* may have descended from a group of australopithecines who ate a greater variety of foods than other ape-humans, allowing them to live in a wider range of habitats.

H. habilis coexisted with and was followed by *Homo erectus* during the Paleolithic Age (**table 16.1**). *H. erectus* left fossil evidence of cooperation, social organization, tools, and use of fire. Fossilized teeth and jaws suggest that these primates ate meat. They were the first to have an angled skull base that permitted them to produce a greater range of sounds, making speech possible. *H. erectus* fossils are widespread. They have been found in China, Java, tropical Africa, and southeast Asia, indicating that these animals could migrate farther than earlier primates. One *Homo erectus* skull was discovered recently in an antique shop in Manhattan! The astute owner took it to the nearby American Museum of Natural History, where paleontologists immediately recognized it. The skull came from Indonesia.

The distribution of *H. erectus* fossils suggests that they lived in families of male-female pairs (most primates have harems). The male hunted, and the female nurtured young. **Figure 16.4** is an artist's rendition of *Homo erectus*. Some anthropologists interpret the fossil record to indicate that *H. erectus* dwelled in different parts of Africa, but others place this hominid only in the far eastern part of the continent, with two other species of *Homo* occupying the west.

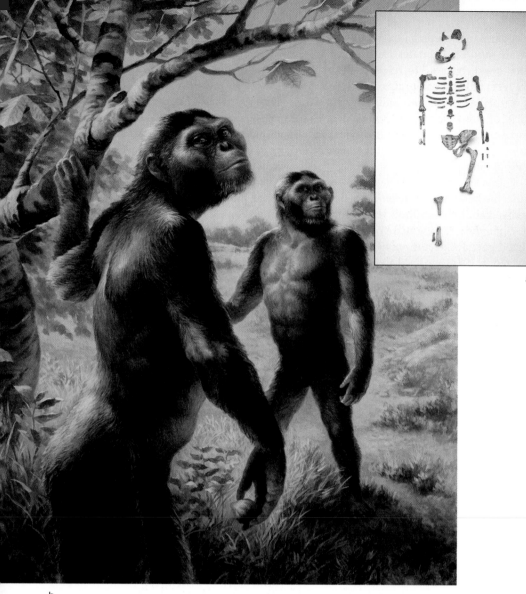

a.

b.

Figure 16.3 Lucy. About 3.6 million years ago, a small-brained human ancestor walked upright in the grasses along a lake in the Afar region of Ethiopia. She skimmed the shores for crabs, turtles, and crocodile eggs to eat. Her discoverers, Donald Johanson of the Cleveland Museum of Natural History and Timothy White of the University of California at Berkeley, named her "Lucy" because they were listening to the Beatles song "Lucy in the Sky with Diamonds" when they found her bones **(a)**. **(b)** shows an artist's interpretation of what this animal on the road to humanity may have looked like.

removed, meat stripped, and the tongue cleanly sliced off.

2. Limb bones from an individual who stood about 1.4 meters (about 4.5 feet) tall. The long legs were like those of a human, but the long arms were more like those of an ape.

3. A partial skull of a different individual, with a small cranium (holding a 450-cubic-centimeter brain, compared to the 1,400-or-so-cc modern human brain) and large teeth, suggesting an apelike lower face.

The *A. garhi* fossil finds are important for many reasons. The evidence is much more complete than the stray teeth and jaw bits of other australopithecines. More importantly, this hominid lived in the right time and place to be, and had characteristics consistent with, the long-sought bridge between *Australopithecus* and *Homo*.

Table 16.1

Cultural Ages

Age	Time (years ago)	Defining Skills
Paleolithic	750,000 to 15,000	Earliest chipped tools
Mesolithic	15,000 to 10,000	Cutting tools, bows and arrows
Neolithic	10,000 to present	Complex tools, agriculture

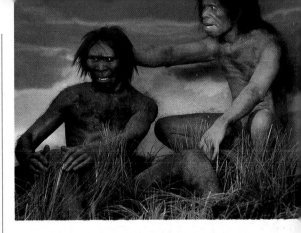

Figure 16.4 *Homo erectus.* This artist's rendition is based on many fossils.

We have a glimpse of our ancestors who lived about 160,000 years ago from skulls discovered near the town of Herto in Ethiopia (**figure 16.5**). The finding was largely due to luck and the power of observation. Driving by Herto in 1997, after a season of punishing rains, paleoanthropologist Tim White of the University of California, Berkeley, spotted a skull emerging from the sand near the Awash River. The skull came from a hippo, and it bore evidence of butchering. Returning a few days later with helpers, White quickly uncovered three human skulls, smashed and in pieces. These and other fossils had survived because the El Niño rains had driven the modern-day residents and their cattle from Herto; otherwise they would have inadvertently trampled the evidence.

One adult skull was from a young man; the other was damaged beyond recognition. The third skull was from a child about seven years of age. All were smooth, with decorative cutmarks, and found alone, with no other body parts. These clues suggest a ritualistic burial. The team also found hundreds of stone blades, axes, and flaking tools, and other human remains. From the scene, the researchers envisioned a band of early humans, with some features much like our own, that lived near a shallow lake that formed when the river overflowed. The lake was home to hippos and fish, and cattle lived near lush vegetation nearby. It isn't clear whether our forebears had the hunting skills to capture a hippo, or simply prepared carcasses that they found to eat.

It took an international team three years to assemble the skulls, and another three years to analyze them sufficiently to publish the results. The people, named *H. sapiens idaltu*, which means "elder" in the local Afar language, are our oldest known ancestors, their faces much more like our own than like the Neanderthals, long an enigma. The *H. sapiens idaltu* fossils provide evidence that the Neanderthals split off from the line leading to us at least 300,000 years ago. The fossils are also consistent with other evidence of humans having originated in Africa, a point we return to soon.

By 70,000 years ago, humans used more intricately carved tools made of bones, and red rock that bore highly symmetrical hatchmarks which may indicate early counting. *H. erectus* may have lived as recently as 35,000 years ago and coexisted with *H. sapiens idaltu.*

The Neanderthals, also contemporaries of *H. erectus* and members of genus *Homo,* appeared in Europe about 150,000 years ago, but may have lived elsewhere long before that. Neanderthals and modern people may have coexisted in what is now Israel about 90,000 years ago. By 70,000 years ago, the Neanderthals had spread to western Asia. They had slightly larger brains than we do, prominent brow ridges, gaps between certain teeth, very muscular jaws, and large, barrel-shaped chests.

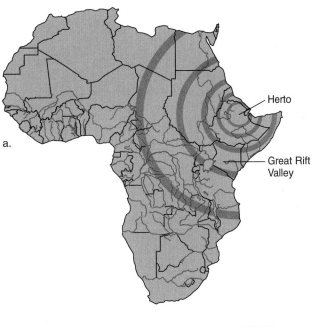

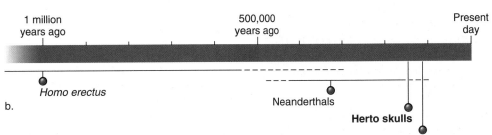

Figure 16.5 *Homo sapiens idaltu.* **(a)** *H. sapiens idaltu* lived in Herto, Ethiopia, an area rich in hominid fossils, about 160,000 years ago. **(b)** Many paleontologists think that if a member of this group were to walk down a street today, dressed normally, he or she would fit right in.

The Neanderthals take their name from Neander Valley, Germany, where quarry workers blasting in a limestone cave on a summer day in 1856 discovered the first preserved bones of this hominid that may or may not have been a member of our species. A Neanderthal discovered in France fifty years later, the "Old Man" of La Chapelle-aux-Saints, led to the common depiction of these people as primitive and slow-witted, stooped perhaps due to arthritis. When paleoanthropologists at the American Museum of Natural History in New York recently reconstructed a complete Neanderthal skeleton from fossils collected all over the world and compared it to that of a modern human, the differences were stark (**figure 16.6**). A Neanderthal had a wider pelvis, shoulders, and ribcage, and shorter forearms and shins; prominent brow ridges, a forward pointing face, and a sloping forehead. The characteristic heavy brow bones might have resulted from genetic drift acting over time on populations isolated in cave systems, not breeding with others. The stocky skeletons might reflect natural selection in a persistently cold climate. Anthropologists still debate whether the Neanderthals were truly different from us, or had a few exaggerated features of humanity. A fossilized, deformed skeleton buried with flowers in Shanidar Cave, Iraq, reveals that the Neanderthals may have been religious hunter-gatherers that were either clever enough or lucky enough to have survived a brutal ice age.

Fossil evidence indicates that from 30,000 to 40,000 years ago, the Neanderthals coexisted with the lighter-weight, finer-boned Cro-Magnons. The newcomers had high foreheads and well-developed frontal brain regions, and signs of culture that we do not see for Neanderthals. The first Cro-Magnon fossils were found in a French cave. Five adults and a baby were arranged in what appeared to be a communal grave. Nearby were pierced seashells that may have been used as jewelry. Intricate art decorated the cave walls. In contrast, the few Neanderthal graves show no evidence of ritual, just quick burial.

We don't know how it happened, but by about 28,000 years ago, the Neanderthals were gone, and the Cro-Magnons presumably continued on the path to humanity. Fossil evidence suggests that it wasn't the weather that felled the Neanderthals, so perhaps the Cro-Magnons outcompeted them for resources. We return to Neanderthals later in the chapter to examine DNA evidence of their relationship to us.

Modern Humans

Cave art from about 14,000 years ago indicates that by that time, our ancestors had developed fine hand coordination and could use symbols—milestones in cultural evolution. By 10,000 years ago, people had migrated from the Middle East across Europe, bringing agricultural practices.

In 1991, hikers in the Ötztaler Alps of northern Italy discovered an ancient man frozen in the ice (**figure 16.7**). After amateurs hacked away at him, causing much damage,

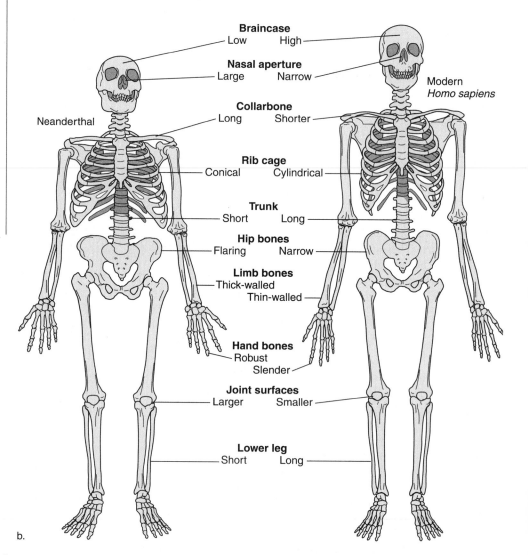

a.

b.

Figure 16.6   A new view of Neanderthals.   (a) A Neanderthal dressed as one of us might not be very noticeable, his features resembling exaggerated versions of our own. (b) Comparison of skeletons, however, reveals many subtle distinctions.

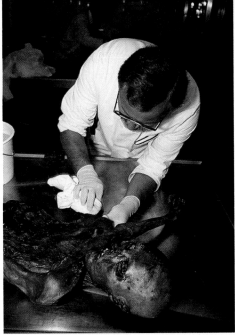

a.

Figure 16.7   A 5,300-year-old man.
(a) Hikers discovered Ötzi, the Ice Man, in the Austrian/Italian Alps in 1991. He lived 5,300 years ago, recently enough to belong to the same gene pool as people living in the area today. **(b)** Ötzi wore well-made clothing, including a hat; used intricate arrows that demonstrate familiarity with ballistics and engineering; and carried mushrooms with antibiotic properties. He had tattoos, indentations in his ears that suggest he wore earrings, and evidence of a haircut. This depiction is derived from the evidence found on and near Ötzi's preserved body.

b.

a microsatellite is a short, repeated DNA sequence, and is therefore not subject to natural selection because it does not affect the phenotype. An "allele" of a microsatellite is simply the number of repeats. The total number of such alleles corresponding to the 377 microsatellites is 4,682. Computer algorithms searched for similarities in allele patterns, without considering other characteristics, and revealed that the people fell into five clusters—which corresponded exactly with what is known about ancient human migration patterns, from Africa to Europe, then across Asia to Oceania and finally to the Americas. This genetic look into the past adds to the abundant and growing evidence that humans originated in Africa.

Key Concepts

Monkeylike *Aegyptopithecus* lived about 30 to 40 million years ago and was ancestral to gibbons, apes, and humans. The first hominoid (ape and human ancestor), *Dryopithecus*, lived 22 to 32 million years ago and may have walked onto grasslands. Hominids (human ancestors) appeared about 19 million years ago. • About 4 million years ago, bipedalism opened up new habitats for *Australopithecus*, who walked upright and used tools. There were several types of australopithecines, and one, *A. garhi*, may have been a direct forebear of *Homo*. By 2 million years ago, *Australopithecus* coexisted with the more humanlike *Homo habilis*. • Later, *H. habilis* coexisted with *H. erectus*, who used tools in more complex societies. *H. erectus* then coexisted with *H. sapiens*. *H. sapiens idaltu* lived 160,000 years ago, and looked remarkably like us. The Neanderthals preceded the Cro-Magnons, and were a side branch from modern humans. • Modern humans appeared about 40,000 years ago. A preserved man from 5,300 years ago is genetically like us.

the Ice Man, named Ötzi, ended up in the hands of several research groups. The Ice Man was on a mountain more than 10,000 feet high 5,300 years ago when he perished. He was dressed for the weather, with a bearskin cap and cloak, and shoes. Berries found with him place the season as late summer or early fall.

Ötzi may have died following a fight. When found he had a knife in one hand, cuts and bruises, and an arrowhead embedded in his left shoulder from the rear. The wound bore blood from two other individuals, according to DNA profiling. His bearskin cloak had the blood of a third person on it. One interpretation is that he killed or wounded two people, and perhaps carried a wounded comrade on his back. Suffering from blood loss or an infected wound, he probably fell into a ditch, where he froze to death and was soon covered by snow. After this safe burial, which preserved his body intact, a glacier sealed the natural tomb. DNA analyses on Ötzi's tissues suggest that he belonged to the same

gene pool as modern people living in the area, which is near the Italian-Austrian border. Researchers are hoping that the heat wave in Europe in the summer of 2003 may reveal other frozen individuals.

Another way that anthropologists try to glimpse what humans were like a few thousand years ago is by studying vanishing indigenous peoples, such as the San (bushmen) and pygmies of Africa, the Basques of Spain, the Etas of Japan, the Hill People of New Guinea, the Yanomami of Brazil, and another Brazilian tribe, the Arawete, who number only 130 individuals. Studying DNA sequences within these populations provides information on their origins, as we'll see later in the chapter.

Yet another way to look back in time is to compare genetic diversity in modern human populations. In one landmark study, researchers determined the pattern of alleles at 377 microsatellite sites distributed on all the autosomes in 1,056 people representing 52 populations defined by geography, language, or culture. Recall that

16.2   Molecular Evolution

Fossils paint an incomplete picture of the past because only certain parts of certain organisms were preserved, and very few have been discovered. Additional information on the past comes from within the cell, where the informational molecules of life change over time. That is, they evolve.

Determining and comparing genome, DNA or protein sequences, and chromosome banding patterns is the field of **molecular evolution.** The premise is that DNA and amino acid sequences change over time as mutations occur. The fewer differences between a gene or protein sequence in two species, the more closely related the two species are presumed to be—that is, the more recently they diverged from a shared ancestor. Molecular evolution analyses are based on the assumption that it is highly unlikely that two unrelated species would evolve precisely the same sequence of DNA nucleotides or amino acids simply by chance.

Comparing Genes and Genomes

We can assess similarities in DNA sequences between two species for a piece of DNA, a single gene, a chromosome segment, or even an entire genome. Most such efforts address evolutionary questions, but they can have practical applications, too. Animal models of human disease provide an example of the utility of knowing our closest genetic relatives.

Animal Models

Identifying corresponding genes in different species is very important in medical research; animal models of human disease are used to test experimental treatments. It is important that an animal model of a human disease have the same signs and symptoms. Because of differences in physiology, development, and lifespan, another mammal might not have the same phenotype as a human with a mutation in the same gene. However, corresponding genes can reveal basic abnormalities at the cell or molecular level. For example, two-thirds of the genes known to cause Mendelian disorders in humans have counterparts in fruit flies!

For some genes, a close correspondence in phenotype can be seen among species. People with Waardenburg syndrome, for example, have a characteristic white forelock of hair; wide-spaced, light-colored eyes; and hearing impairment (**figure 16.8**). The gene responsible is very similar in sequence to one in cats who have white coats and blue eyes and who are deaf. Horses, mice, and minks also have this combination of traits, which is thought to stem from abnormal movements of pigment cells in the embryo's outermost layer.

Targeted Comparative Sequencing

Comparing completely sequenced genomes among different species could, of course, reveal much about evolutionary relationships, but is very time-consuming. A shortcut is a technique called targeted comparative sequencing, which aligns representative sections from the genomes of different species—a little like reading excerpts rather than whole books to get an idea of how similar two books are.

In general, DNA sequences that encode protein tend to be very similar among closely related species. Such sequences are considered "highly conserved." Sequences that are similar in different, closely related species but that do not encode protein often control transcription or translation. In contrast, genome regions that vary widely typically do not affect the phenotype, and are therefore not subject to natural selection. Thus, within a protein-encoding gene, the exons tend to be highly conserved, but the introns, which are spliced out, are not.

The type of information gleaned from targeted comparative sequencing depends upon the species probed. Eric Green, a researcher at the National Institutes of Health, had been working on the cystic fibrosis region of human chromosome 7 for many years, when he decided to investigate corresponding sequences in 17 other vertebrate species. These species spanned our closest relatives, from chimps and baboons, through the familiar cat, dog, cow, mouse, and rat, to chickens and pufferfish. As expected, the DNA sequence similarities paralleled phenotypic similarities and presumably evolutionary relationships. For example, for a 20,000 base portion of the *CFTR* gene, humans had 94 percent in common with baboons, and

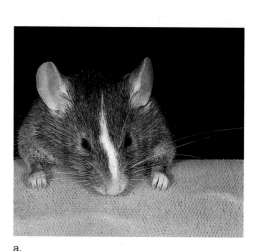
a.

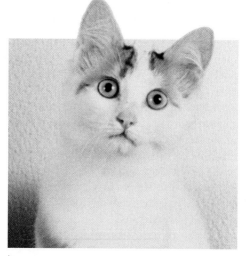
b.

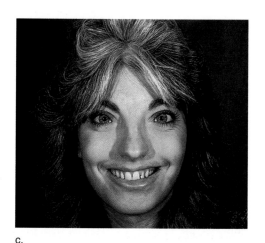
c.

Figure 16.8 One mutation can cause a similar spectrum of effects in different species.   A mutation in mice **(a)**, cats **(b)**, humans **(c)**, and other types of mammals causes light eye color, hearing or other neurological impairment, and a fair forelock in the center of the head.

increasingly less in common with cows, mice, and pufferfish.

Ironically, targeted comparative sequencing is not very informative when restricted to humans and chimps, because our genomes are so similar. The two genomes are like two introductory biology textbooks, presenting basically the same information overall, perhaps in different order. To highlight the differences between us, Edward Rubin, at the U.S. Department of Energy Joint Genome Institute, compared four genome regions among a different set of eighteen vertebrates, but included only primates and hominoids, our closest relatives. The reasoning: Those sequences that all primates, but not other vertebrates, share reveal the functions necessary to be a primate. The DNA sequences that are unique to humans help to define us at the genetic level. Green's work is like comparing excerpts from a dictionary, a science fiction novel, a cookbook and a children's story; Rubin's approach is like comparing only mystery novels. **Figure 16.9** depicts one way to display similarities and differences among the genomes of different species.

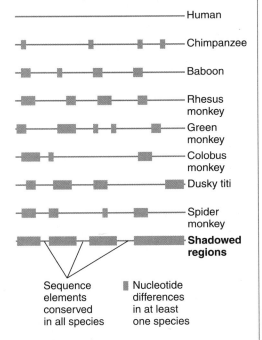

Figure 16.9 Comparing humans to their closest relatives. For this section of a chromosome, the thin lines represent regions where the DNA sequences correspond among species.

Solving a Problem: Comparing Chimps and Humans

There is little question that we have more in common with chimpanzees than with any other animals, but just how similar we are at the genome level depends upon the types of DNA sequences considered. The commonly repeated estimate of 98.7 percent similarity at the genome level between human and chimp originated from studies conducted in the 1970s using a technique called DNA hybridization. DNA from two species is cut and mixed. Complementary pieces bind, and some hybrid molecules form, with one side of the double helix from one species, the other from the other species. The higher the temperature required to separate hybrid double helices, the more of the sequence they share, because they bind more tightly (**Figure 16.10**). These studies used DNA segments present in single copies, indicating that they likely encode protein. Protein comparisons support the 98.7 percent sequence identity.

The chimp genome sequence was published in 2003, with most comparisons between human and chimp of protein-encoding genes. Roy Britten, a researcher at the California Institute of Technology who coinvented DNA hybridization technology, took a different view—he included "indels," for "insertions and deletions," in the calculations. If small insertions and deletions that distinguish the human and chimp versions of the same gene are counted, then our degree of genome similarity diminishes to about 96.6 percent. A simple calculation on a short, hypothetical DNA sequence demonstrates how this happens.

Consider an ancestral sequence of 15 bases:

GATACGAGCTCTAAC

"Ancestral" means that the most recent common ancestor of humans and chimps had this sequence. If a single-base substitution occurred after the divergence from the shared ancestor, then the correspondence would be less than 100 percent:

Chimp: GATACGAGCTCTAAC
Human: GATACGAGCT**A**TAAC

After the C-to-A point mutation occurs, humans and chimps share 14 of these 15 bases, for a correspondence of 93.3 percent, rather than 100 percent identity. But what happens when three bases at a time (so as not to offset the reading frame) are added or deleted in one of the evolutionary lines? Imagine that three bases insert into the human lineage as follows:

Chimp GATACGAGCTCTAAC
Human GAT**GCA**ACGAGCTCTAAC

The correspondence is now 15 out of 18 bases, or 83.3 percent.

If the human lineage lost three bases, the correspondence would also diminish:

Chimp GATACGAGCTCTAAC
Human GATAGCTCTAAC

The sequence now shares 12 out of 15 bases, or 80 percent.

The similarity between the human and chimp genome decreases even more if

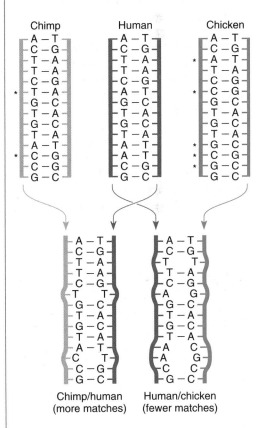

Figure 16.10 The rate of DNA hybridization reflects the degree of evolutionary relatedness. This highly schematic diagram shows why DNA from a human hybridizes more rapidly with chimpanzee DNA than with chicken DNA. Each * refers to a site where chimp or chicken DNA differs from human DNA.

noncoding regions, such as introns and repeats, are considered. However, differences in indels and repeats do not explain how we differ from chimps on a whole organism level. To assess phenotypic distinctions, it is more helpful to look at individual traits, sometimes determined by single genes.

Uniquely human traits include spoken language, abstract reasoning ability, highly opposable thumbs, and larger frontal lobes of the brain. Individual genes can actually have great effects on appearance, physiology, and development. Consider one stark difference between chimp and human that could stem from a single gene is hairiness. Chimpanzees and gorillas express a keratin gene whose counterpart in humans has been silenced into pseudogene status by a nonsense mutation. Natural selection might have favored loss of body hair to provide more efficient cooling when our ancestors left the forests, or as a way to shed skin parasites such as lice. Speech may also be a single gene difference between humans and chimps. A family in London whose members have unintelligible speech led to discovery of a single gene that controls speaking ability—and is present, but different, in chimps.

Another single gene that accounts for great differences among primates controls the switch from embryonic to fetal hemoglobin (see figure 11.2). More primitive primates lack or have very little fetal hemoglobin. In more recently evolved and more complex primates, fetal hemoglobin lengthened the fetal period, which maximized brain growth—and with larger brains came greater skills. Single genes can also explain longer childhood and adolescence in humans compared to chimpanzees.

Single genes that distinguish humans from chimps appear to be few, but they tend too be implicated in Mendelian disorders. Perhaps this reflects the fact that the genes that distinguish us have recently taken on their new functions, and the genome has not yet had time for redundancies to have evolved.

In 1975, Mary-Claire King and the late Allan Wilson, at the University of California, Berkeley, developed the "regulatory hypothesis" to explain why humans and chimps are genetically so similar, but look and behave so differently. They sug-

gested that the key underlying difference is in gene expression, not in genome sequence. Today, DNA gene expression microarrays are providing data that backs up their hypothesis. One study contrasted gene expression in the liver and brain in the two species. The differences in the brain were far greater than in the liver, which is consistent with the cognitive and behavioral distinctions between human and chimpanzee—presumably, our livers are more alike.

Comparisons of the human genome sequence to those of other species are interesting too. Overall, the human genome has a more complex organization of the same basic parts as the fruit fly and roundworm genomes. For example, the human genome harbors thirty copies of the gene that encodes fibroblast growth factor, compared to two copies in the fly and worm genomes. This growth factor is important for the development of highly complex organs. Reading 22.1 explores comparative genomics further.

Genome studies indicate that over deep evolutionary time, genes and gene pieces provided vertebrates, including humans, with defining characteristics of complex neural networks, blood clotting pathways, and acquired immunity. In addition, the genomes of vertebrates make possible refined apoptosis, greater control of transcription, complex development, and more intricate signaling both within and between cells.

Did the Human Genome Duplicate?

Comparing the human genome to itself provides clues to evolution, too. The many duplicated genes and chromosome segments in the human genome suggest that it doubled, at least once, since diverging from a vertebrate ancestor about 500 million years ago. Researchers infer what might have happened from the number and organization of such sequences. The duplications that riddle the genome are consistent with either a double doubling, followed by the loss of some genes, or, more likely, a single doubling followed by additional duplication of certain DNA sequences, a scenario one investigator calls "the big bang" followed by "the slow shuffle."

Sequence information from gene families, which are clusters of genes with similar sequences and functions, supports the lone complete doubling at the dawn of vertebrate life, followed by a continual turnover of about 5 to 10 percent of the genome beginning 30 to 50 million years ago. (Section 16.3 explains how approximate dates are assigned to genetic changes.)

The extensive duplication within the human genome distinguishes us from other primates. Some of the doublings are vast. Half of chromosome 20 repeats, rearranged, on chromosome 18. Much of chromosome 2's short arm reappears as almost three-quarters of chromosome 14, and a block on its long arm is echoed on chromosome 12. The gene-packed yet tiny chromosome 22 includes eight huge duplications and several gene families. The human genome is riddled with redundancy.

Duplications in a genome provide raw material and flexibility for future evolution. A copy of a DNA sequence can mutate, allowing a cell to "try out" a new function while the old one carries on. More often, though, the twin mutates into a silenced pseudogene, leaving a ghost of the gene behind as a similar but untranslated DNA sequence. A duplication can be located near the original DNA sequence, or away from it. A sequence repeated right next to itself is called a tandem duplication, and it usually results from mispairing during DNA replication. A copy of a gene on a different chromosome may arise when messenger RNA is copied (reverse transcribed) into DNA, which then inserts elsewhere among the chromosomes.

Duplication of an entire genome is polyploidy, discussed in chapter 13, and it is common in plants, but not animals. (Polyploidy versus duplications can be compared to burning an entire CD versus copying only certain songs.) If a polyploid event was followed by the loss of some genes, then peppered with additional gene duplications, the result would look much like the modern human genome. The picture became further muddled with time, as inversions and translocations altered the ancestral pattern.

Ancient DNA

When comparing DNA of modern species, a researcher can easily repeat an experiment—

ample samples of chimp or human DNA are available directly from the sources. This isn't so for ancient DNA, such as genetic material from insects preserved in amber, which is hardened resin from pine trees. The mix of chemicals in amber entombed whatever fell into it when it was the consistency of maple syrup. Alcohols and sugars in the resin dried out the specimen, and other organic molecules acted as fixatives, keeping cellular contents in place. The resin itself sealed out oxygen and bacteria, which would otherwise have decomposed tissue before it could be preserved. Finally, organic molecules called tarpenes linked, hardening the resin over a period of 4 to 5 million years. Today, the DNA is extracted and amplified using PCR (see figure 9.16).

Probing ancient, preserved DNA for clues to past life is an exciting field, but one that is subject to romanticization by the media. The novel and film *Jurassic Park* for example, described cloning dinosaurs from blood in mosquitoes trapped in amber—not a very likely scenario. In reality, researchers are exploring how to bring back a mammoth from preserved DNA in mammoths that were flash-frozen at high altitudes. These elephant ancestors roamed the grasslands of Siberia from 1.8 million years ago until about 11,000 years ago. Starvation following the last ice age drove their extinction, although a few isolated populations survived until about 3,800 years ago.

Biologists are searching frozen mammoth remains to see if cell nuclei that could yield DNA might have been preserved. If so, researchers may attempt to recreate a mammoth by cloning, using a mammoth somatic cell nucleus to direct development in an enucleated elephant oocyte. Judging from attempts to clone modern mammals, success isn't likely. An alternative strategy is to use mammoth sperm bearing X chromosomes to artificially inseminate an elephant, which may give birth to a female that is half elephant, half mammoth. Some 13 or so years later, she can then be inseminated by more mammoth sperm, producing a baby that is three-quarters mammoth, and so on.

The first successful extraction of bits of ancient DNA occurred in 1990, from a 17-million-year-old magnolia leaf entombed in amber (**figure 16.11**). The quest to probe ancient DNA has sent researchers into the back rooms of museums, dusting off specimens of pressed leaves, insects stuck with pins into Styrofoam, and old bones and pelts, in search of nucleic acid clues to life in the past.

Comparing Chromosomes

Before gene and genome sequencing, researchers recognized that similarities in chromosome banding patterns reflect evolutionary relatedness. Human chromosome banding patterns match most closely those of chimpanzees, then gorillas, and then orangutans (**table 16.2**). The karyotypes of humans, chimpanzees, and apes differ from each other mostly by inversions, which are changes that occur within chromosomes. Karyotype differences between these three primates and more primitive primates are predominantly translocations between chromosome types.

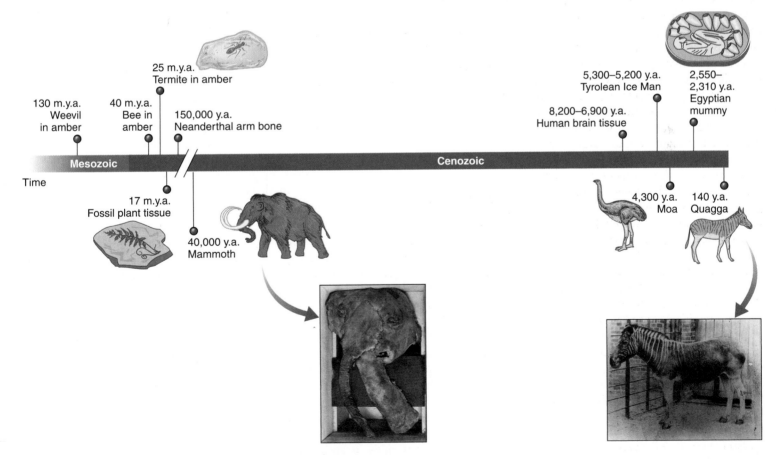

Figure 16.11 Ancient DNA. Researchers have extracted DNA from these organisms.

Table 16.2

Percent of Common Chromosome Bands Between Humans and Other Species

Chimpanzees	99⁺%
Gorillas	99⁺%
Orangutans	99⁺%
African green monkeys	95%
Domestic cats	35%
Mice	7%

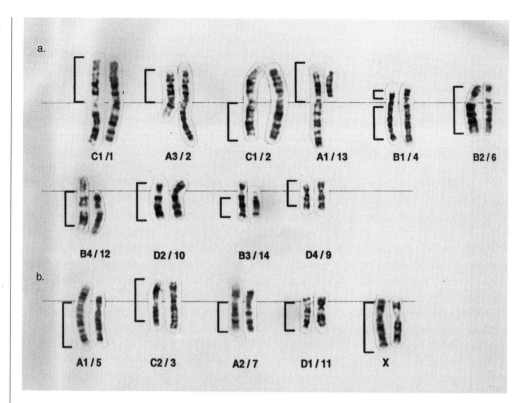

Figure 16.12 Conserved regions of human and cat chromosomes.
In each pair, the chromosome on the left is from a cat, and the chromosome on the right is from a human. The brackets indicate areas that appear to correspond. The chromosomes in **(a)** have similar banding patterns generated from traditional stains that target chromosome regions with generally similar DNA base content. The chromosomes in **(b)** do not look alike, but DNA probes indicate that specific gene pairs do indeed share DNA sequences.

If both copies of human chromosome 2 were broken in half, we would have 48 chromosomes, as the three species of apes do, instead of 46. The banding pattern of chromosome 1 in humans, chimps, gorillas, and orangutans matches that of two small chromosomes in the African green monkey, suggesting that this monkey was ancestral to the other primates. Reading 16.1 describes the evolution of a gene that duplicated, traveled, and then duplicated again, in the genomes of various primates.

We can also compare chromosome patterns between species not as closely related. All mammals, for example, have identically banded X chromosomes. One section of human chromosome 1 that is alike in humans, apes, and monkeys is also remarkably similar to parts of chromosomes in cats and mice. A human even shares several chromosomal segments with a cat (**figure 16.12**), but our karyotype is much less like that of the aardvark, the most primitive placental mammal.

Chromosome band pattern similarities, obtained with stains, although striking, are not ideal measures of species relatedness because a band can contain many genes that differ from those within a band at a corresponding locus in another species. DNA probes used as part of a FISH analysis are more precise because they mark particular genes. Direct correspondence of known gene order, or **synteny,** between species is better evidence of close evolutionary relationships. For example, 11 genes are closely linked on the long arm of human chromosome 21, mouse chromosome 16, and on a chromosome called U10 in cows. However, several genes

on human chromosome 3 are found near the human chromosome 21 counterpart in mice and cows. One possible explanation for this finding is that a mammal ancestral to these three species had all of these genes together, and the genes dispersed to an additional chromosome in humans. It will be enlightening to see how genome sequence information supports or refutes chromosome-level similarities studied with older techniques.

Comparing Proteins

Many different types of organisms use the same proteins, with only slight variations in amino acid sequence. The similarities of protein sequences is compelling evidence for descent from shared ancestors—that is, evolution. The keratin genes that encode a sheep's wool protein, for example, have counterparts on chromosome 11 in humans. The similarities in amino acid sequences in human and chimpanzee pro-

teins are astounding—many proteins are alike in 99 percent of their amino acids. Several are virtually identical. When analyzing a gene's function, researchers routinely consult databases of known genes in many other organisms. Two of the most highly conserved proteins are cytochrome c and homeobox proteins.

Cytochrome c

One of the most ancient and well-studied proteins is cytochrome c, which helps to extract energy from nutrients in the mitochondria for use in the reactions of cellular respiration. Twenty of 104 amino acids occupy identical positions in the cytochrome c of all eukaryotes. The more closely related two species are, the more alike their cytochrome c amino acid sequence is (**figure 16.13**). Human cytochrome c, for example, differs from horse cytochrome c by 12 amino acids, and from kangaroo cytochrome c by 8 amino acids. The human protein is identical to chimpanzee cytochrome c.

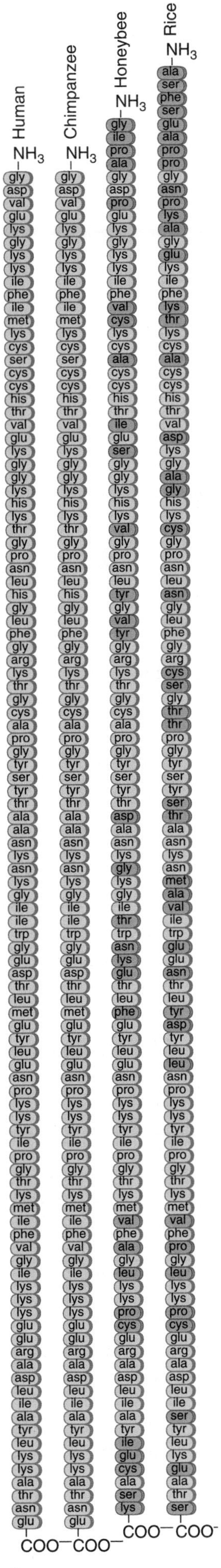

Homeobox Proteins

Another gene that has changed little across evolutionary time is a **homeobox** or HOX gene. It encodes a transcription factor that controls the order in which an embryo turns on genes. This cascade of gene action ultimately ensures that anatomical parts—whether a leg, petal, or segment of a larva—develop in the appropriate places. The highly conserved portion of a homeobox protein is a 60-amino-acid sequence called the homeodomain encoded by a 180-base DNA sequence called the homeobox. (Genes that include homeobox sequences are also termed *homeotic.*) In multicellular species, these genes organize body parts. Humans and most other vertebrates have 39 HOX genes in four clusters called A, B, C, and D. The genes have very few introns. Another intriguing aspect of HOX gene clusters is that the individual genes are expressed in a sequence, in developmental time or anatomical position, that mirrors their order on the chromosome.

The terms *homeobox* and *homeodomain* derive from the homeotic mutants of the fruit fly *Drosophila melanogaster,* which have mixed-up body parts. *Antennapedia,* for example, has legs in place of its antennae; *proboscipedia* grows legs on its mouthparts. Geneticists have studied homeotic fruit flies for half a century. Researchers sequenced the fly homeobox gene in 1983 and then found it in frogs, mice, beetles, mosquitoes, slime molds, chickens, roundworms, corn, humans, petunias, and many other species. Because the homeobox protein is a transcription factor (see chapter 10), it controls the activities of other genes.

Mutations in homeobox genes cause human illnesses. In a form of leukemia, a homeobox mutation shifts certain white blood cell progenitors onto the wrong developmental pathway. The misguided cells retain the rapid cell division characteristic of progenitor cells, causing the cancer. DiGeorge syndrome is another condition that is caused by a homeobox gene. Although affected individuals hardly sprout legs from their heads as do *Antennapedia* flies, the signs and symptoms of DiGeorge syndrome are reminiscent of the flies. These include missing thymus and parathyroid glands and abnormal development of the ears, nose, mouth, and throat—structures corresponding to anatomical regions similar to the sites of abnormalities in the flies. **Figure 16.14** on p. 318 shows another human disorder caused by a mutation in a HOX gene, synpolydactyly.

Experiments that transfer genes of one species into cells of another reveal how highly conserved the homeobox is, implying it is essential and ancient. If a mouse version of the *Antennapedia* gene is placed into the fertilized egg of a normal fly, the adult fly grows legs on its head, expressing the mouse gene as if it were the fly counterpart. The human version of the gene, placed into a mouse's fertilized egg, disrupts the adult mouse's head development. Homeotic genes and the proteins they encode, therefore, provide instructions for development of organisms whose bodies have many parts.

Cytochrome *c* Evolution	
Organism	**Number of amino acid differences from humans**
Chimpanzee	0
Rhesus monkey	1
Rabbit	9
Cow	10
Pigeon	12
Bullfrog	20
Fruit fly	24
Wheat germ	37
Yeast	42

b.

Figure 16.13 Amino acid sequence similarities reflect evolutionary relatedness.
Similarities in amino acid sequence for the respiratory protein cytochrome *c* in humans and other species parallel the degree of species relatedness. **(a)** These chains show the differences in cytochrome *c* sequence among four species. Amino acids that differ from those in the human sequence are highlighted purple. **(b)** This chart compares the sequence differences in nine species for this highly conserved protein.

a.

Figure 16.13a — Cytochrome c amino acid sequences

Human (NH₃–...–COO⁻):
gly-asp-val-glu-lys-gly-lys-ile-phe-ile-met-lys-cys-ser-cys-his-thr-val-glu-lys-gly-gly-lys-his-lys-thr-gly-pro-asn-leu-his-gly-leu-phe-gly-arg-lys-thr-gly-cys-ala-pro-gly-tyr-ser-tyr-thr-ala-ala-asn-lys-asn-lys-gly-ile-ile-trp-gly-glu-asp-thr-leu-met-glu-tyr-leu-glu-asn-pro-lys-lys-tyr-ile-pro-gly-thr-lys-met-ile-phe-val-gly-ile-lys-lys-glu-glu-arg-ala-asp-leu-ile-ala-tyr-leu-lys-lys-thr-asn-glu

Chimpanzee (NH₃–...–COO⁻):
gly-asp-val-glu-lys-gly-lys-ile-phe-ile-met-lys-cys-ser-cys-his-thr-val-glu-lys-gly-gly-lys-his-lys-thr-gly-pro-asn-leu-his-gly-leu-phe-gly-arg-lys-thr-gly-cys-ala-pro-gly-tyr-ser-tyr-thr-ala-ala-asn-lys-asn-lys-gly-ile-ile-trp-gly-glu-asp-thr-leu-met-glu-tyr-leu-glu-asn-pro-lys-lys-tyr-ile-pro-gly-thr-lys-met-ile-phe-val-gly-ile-lys-lys-glu-glu-arg-ala-asp-leu-ile-ala-tyr-leu-lys-lys-thr-asn-glu

Honeybee (NH₃–...–COO⁻):
gly-ile-pro-ala-gly-asp-pro-glu-lys-gly-lys-ile-phe-val-cys-lys-cys-ala-cys-his-ile-ser-ser-gly-gly-lys-his-val-gly-pro-asn-leu-tyr-gly-val-tyr-gly-arg-lys-thr-gly-cys-ala-pro-gly-tyr-ser-tyr-thr-asp-ala-asn-lys-gly-lys-ile-thr-trp-asn-lys-glu-thr-leu-phe-glu-tyr-leu-glu-asn-pro-lys-lys-tyr-ile-pro-gly-thr-lys-met-val-phe-ala-gly-leu-lys-lys-pro-cys-glu-arg-ala-asp-leu-ile-ala-tyr-ile-lys-lys-ala-thr-asn-glu

Rice (NH₃–...–COO⁻):
ala-ser-phe-glu-ala-pro-pro-gly-asn-pro-ala-gly-glu-lys-ile-phe-lys-thr-lys-cys-ala-cys-his-val-asp-lys-gly-ala-gly-his-lys-cys-gly-pro-asn-leu-asn-gly-leu-phe-gly-arg-cys-ser-gly-thr-thr-pro-gly-tyr-ser-tyr-ser-thr-ala-asn-lys-asn-met-ala-val-ile-trp-glu-glu-asn-thr-leu-tyr-asp-tyr-leu-leu-asn-pro-lys-lys-tyr-ile-pro-gly-thr-lys-met-val-phe-pro-gly-leu-lys-lys-pro-glu-arg-ala-asp-leu-ile-ser-tyr-leu-glu-lys-glu-thr-ser-ser

Tracing the Evolution of a Gene in Primates

Tracking the DNA sequence that encodes a specific protein found in the genomes of our closest relatives—other primates—provides a powerful tool to reconstruct evolution. Consider two genes called *PMCHL1* and *PMCHL2*. These genes in the human genome reflect past events that moved, mutated, and duplicated an ancestral DNA sequence. Along the way, the newly created genes acquired functions—still unknown—that natural selection retained.

French researchers Anouk Courseaux and Jean-Louis Nahon had not been planning an evolutionary study when they began to look at the *PMCHL* genes, which are on chromosome 5. The initials stand for "pro *MCH*-like" because the two genes include much of the sequence of a gene called *MCH* that resides on chromosome 12. *MCH* encodes a precursor to a neuropeptide, and it functions in the brain. The researchers hunted for *MCH*-like DNA sequences in the genomes of several primates and superimposed the genetic changes along a timeline to indicate when each type of primate diverged from the ancestral lineage (**figures 1 and 2**).

When the pieces of genetic evidence were assembled, a story began to emerge. Before 35 million years ago, when primates were limited to the prosimians (such as lorises and tarsiers) that looked more like rodents than monkeys, a DNA sequence very similar to the human *MCH* gene resided on a chromosome that corresponds to human chromosome 12. Gradually the New World monkeys, with their long, grasping tails and agility in the trees, flourished. Around 35 million years ago, the ancestral *MCH* gene moved to the counterpart to the short arm of human chromosome 5. This was a retrotransposition

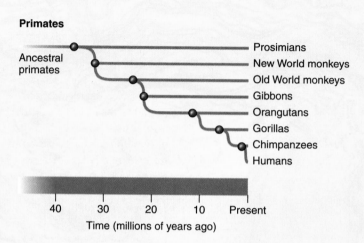

Primates

Prosimians
New World monkeys
Old World monkeys
Gibbons
Orangutans
Gorillas
Chimpanzees
Humans

Ancestral primates

40   30   20   10   Present

Time (millions of years ago)

Figure 1   Evolutionary relationships among modern primates.

event—that is, an mRNA transcribed from the original *MCH* gene was reverse transcribed into a DNA sequence that then inserted itself back into a chromosome—but chromosome 5, not 12. At this time, as evidenced by the present-day genomes of New World monkeys, the early version of the *PMCHL* gene lacked introns.

By about 26 million years ago, the Old World monkeys appeared, with their characteristic grasping thumb and specialized teeth, but shorter tails. The *PMCHL* gene then underwent mutations that introduced a pair of splice sites, adding an intron. By the time gibbons had evolved, the *PMCHL* gene had more introns, had undergone further mutations, and a part of the original gene that did not encode protein was included in the gene, and now did encode protein. The gene grew. Finally, between origin of the gibbon about 14 million years ago and the chimpanzee about 4 million years ago, the *PMCHL* gene underwent two profound events—it duplicated itself, and one copy jumped over the

centromere to land in the long arm of chromosome 5. This is the gene organization that persists in humans today: an ancestral *MCH* gene on chromosome 12 and two *PMCHL* genes on either side of the centromere of chromosome 5. The functions of these two genes are still unknown. However, *PMCHL1* is expressed in fetal, newborn, and adult brain, and *PMCHL2* is expressed in the testis. These genes may illustrate exaptation, which is the arising of a new function from an existing DNA sequence that had a different original function.

The evolution of the *PMCHL* genes tells a broader tale, getting to the heart of what makes us human. We like to consider ourselves very different from the other primates, although to an observer from another world, we might just appear to be hairless, upright apes. Yet DNA sequences among the primates are remarkably alike. Moving and duplicating genes can explain how we can simultaneously be genetically alike yet genetically different.

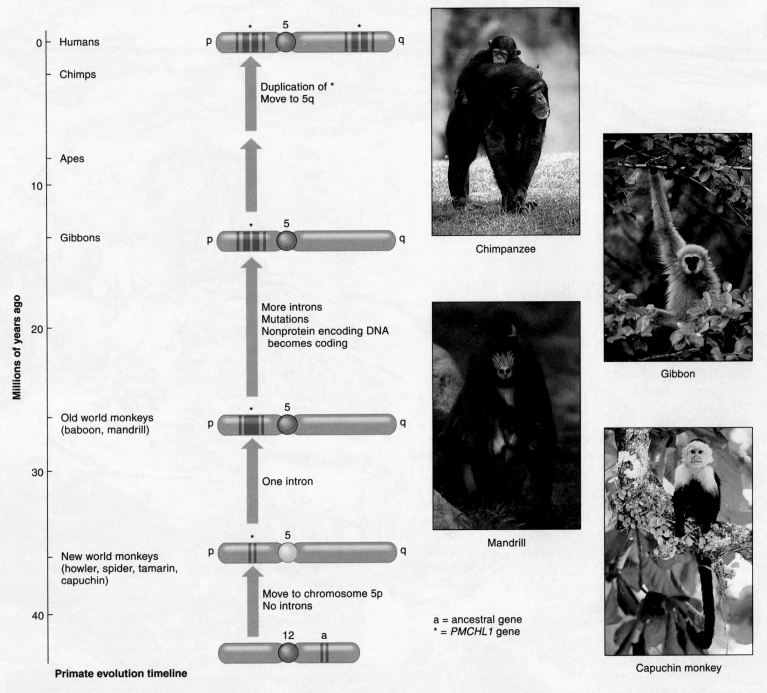

Figure 2 **Gene evolution.** Comparing the same gene among primate species reveals how parts of the human genome arose from gene mutation, movement, and duplication.

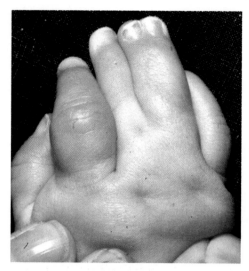

a.

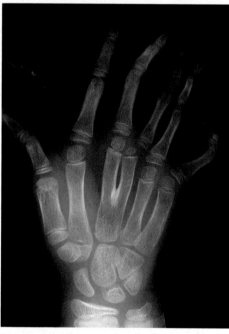

b.

Figure 16.14 A human *HOX* gene mutation causes synpolydactyly.
Mutation in the *HOXD 13* gene disrupts development of fingers and toes, causing a very distinctive phenotype shown in this photograph **(a)** and X-ray image **(b)**. The third and fourth fingers are partially fused with an extra digit within the webbed material. Other digits may be affected to lesser degrees. Researchers discovered the mutation in 182 members of an isolated family living in Turkey. The gene is on chromosome 2q. It has a type of mutation not seen before. The normal protein has a section of 15 alanines. In affected individuals, this polyalanine stretch is expanded by as many as 14 additional alanines.

Key Concepts

Molecular evolution investigations assume that the more recently two species shared an ancestor, the more alike their DNA and protein sequences and chromosome banding patterns. • Because of DNA sequence similarities, human genetic disease can be studied in other species. Targeted comparative sequencing aligns corresponding DNA sequences in different species to reveal evolutionary relationships. The technique identifies genes unique to primates and humans. • Chimps and humans share about 98.7 percent of protein-encoding DNA, but the proportion decreases when we consider insertions, deletions, introns, and repeats. Single-gene differences between the species may be more functionally important. Gene expression patterns also distinguish humans from chimps. The human genome likely duplicated. • Rarely, scientists can obtain DNA from preserved extinct organisms, amplify it, and compare it to sequences in modern species. • Chromosome banding pattern similarities reflect species relationships. Amino acid sequences of highly conserved proteins also reflect species relationships.

16.3 Molecular Clocks

A clock measures the passage of time by moving its hands through a certain degree of a circle in a specific and constant interval of time—a second, a minute, or an hour. Similarly, a polymeric molecule can be used as a **molecular clock** if its building blocks are replaced at a known and constant rate.

The similarity of nuclear DNA sequences in different species can help scientists estimate the time when the organisms diverged from a common ancestor, if the rate of base substitution mutation is known. For example, many nuclear genes studied in humans and chimpanzees differ in 5 percent of their bases, and substitutions occur at a rate of 1 percent per 1 million years. Therefore, 5 million years have presumably passed since the two species diverged. Mitochondrial DNA sequences may also be tracked in molecular clock studies, as we will soon see.

Time scales based on fossil evidence and molecular clocks can be superimposed on evolutionary tree diagrams constructed from DNA or protein sequence data.

However, evolutionary trees can become complex when a single set of data can be arranged into a large number of different tree configurations. A tree for 17 mammalian species, for example, can be constructed in 10,395 different ways! The sequence in which the data are entered into tree-building computer programs influences the tree's shape, which is vital to interpreting species relationships. With new sequence information, the tree possibilities change.

Parsimony analysis is a statistical method used to identify an evolutionary tree likely to represent what really happened. A computer connects all evolutionary tree sequence data using the fewest possible number of mutational events to account for observed DNA base sequence differences. For the 5-base sequence in **figure 16.15,** for example, the data can be arranged into two possible tree diagrams. Because mutations are rare events, the tree that requires the fewest mutations is more likely to reflect reality.

Neanderthals Revisited

Molecular clock data can provide clues to relationships among modern organisms and also compensate for deficiencies in the fossil record. Consider our knowledge of Neanderthals.

Two molecular technologies—analyzing ancient DNA and using mtDNA clocks—indicate that Neanderthals were a side branch on our family tree and diverged from us more than half a million years ago. This is much farther back than the 300,000 years ago that the fossil evidence indicates.

In 1997, a graduate student, Matthias Krings, ground up a bit of arm bone from the original French Neanderthal skeleton. He then amplified several 100-base-pair-long pieces of mtDNA that do not encode protein and mutate very rapidly, perhaps because they do not affect the phenotype and are therefore not under selective pressure. The DNA pieces were sequenced and compared to corresponding sequences from 986 modern *Homo sapiens.* The Neanderthal DNA differed at 26 positions. Not only is this three times the number of differences seen between pairs of the most unrelated modern humans, but the locations of the base differences were completely different from the places where

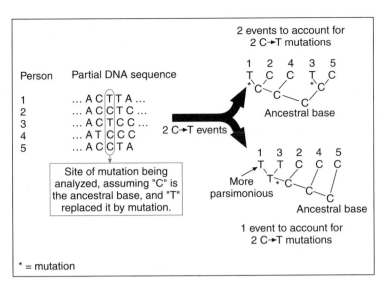

Figure 16.15 Parsimony analysis. Even a computer has trouble arranging DNA differences into an evolutionary tree showing species, population, or individual relationships. A parsimonious tree accounts for all data with the fewest number of mutations. Here, the two individuals who have a T in place of the ancestral C could have arisen in two mutational events or one, assuming that these individuals had a common ancestor. Since mutations are rare events, the more realistic scenario is one mutation.

modern genes vary (SNPs). Analysis of other Neanderthal bones has since supported the 1997 results. This genetic distinction suggests that it is highly unlikely that Neanderthals and modern humans ever interbred. In addition, sequences of mtDNA in the rib and leg bones of two Cro-Magnons from a cave in southern Italy, dating back 25,000 years, are unlike Neanderthal DNA but very similar to DNA from modern humans.

Extrapolations from mutation rates of genes in modern humans and chimps indicate the last shared ancestor between Neanderthals and humans lived from 690,000 to 550,000 years ago. On a more philosophical level, the DNA evidence distancing us from Neanderthals suggests that at one time two types of humans roamed the planet.

Tracking the Sexes: mtDNA and the Y Chromosome

It can be difficult to know which genes to study to trace human origins. Genes mutate at different rates. Therefore, different conclusions can be drawn from deciphering and comparing different DNA sequences. It is a challenge to assemble clues to human origins into a coherent explanation of real events.

Comparing DNA sequences on autosomes and the X chromosome can provide information on groups of people. However, analyzing mitochondrial DNA and sequences on the Y chromosome can reveal which parent passed on a particular DNA sequence in females and males, respectively.

MtDNA reveals maternal lineages because this DNA passes almost exclusively from mothers to offspring, in the oocyte. Only about one hundred mitochondria enter an oocyte from sperm, and usually these are destroyed by the 8-cell embryo stage. MtDNA serves as a clock of recent events, because mutations accumulate faster in mtDNA than in nuclear DNA, because mtDNA lacks repair systems. Also, mtDNA is much more abundant in cells and therefore easier to extract for study—a cell has only one nucleus, but typically thousands of mitochondria and their small genomes (see section 5.2 in chapter 5). However, a drawback to mtDNA dating is that paternal mtDNA can enter an oocyte and recombine with the maternal mtDNA, which obscures conclusions. This is rare, though.

Y chromosome sequences are used to trace paternal lineages. Much of the Y chromosome is identical in males from all population groups, but several sites in the part of the chromosome that does not recombine with the X have been used for molecular

clock studies. In both mtDNA and Y chromosome investigations, researchers compare haplotypes as well as DNA sequences.

Researchers have been using mtDNA analysis longer than they have Y chromosome techniques. Interestingly, when Y chromosome data are added to existing mtDNA information, the interpretations sometimes change. This has been the case, for example, in clarifying the origin of native Americans.

The logic behind mtDNA and Y chromosome analysis is that the more alike DNA sequences are between two individuals, the more recently they presumably shared a common ancestor. Put the reverse way, the greater the genetic differences between two individuals, the less closely related they are, and the more time has passed for those differences to have accrued. Researchers consider DNA sequence differences along with known mutation rates for those sequences to construct evolutionary tree diagrams that point to times and places of origin, or dispersal patterns, among groups of people.

Out of Africa

Theoretically, if a particular sequence of mtDNA could have mutated to yield the mtDNA sequences in modern humans, then that ancestral sequence may represent a very early human or humanlike female— a mitochondrial "Eve," or first woman. **Figure 16.16** shows how one maternal line may have come to persist.

When might this theoretical first woman, the most recent female ancestor to us all, have lived? Berkeley researchers led by the late Allan Wilson compared mtDNA sequences for protein-encoding as well as noncoding DNA regions in a variety of people, including Africans, African Americans, Europeans, New Guineans, Australians, and others. They concluded from several methods that the hypothesized ancestral woman lived about 200,000 years ago, in Africa. The locations of fossil evidence, such as *H. sapiens idaltu* skulls, support an African origin, and Charles Darwin suggested it, too.

One way to reach this time estimate is by comparing how much the mtDNA sequence differs among modern humans to how much it differs between humans and chimpanzees. The differences in mtDNA

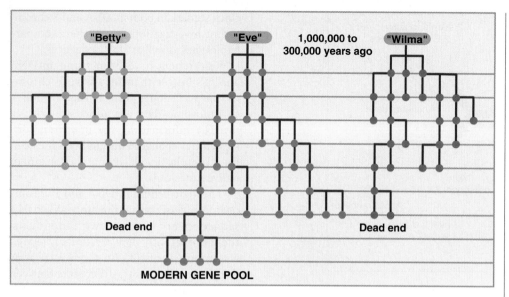

Figure 16.16   Mitochondrial Eve. According to the mitochondrial Eve hypothesis, modern mtDNA retains some sequences from a figurative first woman, "Eve," who lived in Africa 300,000 to 100,000 years ago. In this schematic illustration, the lines represent generations, and the circles, females. Lineages cease whenever a woman does not have a daughter to pass on the mtDNA.

sequences among contemporary humans amount to 1/25 the difference between humans and chimpanzees. The two species diverged about 5 million years ago, according to extrapolation from fossil and molecular evidence. Multiplying 1/25 by 5 million gives a value of 200,000 years ago, assuming that the mtDNA mutation rate is constant over time.

Where did Eve live? Mitochondrial DNA comparisons consistently find that African people have the most numerous and diverse mtDNA mutations. The same is true for other regions of the genome. Therefore Africans have existed longer than other modern peoples, because it takes time for mutations to accumulate. In many evolutionary trees constructed by parsimony analysis, the individuals whose DNA sequences form the bases are from Africa. That is, gene variants in other modern human populations are subsets of an ancestral African genome.

The idea of mitochondrial Eve is part of the "out of Africa" view, or **replacement hypothesis** of human origins. It states that about 200,000 years ago, *H. sapiens* evolved from an *H. erectus* population in Africa. What isn't known is whether this occurred quickly, in small, isolated pockets, or gradually across a broader swath of the continent. However it happened, eventually

descendants of these early *H. sapiens* migrated to the Middle East, Asia, and Europe. An alternate view, largely disproven, is the **multiregional hypothesis,** which maintains that human traits originated in several places, and *H. erectus* migrated, mixing and sharing genes, gradually evolving into *H. sapiens.* The "out of Africa" and multiregionalism hypotheses were once so contentious that scientists fought over them at meetings and in print.

A Native American Tale

The ancestors of native Americans came to North America across the Bering Strait land bridge that formed between Siberia and Alaska during low glacial periods (**figure 16.17**). Anthropologists traditionally dated three waves of migration based on evidence of ancient human habitation and language differences among modern native populations—the Amerindians about 33,000 years ago, the Nadene 15,000 to 12,000 years ago, and the Eskimo-Aleuts from 7,000 to 5,000 years ago. But DNA evidence indicates one migration of people bringing in diverse genes—and they didn't originate in Siberia, as has been long suspected, but in Mongolia.

One of four major mtDNA haplotypes, B, is widespread in the New World but is

not present in Siberians. Haplotype B is present, however, in people who live in Ulan Bator, the capital city of north central Mongolia. According to mtDNA evidence, they were more likely the people who trekked across the land bridge to populate the New World—not the Siberians.

Y chromosome analysis generally supports the Mongolian origin, but it also counters the anthropological evidence indicating three waves of migration. Instead, Y chromosome sequences reveal that all native Americans descended from one founder population that came from the Mongolian/Chinese border in a nearly continuous migration between 37,000 and 23,000 years ago. Because the members of this population brought with them a variety of DNA sequences on their Y chromosomes, it appears that they included different groups.

Another study compared mtDNA from modern Mongolians, Tibetans, and Chinese to remains from a 700-year-old Amerindian graveyard in Illinois. All four of the mtDNA haplotypes common to native Americans were identified among all of these groups, although the Asian peoples had several others as well and the four native American haplotypes were unusual among the Asians. This evidence suggests that a subset of people, carrying the four haplotypes, left Asia long ago to populate the Americas. The fact that the four haplotypes are very rare among Asians today argues for a single long-ago migration to America that brought in the subset. Since each haplotype is rare in Asia, the three-migration hypothesis requires a rare event to have happened three times. One event that introduced all four haplotypes seems more likely.

A study of different Y chromosome haplotypes indicates traces of an ancient Siberian group called the Kets among modern native Americans. The Kets today number fewer than 100, and they still have their own language. It is possible, then, that some Siberians also contributed to the native American gene pool. The emerging picture of native American origins is that many small groups of people wandered over the land bridge, in search of food, and introduced diverse genes to the Americas. Their numbers grew between 37,000 and 23,000 years ago, when a rising sea blocked the land bridge and isolated the native American gene pool.

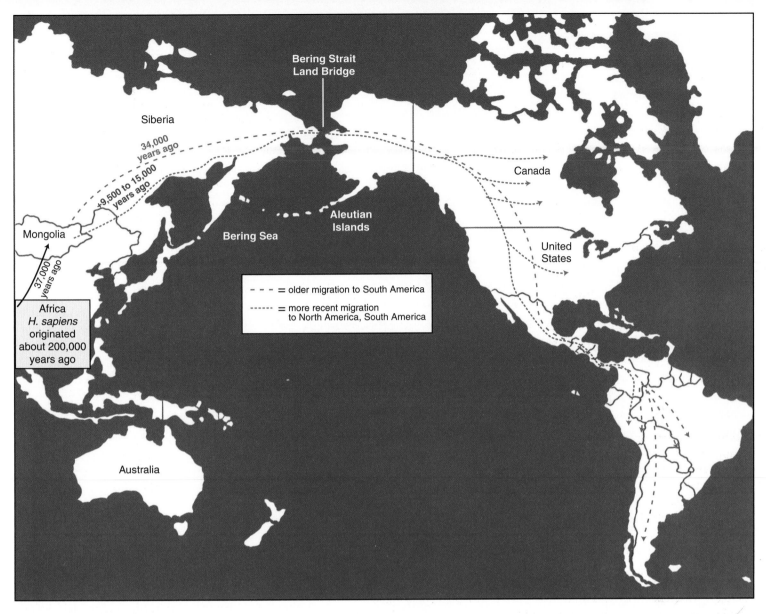

Figure 16.17 Tracing human origins. Analyses of mitochondrial DNA and Y chromosome DNA sequences reveal that the ancestors of native Americans probably came from Mongolia in one migration.

Map labels:
- Bering Strait Land Bridge
- Siberia
- 34,000 years ago
- +9,500 to 15,000 years ago
- Mongolia
- 37,000 years ago
- Africa *H. sapiens* originated about 200,000 years ago
- Bering Sea
- Aleutian Islands
- Canada
- United States
- Australia
- - - - = older migration to South America
- ...... = more recent migration to North America, South America

Key Concepts

Molecular clocks apply mutation rates to time scales to estimate when two individuals or types of organisms most recently shared ancestors. Different genes evolve at different rates. Parsimony analysis selects likely evolutionary trees from DNA data.
• Mitochondrial DNA clocks trace maternal lineages, and Y chromosome sequences trace paternal lineages.
• Molecular clocks have been used to examine the relationship of Neanderthals to modern humans and the origin of modern humans.
• Molecular clock data illuminate migration patterns of native Americans from Asia.

16.4 Eugenics

Fossil evidence, ancient DNA, and molecular clocks are useful in studying our past. We can control the future, to an extent, through reproductive choices that affect the gene pool. Some people try to control the genes in their offspring by seeking mates with high intelligence or certain physical characteristics. This idea was taken to an absurd extreme in a sperm bank in California where the donors are all Nobel Prize winners, and in a website advertising eggs donated by supermodels or young women with high scores on college entrance exams. The ability to control reproductive choices raises many bioethical issues.

Eugenics is the control of individual human reproductive choices to achieve a societal goal. Sir Francis Galton coined the term, meaning "good in birth," in 1883 (**table 16.3**). He defined eugenics as "the science of improvement of the human race germplasm through better breeding." The 2,500-year-old caste system in India and the antimiscegenation laws in the United States that banned marriage between people of different races from 1930 to 1967 were clearly eugenic because they sought to control reproduction to change society.

Galton's ideas were popular for a time. Eugenics societies formed in several nations and attempted to practice his ideas in various ways. Creating incentives for reproduction among those considered superior constitutes

Table 16.3

A Chronology of Eugenics

1883	Sir Francis Galton coins the term *eugenics*.
1889	Sir Francis Galton's writings are published in the book *Natural Inheritance*.
1896	Connecticut enacts law forbidding sex with a person who has epilepsy or is "feebleminded" or an "imbecile."
1904	Galton establishes the Eugenics Record Office at the University of London to keep family records.
1907	First eugenic law in the United States orders sterilization of institutionalized mentally retarded males and criminal males when experts recommend it.
1910	Eugenics Record Office founded in Cold Spring Harbor, New York, to collect family and institutional data.
1924	Immigration Act limits entry into the United States of "idiots, imbeciles, feebleminded, epileptics, insane persons," and restricts immigration to 7 percent of the U.S. population from a particular country according to the 1890 census—keeping out those from southern and eastern Europe.
1927	Supreme Court (*Buck vs. Bell*) upholds compulsory sterilization of the mentally retarded by a vote of 8 to 1, leading to many state laws.
1934	Eugenic sterilization law of Nazi Germany orders sterilization of individuals with conditions thought to be inherited, including epilepsy, schizophrenia, and blindness, depending upon rulings in Genetic Health Courts.
1939	Nazis begin killing 5,000 children with birth defects or mental retardation, then 70,000 "unfit" adults.
1956	U.S. state eugenic sterilization laws are repealed, but 58,000 people have already been sterilized.
1965	U.S. immigration laws reformed, lifting many restrictions.
1980s	California's Center for Germinal Choice is established, where Nobel Prize winners can deposit sperm to inseminate carefully chosen women.
1990s	Laws passed to prevent health insurance or employment discrimination based on genotype.
2000	Human genome sequenced.
2003	Many governments recommend certain genetic tests, and have legislation to prevent genetic discrimination. In the U.S., protective legislation is still in discussion.

positive eugenics. Interfering with reproduction among those judged inferior is an example of negative eugenics.

One vocal supporter of the eugenics movement was Sir Ronald Aylmer Fisher. In 1930, he published a book, *The Genetical Theory of Natural Selection*, which connected the concepts of Charles Darwin and Gregor Mendel and listed the basic tenets of population genetics. Natural selection and Mendelian inheritance provided a framework for eugenics. The final five chapters of Fisher's otherwise highly regarded work tried to apply the principles of population genetics to human society. Fisher maintained that those at the top of a society tend to be "genetically infertile," producing fewer children than the less-affluent classes. This, he claimed, was the reason why civilizations ultimately topple. He offered several practical suggestions to remedy this, including state monetary gifts to high-income families for each child born to them.

Early in the twentieth century, eugenics focused on maintaining purity. One promi-

nent geneticist, Luther Burbank, realized the value of genetic diversity at the beginning of a eugenic effort. Known for selecting interesting plants and crossing them to breed plants with useful characteristics, such as less prickly cacti and a small-pitted plum, Burbank in 1970 applied his agricultural ideas to people. In a book called *The Training of the Human Plant*, he encouraged immigration to the United States so that advantageous combinations of traits would appear as the new Americans interbred. Burbank's plan ran into problems, however, at the selection stage, which allowed only those with "desirable" trait combinations to reproduce.

On the East Coast of the United States, Charles Davenport led the eugenics movement. In 1910, he established the Eugenics Record Office at Cold Spring Harbor, New York. There he headed a massive effort to compile data from institutions, prisons, and the general society. In the rather simplistic view of genetics at the time, he attributed nearly every trait to a single gene. "Feeblemindedness," he

thought, was inherited as an autosomal recessive trait.

Other nations practiced eugenics. From 1934 until 1976, the Swedish government forced certain individuals to be sterilized as part of a "scientific and modern way of changing society for the better," according to one historian. At first, only mentally ill people were sterilized, but poor, single mothers were later included. Revelation of the Nazi atrocities did not halt eugenics in Sweden, but the women's movement in the 1970s pushed for an end to forced sterilizations.

Seeking information on human genetics does not necessarily have anything to do with eugenics, although genetic tests can alter allele frequencies (see Bioethics: Choices for the Future on p. 323). In chapter 1, Bioethics: Choices for the Future describes how some nations are acquiring genetic information on citizens. These projects are not eugenic, however, because the information is used to improve health, not to make reproductive decisions. Eugenics, in contrast, uses such information to maximize the

Two Views of Neural Tube Defects

Genetic technologies permit people to make reproductive choices that can alter allele frequencies in populations. Identifying carriers of a recessive illness, who then may decide not to have children together, is one way to remove some disease-causing alleles from a population, by decreasing the number of homozygous recessive individuals. Screening pregnant women for fetal anomalies, then terminating affected pregnancies, also alters disease prevalence and, if the disorder has a genetic component, allele frequencies. This is the case for neural tube defects (NTDs), which are multifactorial.

An NTD forms at the end of the first month, when the embryo's neural tube does not completely close. If the opening is in the head, the condition is called anencephaly, and usually ends in miscarriage, stillbirth, or a newborn who dies within days. If the opening is in the spinal cord, the condition is called spina bifida. Usually the individual is paralyzed from the point of the lesion down, but can live into adulthood and have normal intelligence. Sometimes surgery can improve functioning in people with mild cases of spina bifida. People with spina bifida often also have hydrocephalus, or "water on the brain."

In 1992, the Centers for Disease Control and Prevention summarized studies indicating that taking the vitamin folic acid in pregnancy lowers the risk of NTD recurrence by 50 percent, from 3 to 4 percent to 1.5 to 2 percent. Women who had had an affected child began taking large doses of the vitamin in the months before conception. But when epidemiologists tried to monitor how well folic acid supplementation was working, they faced a problem—the prevalence values of NTDs were greatly underestimated. This happened because the statistics on NTD prevalence—vital to discovering whether folic acid was actually preventing the defect—included only newborns, stillborns, and older fetuses. Most reports did not account for pregnancies terminated following a prenatal diagnosis of an NTD. These pregnancies caused the underreporting of anencephaly by 60 to 70 percent, and of spina bifida, by 20 to 30 percent in some states. NTD screening and subsequent termination of affected pregnancies alters the allele frequencies by preventing causative genes from passing to new generations.

A Personal View

Blaine Deatherage-Newsom has a different view of population screening for neural tube defects because he has one (**figure 1**). Blaine was born in 1979 with spina bifida. Paralyzed from the armpits down, he has endured much physical pain, but he has also achieved a great deal. He put the question, "If we had the technology to eliminate disabilities from the population, would that be good public policy?" on the Internet—initiating a global discussion. His view on NTD screening is one we do not often hear:

> I was born with spina bifida and hydrocephalus. I hear that when parents have a test and find out that their unborn child has spina bifida, in more than 95 percent of the cases they choose to have an abortion. I also went to an exhibit at the Oregon Museum of Science and Industry several years ago where the exhibit described a child born with spina bifida and hydrocephalus, and ... asked people to vote on whether the child should live or die. I voted that the child should live, but when I voted, the child was losing by quite a few votes.
>
> When these things happen, I get worried. I wonder if people are saying that they think the world would be a better place without me. I wonder if people just think the lives of people with disabilities are so full of misery and suffering that they think we would be better off dead. It's true that my life has suffering (especially when I'm having one of my 11 surgeries so far), but most of the time I am very happy and I like my life very much. My mom says she can't imagine the world without me, and she is convinced that everyone who has a chance to know me thinks that the world is a far better place because I'm in it.

Is eliminating disabilities good public policy? It depends on your point of view.

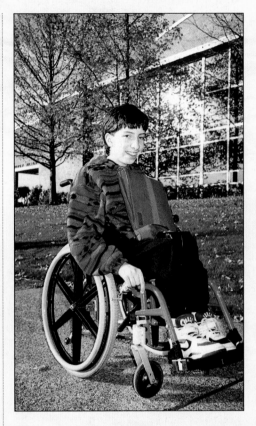

Figure 1 Blaine Deatherage-Newsom.

Excerpt by Blaine Deatherage-Newsom, "If we could eliminate disabilities from the population, should we? Results of a survey on the Internet." Reprinted by permission.

genetic contribution from those deemed desirable and minimize the contribution from those considered unacceptable. A major fallacy of eugenics is its subjectivity. Who decides which traits are desirable or superior?

Eugenic thinking arises from time to time, even today. In 1994, for example, China passed the Maternal and Infant Health Care Law, which proposes "ensuring the quality of the newborn population" and forbids procreation between two people if physical exams show "genetic disease of a serious nature . . . that may totally or partially deprive the victim of the ability to live independently, that [is] highly possible to recur in generations to come, and that [is] medically considered inappropriate for reproduction." Such "genetic diseases" include mental retardation, mental illness, and seizures, conditions that are ill-defined in the law and are not necessarily inherited.

Dor Yeshorim, the organization that identifies carriers of a dozen genetic diseases in Ashkenazi Jewish populations, is eugenic because people use the information to prevent reproduction between certain individuals. The program most definitely alters the gene pool—today, Tay-Sachs disease, once seen nearly entirely in Jewish people, is actually more common in other populations.

Because genetic technologies may affect reproductive choices and can influence which alleles are passed to the next generation, modern genetics has sometimes been compared to eugenics. Medical genetics and eugenics differ in their overall goals. Eugenics aims to skew allele frequencies in future generations by allowing only people with certain "valuable" genotypes to reproduce, for the supposed benefit of the population as a whole. The goal of medical genetics, in contrast, is usually to skew allele frequencies in order to prevent suffering on a family level.

One particularly frightening aspect of the eugenics movement early in the twentieth century was the vague nature of the traits considered hereditary and undesirable, such as "feeblemindedness," "criminality," and "insanity." Now, as a new century dawns and the human genome is analyzed, will eugenics resurge? Will we use new genetic information to choose the traits of the next generation?

Many people fear that tests to identify carriers or disease susceptibility will be used eugenically, particularly in nations where the government does not underwrite health care. Laws are being implemented in many nations to prevent genetic discrimination. Let's hope that in addition to deciphering our genetic blueprints, we also learn how to apply that information wisely. Unlike other species, we have the ability to affect our own evolution.

Key Concepts

Eugenics is the control of individual human reproduction for societal goals, maximizing the genetic contribution of those deemed acceptable (positive eugenics) and minimizing the contribution from those considered unacceptable (negative eugenics). Some people consider modern genetic screening practices eugenic, but genetic testing usually aims to prevent or alleviate human suffering.

Summary

16.1 Human Origins

1. The first primates were rodentlike insectivores that lived about 60 million years ago. By 30 to 40 million years ago, monkeylike *Aegyptopithecus* lived. **Hominoids,** ancestral to apes and humans, lived 22 to 32 million years ago. They include *Dryopithecus* and other primates who began to walk upright.

2. **Hominids,** ancestral to humans only, appeared about 19 million years ago. These animals were more upright, dwelled on the plains, and had smaller brains than their forebears. The *Australopithecines* preceded and then coexisted with *Homo habilis,* who lived in caves, had strong family units, and used tools extensively. *Homo erectus* was a contemporary who outsurvived *H. habilis,* lived in societies, and used fire. *Homo sapeins idaltu* lived about 160,000 years ago, and looked like us. Evidence of tool use dates to 70,000 years ago. *H. erectus* overlapped in time with our own species.

3. Early *Homo sapiens* also included the Neanderthals and Cro-Magnons, although Neanderthals were a dead end. Modern humans appeared about 40,000 years ago, and culture was apparent by 14,000 years ago. Today, microsatellite diversity patterns correspond to geography.

16.2 Molecular Evolution

4. **Molecular evolution** considers differences at the genome, chromosome, protein, or DNA sequence levels with mutation rates to estimate species relatedness. Animal models are possible because of similarities in DNA sequence among species.

5. Targeted comparative sequencing aligns corresponding DNA sequences in different species.

6. Humans and chimps share 98.7 percent of their protein-encoding gene sequences. Indels, introns, and repeats create genome differences between humans and chimps.

7. Single genes and differences in gene expression can account for great distinctions between chimps and humans.

8. The human genome shows many signs of past duplication.

9. Amplifying ancient DNA is difficult because contamination may occur.

10. Closely related species have similar chromosome banding patterns. Genes in the same order on chromosomes in different species are **syntenic.**

11. Cytochrome *c* and homeobox proteins are highly conserved.

16.3 Molecular Clocks

12. Gene sequence information from several species may be used to construct evolutionary tree diagrams, and a **molecular clock** based on the known mutation rate of the gene may then be applied. Different genes mutate at different rates. Molecular trees indicate when species diverged from shared ancestors.

13. **Parsimony analysis** selects the evolutionary trees requiring the fewest mutations, which are therefore the most likely.

14. Molecular clocks based on mitochondrial DNA are used to date recent events through the maternal line because this DNA mutates faster than nuclear DNA. Y chromosome genes are used to trace paternal lineage. Both types of evidence are used to study human origins and migrations.

16.4 Eugenics

15. **Eugenics** is the control of individual reproduction to serve a societal goal.

16. Positive eugenics encourages those deemed acceptable or superior to reproduce. Negative eugenics restricts reproduction of those considered inferior. Eugenics extends the concept of natural selection and Mendel's laws but does not translate well into practice.

17. Some aspects of genetic technology also affect reproductive choices and allele frequencies, but the goal is to alleviate or prevent suffering, rather than to change society.

Review Questions

1. What is the difference between a hominoid and a hominid?

2. Some anthropologists classify chimpanzees along with humans in genus *Homo.* How does this conflict with fossil evidence of the *Australopithecus* species?

3. Give an example of how a single gene difference can have a profound effect on the phenotypes of two species.

4. What is the evidence that *Australopithecus garhi* may have been a direct forebear of *Homo*?

5. Give an example of molecular evidence that is consistent with fossil or other evidence, and an example of molecular evidence that conflicts with other information.

6. How does the information provided by Y chromosome and mitochondrial DNA sequences differ from the information obtained from nuclear DNA sequences?

7. List three aspects of development, anatomy, or physiology that were important in human evolution.

8. Why are exons highly conserved, but introns are not?

9. Explain how indels could cause the divergence of our genome sequence from that of chimpanzees, yet not contribute to observable differences between the two species.

10. Protein-encoding genes have different mutation rates. How might this complicate the interpretation of targeted comparative sequencing experiments?

11. Cite two ways that humans and chimps can differ greatly at the genetic level, but still be very alike in terms of DNA sequence.

12. Why does comparing gene sequences offer more information for molecular evolution studies than comparing protein sequences?

13. Why can comparing the sequences of different genes or proteins lead to different conclusions about when two groups diverged from a common ancestor?

14. Why is comparing the DNA sequence of one gene a less accurate estimate of the evolutionary relationship between two species than a DNA hybridization experiment that compares large portions of the two genomes?

15. Cite a limitation of comparing chromosome banding patterns to estimate species' relationships.

16. What types of information are needed to construct an evolutionary tree diagram? What assumptions are necessary? What are the limitations of these diagrams?

17. Cite three examples of eugenic actions or policies.

18. How can the human and chimp genomes be 99 percent alike in DNA sequence, yet still be different?

Applied Questions

1. A geneticist aboard a federation starship is given the task of determining how closely related Humans, Klingons, Romulans, and Betazoids are. Each organism walks on two legs, lives in complex societies, uses tools and technologies, looks similar, and reproduces in the same manner. Each can interbreed with any of the others. The geneticist finds the following data:

• Klingons and Romulans each have 44 chromosomes. Humans and Betazoids have 46 chromosomes. Human chromosomes 15 and 17 resemble part of the same large chromosome in Klingons and Romulans.

• Humans and Klingons have 97 percent of their chromosome bands in common. Humans and Romulans have 98 percent of their chromosome bands in common, and Humans and Betazoids show 100 percent correspondence. Humans and Betazoids differ only by an extra segment on chromosome 11, which appears to be a duplication.

- The cytochrome *c* amino acid sequence is identical in Humans and Betazoids, differs by one amino acid between Humans and Romulans, and differs by two amino acids between Humans and Klingons.

- The gene for collagen contains 50 introns in Humans, 50 introns in Betazoids, 62 introns in Romulans, and 74 introns in Klingons.

- Mitochondrial DNA analysis reveals many more individual differences between Klingons and Romulans than between Humans and Betazoids.

a. Hypothesize the chromosomal aberrations that might explain the karyotypic differences among these four types of organisms.

b. Which are our closest relatives among the Klingons, Romulans, and Betazoids? What is the evidence for this?

c. Are Klingons, Romulans, Humans, and Betazoids distinct species? What information reveals this?

d. Which of the evolutionary tree diagrams is consistent with the data?

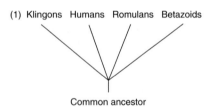

(1) Klingons   Humans   Romulans   Betazoids

Common ancestor

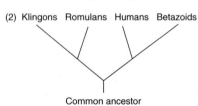

(2) Klingons   Romulans   Humans   Betazoids

Common ancestor

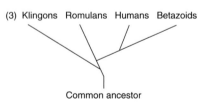

(3) Klingons   Romulans   Humans   Betazoids

Common ancestor

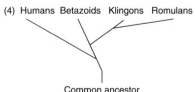

(4) Humans   Betazoids   Klingons   Romulans

Common ancestor

2. Give three examples of negative eugenic measures and three examples of positive eugenic measures.

3. A molecular anthropologist who is studying diabetes in native Americans feels that he can obtain information on why certain groups are prone to the disorder by analyzing genetic variants in small, isolated populations around the world. Do you think that the goal of understanding disease and alleviating suffering in one group of people justifies obtaining and studying the DNA of other people who have had little contact with cultures outside their own, even if they might be frightened by such attempts? Can you suggest a compromise intervention that might benefit everyone concerned?

4. In 1997, law schools in two states reversed their affirmative action policies and began evaluating all applicants on an equal basis—that is, applying the same admittance requirements to all. In fall 1997, classrooms of new law students had few, if any, nonwhite faces. How was this action eugenic, and how was it not?

5. Several women have offered to be artificially inseminated with sperm from the Ice Man, the human who died 5,300 years ago and was recently found in the Alps. However, he had been castrated. If sperm could have been recovered, and a woman inseminated, what do you think the child would be like?

6. The Human Genome Diversity Project is sampling DNA from white blood cells collected from 1,000 people that represent 40 to 50 populations in order to learn about their differences. Suggest a plan for utilizing this information yet avoid eugenics.

7. Anthropologist Daniel E. Lieberman wrote in *Nature* magazine of the paper describing the discovery of the partial skull of *Kenyanthropus platyops,* "I suspect the chief role of *K. platyops* in the next few years will be to act as a sort of party spoiler, highlighting the confusion that confronts research into evolutionary relationships among hominins."

a. What are the classification problems that *K. platyops* poses?

b. What do you think are the limitations of attempting to classify pre-humans on the basis of skeletal remains?

Web Activities

8. Researchers select organisms to help them study versions of human diseases based on ease of cultivation. Mice, rats, fruit flies, and roundworms are examples of such "model" organisms. Do you think that when researchers choose model organisms, they should consider genome similarities? Cite a reason for your answer.

9. Go to the website for the National Institutes of Health Intramural Sequencing Center at http://www.nisc.nih.gov. Under Scientific Projects, click Comparative Vertebrate Sequencing (first choice). Scroll down. Locate one where the red bars align for humans and chimps and/or another species. Read "gene name" at the bottom of the screen, and then look up this name on OMIM. Describe a human trait or condition that this gene confers.

10. Imagine you were asked to conduct targeted comparative sequencing for ten genome regions among the following organisms. List them in decreasing order of how similar you expect them to be to humans:

Ötzi the Ice Man

A Neanderthal

Australopithecus afarensis

A modern baboon

Homo habilis

H. sapiens idaltu

Case Studies

11. In the 1870s, a prison inspector and self-described sociologist named Richard Dugdale noticed that a disproportionate number of inmates at his facility in Ulster County, New York, were related. He began studying them, calling the family the "Jukes," although he kept records of their real names. Dugdale traced the family back seven generations to a son of Dutch settlers, a man named Max, a pioneer who lived off the land. Margaret, "the mother of criminals," as Dugdale would write in his 1877 book *The Jukes: A Study in Crime, Pauperism, Disease and Heredity,* married one of Max's sons, and the couple presumably gave rise to 540 of the 709 criminals on Dugdale's watch. Dugdale attributed the Jukes' less desireable

characteristics to heredity. He wrote, among many conclusions, that "harlotry may become a hereditary characteristic and be perpetuated without any specially favoring environment to call it into activity."

The Jukes study influenced social scientists to probe other families seemingly riddled with misfits—they were all caucasian, descended from colonial settlers, and poor. Poverty was not seen as an economic problem, but as a reflection of an inner, inborn, hard-to-define degeneracy, that if left unchecked would cost society dearly. Dugdale's book eventually became fodder for the fledgling eugenics movement. In 1911, researchers at the Eugenics Record Office in Cold Spring Harbor updated the Dugdale

account, describing the Jukes' phenotype as "feeblemindedness, indolence, licentiousness, and dishonesty." Criminality, too, was considered an inherited trait. The evidence from the Jukes family and others was used to argue for compulsory sterilization of those deemed unfit. But the original research on the Jukes family was flawed, and its accuracy was never questioned. Less notorious Jukes family members served in respected professions, some even holding public office. The Jukes' were vindicated in 2003, when archives at the State University of New York at Albany revealed the original names of the people in Dugdale's account; most were not even related. The Jukes family curse was more legend than fact.

a. What would have had to have happened to the original jailed Jukes family members or their descendants to be considered eugenic?

b. How could studies on one family harm others?

c. Cite an example of an idea based on eugenics today or in the recent past.

d. If you were a contemporary of Dugdale's, what type of evidence would you have sought to counter his ideas?

Learn to apply the skills of a genetic counselor with this additional case found in the *Case Workbook in Human Genetics:*

Novelty seeking and ADHD

Suggested Readings

Balter, Michael. January 11, 2002. From a modern human's brow—or doodling? *Science* 295:247–48. Do hatchmarks on red rocks found in South Africa set the origin of modern human behavior back to 77,000 years ago?

Bear, Greg. 1999, 2003. *Darwin's radio* and *Darwin's Children.* New York: The Ballantine Publishing Group. Two novels about modern humans evolving into a new species.

Boffelli, Dario, et al. February 28, 2003. Phylogenetic shadowing of primate sequences to find functional regions of the human genome. *Science* 299:1391–94. To understand our evolution, we must look at the genomic differences between humans and other primates.

Britten, R. J. October 15, 2002. Divergence between samples of chimp and human DNA sequence is 5 percent, counting indels. *Proceedings of the National Academy of Sciences* 99(21):13633–35. How closely related we are to chimps at the genome level depends upon how the genomes are compared.

Caramelli, David, et al. May 27, 2003. Evidence for a genetic discontinuity between Neanderthals and 24,000-year-old anatomically modern Europeans. *Proceedings*

of the National Academy of Sciences 199(11):6593–97. Sequencing mtDNA from Cro-Magnon bones adds to the evidence that Neanderthals are not our direct ancestors.

Carlson, Elof Axel. 2001. *The Unfit: The History of a Bad Idea.* New York: Cold Spring Harbor Press. Within eugenics lay the seeds of Naziism.

Courseaux, Anouk, and Jean-Louis Nahon. February 16, 2001. Birth of two chimeric genes in the Hominidae lineage. *Science* 291:1293–97. Through evolutionary time, as the primates evolved, genes duplicated, diverged, and moved.

Christianson, Scott. February 8, 2003. Bad seed or bad science: The story of the notorious Jukes family. *The New York Times,* p.F1. A flawed study helped found eugenics in the United States.

Fowler, Brenda. August 7, 2001. For 5,300-year-old ice man, extra autopsy tells the tale. *The New York Times,* p. D2. Ötzi was in a fight before he perished.

Gibbon, Ann. May 11, 2001. Modern men trace ancestry to African migrants. *Science* 292:1051–52. Most genetic evidence supports the replacement hypothesis of human origins.

Gillham, Nicholas Wright. 2001. *A Life of Sir Francis Galton: From African Exploration to the Birth of Eugenics.* New York: Oxford University Press. A history of eugenics, and other topics.

Gorman, James. March 11, 2003. The unbearable loneliness of being *Homo sapiens. The New York Times,* p. F1. The writer laments humans as a one-of-a-kind species—at least for now.

King, Mary-Claire, and Arno G. Motulsky. December 20, 2002. Mapping human history. *Science* 298:2342–43. Allele frequencies reflect geography.

Lewis, Ricki. January 27, 2003. First a bang, then a shuffle. *The Scientist* 17(2):18–20. The human genome doubled—at least once.

Lewis, Ricki. December 9, 2002. Targeted comparative sequencing illuminates vertebrate evolution. *The Scientist* 16(24):36–37. Comparing genome segments can reveal control regions.

Muller, Wolfgang, et al. October 31, 2003. Origin and migration of the Alpine Iceman. *Science* 302:862–66. The Iceman did not wander far during his lifetime from where his body was found.

Pennisi, Elizabeth. December 12, 2003. Genome comparisons hold clues to human evolution. *Science* 302:1876–77. Very few genes separate chimps from humans.

Pray, Leslie. August 19, 2002. Evolutionists present their 1.3 percent solution. *The Scientist* 16(16):36–37. Differing gene expression patterns may explain why humans and chimps are so similar genetically.

Stringer, Chris. June 12, 2003. Out of Ethiopia. *Nature* 423:692–95. Reconstructions of *H. sapiens idaltu* look eerily familiar.

Wade, Nicholas. August 19, 2003. Why humans and their fur parted ways. *The New York Times,* p. F1. Can single genes control our lack of fur and use of clothing?

Wilford, John Noble. December 31, 2002. Fully assembled at last, Neanderthal strides onstage. *The New York Times,* p. D1. A Neanderthal skeleton has marked differences from ours.

Wong, Kate. November 2003. Stranger in a new land. *Scientific American* 284(5):74–83. A look at *Homo* fossils in the Republic of Georgia, some of the earliest in our genus to leave Africa.

Weekly updates of current news related to human genetics are available through Power Web on your Online Learning Center.

VISIT YOUR ONLINE LEARNING CENTER

Visit your online learning center for additional resources and tools to help you master this chapter. See us at

www.mhhe.com/lewisgenetics6.

Genetics of Immunity

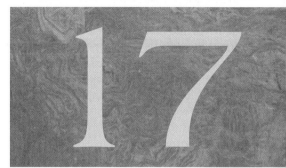

CHAPTER CONTENTS

17.1   The Importance of Cell Surfaces
Our cell surfaces are marked with molecules that indicate "self" as well as tissue type. The immune system is a vast army of cells, biochemicals, and associated vessels and organs that protects the body against "nonself" cells and molecules. It guards against infection and cancer—but can malfunction.

17.2   The Human Immune System
A pathogen faces a daunting task when it attempts to penetrate the human body's immune defenses. It must first breach physical barriers and torrents of body fluids, then overcome the broad defenses of innate immunity. Meanwhile, the antibodies and cytokines of the adaptive immune response are readying for attack. The adaptive part of the immune system "remembers" encounters and rapidly combats future infections.

17.3   Abnormal Immunity
When the immune system malfunctions, the effects on health can be disastrous. Deficient immunity, whether inherited or acquired, opens the body to rampant infection and cancers. Autoimmunity sets the immune system against the body, and allergies represent misguided attacks against harmless substances.

17.4   Altering Immune Function
Understanding the immune response enables medical science to alter and direct it. Vaccines prevent infections by inducing a false first infection. Monoclonal antibodies and cytokines boost immunity to treat a variety of conditions. Conversely, immune function must be subdued for transplants to replace body parts.

17.5   A Genomic View of Immunity—The Pathogen's Perspective
Infectious disease is a consequence of specific interactions between the human genome and that of the pathogen. Sequencing the genomes of infectious organisms and viruses can suggest new ways to treat illness.

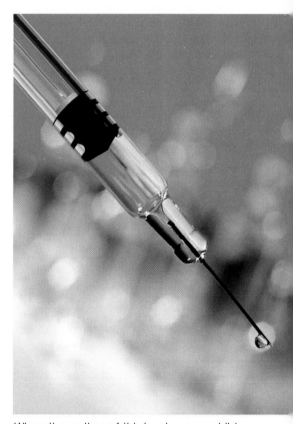

When the author of this book was a child, suffering with measles, mumps, chickenpox, and rubella was routine. She was one of the first to receive the vaccine against polio. Today, vaccines have vanquished these five illnesses, at least in developed nations. Today, children also receive vaccines against infection by hepatitis B virus and *Haemophilus influenzae,* a bacterium.

Leslie Hancock was born with cystic fibrosis. At age six, her liver hardened as a complication, and the little girl desperately needed a new one. But because of a shortage of donor organs, a third of the children awaiting livers die before a transplant can be performed. Fortunately, Leslie's father, Jim, was able to donate part of his liver because his and Leslie's cell surfaces are so similar that her body accepted part of his. "When the subject of a living-relative transplant came up, I never had to think about it. It was just something I wanted to do," Jim recalls (**figure 17.1**).

After the surgery, Leslie took drugs to suppress her immune system, and two months later, she was back in kindergarten. Transplants between blood relatives succeed in about 90 percent of cases, compared to 80 percent for unrelated people whose cell surfaces are similar by chance. In the future, gene expression profiling will help physicians to better match donors to recipients.

In the case of an organ transplant, the immune system is an obstacle. More often, this organ system protects the body against infection-causing viruses and microorganisms (collectively called pathogens) as well as cancer cells. Because immune system cells produce proteins, immunity is a genetic matter, although environmental cues trigger many components of the immune response.

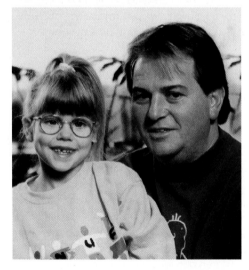

Figure 17.1 **The importance of cell surfaces.** Jim Hancock, of Dubuque, Iowa, gave his six-year-old daughter, Leslie, part of his liver. The transplant worked because the cell surfaces of this father and daughter are very similar. The little girl's immune system accepted the new tissue as part of her body.

17.1 The Importance of Cell Surfaces

We share the planet with plants, microbes, fungi, and other animals. The human immune system has evolved to keep potentially harmful organisms out of our bodies. This system is a mobile army of about 2 trillion cells and the biochemicals they produce. Protection is based upon the ability of the immune system to recognize "foreign" or "nonself" surfaces, which include those of microbes such as bacteria (see figure 2.2) and yeast (see figure 17.8), nonliving "infectious agents" such as viruses, and even tumor cells and transplanted cells. Then, the system launches a highly coordinated, multipronged attack.

Pathogens

Organisms and infectious agents (such as viruses and prions) that cause disease are termed pathogens. Bacteria and viruses cause most infections in humans.

Bacteria are prokaryotic cells, which means that they lack membrane-bounded, complex organelles, but they are nonetheless cells. Antibiotic drugs treat bacterial infections. Much of the action of the immune system is directed against viruses, which are simpler than cells and straddle the boundary between the nonliving and the living. Few drugs can treat viral infections, which is why outbreaks of unknown types, or those that invade a new geographic region—such as the SARS and monkeypox viruses—raise high health alerts.

A **virus** is a single or double strand of RNA or DNA wrapped in a protein coat, and in some types, in an outer envelope, too. A virus can reproduce only if it enters and uses a host cell's energy resources, protein synthetic machinery, and secretion pathway.

A virus is a stunningly streamlined structure. It may have only a few protein-encoding genes, but many copies of the same protein can assemble to form an intricate covering, like the panes of glass in a greenhouse. Ebola virus, for example, is an extremely simple, but deadly virus, encoding just seven proteins (**figure 17.2a**). The SARS virus produces nine different proteins. In contrast, the smallpox virus has more than 100 different types of pro-teins. HIV also has a complex structure (figure 17.2b).

Human chromosomes harbor viral DNA sequences that are vestiges of past infections, perhaps in distant ancestors. Many DNA viruses reproduce by inserting DNA into the host cell's genetic material. In contrast, it takes several steps for an RNA virus to insert DNA into a human chromosome, because the DNA must first be copied from the RNA by a viral enzyme called reverse transcriptase. The DNA that represents the RNA virus then inserts into the host cell's chromosome. (In some viruses, the invading DNA is replicated separately from a host chromosome.) Certain RNA viruses are called "retro" because they transmit genetic information opposite the usual direction—from DNA to RNA to protein. HIV is a retrovirus.

Once viral DNA integrates into the host cell's DNA, it can either remain and replicate along with the host's DNA without causing harm, or it can take over and kill the cell. Viral genes direct the host cell to replicate viral DNA and then use it to manufacture viral proteins at the expense of the cell's normal activities. The cell fills with viral DNA and protein, which assemble into new viruses. The cell bursts, releasing many new virus copies into the body.

Diverse viruses infect all types of organisms. They were discovered in tobacco plants, but also infect microorganisms, fungi, and, of course, animals. Their genetic material cannot repair itself, so the mutation rate may be high—which is one reason why we cannot develop an effective vaccine against HIV or the common cold, and why new influenza vaccines must be developed each year. The immune system does not recognize infectious prions. This is because unlike viruses, prions are variants of proteins normally in the body that have the same amino acid sequence.

Genetic Control of Immunity

Genes that affect immunity may confer susceptibilities or resistances to certain infectious diseases, or raise the risk of developing an allergic or **autoimmune** condition, in which the immune system attacks an individual's own tissues. Most such effects are polygenic. However, a few single genes exert powerful effects on immunity.

Certain classes of genes oversee immunity by encoding **antibodies** and **cytokines,** proteins that directly attack foreign antigens. An **antigen** is any molecule that elicits an immune response, and is usually a protein or carbohydrate. Genes specify the cell surface antigens that mark the body's cells as "self."

Because genes control immunity, mutations can impair immune function, causing immune deficiencies, autoimmune disorders, allergies, and cancer. But understanding how genes control immunity also makes it possible to enhance or redirect the system's ability to fight disease. We begin our look at normal immunity with some familiar examples of our personal cellular landscapes.

Blood Groups

Transplanting an organ as complex as a liver is a major and risky medical procedure. A far simpler type of transplant, although still very dependent on matching cell surfaces, is a blood transfusion. Using one person's blood to restore another's health was proposed centuries ago. To do so safely and successfully, however, it was necessary to understand the genetics of blood types.

ABO Blood Groups

The first transfusions, performed in the late 1600s, used lamb's blood. By the 1800s, physicians were trying to use human blood. Results were unpredictable—some recipients recovered, but others died. So poor was the success rate that, by the late 1800s, many nations banned transfusions.

Then Austrian physician Karl Landsteiner began investigating why transfusions sometimes worked and sometimes didn't. In 1900, he determined that human blood was of differing types, and only certain combinations were compatible. In 1910, identification of the ABO blood antigen locus explained the blood type incompatibilities (**figure 17.3**). Today, we know of more than 20 different genes whose protein products are part of the surface topography of red blood cells.

Recall from chapter 5 that the *I* gene alleles encode enzymes that place antigens A, B, both A and B, or neither antigen on sugar chains on red blood cells (see table 5.1). Blood type incompatibility occurs when a person's immune system manufactures antibodies that attack the antigens his or her cells do not carry. A person with blood type A, for example, has antibodies against type B antigen. If he or she is transfused with type B blood, the anti-B antibodies clump the transfused red blood cells, blocking circulation and depriving tissues of oxygen. A person with type AB blood doesn't manufacture antibodies against either antigen A or B,

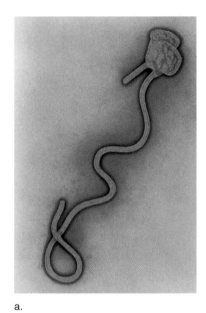

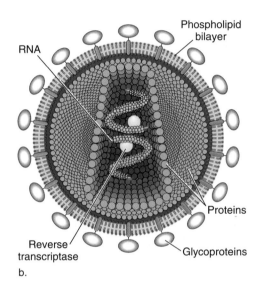

Figure 17.2 Virus structure.   Viruses are nucleic acids in protein coats. **(a)** Ebola virus is a single strand of RNA and just seven proteins. People become infected when they touch the body fluids of those who have died of the infection. Symptoms progress rapidly, from headache and fever, to vomiting blood, to tearing apart of the internal organs. **(b)** The human immunodeficiency virus (HIV), which causes AIDS, consists of RNA surrounded by several protein layers. Once inside a human cell, the virus uses an enzyme it encodes, reverse transcriptase, to make a DNA copy of its RNA. The virus then inserts this copy into the host cell's DNA. The infected cell not only dies, but produces and releases many viral particles.

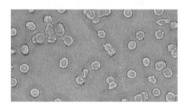
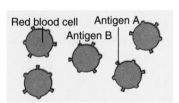
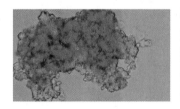
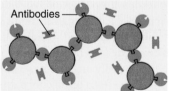

Compatible Blood Types (no clumping)	
Donor	*Recipient*
O	O, A, B, AB
A	A, AB
B	B, AB
AB	AB

Incompatible Blood Types (clumping)	
Donor	*Recipient*
A	B, O
B	A, O
AB	A, B, O

Figure 17.3 ABO blood types.   Genetics explains blood incompatibilities.

because if he or she did, the person's own blood would clump. Therefore, someone with type AB blood can receive any ABO blood type. Type O blood has neither A nor B antigens, so it cannot stimulate an immune response in a transfusion recipient; people with type O blood can thus donate to anyone. However, the idea that a person with AB blood is a "universal recipient" and one with type O blood is a "universal donor" is more theoretical than practical, because antibodies to other donor blood antigens (for example, the Rh factor, discussed next) can cause slight incompatibilities. For this reason, blood is as closely matched as possible.

A person who receives mismatched blood quickly feels the effects—anxiety, difficulty breathing, facial flushing, headache, and severe pain in the neck, chest, and lower back. Red blood cells burst, releasing free hemoglobin that can damage the kidneys.

The Rh Factor

ABO blood type is often further differentiated by a $^+$ or $^-$, which refers to another blood group antigen called the Rh factor. Whether a person has the Rh factor (Rh^+) or not (Rh^-) is determined by a combination of alleles of three genes. The antigens were originally identified in rhesus monkeys, hence the name.

Rh type is important when an Rh^+ man and an Rh^- woman conceive a child who is Rh^+. The pregnant woman's immune system reacts to the few fetal cells that enter her bloodstream by manufacturing antibodies against them (**figure 17.4**). Not enough antibodies form to harm the first fetus, but if she carries a second Rh^+ fetus, the woman's now plentiful antibodies attack the fetal blood supply. In the fetus, bilirubin, a breakdown product of red blood cells, accumulates, damaging the brain and turning the skin and whites of the eyes yellow. The fetal liver and spleen swell as they rapidly produce new red blood cells. If the fetus or newborn does not receive a transfusion of Rh^- blood and have some of its Rh^+ blood removed, then the heart and blood vessels collapse and fatal respiratory distress sets in. Rh disease that progresses this far is called hydrops fetalis.

Fortunately, natural and medical protections make hydrops fetalis rare today, although exchange blood transfusions were once common. Determining parental ABO blood types indicates whether an immune reaction against the fetus of an Rh-incompatible couple will take place. If the woman has type O blood and the fetus is A or B, then her anti-A or anti-B antibodies attack the fetal blood cells in her circulation before her system has a chance to manufacture the anti-Rh antibodies. This blocks the anti-Rh reaction.

Obstetricians routinely determine a pregnant woman's blood type. If she and her partner are Rh incompatible, doctors inject a drug (called RhoGAM) during pregnancy and after the birth. The drug covers antigens on fetal blood cells in the woman's circulation so that she does not manufacture anti-Rh antibodies. However, events other than pregnancy and childbirth can expose an Rh^- woman's system to Rh^+ cells, placing even her first child at risk. These include amniocentesis, a blood transfusion, an ectopic (tubal) pregnancy, a miscarriage, or an abortion.

Other Blood Groups

Another way of distinguishing red blood cells is by the *L* gene, whose codominant alleles *M*, *N*, and *S* combine to form six different genotypes and phenotypes (glycoprotein cell surface patterns). Another blood-type determining gene is called Lewis. It encodes an enzyme that adds an antigen to the sugar fucose, which the product of the *H* gene then places on red blood cells. (Recall from section 5.1 that the *H* gene is necessary for ABO expression.) Individuals with genotype *LeLe* or *Lele* have the Lewis antigen on red blood cell plasma membranes and in saliva, whereas *lele* people do not produce the antigen. Another interesting gene that affects the blood is the secretor gene. People who have the dominant allele *Se* secrete the A, B, and H antigens in body fluids, including semen, saliva, tears, and mucus.

Cell surfaces are dotted with many molecules other than those that confer blood type. Many of these protein surface features are encoded by genes that are part of a 6-million-base-long cluster on the short arm of chromosome 6 called the **major histocompatibility complex** (MHC). The MHC includes about 70 genes.

The Human Leukocyte Antigens

The genes of the MHC are classified into three functional groups. Class III MHC

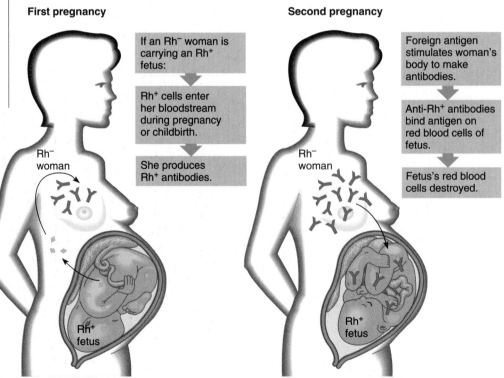

First pregnancy

Rh$^-$ woman

Rh$^+$ fetus

If an Rh$^-$ woman is carrying an Rh$^+$ fetus:

Rh$^+$ cells enter her bloodstream during pregnancy or childbirth.

She produces Rh$^+$ antibodies.

Second pregnancy

Rh$^-$ woman

Rh$^+$ fetus

Foreign antigen stimulates woman's body to make antibodies.

Anti-Rh$^+$ antibodies bind antigen on red blood cells of fetus.

Fetus's red blood cells destroyed.

Figure 17.4 Rh incompatibility. Fetal cells entering the pregnant woman's bloodstream can stimulate her immune system to make anti-Rh antibodies, if the fetus is Rh$^+$ and she is Rh$^-$. A drug called RhoGAM prevents attacks on subsequent fetuses.

genes encode proteins that are in blood plasma and that carry out some of the innate immune functions discussed here. The class I and II genes of the MHC encode the **human leukocyte antigens** (HLA), first studied in leukocytes, a broad term for white blood cells. The HLA proteins link to sugars to form branchlike glycoproteins that emanate from cell surfaces. Some of these HLA glycoproteins latch onto bacterial and viral proteins, displaying them like badges to alert other immune system cells. This action, called **antigen processing,** is often the first step in an immune response. The cell that displays the foreign antigen an HLA protein holds is an **antigen-presenting cell. Figure 17.5** shows how a large cell called a **macrophage** displays bacterial antigens. Certain white blood cells called T cells (or T lymphocytes) also function as antigen-presenting cells. Class I and II HLA proteins differ in the types of immune system cells they alert.

All cells with nuclei (that is, all cells except red blood cells) have some HLA antigens, which identify them as "self," or belonging to the same individual. In addition to these common HLA markers are more specific markers that distinguish particular tissue types. Class I includes three genes, called *A, B,* and *C,* that are very variable and are found on all cell types, and three other genes, *E, F,* and *G,* that are more restricted in their distribution. Class II includes three major genes whose encoded proteins are found mostly on antigen-presenting cells.

Because the HLA classes consist of several genes that have many alleles, individuals have an overall HLA "type." Only 2 in every 20,000 unrelated people match for the six major HLA genes by chance. When transplant physicians attempt to match donor tissue to a potential recipient, they determine how alike the two individuals are at these six loci. Usually at least four of the genes must match for a transplant to have a reasonable chance of success. Before DNA profiling, HLA typing was the predominant type of blood test used in forensic and paternity cases to rule out involvement of certain individuals. However, HLA genotyping has become very complex because hundreds of alleles are now known, and HLA genotype and disease associations differ in different populations.

About 50 percent of the genetic influence on immunity stems from HLA genes. However, a few disorders are very strongly associated with particular HLA types. This is the case for ankylosing spondylitis, which inflames and deforms vertebrae. A person with either of two particular subtypes of an HLA antigen called B27 is 100 times as likely to develop the condition as someone who lacks either form of the antigen. HLA-associated risks are not absolute. More than 90 percent of people who suffer from ankylosing spondylitis have the B27 antigen, which occurs in only 5 percent of the general population. However, 10 percent of people who have ankylosing spondylitis do *not* have the B27 antigen, and some people who have the antigen never develop the disease.

Key Concepts

The immune system consists of cells and biochemicals that distinguish self from nonself antigens. • Pathogens inlcude microbes and infectious agents, such as viruses, which take over a host cell's protein synthesis machinery to reproduce. • Blood types result from self antigen patterns on red blood cells. • The HLA complex is a highly diverse group of cell surface proteins, some of which display foreign antigens to other parts of the immune system, triggering a response.

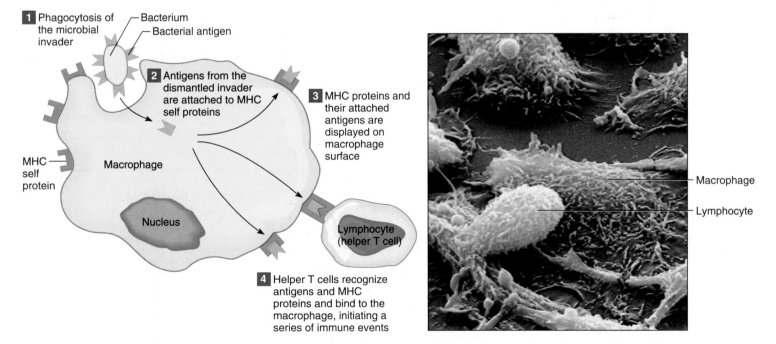

Figure 17.5 Macrophages are antigen-presenting cells. A macrophage engulfs a bacterium, then displays foreign antigens on its surface, held in place by major histocompatibility complex (MHC) self proteins. This event sets into motion many immune reactions.

17.2 The Human Immune System

On a macroscopic level, the immune system includes a network of vessels called lymphatics, which transport lymph, a watery fluid, to bean-shaped structures called lymph nodes. The spleen and thymus gland are also part of the immune system (**figure 17.6**). On a microscopic level, the immune system consists of white blood cells called **lymphocytes** and the wandering, scavenging macrophages that capture and degrade bacteria, viruses, and cellular debris. **B cells** and **T cells** are the two major types of lymphocytes.

The immune response consists of two lines of defense—an immediate generalized **innate immunity,** and a more specific, slower **adaptive immunity.** These defenses act after various physical barriers keep pathogens out. **Table 17.1** and **figure 17.7** summarize these basic components of immunity.

Physical Barriers and the Innate Immune Response

Several familiar structures and fluids keep pathogens from entering the body in the innate immune response. Unbroken skin and mucous membranes such as the lining inside the mouth are part of this first line of defense, as are earwax and the waving cilia that push debris and pathogens up and out of the respiratory tract. Most microbes that make it to the stomach perish in a vat of churning acid—though a notable exception is the bacterium that causes peptic ulcers. Other microbes are flushed out in diarrhea. These

barriers are nonspecific—they keep out anything foreign, not just particular pathogens.

If a pathogen breaches these physical barriers, innate immunity provides a rapid, broad defense. The term *innate* refers to the fact that these general defenses are in the body, ready to function should infection begin. A process called **inflammation** is a central part of the innate immune response. Inflammation creates a hostile environment for pathogenss at an injury site, sending in cells that engulf and destroy them. Such cells are called phagocytes, and their engulfing action is **phagocytosis (figure 17.8)** Certain blood cells, such as neutrophils, are phagocytes, as are the large, wandering

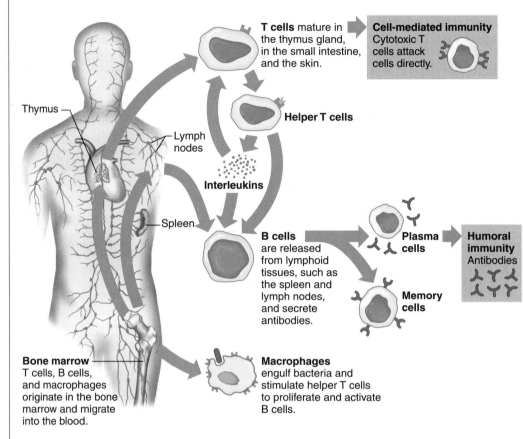

T cells mature in the thymus gland, in the small intestine, and the skin.

Cell-mediated immunity Cytotoxic T cells attack cells directly.

Helper T cells

Interleukins

B cells are released from lymphoid tissues, such as the spleen and lymph nodes, and secrete antibodies.

Plasma cells

Humoral immunity Antibodies

Memory cells

Thymus

Lymph nodes

Spleen

Bone marrow T cells, B cells, and macrophages originate in the bone marrow and migrate into the blood.

Macrophages engulf bacteria and stimulate helper T cells to proliferate and activate B cells.

Figure 17.6 Immune cells are diverse. T cells, B cells, and macrophages build an overall immune response. All three types of cells originate in the bone marrow and circulate in the blood.

Table 17.1		
Major Components of the Immune Response		
First Line of Defense: Physical Barriers	**Second Line of Defense: Nonspecific, Innate Immunity**	**Third Line of Defense: Specific, Adaptive Immunity**
Unbroken skin	Phagocytosis (engulfing cells)	Humoral immune response
Mucous membranes and their secretions	Antimicrobial proteins	B cells, antibodies, memory cells
Infection-fighting chemicals in tears, saliva, and other body fluids	Complement system	Cellular immune response
Flushing effect of tears, saliva, urination, and diarrhea	Collectins	T cells, cytokines, memory cells
	Cytokines	
	Inflammatory response	
	Fever	

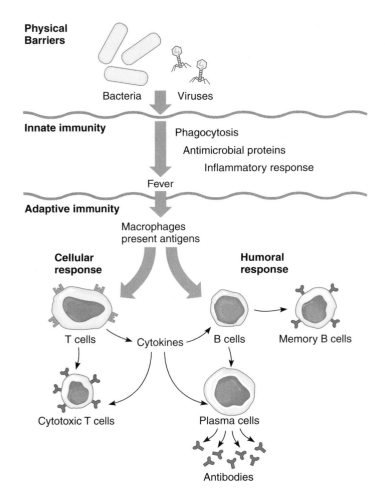

Physical Barriers

Bacteria   Viruses

Innate immunity

Phagocytosis
Antimicrobial proteins
Inflammatory response

Fever

Adaptive immunity

Macrophages present antigens

Cellular response   **Humoral response**

T cells   Cytokines   B cells   Memory B cells

Cytotoxic T cells   Plasma cells

Antibodies

Figure 17.7 **Levels of immune protection.** Disease-causing organisms and viruses (pathogens) first encounter barriers that prevent their entry into the body. If the pathogens breach these barriers, an array of nonspecific cells and molecules attack the pathogen in the innate immune response. If this is ineffective, the adaptive immune response begins: antigen-presenting cells stimulate T cells to produce cytokines, which activate B cells to differentiate into plasma cells, which secrete antibodies. Once activated, these specific cells retain a memory of the pathogen, allowing faster responses to subsequent attacks.

macrophages. At the same time, plasma (the liquid portion of blood) accumulates, diluting toxins and bringing in antimicrobial chemicals. Increased blood flow warms the area, turning it swollen and red. The person may not be very comfortable, but often, the pathogen does not survive. Inflammation at the site of an injury can prevent infection.

Three major classes of proteins participate in the innate immune response—the complement system, collectins, and cytokines. Mutations in the genes that encode these proteins can produce disorders that increase susceptibility to infection. Yet, some mutations have no effect; perhaps other proteins provide the function.

The **complement system** consists of plasma proteins that assist, or complement, several of the body's other defense mecha-

nisms. Some complement proteins puncture bacterial plasma membranes, bursting the cells. Others dismantle viruses. Yet other complement proteins assist inflammation by triggering the release of **histamine** from **mast cells,** another type of immune system cell that is involved in allergies. Histamine dilates blood vessels, enabling fluid to rush to the infected or injured area. Still other complement proteins attract phagocytes to an injury site.

Collectins are proteins that broadly protect against bacteria, yeasts, and some viruses by detecting slight differences from human cells in their surfaces. Groups of human collectins correspond to the surfaces of different types of pathogens, such as the distinctive sugars on infecting yeast, the linked sugars and lipids of certain bacteria, and the surface features of some RNA viruses.

Cytokines play many roles in immunity. As part of the innate immune response, cytokines called **interferons** alert other components of the immune system to the presence of cells infected with viruses. These cells are then destroyed, which limits the spread of infection. **Interleukins** are cytokines that cause fever, temporarily maintaining a higher body temperature that directly kills some infecting bacteria and viruses. Fever also counters microbial growth indirectly, because higher body temperature reduces the iron level in the blood. Bacteria and fungi require more iron as the body temperature rises; therefore, a fever-ridden body stops their growth. Phagocytes also attack more vigorously when the temperature rises. **Tumor necrosis factor** is another type of cytokine that activates other protective biochemicals, destroys certain bacterial toxins, and also attacks cancer cells. Many of the more unpleasant aspects of suffering from an infection are actually due to the immune response, rather than to the actions of the pathogens.

The Adaptive Immune Response

Adaptive immunity must be stimulated into action, taking days to respond, compared to minutes for innate immunity. Adaptive immunity is highly specific and directed.

B cells and T cells carry out adaptive immunity. B cells produce antibodies in response to activation by T cells in the **humoral immune response.** T cells produce cytokines and activate other cells in the **cellular immune response.** Lymphocytes differentiate in the bone marrow and migrate to the lymph nodes, spleen, and thymus gland, as well as circulate in the blood and tissue fluid.

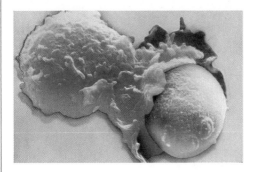

Figure 17.8 **Nature's garbage collectors.** A human phagocyte engulfs a yeast cell.

The adaptive arm of the immune system has three basic characteristics. It is *diverse*, vanquishing many types of pathogens. It is *specific*, distinguishing the cells and molecules that cause disease from those that are harmless. The immune system also *remembers*, responding faster to a subsequent encounter with a foreign antigen than it did the first time. The first assault initiates a **primary immune response.** The second assault, based on the system's "memory," is a **secondary immune response.** This is why we get some infections, such as chickenpox, only once. However, upper respiratory infections and influenza recur because the causative viruses mutate, presenting a different face to our immune systems each season. In addition, different viruses can cause the same respiratory symptoms.

The Humoral Immune Response—B Cells and Antibodies

B cells secreting antibodies into the bloodstream constitute the humoral immune response. (*Humor* means fluid.) An antibody response begins when an antigen-presenting macrophage activates a T cell, which in turn contacts a B cell that has surface receptors that can bind the same type of foreign antigen. The immune system has so many B cells, each with different combinations of surface antigens, that there is almost always one or more available that corresponds to a particular foreign antigen. Turnover of these cells is high. Each day, millions of B cells perish in the lymph nodes and spleen, while millions more form in the bone marrow, each with a unique combination of surface molecules.

Once the activated T cell finds a B cell match, it releases cytokines that stimulate the B cell to divide. Soon the B cell gives rise to two types of cells (**figure 17.9**). The first, **plasma cells,** are antibody factories, secreting up to 2,000 identical antibodies each per second at the height of their few-day lifespan. These cells provide the primary immune response. Plasma cells derived from different B cells secrete different antibodies, with each type corresponding to a specific portion of the pathogen in what is called a polyclonal antibody response (**figure 17.10**). This response is like hitting a person in different parts of the body. The second type of B cell descendant, **memory cells,** are far fewer and usually are dormant. They respond to the foreign antigen faster and with more force should it appear again. This is a secondary immune response.

Antibodies are constructed of several polypeptides and are therefore encoded by several genes. The simplest antibody molecule is four polypeptide chains connected by disulfide (sulfur-sulfur) bonds, forming a

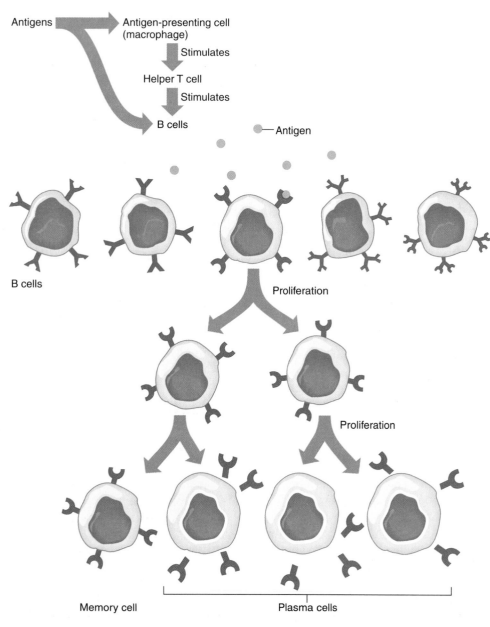

Figure 17.9 Production of antibodies. The humoral immune response involves B cell proliferation and maturation into antibody-secreting plasma cells. Note that only the B cell that binds the antigen proliferates; its descendants may develop into memory cells or plasma cells.

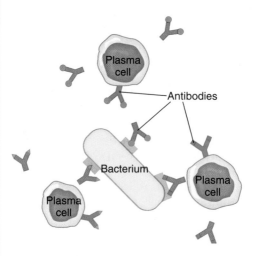

Figure 17.10 An immune response recognizes many targets. A humoral immune response is polyclonal, which means that different plasma cells produce antibody proteins that recognize and bind to different features of a foreign cell's surface.

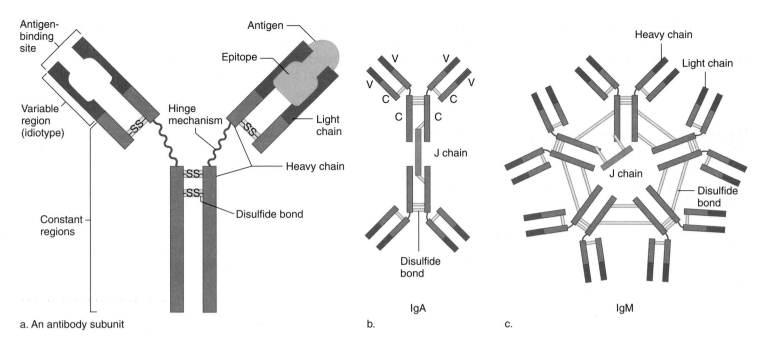

Figure 17.11 **Antibody structure.** The simplest antibody molecule **(a)** consists of four polypeptide chains, two heavy and two light, joined by two sulfur atoms that form a disulfide bond. Part of each polypeptide chain has a constant sequence of amino acids, and the remainder varies. The tops of the Y-shaped molecules form antigen binding sites. **(b)** IgA consists of two Y-shaped subunits, and IgM **(c)** consists of five subunits. J chain proteins connect the units.

shape like the letter Y (**figure 17.11**). A large antibody molecule might consist of three, four, or five such Ys joined.

In a Y-shaped antibody subunit, the two longer polypeptides are called **heavy chains,** and the other two **light chains.** The lower portion of each chain is an amino acid sequence that is very similar in all antibody molecules, even in different species. These areas are called **constant regions.** The amino acid sequence of the upper portions of each polypeptide chain, the **variable regions,** can differ greatly among antibodies.

Antibodies can bind certain antigens because of the three-dimensional shapes of the tips of the variable regions. These specialized ends are called **antigen binding sites,** and the parts that actually contact the antigen are called **idiotypes.** The parts of the antigens that idiotypes bind are **epitopes.** An antibody contorts to form a pocket around the antigen.

Antibodies have several functions. Antibody-antigen binding may inactivate a pathogen or neutralize the toxin it produces. Antibodies can also clump pathogens, making them more visible to macrophages, which then destroy them. Antibodies also activate complement, extending the innate immune response.

Antibodies come in five major types, distinguished by location and function

Table 17.2

Types of Antibodies

Type*	Location	Functions
IgA	Milk, saliva, urine, and tears; respiratory and digestive secretions	Protects against pathogens at points of entry into body
IgD	On B cells in blood	Stimulates B cells to make other types of antibodies, particularly in infants
IgE	In secretions with IgA and in mast cells in tissues	Acts as receptor for antigens that cause mast cells to secrete allergy mediators
IgG	Blood plasma and tissue fluid; passes to fetus	Protects against bacteria, viruses, and toxins, especially in secondary immune response
IgM	Blood plasma	Fights bacteria in primary immune response; includes anti-A and anti-B antibodies of ABO blood groups

*The letters *A, D, E, G,* and *M* refer to the specific conformation of heavy chains characteristic of each class of antibody.

(**table 17.2**). (Antibodies are also called immunoglobulins, abbreviated *Ig*.) Different antibody types predominate in different stages of an infection.

The human body can manufacture a seemingly limitless number of different antibodies, though the genome of course has a limited number of antibody genes. This great diversity is possible because parts of different antibody genes combine. During the early development of B cells, sections of their antibody genes move to other chromosomal locations, creating new genetic instructions for antibodies. In this way, 200 genes generate about 100 trillion different antibody types. Because of this tremendous diversity, a human body can respond to nearly any infection. A single stimulated B cell is said to give rise to a clone of plasma and memory cells because all of its descendants express the same antibody gene combinations.

The Cellular Immune Response—T cells and Cytokines

T cells provide the cellular immune response, so-called because the cells themselves travel to where they act, unlike B cells, which secrete antibodies into the bloodstream. T cells begin as stem cells in the bone marrow, then travel to the thymus gland ("T" refers to thymus). As the immature T cells, called thymocytes, migrate toward the interior of the thymus, they display diverse cell surface receptors. An extensive selection process unfolds. As the wandering thymocytes touch lining cells in the gland that are studded with "self" antigens, thymocytes that do not attack the lining cells begin maturing into T cells, whereas those that harm the lining cells die by apoptosis—in great numbers. Gradually, T-cells-to-be that recognize self are selected and persist.

Several types of T cells are distinguished by the types and patterns of receptors on their surfaces, and by their functions. **Helper T cells** recognize foreign antigens on macrophages, stimulate B cells to produce antibodies, secrete cytokines, and activate another type of T cell called a **cytotoxic T cell,** also called a killer T cell. Certain T cells may help to suppress an immune response when it is no longer required. The cytokines that helper T cells secrete include interleukins, interferons, tumor necrosis factor, and **colony stimulating factors,** which stimulate white blood cells in bone marrow to mature (**table 17.3**). Cytokines interact with and signal each other.

Distinctive surfaces distinguish subsets of helper T cells. Certain antigens called cluster-of-differentiation antigens, or CD antigens, enable T cells to recognize foreign antigens displayed on macrophages. One such cell type, called a CD4 helper T cell, is an early target of HIV. Considering the critical role helper T cells play in coordinating immunity, it is little wonder that HIV infection ultimately topples the entire system, a point we will return to soon.

Cytotoxic T cells lack CD4 receptors but have CD8 receptors. These cells attack virally infected and cancerous cells by attaching to them and releasing chemicals. They do this by linking two surface peptides to form structures called T cell receptors that bind foreign antigens. When a cytotoxic T cell encounters a nonself cell—a cancer cell, for example—the T cell recep-

tors draw the two cells into physical contact. The T cell then releases a protein called perforin, which drills holes in the cancer cell's plasma membrane, killing it (**figure 17.12**). Cytotoxic T cell receptors also attract body cells that are covered with certain viruses, destroying the cells before

the viruses on them can enter, replicate, and spread the infection. Cytotoxic T cells continually monitor body cells, recognizing and eliminating virally infected and tumor cells.

Table 17.4 summarizes immune system cell types.

Table 17.3

Types of Cytokines

Cytokine	Function
Colony stimulating factors	Stimulate bone marrow to produce lymphocytes
Interferons	Block viral replication, stimulate macrophages to engulf viruses, stimulate B cells to produce antibodies, attack cancer cells
Interleukins	Control lymphocyte differentiation and growth, cause fever that accompanies bacterial infection
Tumor necrosis factor	Stops tumor growth, releases growth factors, stimulates lymphocyte differentiation, dismantles bacterial toxins

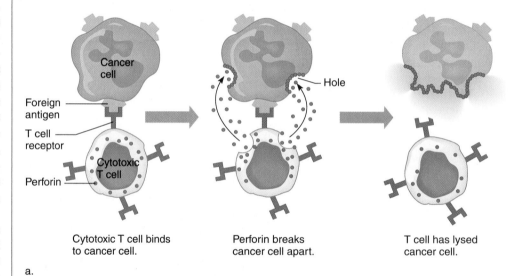

Cytotoxic T cell binds to cancer cell.

Perforin breaks cancer cell apart.

T cell has lysed cancer cell.

a.

b.

Figure 17.12 Death of a cancer cell. (a) A cytotoxic T cell binds to a cancer cell and injects perforin, a protein that pokes holes in the cancer cell's plasma membrane. As holes form, the cancer cell dies, leaving behind debris that macrophages clear away. (b) The smaller cell is a cytotoxic T cell, which homes in on the surface of the large cancer cell above it. The cytotoxic T cell will shatter the cancer cell, leaving behind scattered fibers.

Table 17.4

Types of Immune System Cells

Cell Type	Function
Macrophage	Presents antigens
	Performs phagocytosis
Mast cell	Releases histamine in inflammation
	Releases allergy mediators
B cell	Matures into antibody-producing plasma cell or into memory cell
T cells	
Helper	Recognizes nonself antigens presented on macrophages
	Stimulates B cells to produce antibodies
	Secretes cytokines
	Activates cytotoxic T cells
Cytotoxic	Attacks cancer cells and cells infected with viruses

Key Concepts

The immune system consists of physical barriers; an innate immune response of inflammation, phagocytosis, complement, collectins, and cytokines; and a more directed adaptive immune response. Adaptive immunity is diverse and specific, and it remembers. It has two components. • In the humoral immune response, stimulated B cells divide and differentiate into plasma cells and memory cells. A plasma cell secretes abundant antibodies of a single type. Antibodies are made of Y-shaped polypeptides, each consisting of two light and two heavy chains. Each chain consists of a constant and a variable region, and the tips of the Y form an antigen binding site with a specific idiotype. Antibodies make foreign antigens more visible to macrophages and stimulate complement. Shuffling gene pieces generates astounding antibody diversity. • In the cellular immune response, helper T cells stimulate B cells to manufacture antibodies and cytotoxic T cells to secrete cytokines. Using T cell receptors, cytotoxic T cells bind to nonself cells and virus-covered cells and cause them to burst.

17.3 Abnormal Immunity

The immune system continually adapts to environmental change. Because the immune response is so diverse, its breakdown affects health in many ways. Immune system malfunction may be inherited or acquired, and immunity may be too strong, too weak, or misdirected.

Inherited Immune Deficiencies

Scientists recognize more than 20 types of inherited immune deficiencies, affecting both innate and adaptive immunity. In chronic granulomatous disease, neutrophils can engulf bacteria, but, due to deficiency of an enzyme called oxidase, they cannot produce the activated oxygen compounds that kill bacteria. Because this enzyme is made of four polypeptide chains, four genes encode it, and there are four ways to inherit the disease, all X-linked. A very rare autosomal recessive form is caused by a defect in the vacuole that encloses bacteria. Antibiotics and gamma interferon are used to prevent bacterial infections in these patients, and the disease can be cured with a bone marrow or an umbilical cord stem cell transplant.

Mutations in genes that encode cytokines or T cell receptors impair cellular immunity, which primarily targets viruses and cancer cells. But because T cells activate the B cells that manufacture antibodies, abnormal cellular immunity (T cell function) disrupts humoral immunity (B cell function). Mutations in the genes that encode antibody segments, that control how the segments join, or that direct maturation of B cells mostly impair immunity against bacterial infection. Inherited immune deficiency can also result from defective B cells. In one condition, B cells lack B cell linker protein, which normally signals the cells to mature into plasma cells. A person with this type of immune deficiency is highly vulnerable to certain bacterial infections, particularly of the ear and sinuses.

Severe combined immune deficiencies (SCID) affect both humoral and cellular immunity. About half of SCID cases are X-linked. In a less severe form, the individual lacks B cells but has T cells. Before antibiotic drugs became available, individuals with this form of SCID died before the age of 10 years of overwhelming bacterial infection. In a more severe form of X-linked SCID, lack of T cells too causes death by 18 months of age, usually of severe and diverse infections. Gene therapy for X-linked SCID is effective, but can cause leukemia. Ironically, an autosomal recessive form of SCID, called adenosine deaminase deficiency, became the first illness successfully treated with gene therapy. Both are discussed further in chapter 20.

A young man named David Vetter taught the world about the difficulty of life without immunity years before AIDS appeared. David had an autosomal form of SCID that caused him to be born without a thymus gland. His T cells could not mature and activate B cells, leaving him defenseless in a germ-filled world. Born in Texas in 1971, David spent his short life in a vinyl bubble, awaiting a treatment that never came. As he reached adolescence, David wanted to leave his bubble. An experimental bone marrow transplant was unsuccessful— soon afterward, David began vomiting and developed diarrhea, both signs of infection. David left the bubble, but died within days of a massive infection.

Acquired Immune Deficiency Syndrome

AIDS is not inherited, but acquired by infection with HIV, a virus that gradually shuts down the immune system (see figure 17.2b). First, HIV enters macrophages, impairing this first line of defense. In these cells and later in helper T cells, the virus adheres with its surface protein, called gp120, to two coreceptors on the host cell

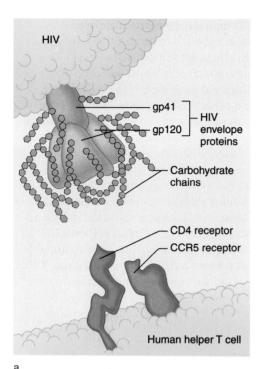

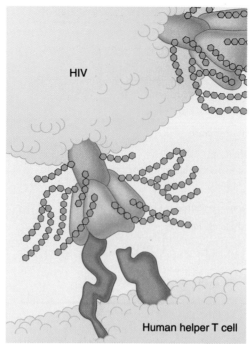

a.

b.

Figure 17.13 HIV binds to a helper T cell. **(a)** The part of HIV that binds to helper T cells is called gp120 (gp stands for glycoprotein). **(b)** When the carbohydrate chains that shield the protein portion of gp120 move aside as they approach the cell surface, the viral molecule can bind to a CD4 receptor. Binding to a receptor called CCR5 is also necessary for HIV to dock at a helper T cell. Once bound to the cell surface, the viral envelope fuses with the plasma membrane, enabling the virus to enter. A few lucky individuals lack CCR5 and thus cannot be infected by HIV. New types of drugs to fight HIV infection block the steps of viral entry. (The size of HIV here is greatly exaggerated.)

surface, CD4 and CCR5 (**figure 17.13**). Another glycoprotein, gp41, anchors gp120 molecules into the viral envelope. When the virus binds both coreceptors, virus and cell surface contort in a way that enables viral entry into the cell. Once in the cell, reverse transcriptase catalyzes construction of a DNA strand complementary to the viral RNA, which replicates to form a DNA double helix. This enters the nucleus and inserts into a chromosome. The viral DNA sequences are transcribed and translated, and the cell fills with viral pieces, which are assembled into complete new viral particles that eventually burst from the cell (**figure 17.14**).

Once helper T cells start to die at a high rate, bacterial infections begin, because B cells aren't activated to produce antibodies. Much later in infection, HIV variants arise that can bind to a receptor called CXCR4 on cytotoxic T cells, killing them. Loss of these cells renders the body very vulnerable to viral infections and cancer.

HIV has an advantage over the human immune system because it replicates quickly, changes quickly, and can hide. The virus is very prone to mutation, both because it cannot repair replication errors, and because those errors happen frequently—1 per every 5,000 or so bases—because of the "sloppiness" of reverse transcriptase. The immune system simply cannot keep up; antibodies against one viral variant are useless against the next. For several years, the bone marrow produces 2 billion new T and B cells a day to counter the million to a billion new HIV particles that burst daily from shattered cells.

So genetically diverse is the population of HIV in a human host that, within days of the initial infection, variants arise that resist the drugs used to treat AIDS. HIV's changeable nature has important clinical implications. Combining drugs with different actions provides the greatest chance of slowing the disease process, so that AIDS becomes a chronic, lifelong, but treatable illness, instead of a killer.

Three types of drugs have cut the death rate from AIDS dramatically. Reverse transcriptase inhibitors block the copying of

viral RNA into DNA. Protease inhibitors block the trimming of certain viral proteins, which is required for new viral particles to assemble. Entry inhibitors block the ability of the virus to bind to a cell, fuse with the plasma membrane, and enter.

Clues to developing new drugs to treat AIDS come from people at high risk who resist infection. For example, researchers have identified four receptors or the molecules that bind to them that are altered by mutation in ways that keep HIV out of cells in resistant individuals. To find these receptors, researchers scrutinized the DNA of people who had unprotected sex with many partners, and people with hemophilia who had received HIV-tainted blood in the 1980s—but who were not infected. Some of them were homozygous recessive for a 32-base deletion in the CCR5 gene. Their CCR5 coreceptors were too stunted, thanks to a premature "stop" codon, to reach the cell's surface (see figure 17.13). Like a ferry arriving at shore to find no dock, HIV has nowhere to bind on the cells of these fortunate individuals. Heterozygotes, with one copy of the deletion, can become infected with HIV, but they remain healthy for several years longer than people who do not have the deletion. Curiously, the same *CCR5* mutation may have enabled people to survive plague in Europe during the middle ages. Apparently both the virus that causes AIDS and the bacterium that causes plague use the same portal into a human cell.

Autoimmunity

Autoimmunity is a reaction that occurs when the immune system produces antibodies, called **autoantibodies,** that attack the body's own healthy tissues. The signs and symptoms of autoimmune disorders reflect the cell types under attack. For example, autoimmune ulcerative colitis affects colon cells, causing severe abdominal pain.

A mutation in a single gene can cause varied symptoms of an autoimmune disorder. For example, a mutation in a gene on chromosome 21q causes "autoimmune polyendocrinopathy syndrome type I." Malfunction of various endocrine glands occurs in a similar sequence in patients. Children under 5 develop candidiasis, a fungal infection (not an autoimmune disorder). By age 10, the individual's parathyroid

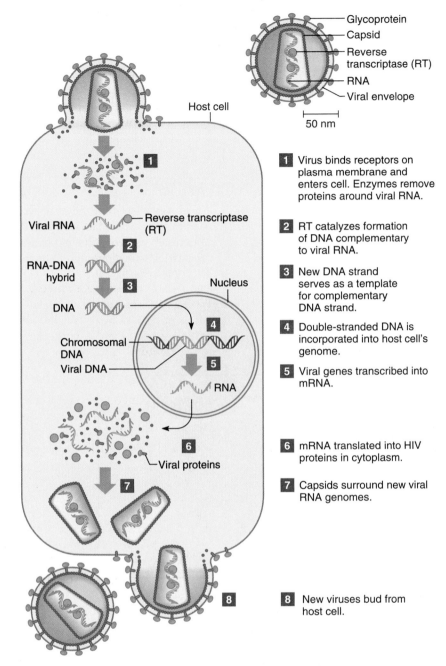

Host cell

Glycoprotein
Capsid
Reverse transcriptase (RT)
RNA
Viral envelope

50 nm

Viral RNA

Reverse transcriptase (RT)

RNA-DNA hybrid

DNA

Nucleus

Chromosomal DNA
Viral DNA

RNA

Viral proteins

1 Virus binds receptors on plasma membrane and enters cell. Enzymes remove proteins around viral RNA.

2 RT catalyzes formation of DNA complementary to viral RNA.

3 New DNA strand serves as a template for complementary DNA strand.

4 Double-stranded DNA is incorporated into host cell's genome.

5 Viral genes transcribed into mRNA.

6 mRNA translated into HIV proteins in cytoplasm.

7 Capsids surround new viral RNA genomes.

8 New viruses bud from host cell.

Figure 17.14 How HIV infects. HIV integrates into the host chromosome, then commandeers transcription and translation, ultimately producing more virus particles.

glands begin to fail, affecting calcium metabolism. By age 15, most affected individuals also develop Addison disease, reflecting a deficiency in adrenal gland hormones. Other associated conditions include thyroid deficiency, diabetes mellitus, vitiligo (skin whitening), and alopecia (hair loss).

The symptoms of many autoimmune conditions can arise by other mechanisms, making diagnosis difficult. Hemolytic anemia, for example, may be autoimmune, inherited, or a reaction to toxin exposure.

Autoimmunity may arise in several ways:

• A virus replicating within a cell incorporates proteins from the cell's surface onto its own. When the immune system "learns" the surface of the virus to destroy it, it also learns to attack human cells that normally bear the protein.

• Some thymocytes that should have died in the thymus somehow escape the massive die-off, persisting to attack "self" tissue later on.

• A nonself antigen coincidentally resembles a self antigen, and the immune system attacks both. In rheumatic fever, for example, antigens on heart valve cells resemble those on *Streptococcus* bacteria; antibodies produced to fight a strep throat also attack the heart valve cells. Some cases of insulin-dependent diabetes mellitus may also be due to this type of autoimmunity. Part of a protein on insulin-producing pancreatic cells resembles part of bovine serum albumin (BSA), a protein in cow's milk. Children who are allergic to cow's milk may develop antibodies against BSA, which later attack the similar-appearing pancreas cells, causing diabetes.

Some disorders traditionally thought to be autoimmune in origin may in fact have a more bizarre cause—fetal cells persisting in a woman's circulation, even decades after the fetus has grown up! In response to an as yet unknown trigger, the fetal cells, perhaps "hiding" in a tissue such as skin, emerge, stimulating antibody production. The resulting antibodies and symptoms appear to be an autoimmune disorder. This mechanism, called microchimerism ("small mosaic"), may explain the higher prevalence of autoimmune disorders among women. It was discovered in a disorder called scleroderma, which means "hard skin" (**figure 17.15**).

Patients describe scleroderma, which typically begins between ages 45 and 55, as

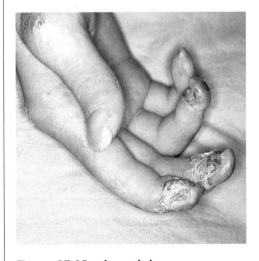

Figure 17.15 An autoimmune disorder—maybe. Scleroderma hardens the skin. Some cases appear to be caused by a long-delayed immune system reaction to cells retained from a fetus decades earlier!

"the body turning to stone." Symptoms include fatigue, swollen joints, stiff fingers, and a masklike face. The hardening may also affect blood vessels, the lungs, and the esophagus. Clues that scleroderma is a delayed response to persisting fetal cells include the following observations:

- It is much more common in women.

- Symptoms resemble those of graft-versus-host disease (GVHD), in which

transplanted tissue produces chemicals that destroy the host's body. Antigens on cells in scleroderma lesions match those that cause GVHD.

- Mothers who have scleroderma and their sons have cell surfaces that are more similar than those of unaffected mothers and their sons. Perhaps the similarity of cell surfaces enabled the fetal cells to escape destruction by the woman's immune system.

- Skin lesions from affected mothers of sons include cells that have Y chromosomes. Mothers can develop scleroderma from daughters too, but

the fetal cells cannot be as easily distinguished because they are XX, like the mothers' cells.

It's possible that other disorders traditionally considered autoimmune and that are more prevalent in women may actually reflect an immune system response to lingering fetal cells.

Allergies

An allergy is an immune system response to a substance, called an **allergen,** that does not actually present a threat. Many allergens are particles small enough to be carried in

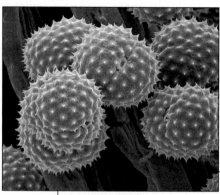

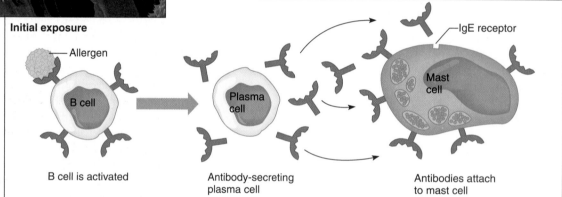

Initial exposure

Allergen

B cell

B cell is activated

Plasma cell

Antibody-secreting plasma cell

IgE receptor

Mast cell

Antibodies attach to mast cell

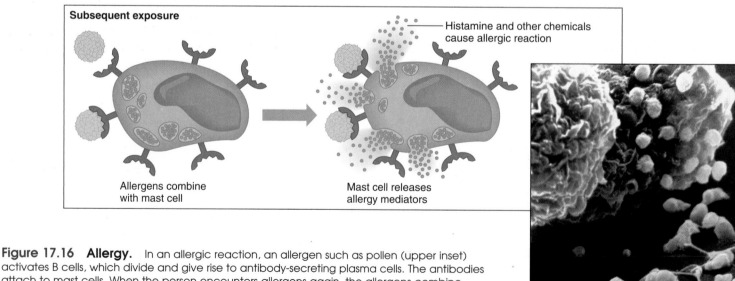

Subsequent exposure

Allergens combine with mast cell

Histamine and other chemicals cause allergic reaction

Mast cell releases allergy mediators

Figure 17.16   Allergy.   In an allergic reaction, an allergen such as pollen (upper inset) activates B cells, which divide and give rise to antibody-secreting plasma cells. The antibodies attach to mast cells. When the person encounters allergens again, the allergens combine with the antibodies on the mast cells, which then burst (lower inset), releasing the chemicals that cause itchy eyes and a runny nose.

the air and into a person's respiratory tract. The size of the allergen may determine the type of allergy. For example, grass pollen is large and remains in the upper respiratory tract, where it causes hay fever. But allergens from house dust mites, cat dander, and cockroaches are small enough to infiltrate the lungs, triggering asthma (**figure 17.16**). Asthma is a chronic disease in which contractions of the airways, inflammation, and accumulation of mucus block air flow.

Both humoral and cellular immunity take part in an allergic response. Antibodies of class IgE bind to mast cells, sending signals that cause the mast cells to open and release allergy mediators such as histamine and heparin. Allergy mediators cause inflammation, with symptoms that may include the runny eyes of hay fever, the narrowed airways of asthma, rashes, or the overwhelming bodywide allergic reaction called anaphylactic shock. Allergens also activate a class of helper T cells that produce a particular mix of cytokines whose genes are clustered on chromosome 5q. Regions of chromosomes 12q and 17q have genes that control IgE production.

The fact that allergies have become very common only during the past century suggests a much stronger environmental than genetic component. Still, people inherit susceptibilities to allergy. Twin studies of various allergies reveal about a 75 percent concordance, and isolated populations with a great deal of inbreeding tend to have a high prevalence of certain allergies.

The allergies that people suffer today may be a holdover of an immune function that was important in the past. Evidence for this hypothesis is that people with allergies have higher levels of white blood cells called eosinophils than do others, and these cells fight parasitic infections that are no longer common. In a more general sense, because allergies are more common in developed nations and have become more prevalent since the introduction of antibiotic drugs, some researchers hypothesize that allergies may result from a childhood relatively free of infection, compared to times past—almost as if the immune system is reacting to being underutilized. This idea that allergies stem from an environment too clean to have stimulated the immune system very much is called the hygiene hypothesis.

Key Concepts

Inherited immune deficiencies affect innate and adaptive immunity. • HIV replicates very rapidly, and T cell production matches it until the immune response is overwhelmed and AIDS begins. HIV is a retrovirus that injects its RNA into host cells by binding coreceptors. Reverse transcriptase then copies viral RNA into DNA. HIV uses the cell's protein synthesis machinery to mass produce itself; then the cell bursts, releasing virus. HIV continually mutates, becoming resistant to drugs. • In autoimmune disorders, autoantibodies attack healthy tissue. These conditions may be caused by a virus that borrows a self antigen, T cells that never learn to recognize self, or healthy cells bearing antigens that resemble nonself antigens. Some conditions considered autoimmune may actually reflect an immune system response to retained fetal cells. • An overly sensitive immune system causes allergies. In an allergic reaction, allergens bind to IgE antibodies on mast cells, which release allergy mediators. A subset of helper T cells secretes cytokines that contribute to allergy symptoms.

17.4 Altering Immune Function

Medical technology can alter or augment immune system functions in various ways. Vaccines trick the immune system into acting early. Antibiotic drugs, which are substances derived from organisms such as fungi and soil bacteria, have been used for decades to assist an immune response. Cytokines and altered antibodies are used as drugs to treat a variety of conditions. Transplants require suppression of the immune system so that the body will accept a nonself body part.

Vaccines

A vaccine is an inactive or partial form of a pathogen that stimulates the immune system to alert B cells to produce antibodies. When the person encounters the pathogen in its natural state later, a secondary immune response ensues, even before symptoms arise. Vaccines consisting of entire viruses or bacteria can, rarely, cause illness if they mutate to a pathogenic form. This is a risk presented by the original smallpox vaccine. A safer type of vaccine uses only the part of the pathogen's surface that elicits an immune response. Vaccines against different illnesses can be combined into one injection, or the genes encoding antigens from several pathogens can be inserted into a harmless virus and delivered as a "super vaccine." **Table 17.5** lists approaches to constructing vaccines.

Vaccine technology dates back to the eleventh century in China. Because people observed that those who recovered from smallpox never got it again, they collected the scabs of infected individuals and crushed them into a powder, which they inhaled or rubbed into pricked skin. In 1796, the wife of a British ambassador to Turkey witnessed the Chinese method of vaccination and mentioned it to an English country physician, Edward Jenner. Intrigued, Jenner had himself vaccinated the Chinese way, and then thought of a different approach.

It was widely known that people who milked cows contracted a mild illness called

Table 17.5

Types of Vaccines

Type	Disease Prevented
Entire weakened (attenuated) pathogen	Polio
Inactivated toxin	Tetanus
Part of pathogen surface	Hepatitis B
Recombinant vaccine (pathogen's gene placed in harmless bacteria or yeast)	Lyme disease
"Naked" DNA from pathogen	Influenza, hepatitis B

cowpox, but did not get smallpox. The cows became ill from infected horses. Since the virus seemed to jump species, Jenner wondered whether exposing a healthy person to cowpox lesions might protect against smallpox. A slightly different virus causes cowpox, but Jenner's approach worked, leading to development of the first vaccine (in fact, the word comes from the Latin *vacca,* for "cow"). Unable to experiment on himself because he'd already taken the Chinese vaccine, Jenner instead tried his first vaccine on a volunteer, 8-year-old James Phipps. Jenner dipped a needle in pus oozing from a small cowpox sore on a milkmaid named Sarah Nelmes, then scratched the boy's arm with it. He then exposed the boy to people with smallpox. Young James never became ill. Eventually, improved versions of Jenner's smallpox vaccine would eradicate a disease that once killed millions (**figure 17.17**), and vaccination became unnecessary. However, several nations have resumed smallpox vaccination programs to counter bioterrorism risks, as section 17.5 discusses.

Polio is another vaccine success story. Many adults recall lining up in the 1950s to receive the first polio vaccines—injections, and a few years later, oral vaccine squirted onto sugar cubes. The 1960s brought vaccines to protect against diseases that were once a normal part of childhood—measles, mumps, and rubella. Several other vaccines are on the list today, including chickenpox and hepatitis B.

People still receive most vaccines as injections, but several new delivery methods include nasal sprays and genetically modified fruits and vegetables. A banana as a vaccine against an infection makes sense in theory, but in practice it is proving difficult to obtain a uniform product. Edible plants are given genes from pathogens that encode the antigens that evoke an immune response in the human body. The foreign antigens stimulate phagocytic cells called dendritic cells beneath the small intestinal lining that "present" the antigens to nearby T cells. From here, the antigens are passed to the bloodstream, where they stimulate B cells to divide to yield plasma cells that produce IgA. These antibodies coat the small intestinal lining, protecting against food-borne pathogens.

Initially, plant-based vaccines were promising in animal studies. Consider a potato given an *E. coli* gene that encodes a toxin that causes a type of infant and traveler's diarrhea. A week after mice eat the raw, shredded potatoes, antibodies against the toxin appear in their circulations. In humans, a trial of hepatitis B vaccine, also given in potatoes, raised antibody levels, but also raised fears that it could backfire, impairing the ability of the immune system to respond to natural hepatitis B virus. Current research focuses on converting plant-based vaccines into powders so that doses can be regulated—but this counters the original perhaps-too-rosy view of easily immunizing Third-World babies with bananas.

Immunotherapy

Immunotherapy amplifies or redirects the immune response. It originated in the nineteenth century. Today, a few immunotherapies are in use, with more in clinical trials.

Monoclonal Antibodies Boost Humoral Immunity

When a B cell recognizes a single foreign antigen, it manufactures a single, or monoclonal, type of antibody. A large amount of a single antibody type would be useful in targeting a particular pathogen or cancer cell because of the antibody's great specificity.

In 1975, British researchers Cesar Milstein and George Köhler devised **monoclonal antibody (MAb) technology,** which massproduces a single B cell, preserving its specificity and amplifying its antibody type. First, they injected a mouse with a sheep's red blood cells (**figure 17.18**). They then isolated a single B cell from the mouse's spleen and fused it with a cancerous white blood cell from a mouse. The fused cell, called a hybridoma, had a valuable pair of talents. Like the B cell, it produced large amounts of a single antibody type. Like the cancer cell, it divided continuously.

Today MAbs are more like human antibodies—the original mouse versions caused allergic reactions. MAbs are used in basic research, veterinary and human health

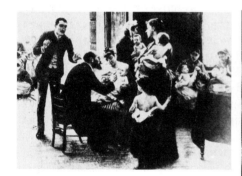

a.

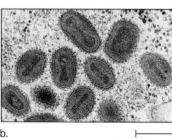

b.

0.1 µm

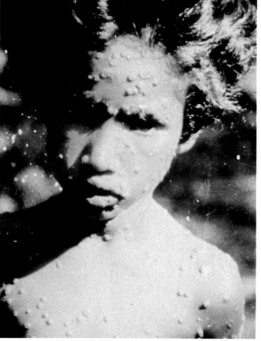

c.

Figure 17.17 Smallpox: gone? (a) Edward Jenner invented the modern version of a smallpox (b) vaccine in 1798. This boy (c) is one of the last victims of smallpox, which has not naturally infected a human since 1977. Because many doctors are unfamiliar with smallpox, and people are no longer vaccinated, an outbreak would be a major health disaster.

Figure 17.18 Monoclonal antibody technology.

Monoclonal antibodies are pure preparations of a single antibody type that recognize a single antigen. They are useful in diagnosing and treating disease because of their specificity.

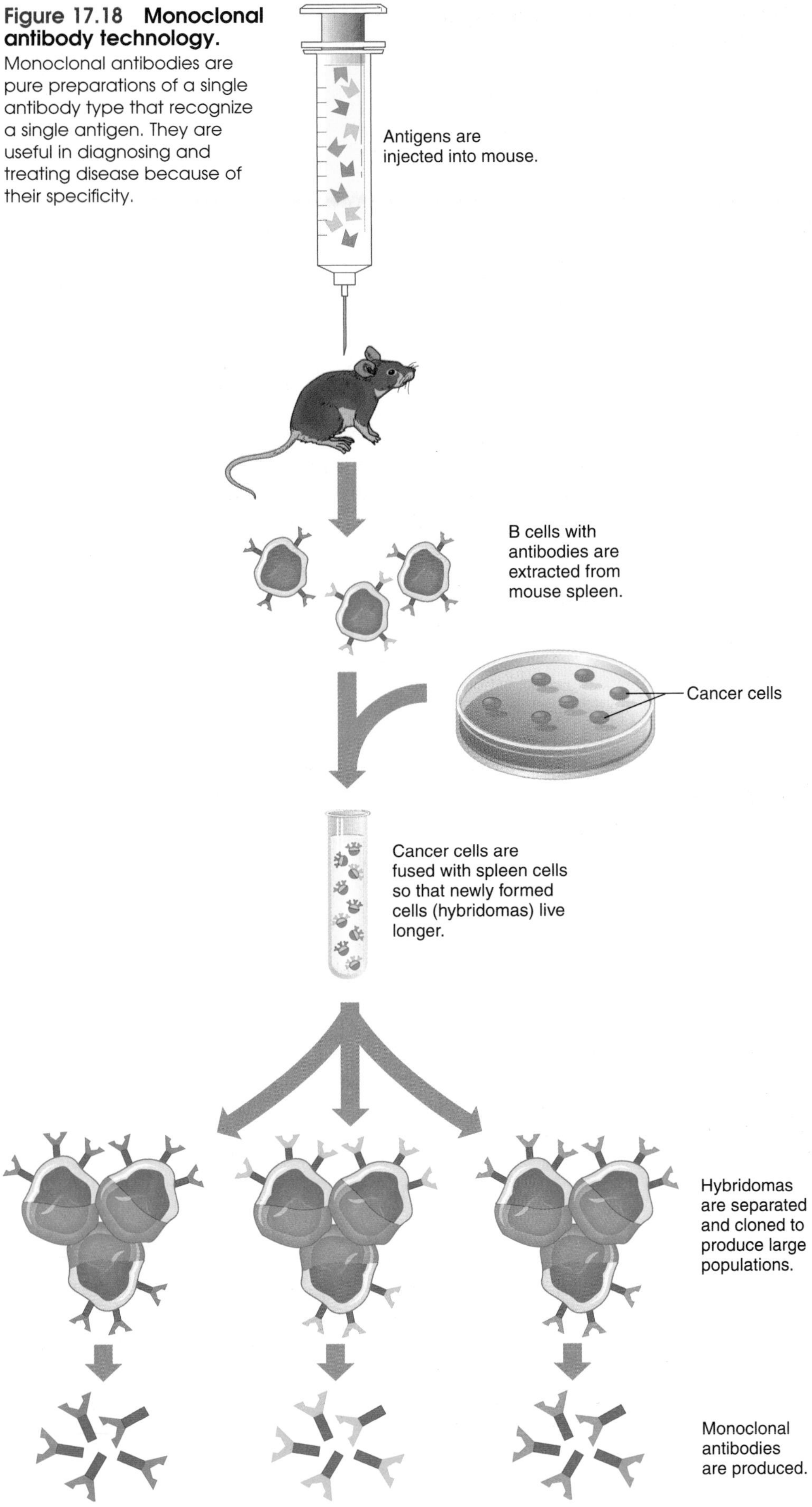

Antigens are injected into mouse.

B cells with antibodies are extracted from mouse spleen.

Cancer cells

Cancer cells are fused with spleen cells so that newly formed cells (hybridomas) live longer.

Hybridomas are separated and cloned to produce large populations.

Monoclonal antibodies are produced.

care, agriculture, forestry, and forensics. MAbs are used to diagnose everything from strep throat to turf grass disease. In a home pregnancy test, a woman places drops of her urine onto a paper strip impregnated with a MAb that binds to hCG, the "pregnancy" hormone. A color change ensues if the MAb binds its target. In cancer diagnosis, if a MAb attached to a fluorescent dye and injected into a patient or applied to a sample of tissue or body fluid binds its target—an antigen found mostly or only on cancer cells—a scanning technology or fluorescence microscope detects the fluorescence, and the disease. MAbs linked to radioactive isotopes or to drugs deliver treatment to cancer cells. A MAb-based drug called Herceptin blocks receptors on breast cancer cell surfaces, preventing them from receiving signals to divide.

Cytokines Boost Cellular Immunity

As coordinators of immunity, cytokines are used to treat a variety of conditions. However, it has been difficult to develop these body chemicals into drugs because they remain active only for short periods, and they must be delivered precisely where they are needed, or overdose or side effects can occur.

Interferon (IF) was the first cytokine tested on a large scale. When researchers discovered it in the 1950s, they hailed it as a potential cure-all wonder drug. Although it did not live up to early expectations, various interferons today treat a few types of cancer, genital warts, and multiple sclerosis.

Interleukin-2 (IL-2) is administered intravenously to treat kidney cancer recurrence. Colony stimulating factors, which cause immature white blood cells to mature and differentiate, boost white blood cell levels in people with suppressed immune systems, such as individuals with AIDS or receiving cancer chemotherapy. This allows a patient to withstand higher doses of a conventional drug.

Because excess tumor necrosis factor (TNF) underlies some disorders, blocking its activity treats some conditions. The drug Enbrel, for example, consists of part of a receptor for TNF, preventing the cytokine from binding to cells that line joints and normally secrete lubricating fluid.

Transplantation

When a car breaks down, replacing the damaged part often fixes the trouble. The same is sometimes true for the human body. Hearts, kidneys, livers, lungs, corneas, pancreases, skin, and bone marrow are routinely transplanted, sometimes several organs at a time. Although transplant medicine had a shaky start (see the Technology Timeline: Transplantation), many problems have been worked out (see figure 17.1). Today, thousands of transplants are performed annually and recipients gain years of life. The challenge to successful transplantation lies in genetics—individual inherited differences in cell surfaces determine whether the body will accept tissue from a particular donor.

Transplant Types

Transplants are classified by the relationship of donor to recipient (**figure 17.19**):

1. An **autograft** transfers tissue from one part of a person's body to another. A skin graft taken from the thigh to replace burned skin on the chest, or a leg vein that replaces a coronary artery, are autografts. The immune system does not reject the graft because the tissue is self. (Technically, an autograft is not a transplant because it involves only one person.)

2. An **isograft** is tissue from a monozygotic twin. Because the twins are genetically identical, the recipient's immune system does not reject the transplant. Ovary isografts have been performed.

3. An **allograft** comes from an individual who is not genetically identical to the recipient, but is a member of the same species. A kidney transplant from an unrelated donor is an allograft.

4. A **xenograft** transplants tissue from one species to another. (See the Bioethics Box on page 347.)

Rejection Reactions— Or Acceptance

The immune system recognizes most donor tissue as nonself and may attempt to destroy it in a tissue rejection reaction that involves T cells, antibodies, and activation of complement. The greater the dif-

Technology Timeline

Transplantation

1899	First allograft—a kidney from dog to dog.
1902	Pig kidney is attached to blood vessels of a woman dying of kidney failure.
1905	First successful corneal transplant, from a boy who lost an eye in an accident to a man whose cornea was chemically damaged. Works because cornea cells lack antigens.
1940s	First kidney transplants on young people with end-stage kidney failure.
1950s	Blood typing predicts success of donor-recipient pairs for organ transplants. Invention of heart-lung bypass machine makes heart transplants feasible.
1960s	First effective immunosuppressant drugs developed. Heart transplants performed in dogs with mixed success.
1967	First human heart transplant. Patient lives 18 days.
1968	Uniform Anatomical Gift Act passes. Requires informed consent from next of kin before organs or tissues can be donated.
1970s	Transplant problems: they extend life only briefly and do not correct underlying disease; surgical complications; rejection reactions. Many hospitals ban transplants.
1980s	Improved immunosuppressant drugs, surgical techniques, and tissue matching, plus the ability to strip antigens from donor tissue, reawaken interest in transplants.
1984	Doctors transplant a baboon's heart into "Baby Fae," who was born with half a heart. She lives 20 days before rejecting the xenograft.
1992	Surgeons transplant a baboon liver into a 35-year-old man with hepatitis. The man lives for 71 days, dying of an unrelated cause.
1997	Pig cell implants used to treat pancreatic failure and Parkinson disease. Pig liver used to maintain liver function for six hours as young man awaited a human liver.
2000	Cloning of pigs brings xenotransplantation closer to reality.
2003	Cloned mini-pigs genetically modified to lack cell surface molecules that provoke human immune response.
2003	DNA gene expression microarrays predict which patients are likely to reject kidney transplants.

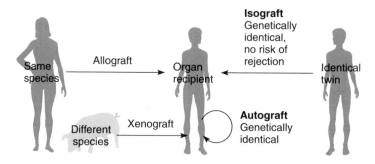

Figure 17.19   Transplant types.   An autograft is within an individual. An isograft is between identical twins. An allograft is between members of the same species, and a xenograft is between members of different species.

Pig Parts

In 1902, a German medical journal reported an astonishing experiment. A physician, Emmerich Ullman, had attached the blood vessels of a patient dying of kidney failure to a pig's kidney set up by her bedside. The experiment failed when the patient's immune system rejected the attachment almost immediately.

Nearly a century later, in 1997, an eerily similar experiment took place. Robert Pennington, a 19-year-old suffering from acute liver failure and desperately needing a transplant, survived for six and a half hours with his blood circulating outside of his body through a living liver removed from a 15-week-old, 118-pound pig named Sweetie Pie. The pig liver served as a bridge until a human liver became available. But Sweetie Pie was no ordinary pig. She had been genetically modified and bred so that her cells displayed a human protein that controlled the complement-mediated hyperacute rejection reaction against tissue transplanted from an animal of another species. Because of this slight but key bit of added humanity, plus immunosuppressant drugs, Pennington's body was able to tolerate the pig liver's help for the few crucial hours. Baboons have also been used as sources of transplant organs, but they have not yet been genetically modified (**figure 1**).

Successful xenotransplants would help alleviate the organ shortage. However, some people object to the idea of intentionally raising animals to use their organs as transplants because it requires killing the donors. One researcher counters such protests by

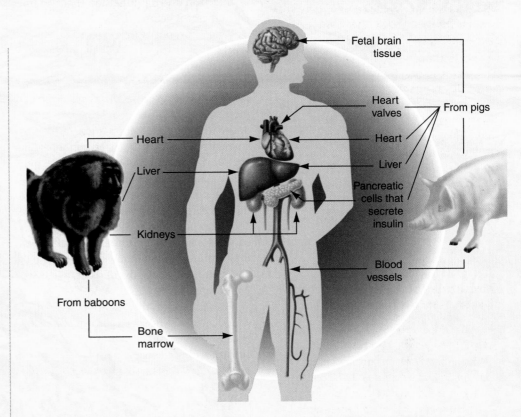

Figure 1 Baboons and pigs can provide tissues and organs for transplant.

comparing the use of animal organs to eating them. Those who eat ham or bacon can hardly justify objecting to a pig-to-human transplant.

A possible danger of xenotransplants is that people may acquire viruses from the organ donors. Viruses can "jump" species, and the outcome in the new host is unpredictable. So far, it is known that a virus called PERV—for "porcine endogenous retrovirus"—can infect human cells in cul-

ture. However, a study of several dozen patients who received implants of pig tissue for a variety of reasons revealed that none showed evidence of PERV years later. That study, though, looked only at blood. We still do not know what effect pig viruses can have on a human body. Because many viral infections take years to cause symptoms, introducing a new infectious disease in the future could be the trade-off for using xenotransplants to solve the current organ shortage.

ference between recipient and donor cell surfaces, the more rapid and severe the rejection reaction. An extreme example is the **hyperacute rejection reaction** against tissue transplanted from another species—the donor tissue is usually destroyed in minutes as blood vessels blacken and cut off the blood supply.

Physicians use several approaches to dampen rejection so that a transplant

recipient can survive. These include closely matching the HLA types of donor and recipient, and stripping donor tissue of antigens. Newer immunosuppressive drugs inhibit production of the antibodies and T cells that specifically attack transplanted tissue, while sparing other components of the immune system. Experiments on transplanted tissues using gene expression microarrays reveal at least three types of

rejection not otherwise obvious. Such profiling will likely be used to avoid rejection reactions.

Graft-versus-host disease is a different type of immune problem that arises sometimes in bone marrow transplants used to correct certain blood deficiencies and cancers. The transplanted bone marrow, which is actually part of the donor's immune system, attacks the recipient—its new body—as foreign.

17.5 A Genomic View of Immunity—The Pathogen's Perspective

Immunity against infectious disease involves interactions of two genomes—ours and the pathogen's. At the same time that human genome information is revealing how the immune system halts infectious disease, information coming from the sequencing of the genomes of pathogens is also useful. Table 1.3 lists some of the pathogens whose genomes have been sequenced.

Knowing the DNA sequence of a pathogen's genome, or the sequences of key genes, can reveal exactly how that organism causes illness in humans, which can suggest new treatment strategies. The sequence for *Streptococcus pneumoniae,* for example, revealed instructions for a huge protein that enables the bacterium to adhere to human cells. Pharmaceutical researchers can now search for compounds that dismantle this previously unknown adhesion protein.

Crowd Diseases

History also provides clues to infectious diseases. Because adaptive immunity responds to an environmental stimulus—a pathogen— epidemics often followed the introduction of an infection into a population that had not encountered it before.

When Europeans first explored the New World, they inadvertently brought bacteria and viruses to which their immune systems had adapted. The immune systems of native Americans, however, had never encountered these pathogens. Many people died. Smallpox decimated the Aztec population in Mexico from 20 million in 1519, when conquistador Hernán Cortés arrived from Spain, to 10 million by 1521, when Cortés returned. By 1618, the Aztec nation had fallen to 1.6 million. The Incas in Peru and northern populations were also dying of smallpox. When explorers visited what is now the southeast United States, they found abandoned towns where natives had died from smallpox, measles, pertussis, typhus, and influenza.

The diseases that so easily killed native Americans are known as "crowd" diseases, because they arise with the spread of agriculture and urbanization and affect many people. Crowd diseases swept Europe and Asia as expanding trade routes spread bacteria and viruses along with silk and spices. More recently, air travel has spread crowd diseases, such as SARS.

Crowd diseases tend to pass from conquerors who live in large, intercommunicating societies to smaller, more isolated and more susceptible populations, and not vice versa. When Columbus arrived in the New World, the large populations of Europe and Asia had existed far longer than American settlements. In Europe and Asia, infectious diseases had time to become established and for human populations to adapt to them. In contrast, an unfamiliar infectious disease can quickly wipe out an isolated tribe, leaving no one behind to give the illness to new invaders.

Fortunately, most crowd diseases vanish quickly. Vaccines or treatments may stop transmission; people may alter their behaviors to avoid contracting the infection, or the disease may kill before individuals can pass it on. Sometimes, we don't know why a disease vanishes or becomes less severe. We may be able to treat and control newly evolving infectious diseases one at a time, with new drugs and vaccines. But the mutation process that continually spawns new genetic variants in microbe populations— resulting in evolution—means that new infectious diseases will continue to arise, and old ones to return or ravage new populations.

Bioweapons

It may seem incomprehensible that anyone would ever use pathogens to intentionally harm people, but it is a sad fact of history— and the present—that such bioweapons exist. Biological weapons have been around since medieval warriors catapulted plague-ridden corpses over city walls to kill the inhabitants. During the French and Indian War, the British gave Indians blankets intentionally contaminated with secretions from smallpox victims. Although international law banned "germ warfare" in 1925, from 1932 until 1942 Japan field-tested bacterial bioweapons in rural China, killing thousands.

In 1973, the Soviet Union established an organization called Biopreparat. Thousands of workers in 50 facilities prepared anthrax bombs and other bioweapons under the guise of manufacturing legitimate drugs, vaccines, and veterinary products. Soviet bioweapons were even more lethal than their natural counterparts. Plague bacteria, for example, were genetically modified to resist sixteen antibiotics and to manufacture a protein that strips nerve cells of their fatty coats, adding paralysis to the natural symptoms.

In 1979, an accident occurred in a Soviet city then called Sverdlovsk. At Military Compound Number 19, a miscommunication among shift workers in charge of changing safety air filters caused the release of a cloud of dried anthrax spores over the city. Within weeks, more than 100 people died of anthrax, mostly young, healthy men who were outside on that Friday night and breathed in enough anthrax spores to give them the inhaled form of the illness. The government, which officially announced that the deaths were due to eating infected meat, worsened matters by spraying jets of water everywhere, reaerosolizing the spores and causing more infections.

The symptoms of inhalation anthrax result from a toxin that consists of three proteins. One protein forms a barrel-like structure that binds to macrophages and admits the other two components of the toxin. One of these components overloads signal transduction and impairs the cell's ability to function as a phagocyte. The other toxin component breaks open macrophages, which release tumor necrosis factor and interleukins. Early symptoms of inhalation anthrax resemble influenza, but the victim rapidly suffers respiratory collapse.

In September 1992, Boris Yeltsin officially halted bioweapon research in the former Soviet Union. Twenty years earlier, political leaders in London, Moscow, and Washington had signed the Biological Weapons Convention, an effort to prevent bioterrorism. Its protocols are being strengthened today.

In the United States, a small-scale bioweapons effort began in 1942. A facility at Fort Detrick in Frederick, Maryland, stored 5,000 bombs loaded with anthrax spores; a production facility for the bombs was located in Terre Haute, Indiana; and Mississippi and Utah had test sites. President Richard Nixon halted the program in 1969; he thought that conventional and nuclear weapons were a sufficient deterrent and defense.

Bioterrorism has come far since smallpox-infested blankets were catapulted over ancient city walls, and the Japanese dropped porcelain containers of plague-ridden fleas over China. Today's bioterrorists not only know how to grow and dry pathogens, but how to control particle size so that they can more easily infect a human body. In addition, genetic modification can alter the characteristics of a virus or bacterium intended for use as a weapon, making it even deadlier, or targeting specific types of victims.

Summary

17.1 The Importance of Cell Surfaces

1. The cells and biochemicals of the immune system distinguish self from nonself, protecting the body against infections and cancer.

2. Most genetic effects on immunity are polygenic, but a few single genes have significant effects.

3. Patterns of cell surface proteins and glycoproteins determine blood types. A blood incompatibility occurs if a blood recipient manufactures **antibodies** against antigens in donor blood. Blood type systems include ABO and Rh.

4. HLA genes are closely linked on chromosome 6 and encode cell surface antigens that present foreign antigens to the immune system.

17.2 The Human Immune System

5. If a pathogen breaches physical barriers, the **innate immune response** produces the redness and swelling of inflammation, plus **complement, collectins,** and **cytokines.** The response is broad and general.

6. The **adaptive immune response** is slower, specific, and has memory. This response is both humoral and cellular.

7. The **humoral immune response** begins when macrophages display foreign antigens near HLA antigens. This activates **helper T cells,** which activate **B cells.** The B cells, in turn, give rise to **plasma cells** and secrete specific antibodies. Some B cells give rise to **memory cells.**

8. An antibody is Y-shaped and made up of four polypeptide chains, two **heavy** and two **light.** Each antibody molecule has regions of **constant** amino acid sequence and regions of **variable** sequence.

9. The tips of the Y of each subunit form **antigen binding sites,** which include the more specific **idiotypes** that bind foreign antigens at their **epitopes.**

10. Antibodies bind antigens to form immune complexes large enough for other immune system components to detect and destroy. Antibody genes are rearranged during early B cell development, providing instructions to produce a great variety of antibodies.

11. T cells carry out the **cellular immune response.** Their precursors, called thymocytes, are selected in the thymus to recognize self. Helper T cells secrete cytokines that activate other T cells and B cells. A helper T cell's CD4 antigen binds macrophages that present foreign antigens. **Cytotoxic T cells** release biochemicals that bore into and kill bacteria and also destroy cells covered with viruses.

17.3 Abnormal Immunity

12. Mutations in antibody or cytokine genes, or in genes encoding T cell receptors, cause inherited immune deficiencies. Severe combined immune deficiencies affect both branches of the immune system.

13. HIV binds to the coreceptors CD4 and CCR5 on macrophages and helper T cells, and, later in infection, triggers apoptosis of cytotoxic T cells. As HIV replicates, it mutates, evading immune attack. Falling CD4 helper T cell numbers allow opportunistic infections and cancers to flourish. People who cannot produce a complete CCR5 protein resist HIV infection.

14. In an **autoimmune disease,** the body manufactures **autoantibodies** against its own cells. Autoimmunity may result from a virus that incorporates and displays a self antigen, from bacteria or cancer cells that have antigens that resemble self antigens, from unselected T cells, or from lingering fetal cells.

15. In susceptible individuals, allergens stimulate IgE antibodies to bind to **mast cells,** which causes the cells to release allergy mediators. Certain helper T cells release selected cytokines. Allergies may be a holdover of past immune function.

17.4 Altering Immune Function

16. A **vaccine** presents a disabled pathogen, or part of one, to elicit a primary immune response.

17. **Immunotherapy** enhances or redirects immune function. **Monoclonal antibodies** are useful in diagnosing and treating some diseases because of their abundance and specificity. To create MAbs, individual activated B cells are fused with cancer cells to form hybridomas. Cytokines are used to treat various conditions.

18. Transplant types include **autografts** (within oneself), **isografts** (between identical twins), **allografts** (within a species), and **xenografts** (between species). A tissue rejection reaction occurs if donor tissue is too unlike recipient tissue.

17.5 A Genomic View of Immunity— The Pathogen's Perspective

19. Infectious disease involves interactions between the host's and the pathogen's genomes. Learning the genome sequences of pathogens can reveal how they infect, which provides clues to developing new treatments.

20. Crowd diseases spread rapidly through a population that has had no prior exposure, passed from members of a population that have had time to adapt to the pathogen.

21. Throughout history, people have used bacteria and viruses as weapons.

Review Questions

1. Match the cell type to the type of biochemical it produces.

   1. mast cell
   2. T cell
   3. B cell
   4. macrophage
   5. all cells with nuclei
   6. antigen-presenting cell

   a. antibodies
   b. HLA class II genes
   c. interleukin
   d. histamine
   e. interferon
   f. heparin
   g. tumor necrosis factor
   h. HLA class I *A, B,* and *C* genes

2. What is the physical basis of a blood type? of blood incompatibility?

3. What would be the consequences of lacking:
   a. helper T cells
   b. cytotoxic T cells
   c. B cells
   d. macrophages

4. State the function of each of the following immune system biochemicals:
   a. complement proteins
   b. collectins
   c. antibodies
   d. cytokines

5. Cite three reasons why developing a vaccine against HIV infection has been challenging.

6. It was once said that thymocytes are "educated" in the thymus, meaning that immature T cells are somehow "taught" to recognize self cell surfaces and refrain from attack. This is not exactly what happens. Why?

7. What part do antibodies play in allergic reactions and in autoimmune disorders?

8. How do each of the following illnesses disturb immunity?
   a. graft-versus-host disease
   b. SCID
   c. scleroderma
   d. AIDS
   e. hayfever

9. Why is a deficiency of T cells more dangerous than a deficiency of B cells?

10. What do a plasma cell and a memory cell descended from the same B cell have in common? How do they differ?

11. Why is a polyclonal antibody response valuable in the body, but a monoclonal antibody valuable as a diagnostic tool?

12. A person exposed for the first time to Coxsackie virus develops a painful sore throat. How is the immune system alerted to the exposure to the virus? When the person encounters the virus again, why doesn't she develop symptoms?

Applied Questions

1. A man is flown to an emergency room of a major medical center, near death after massive blood loss in a car accident. There isn't time to match blood types, so the physician orders type O negative blood. Why did she order this type of blood?

2. Rasmussen's encephalitis is a rare and severe form of epilepsy that causes children to have 100 or more seizures a day. Affected children have antibodies that attack brain cell receptors that normally receive nervous system biochemicals. Is this condition most likely an inherited immune deficiency, an adaptive immune deficiency, an autoimmune disorder, or an allergy? State a reason for your answer.

3. Allergy to a protein in peanuts can cause anaphylactic shock. An experimental vaccine consists of the gene encoding this protein, wrapped in an edible carbohydrate, so it can be eaten and stimulate production of protective antibodies in the small intestine. When this vaccine was fed to rats who have a peanut allergy, their blood showed lowered levels of IgE, but increased levels of IgG. Also, their bowel movements contained higher than usual levels of IgA. Is the vaccine working? How can you tell?

4. In people with a certain HLA genotype, a protein in their joints resembles an antigen on the bacterium that causes Lyme disease, an infection transmitted in a tick bite that causes flulike symptoms followed by arthritis (joint inflammation). When these individuals become infected, their immune systems attack not only the bacteria, but also their joints. Explain why antibiotic therapy helps treat the early phase of the disease, but not the arthritis.

5. Even in overwhelmingly deadly infectious diseases, such as bubonic plague and Ebola hemorrhagic fever, a small percentage of the human population survives. Suggest two mechanisms based on immune system functioning that can account for their survival.

6. A young woman who has aplastic anemia will soon die as her lymphocyte levels drop sharply. What type of cytokine might help her?

7. In Robin Cook's novel *Chromosome Six,* a geneticist places a portion of human chromosome 6 into fertilized ova from bonobos (pygmy chimps). The bonobos that result are used to provide organs for transplant into specific individuals. Explain how this technique would work.

8. Suggest ways that local, state, and federal governments can prepare to handle a bioterrorism attack.

9. Is the heritability of SCID likely to be higher or lower than that for an allergy? Why?

Web Activities

10. Many websites describe products (food supplements) that supposedly "boost" immune system function. Very often, the descriptions are vague, use meaningless jargon or buzzwords, or have misinformation. Locate such a website and identify claims that are unclear, deceptive, or incorrect. Alternatively, identify a claim that *is* consistent with the description of immune system function in this chapter.

Case Studies

11. State whether each of the following situations involves an autograft, an isograft, an allograft, or a xenograft.

a. Jim Hancock (figure 17.1) donating part of his liver to help his daughter, Leslie, who has a damaged liver due to cystic fibrosis.

b. A woman with infertility receiving an ovary transplant from her identical twin sister. (This is the only way this particular transplant works.)

c. A man receiving a heart valve from a pig.

d. A woman who has had a breast removed having a new breast reconstructed using fatty tissue from her thigh.

12. Mark and Louise planning to have their first child, but they are concerned because they think that they have an Rh incompatibility. He is Rh⁻ and she is Rh⁺. Will there be a problem? Why or why not?

Learn to apply the skills of genetic counselor with this additional case found in the *Case Workbook in Human Genetics:*

5 Little Piggies

Suggested Readings

Alibek, Ken. 1999. *Biohazard.* New York: Random House, Inc. The chilling tale of bioweaponry in the Soviet Union.

Bonetta, Laura. February 2002. Edible vaccines: Not quite ready for prime time. *Nature Medicine* 8:94 Plant-based vaccines are difficult to produce.

Ezekowitz, R. Alan. March 22, 2001. What is the best way to treat inherited disorders? *The New England Journal of Medicine* 344, no. 12:926–27. Stem cells from an HLA-matched sibling can cure chronic granulomatous disease, but is risky.

Fahrer, Aude M., et al. February 15, 2001. A genomic view of immunology. *Nature* 409:836. The human genome sequence is revealing genes that provide immunity.

Hill, Adrian V. S. June 23, 2001. Immunogenetics and genomics. *The Lancet* 357:2037–40. The human genome sequence provides insight into immune function.

Kahan, Barry D. October 2003. Individuality: The barrier to optimal immunosuppression. *Nature Reviews Immunology* 3(10):831–38. Transplants require targeted immunosuppression.

Lewis, Ricki. January 19, 2004. TSG101: An antiviral target with a murky past. *The Scientist* 18(1):22. HIV uses the secretion pathway to bud from a cell.

Lewis, Ricki. July 8, 2002. Smallpox vaccination: On hold, but lessons learned. *The Scientist* 16(14):29. The original smallpox vaccine carries risks of serious side effects.

Lewis, Ricki. October 1, 2001. New weapons against HIV. *The Scientist* 15(19):1. Entry inhibitors are new tools against AIDS.

Lewis, Ricki. October 29, 2001. Plague genome: The evolution of a pathogen. *The Scientist* 15(21):1. Will the publication of pathogen genomes give ideas to bioterrorists?

Lewis, Ricki. October 16, 2000. Porcine possibilities. *The Scientist* 14:1. The pros and cons of pig parts as transplants.

Marra, Marco, et al. May 11, 2003. The genome sequence of the SARS-associated coronavirus. www.scienceexpress.com. Researchers sequenced the SARS genome fast.

Nossal, Gustav, J. V. January 23, 2003. The double helix and immunology. *Nature* 421:440–44. The human genome sequence reveals the controls of immunity.

Ridley, Matt. March 2000. Asthma, environment, and the genome. *Natural History,* vol. 109. Asthma may reflect underutilized immunity.

Sarwal, Minnie, et al. July 10, 2003. Molecular heterogeneity in acute renal allograft rejection identified by DNA microarray profiling. *The New England Journal of Medicine,* 349(2):125–38. Genetic clues can predict transplant success.

VISIT YOUR ONLINE LEARNING CENTER

Visit your online learning center for additional resources and tools to help you master this chapter. See us at

www.mhhe.com/lewisgenetics6.

Weekly updates of current news related to human genetics are available through Power Web on your Online Learning Center.

C H A P T E R

The Genetics of Cancer

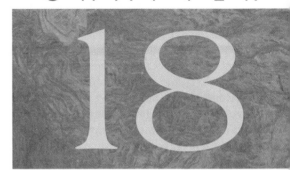

18

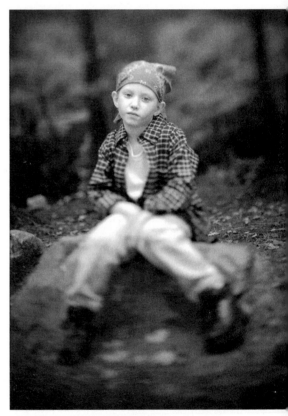

Cancer mostly affects adults, but certain types of cancer, such as leukemias and retinoblastoma, are seen in children.

Cancer has been attributed to environmental insults and to disruptions from within, including excess bile, fermenting lymph, injury, irritation, and simply "melancholia." Today we know that the collection of diseases called cancer reflects a profound derangement of the cell cycle. Not only do sequences of mutations underlie the progression of cancer as it invades and spreads, but changing levels of many proteins accompany the process, too. Although what we know of the genetic underpinnings of cancer is much more complex than it was just a few years ago, our increasing understanding of these illnesses that affect a third of us is already producing new ways to individualize diagnosis and target therapies. Medical science is on the cusp of great changes in how we learn to live with cancer—and the basis is genomics.

18.1 Cancer as a Genetic Disorder

Cancer is a complication of being a many-celled organism. All of our different specialized cell types must follow a schedule of mitosis—the cell cycle—so that organs and other body parts either grow appropriately during childhood, or stay a particular size and shape in an adult. If a cell escapes normal controls on its division rate, it forms a growth called a tumor (**figure 18.1**). In the blood, such a cell divides to take over the population of blood cells. A tumor is benign if it grows in place but does not spread into, or "invade," surrounding tissue; it is cancerous, or malignant, if it infiltrates nearby tissue. The word *cancer* comes from the Greek "karkinos," for "crab"; to Hippocrates, the characteristic grasping growth of a malignant tumor evoked the shape of a crab's body. A malignant tumor not only invades locally, but sends parts of itself into the bloodstream, which transports it to other areas, where the cancer cells form new tumors. This process of spreading is termed **metastasis.** The word means "not standing still."

Cancer is a group of disorders that arise from alterations in genes. Only 10 percent of cases are single-gene disorders, in which the faulty instructions are in every cell at birth. More often, mutations in cancer-causing genes occur in somatic cells over a lifetime. That is, cancer is a genetic disease at the cellular level, rather than at the whole-body level.

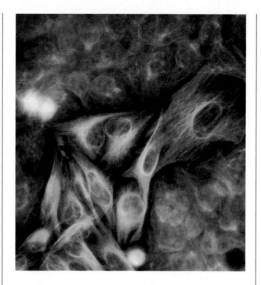

Figure 18.1 Staining highlights cancer cells. The orange cells are a melanoma (skin cancer) that is invading normal skin. Cancer cells, when stained for the presence of gene variants characteristic of cancer cells only, look very different from surrounding healthy tissue.

It is likely that combinations of particular gene variants sum to increase the risk of cancer, which may explain how cancer can "run in families" yet not follow a Mendelian pattern of inheritance. Cancer often takes years to develop, as a sequence of genes mutate in the affected tissue. Then, the cells whose mutations enable them to divide more often than others gradually take over the tissue. At the same time, changes at the gene expression level fuel the disease process. Researchers are finding that even though a cancer may not spread for years, mutations or changes in gene expression that indicate that it will do so can occur early in the course of illness.

It took many years for scientists to view cancer as a genetic phenomenon. When President Richard Nixon declared a "war on cancer" in 1971, the targets were radiation, viruses, and chemicals. These agents cause cancer by interfering with the precise genetic controls of cell division. One noted cancer researcher put it bluntly: "In cancer, the genome is shot to hell."

Researchers first discovered genes that could cause cancer in 1976, but there had been earlier hints. For example, most substances known to be **carcinogens** (causing cancer) are also mutagens (damaging DNA) when placed on cells growing in culture (the Ames test). Did the genetic change

cause the cancer? A second line of evidence came from families in which colon or breast cancer was so prevalent that it fit the inheritance pattern of a Mendelian trait.

From Single Mutations to Sweeping Changes in Gene Expression

In the 1980s and 1990s, searches for cancer-causing genes began with families that had many young members who had the same type of cancer, a rare situation. Researchers then identified parts of the genome that the affected individuals shared, such as a chromosomal aberration or a unique DNA sequence. Next, the search focused on specific genes in the identified region that could affect cell cycle control. This approach led to the discovery of more than 100 **oncogenes,** which cause cancer when they are inappropriately activated, and of more than 30 **tumor suppressor genes,** whose deletion or inactivation causes cancer.

While many researchers continue to study the single genes that can cause or contribute to the development of cancer, a genomics-based approach to understanding cancer uses DNA microarrays that highlight the expression differences in thousands of genes. At first this approach was used to supplement what was known about differences among cancers of the same tissue, such as leukemias and lymphomas (cancers of the blood and lymph systems), based on characteristics that could be seen under a microscope, such as nucleus shape. The technique has become so refined that researchers are discovering entirely new cancer types. **Figure 18.2** highlights one such discovery. Realizing that mixed-lineage leukemia (MLL) is not the same disease as acute lymphoblastic leukemia (ALL) promises to lead to targeted and more effective treatments. MLL usually kills in infancy. The Technology Timeline traces how researchers have studied leukemias.

DNA microarray expression panels will also likely become widely used in cancer diagnosis. Summarized one researcher, "Thousands of individual genes define the molecular portraits of each tumor."

Loss of Cell Cycle Control

Cancer is a consequence of disruption of the cell cycle. It begins when a cell divides

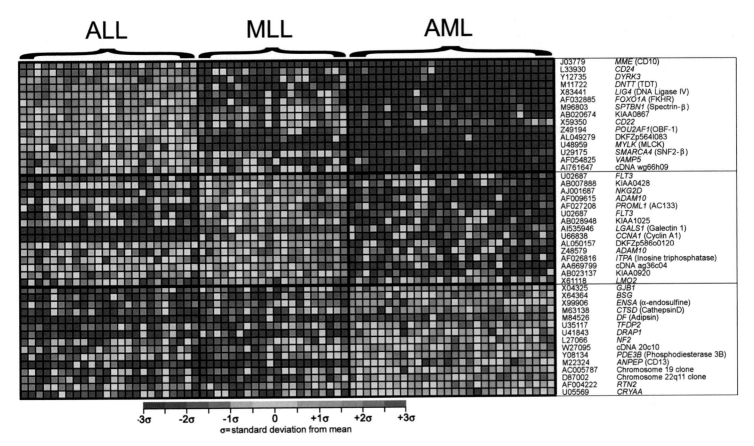

J03779	MME (CD10)
L33930	CD24
Y12735	DYRK3
M11722	DNTT (TDT)
X83441	LIG4 (DNA Ligase IV)
AF032885	FOXO1A (FKHR)
M96803	SPTBN1 (Spectrin-β)
AB020674	KIAA0867
X59350	CD22
Z49194	POU2AF1(OBF-1)
AL049279	DKFZp564I083
U48959	MYLK (MLCK)
U29175	SMARCA4 (SNF2-β)
AF054825	VAMP5
AI761647	cDNA wg66h09
U02687	FLT3
AB007888	KIAA0428
AJ001687	NKG2D
AF009615	ADAM10
AF027208	PROML1 (AC133)
U02687	FLT3
AB028948	KIAA1025
AI535946	LGALS1 (Galectin 1)
U66838	CCNA1 (Cyclin A1)
AL050157	DKFZp586o0120
Z48579	ADAM10
AF026816	ITPA (Inosine triphosphatase)
AA669799	cDNA ag36c04
AB023137	KIAA0920
X61118	LMO2
X04325	GJB1
X64364	BSG
X99906	ENSA (α-endosulfine)
M63138	CTSD (CathepsinD)
M84526	DF (Adipsin)
U35117	TFDP2
U41843	DRAP1
L27066	NF2
W27095	cDNA 20c10
Y08134	PDE3B (Phosphodiesterase 3B)
M22324	ANPEP (CD13)
AC005787	Chromosome 19 clone
D87002	Chromosome 22q11 clone
AF004222	RTN2
U05569	CRYAA

-3σ -2σ -1σ 0 +1σ +2σ +3σ
σ=standard deviation from mean

Figure 18.2 **DNA microarrays reveal a "hidden" type of leukemia.** It is easy to see that these three leukemias—ALL, MLL, and AML—differ in their gene expression patterns. The vertical columns of squares represent tumor samples, and the horizontal rows compare the activities of particular genes. Red tones indicate higher-than-normal expression and blue tones show lower-than-normal expression. The different patterns indicate very distinct cancers, although the cells may look alike under a microscope. For many years, the newly recognized mixed-lineage leukemia (MLL) was considered a subtype of acute lymphoblastic leukemia (ALL), and was treated as such—with little success. Microarray analyses will refine cancer diagnosis and make more effective treatment possible.

more frequently, or more times, than the normal cell type it descended from.

The timing, rate, and number of mitoses depend on protein growth factors and signaling molecules from outside the cell, and on transcription factors from within. Because these biochemicals are under genetic control, so is the cell cycle abnormality that is cancer. Cancer cells probably arise in everyone, because mitosis occurs so frequently that an occasional cell escapes control. However, the immune system destroys most cancer cells after recognizing tumor-specific antigens on their surfaces.

The discovery of the checkpoints that control the cell cycle revealed how cancer can begin (see figure 2.17). A mutation in a gene that normally halts or slows the cell cycle can lift the constraint, leading to inappropriate mitosis. Another cell-cycle-related cause of cancer is failure to pause long enough to repair DNA.

Loss of control over telomere length may also contribute to cancer. Recall from figure 2.18 that telomeres, or chromosome tips, protect chromosomes from breaking. Human telomeres consist of the DNA sequence TTAGGG repeated thousands of times. The repeats are normally lost as a cell matures, at the rate of about 15 to 40 nucleotides per cell division. The more specialized a cell, the shorter its telomeres. The chromosomes in skin, nerve, and muscle cells, for example, have short telomeres. Chromosomes in a sperm cell or oocyte, however, have long telomeres. This makes sense—as the precursors of a new organism, gametes must retain the capacity to divide many times.

Gametes keep their telomeres long, thanks to an enzyme, **telomerase**, that is a complex of RNA and protein. Part of the RNA—the sequence AAUCCC—serves as a template for the 6-DNA-base repeat that builds telomeres **(figure 18.3)**. Telomerase moves down a chromosome tip like a zip-

per, adding six "teeth" at a time. In this way, telomerase repeatedly adds telomere material to the chromosomes of gametes.

In normal, specialized cells, telomerase is turned off, and telomeres shrink, signaling a halt to cell division when they reach a certain size. In cancer cells, telomerase is turned back on. Telomeres extend, and this releases the normal brake on rapid cell division. As daughter cells of the original abnormal cell continue to divide uncontrollably, a tumor forms, grows, and may spread. Usually, the longer the telomeres in cancer cells, the more advanced the disease. However, turning on telomerase production in a cell is not sufficient in itself to cause cancer. Many things must go wrong for cancer to begin.

Inherited Versus Sporadic Cancer

Most cancers are isolated, or sporadic, which means that the causative mutation

A cancer cell is **dedifferenti-ated,** which means that it is less specialized than the normal cell type it arose from. A skin cancer cell, for example, is rounder and softer than the flattened, scaly, healthy skin cells above it in the epidermis. Cancer cell growth also differs. Normal cells placed in a container divide to form a single layer; cancer cells pile up on one another. In an organism, this pileup would produce a tumor. Cancer cells that grow all over one another lack **contact inhibition**—they do not stop dividing when they crowd other cells.

Cancer cells have surface structures that enable them to squeeze into any space, a property called **invasiveness** (**figure 18.5**). They anchor themselves to tissue boundaries, called basement membranes, where they secrete enzymes that cut paths through healthy tissue. Unlike a benign tumor, an invasive malignant tumor grows irregularly, sending tentacles in all directions.

Eventually, unless treatment stops them, cancer cells reach the bloodstream or lymphatic vessels, which take them to other parts of the body. The traveling cancer cells settle into new sites. Once they've grown to the size of a pinhead, interior cells respond to the oxygen-poor environment by secreting a factor, called vascular endothelial growth factor, that stimulates nearby capillaries (the tiniest blood vessels) to sprout new branches that extend toward the tumor, bringing in oxygen and nutrients and removing wastes. This growth of new capillaries is **angiogenesis.** Capillaries may snake into and out of the tumor (**figure 18.6**). Cancer cells wrap around the blood vessels and creep out upon this scaffolding, invading nearby tissue. Cancer cells may also secrete hormones that encourage their own growth, hormones the cells they descend from do not produce.

Once cancer cells move to a new body part, the disease has metastasized. The DNA of secondary tumor cells often mutates, many times causing new chrom-

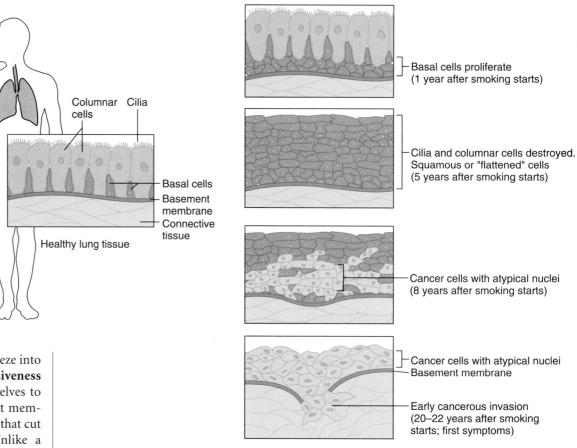

Figure 18.5 Cancers take many years to spread. Lung cancer due to smoking begins with irritation of the lining tissue in respiratory tubes (bronchial epithelium). Ciliated cells die (but can be restored if smoking ceases), basal cells divide, and then, if the irritation continues, cancerous changes may appear.

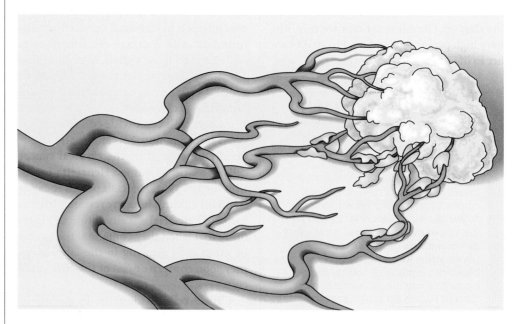

Figure 18.6 Angiogenesis nurtures a tumor. Cells starved for oxygen deep within a tumor secrete vascular endothelial growth factor, which stimulates nearby capillaries to extend branches toward a tumor.

osome aberrations. Many cancer cells are aneuploid. The metastasized cancer thus becomes a new genetic entity, often resistant to treatments that were effective against most cells of the original tumor. Because gene expression patterns associated with metastasis are detectable early, new cancer treatments may actually prevent metastasis.

Table 18.2 summarizes the characteristics of cancer cells.

Table 18.2
Characteristics of Cancer Cells

Oilier, less adherent

Loss of cell cycle control

Heritability

Transplantability

Dedifferentiation

Loss of contact inhibition

Ability to induce local blood vessel formation (angiogenesis)

Invasiveness

Increased mutation rate

Ability to spread (metastasis)

Key Concepts

Cancer occurs when cells divide faster or more times than normal. Cancer cells are heritable, transplantable, and dedifferentiated. They lack contact inhibition, cutting through basement membranes. A cancerous growth is invasive and can metastasize and stimulate angiogenesis, spreading further.

18.3 Genes That Cause Cancer

Mutations in three types of genes can cause cancer (**table 18.3**) Most are oncogenes or tumor suppressor genes. The third category includes DNA repair genes (see section 12.6). Mutations in DNA repair genes allow other mutations to persist unfixed and to accumulate. When such mutations activate oncogenes or inactivate tumor suppressor genes, cancer results. DNA repair disorders are often inherited in a Mendelian fashion, and are quite rare.

Table 18.3
Types of Cancer-Causing Genes

Type of Gene	Mechanism of Carcinogenesis
Oncogene	Actively promotes cancer. Normal version, a proto-oncogene, controls cell cycle. Oncogene activates cell division at inappropriate time or place.
Tumor suppressor gene mutation	Mutation removes normal suppression of cell division.
DNA repair gene mutation	Effect indirect. Faulty DNA repair gene allows many mutations to accumulate, some in proto-oncogenes and tumor suppressor genes.

Oncogenes

Genes that normally trigger cell division are called **proto-oncogenes.** They are active where and when high rates of cell division are necessary, such as in a wound or in an embryo. When proto-oncogenes are turned on at the wrong time or place, they function as oncogenes ("onco" means cancer). This abnormal activation may be the result of a mutation. A single base change in a proto-oncogene causes bladder cancer, for example. Alternatively, a proto-oncogene may be moved near a gene that is highly expressed; then it, too, is rapidly or frequently transcribed. For example, a human proto-oncogene is normally activated in cells at the site of a wound, where it stimulates production of growth factors that cause mitosis to fill the damaged area in with new cells. When that proto-oncogene is activated at a site other than a wound—as an oncogene—it still hikes growth factor production and stimulates mitosis. However, because the site of the action is not damaged tissue, the new cells form a tumor.

Some proto-oncogenes encode transcription factors that, as oncogenes, are too highly expressed. (Recall from chapter 10 that transcription factors bind to specific genes and activate transcription.) The products of these activated genes then contribute to the cancer cell's characteristics.

Increased Expression in a New Location

A proto-oncogene can be transformed into its out-of-control oncogene counterpart when it is placed next to a gene that boosts its expression. A virus infecting a cell, for example, may insert DNA next to a proto-oncogene. When the viral DNA is rapidly transcribed, the adjacent proto-oncogene (now an oncogene) is also rapidly transcribed. Increased production of the oncogene's protein product then switches on the genes that promote mitosis, triggering the cascade of changes that leads to cancer. Kaposi sarcoma and acute T cell leukemia are human cancers caused by viruses.

A proto-oncogene can also be activated when it is moved next to a very active gene that is a normal part of the genome. This can happen when a chromosome is inverted or translocated. For example, a cancer of the parathyroid glands in the neck is associated with an inversion on chromosome 11, which places a proto-oncogene next to a DNA sequence that controls transcription of the parathyroid hormone gene. When the gland synthesizes the hormone, the oncogene is expressed. The cells divide, forming a tumor.

Ironically, the immune system contributes to cancer when a translocation or inversion places a proto-oncogene next to an antibody gene. Recall from chapter 17 that antibody genes normally move into novel combinations when a B cell is stimulated and they are very actively transcribed. Cancers associated with viral infections, such as liver cancer following hepatitis, may be caused when proto-oncogenes are mistakenly activated along with antibody genes. Similarly, in Burkitt lymphoma, a cancer common in Africa, a large tumor develops from lymph glands near the jaw. People with Burkitt lymphoma are infected with the Epstein-Barr virus, which stimulates specific chromosome movements in maturing B cells to assemble antibodies against the virus. A translocation places a proto-oncogene on chromosome 8 next to an antibody gene on

Retinoblastoma—The Two-Hit Hypothesis

Our current understanding of tumor-suppressing genes began with observations by Alfred Knudson. He studied retinoblastoma (RB), a rare childhood eye cancer. Distinct tumors, representing individual original cancerous cells, develop in the eye (**figure 1**). Sometimes RB affects one eye, and sometimes both. Knudson examined the medical records of 48 children with RB admitted to M.D. Anderson Hospital in Houston between 1944 and 1969. He recorded the following information for each child:

1. Whether one eye or two were affected

2. How old the child was at the time of diagnosis

3. Whether any other relatives had RB

4. Sex

5. Number of tumors per eye

The fact that RB occurred in boys and girls told Knudson that any genetic control was autosomal. Pooling data from families with more than one case of RB revealed that approximately 50 percent of the children of an affected parent were also affected, suggesting dominant inheritance. Knudson also noted that in some families, a child with two

affected eyes would have an affected grandparent, but both parents had healthy eyes. A picture of autosomal dominant inheritance with incomplete penetrance began to emerge.

Knudson, however, proposed a different explanation: An initial, inherited recessive mutation had to be followed by a second, somatic mutation in the eye to trigger tumor formation. This idea became known as the "two-hit hypothesis" of cancer causation. Occasionally the second mutation would not occur, and this would explain an unaffected generation between affected ones.

Two mutations explained another observation Knudson gleaned from medical records. Children with tumors in both eyes become affected much earlier than children with tumors in only one eye—generally before the age of five. This would make sense if a hereditary, bilateral (two-eye) form of RB requires a germline mutation followed by a somatic mutation, but a nonhereditary, unilateral (one-eye) form results from two somatic mutations in the same gene in the same cell. That is, in inherited RB, a newborn is halfway on the road to tumor development—just one somatic mutation in the eye is needed. The unilateral, noninherited form appears later in childhood

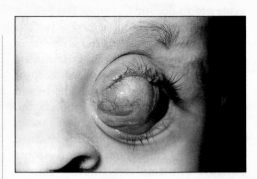

Figure 1 Retinoblastoma. In inherited retinoblastoma, all of the person's cells are heterozygous for a mutation in the *RB* gene. A second mutation, occurring in the original unmutated allele in cone cells in the retina, releases controls on mitosis, and a tumor develops.

because it takes longer for two somatic mutations in the same gene to occur in the same cell. Knudson used mathematics to show that the average number of tumors per eye—three—was consistent with two "hits."

Although it would be another 15 years before researchers identified the *RB* gene on chromosome 13, and longer still before its role in controlling the cell cycle was identified, Knudson's insights paved the way for those discoveries and for recognizing the widespread action of tumor suppressors in general.

More than half of human cancers involve a point mutation or deletion in the *p53* gene. The precise locations and types of mutations—a transition (purine to purine or pyrimidine to pyrimidine) or transversion (purine to pyrimidine or vice versa)—are different in different cancers. Cancers of the colon, breast, bladder, lung, liver, blood, brain, esophagus, and skin show distinct types of *p53* mutations.

Mutational analysis and epidemiological observations reveal that p53 protein may be a genetic mediator between environmental insults and development of cancer (**figure 18.9**). Consider a type of liver cancer prevalent in populations in southern Africa and Qidong, China. These two groups have in

common exposure to the hepatitis B virus and to a food contaminant called aflatoxin B1. Most of the people with the liver cancer have the same point mutation in the *p53* gene that substitutes a T for a G. Could the food toxin, hepatitis virus, or both cause the mutation? Alternatively, the virus or toxin might trigger expression of an existing *p53* gene variant.

In most *p53*-related cancers, mutations occur only in somatic cells. However, about 100 families worldwide suffer from a germline condition called the Li-Fraumeni family cancer syndrome. Family members who inherit a mutation in the *p53* gene have a very high risk of developing cancer—50 percent by age 30, and 90 percent by age 70. The risk of breast cancer is near 100 per-

cent (see In Their Own Words on page 364). A somatic mutation in the affected tissue is necessary for cancer to develop, as is true for inherited retinoblastoma. Li-Fraumeni patients also develop cancers of the brain, blood, bone, adrenal glands, or soft solid tissues, such as muscle or connective tissue.

BRCA1—A Genetic Counseling Challenge

Breast cancer that recurs in families can reflect the inheritance of a germline mutation (familial), or be caused by two-hit somatic mutations that happen more than once in a family due to chance (sporadic). Familial breast cancer touches on many of the complications of Mendel's laws discussed in chapter 5—multiple alleles, incomplete penetrance, variable expressivity, environmental influences, genetic heterogeneity, and polygenic inheritance and epistasis. Only 5 percent of breast cancers are familial, and of these, 15 to 20 percent are caused by mutations in the genes *BRCA1* or *BRCA2*. Because breast cancer is so common, some women seeking genetic counseling may have sporadic cases that appear to be inherited—or the reverse. **Table 18.4** highlights some of the challenges encountered in genetic counseling for breast cancer.

The *BRCA1* gene, which stands for "breast cancer predisposition gene 1," greatly increases the lifetime risk of inheriting breast and ovarian cancer. It is a tumor suppressor gene, because the phenotype results from a loss of function. In the most common mutation, two adjacent bases are deleted, altering the reading frame and shortening the protein. The mutation is inherited as an autosomal dominant trait, but with late onset of symptoms and incomplete penetrance.

The *BRCA1* gene encodes a large protein that normally resides in the nucleus, where it activates transcription of the genes that respond to p53 protein. Therefore, BRCA1 protein is necessary for DNA repair—specifically, mending double-stranded breaks that could threaten the stability of chromosomes.

BRCA1 mutations have different incidences in different populations, and the risk of cancer varies in different populations, indicating that the BRCA1 protein interacts with other proteins and perhaps with environmental factors, too (**Table 18.5**). Only 1 in 833 people in the general U.S. population has a mutant *BRCA1* allele. But among the Ashkenazi Jewish population, slightly more than 2 percent of all individuals have one mutant *BRCA1* allele. It was in such families that the *BRCA1* gene was discovered—several members became ill at very young ages. In this group, a woman who inherits a *BRCA1* mutation faces a greater than 80 percent risk of developing breast cancer over her lifetime and a 50 percent risk of developing ovarian cancer. Some still-healthy relatives with the mutant gene have had the affected organs removed to prevent the cancers. But risk, even if a *BRCA1* or *BRCA2* mutation is inherited, is difficult to predict because of environmental factors. Women with such a mutation born after 1940 have a higher risk than those born earlier, suggesting a non-genetic influence.

BRCA2 breast cancer is also common among the Ashkenazim. This gene encodes a nuclear protein that is even larger than the BRCA1 protein. Ashkenazi women who inherit a mutation in *BRCA2* face a 60 to 85 percent lifetime risk of developing breast cancer and a 10 to 20 percent risk of developing ovarian cancer. Men who inherit a *BRCA2* mutation have a 6 percent lifetime risk of developing breast cancer, which is 100 times the risk for men in the general population. Inheriting a *BRCA2* mutation also increases the risk of developing cancers of the colon, prostate, pancreas, gallbladder or stomach, as well as malignant melanoma. The fact that p53, BRCA1 and BRCA2 proteins all bind to each other in the nucleus suggests that they interact to enable a cell to repair double-stranded DNA breaks.

Still other genes that affect these three (*BRCA1, BRCA2,* and *p53*) can cause breast cancer. For example, the product of a gene called *ATM* adds a phosphate to the product of a gene called *CHEK2*, which then adds a phosphate to the BRCA1 protein. Mutations in *ATM* and *CHEK2* also cause

Figure 18.9 *p53* **cancers reflect environmental insults.** The environment triggers mutations or changes in gene expression that lead to cancer. The *p53* gene may be a mediator.

Table 18.4

The Complexities of Providing Genetic Counseling for Familial Breast Cancer

1. Many mutations and polymorphisms are known in breast cancer genes.

2. Breast cancer can occur in other ways. When more than one case occurs in a family, it can be either familial or sporadic. A woman who does not have a *BRCA1* or *BRCA2* mutation can still develop breast cancer. A woman with no affected relatives can have a *BRCA1* or *BRCA2* mutation.

3. *BRCA1* and *BRCA2* are incompletely penetrant—that is, inheriting a disease-causing allele does not always mean developing cancer.

4. The risk associated with *BRCA1* or *BRCA2* mutations varies depending upon interactions with other genes as well as environmental exposures.

p53: A Family's View

To a family with Li-Fraumeni cancer syndrome, *p53* is more than a transcription factor that lies at the crossroads of the cell cycle. A germline mutation sets the stage for multiple, early cancers. Patricia Holm's family is one of only about 100 known to have the condition. Here is her story:

At 25 years old Timothy Whittaker, my husband, developed liposarcoma, a rare cancer of the fat cells. He suffered greatly and weighed at the time of his death 55 pounds—eight months after diagnosis.

The younger of our girls, Jennifer Leigh, was born in 1973. She was perfectly healthy throughout her childhood, but as her school career began, she had trouble in her studies. I have since wondered if the tumor was growing even then. The summer between her junior and senior years, when she was 17, Jennifer developed a headache that sent us three times in four days to the E.R. On the fourth day, a CT scan revealed a lemon-sized tumor in her left parietal lobe. The first resection pathology revealed a pleomorphic xanthoastrocytoma. Four months later, pathology revealed anaplastic astrocytoma. After nine months of chemotherapy and radiation, the tumor was back, the pathology report glioblastoma multiforme—a death sentence. In the 27 months from diagnosis to death, every approved and unapproved method of treatment was used, and nothing ever helped . . . we went to four states and two countries seeking a cure. There wasn't one, and exactly 19 years after the death of Timothy, Jennifer died at the age of 20.

Doctors assured me that liposarcoma and brain tumors have absolutely no connection. Bad luck? A witch's curse? What was going on? The answer would come much later.

In August 1998 our daughter, Kimberly, gave birth to a baby girl, Grace. Shortly thereafter she felt a thickening in her left breast. Repeated attempts to alarm her ob/gyn failed, as he saw this as normal breast change, probably a clogged milk duct. In May 2000, Kim felt a lump under her arm that in three weeks became the size of a golf ball. She then had her general medical doctor take a look and he sent her for a mammogram the same day. A lump was not seen on the mammogram, but her breast was full of microcalcifications and looked like a starry night! An ultrasound was done, and there on the screen was an enormous black mass. Oh my God, not again.

The next year and a half consisted of chemotherapy, radiation, double mastectomies and 40 weekly treatments of Herceptin. Pathology was intraductal carcinoma. After all her treatments, the pathology on the removed breasts was ductal carcinoma *in situ* only; she had a complete response to chemotherapy. Finally, a victory over cancer! Today Kim is doing very well.

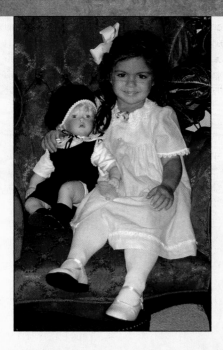

Shortly after diagnosis, a genetic workup revealed that Kim had Li-Fraumeni family cancer syndrome. Grace, who had a 50/50 chance of inheriting the mutation and is now 4 years old, has not been tested. But as you can imagine, for both Grace and her mother there is no such thing as a simple headache, no harmless sore throat, no lymph node that loving fingers don't glide over in hopes that there will be no knot under the skin. It can be a daily struggle to live with the knowledge that there is a bomb ticking in every cell of your body that is lying in wait for the right stimulus to set it off.

Patricia Holm

Table 18.5

Lifetime Risk That Inheriting a *BRCA1* Mutation Will Lead to Breast Cancer

Group	Risk (%)
Ashkenazim with confirmed strong family history of early-onset cases	87
Ashkenazim with family history of breast cancer, but not early onset or many affected members	56
Ashkenazim with no family history of breast cancer	36
General population	8–10

breast cancer. Another form of breast cancer results from mutations in any of five genes known to cause Fanconi anemia, a fatal blood disorder. Five of the Fanconi anemia proteins form a cluster that activates a sixth protein, which in turns binds to and inactivates the BRCA2 protein.

The many ways to develop breast cancer indicate that this isn't one illness, but probably ten to twenty different types. In each type, disruptions of a signal transduction pathway or DNA repair mechanism accelerates the cell cycle in the affected tissue, usually a milk duct.

Table 18.6 lists some oncogenes and tumor suppressor genes.

Table 18.6
Cancer Genes

Oncogenes	Cancer Location/Type	Mechanism
myc	Blood, breast, lung, brain, stomach	Alters transcription factor
PDGF	Brain	Alters growth factors or growth factor receptors
RET	Thyroid	Alters growth factors or growth factor receptors
erb-B	Brain, breast	Alters growth factors or growth factor receptors
Her-2/neu	Breast, ovarian, salivary glands	Alters growth factors or growth factor receptors
ras	Blood, lung, colon, ovary, pancreas	Affects signal transduction
bcl-2	Blood	Releases brake on apoptosis
PRAD1	Breast, head, and neck	Disrupts cell cycle protein (cyclin)
abl	White blood cells	Translocation alters proto-oncogene and stimulates cell division

Tumor Suppressors		
MTS1	Many sites	Releases brake on cell cycle
RB	Eye, bone, breast, lung, bladder	Releases brake on cell cycle
WT1	Kidney	Releases brake on cell cycle
p53	Many sites	Disrupts p53 protein, which normally determines whether DNA is repaired or cell dies
DPC4	Pancreas	Affects signal transduction
NF1	Peripheral nerves	Disrupts inhibition of normal *ras*, which stimulates cell division
APC	Colon, stomach	Makes nearby DNA more susceptible to replication errors
BRCA1, BRCA2	Breast, ovary, prostate	Faulty repair of double-stranded DNA breaks
hMSH2, hMLH1, hPMS1, hPMS2	Colon, uterus, ovary	Disrupts DNA mismatch repair
Lkb1	Peutz-Jeghers syndrome (many sites)	After birth, fails to block expression of vascular endothelial growth factor, normally active in embryo

Key Concepts

Proto-oncogenes normally control the cell cycle. They can become oncogenes when they mutate, when they move next to a gene that is highly expressed, or when they are transcribed and translated along with another gene, resulting in a fusion protein that triggers cancer. • Mutations in tumor suppressor genes usually are deletions that cause a cell to ignore extracellular constraints on cell division. The *RB, p53,* and *BRCA1* genes encode tumor suppressors. Other genes cause breast cancer, too.

18.4 A Series of Genetic Changes Causes Some Cancers

Some cancers are the culmination of a series of changes in several genes. To identify the steps, researchers examine tumor cell DNA from people in various stages of the same type of cancer. The older the tumor, the more genetic changes accumulate. Therefore, a mutation present in all stages acts early in carcinogenesis, whereas a mutation seen only in the tumor cells of people near the end stages functions late in the process. Each step provides a potential point of treatment. Following is a closer look at two types of cancer that reflect a series of genetic changes.

A Rapidly Growing Brain Tumor

Astrocytomas, the most common types of brain tumors, affect cells called astrocytes. These tumors grow quickly. The man whose brain is shown in **figure 18.10** died just three months after noticing twitching in an eye. During that time, a series of single-gene and chromosomal changes occurred. Loss of both *p53* alleles came early because this appears in many early-stage tumor cells, as well as in later ones.

By the time an astrocytoma has grown into a small tumor, another genetic change is apparent—loss of both alleles of several genes on chromosome 9. Some of the missing genes encode interferons, so the loss probably disrupts immune protection against the developing cancer. Two other deleted genes encode tumor suppressors.

At least two additional mutations speed the tumor's growth. First, an oncogene on chromosome 7 is activated, overexpressing a gene that encodes a cell surface receptor for a growth factor. The cancer cells bear too many growth factor receptors and receive too many messages to divide. Finally, the cancer cells lose one or even both copies of chromosome 10. This is a final change, because it is seen in all end-stage tumors, but not in early ones.

Colon Cancer

Colon (large intestine) cancer does not usually occur in families with the frequency or pattern expected of a single-gene disorder.

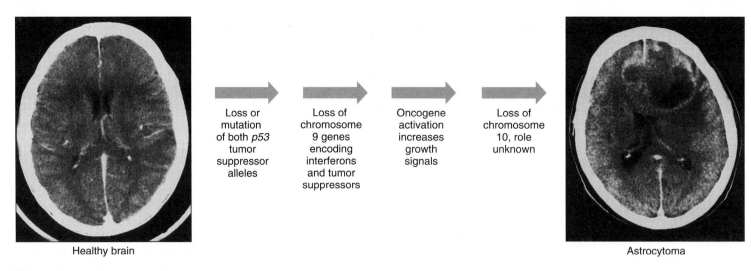

Loss or mutation of both *p53* tumor suppressor alleles → Loss of chromosome 9 genes encoding interferons and tumor suppressors → Oncogene activation increases growth signals → Loss of chromosome 10, role unknown

Healthy brain

Astrocytoma

Figure 18.10   Several genes can contribute to a cancer.   A series of genetic changes transforms normal astrocytes, which support nerve cells in the brain, into a rapidly growing cancer.

However, when family members with noncancerous growths (polyps) in the colon are considered with those who have colon cancer, a Mendelian pattern emerges. Five percent of cases are inherited. One in 5,000 people in the United States has precancerous colon polyps, a condition called familial adenomatous polyposis (FAP).

FAP begins in early childhood with tiny polyps, often hundreds, that progress over many years to colon cancer. Colon lining cells typically live three days. In FAP, they fail to die on schedule and instead build up, forming polyps. Connecting FAP to the development of colon cancer enabled researchers to view the stepwise progression of a cancer (**figure 18.11**). Several genes, including both oncogenes and tumor suppressors, take part.

The study of the hereditary nature of some colon cancers began at the University of Utah in Salt Lake City in the fall of 1947, when young professor Eldon Gardner stated that he thought cancer might be inherited. A student, Eugene Robertson, excitedly told the class that he knew of a family in which a grandmother, her three children, and three grandchildren had colon cancer.

Intrigued, Gardner delved into the family's records and began interviewing relatives. He eventually found 51 family members and arranged for each to be examined with a colonoscope, a lit instrument passed into the rectum to view the wall of the colon. The colons of 6 of the 51 people were riddled with the gobletlike precancerous polyps, although none of the 6 had symp-

toms. Removal of their colons probably saved their lives.

In the years that followed, researchers identified other families with more than one case of colon polyps. Individuals with only polyps were diagnosed with FAP. If a person with colon polyps had cancer elsewhere, extra teeth, and pigment patches in the eye, the condition was called Gardner syndrome, named for the professor. Researchers identified the chromosomal defect that causes Gardner syndrome in 1985 with the help of a 42-year-old man at the Roswell Park Cancer Institute in Buffalo, New York. He had several problems—no gallbladder, an incomplete liver, an abnormal kidney, mental retardation, and Gardner syndrome. To a geneticist, a seemingly unrelated combination of symp-

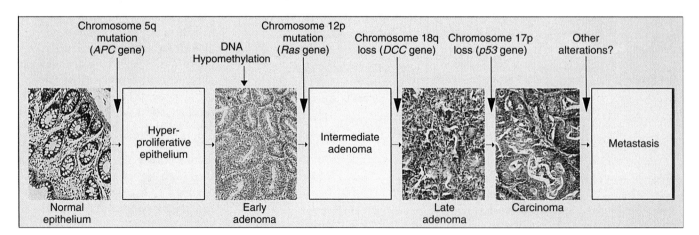

Chromosome 5q mutation (*APC* gene) → DNA Hypomethylation → Chromosome 12p mutation (*Ras* gene) → Chromosome 18q loss (*DCC* gene) → Chromosome 17p loss (*p53* gene) → Other alterations?

Normal epithelium → Hyper-proliferative epithelium → Early adenoma → Intermediate adenoma → Late adenoma → Carcinoma → Metastasis

Figure 18.11   Several genes contribute to FAP colon cancer.   Cells lining the colon begin to divide more frequently when the *APC* gene on chromosome 5q undergoes a point mutation. This causes replication errors that disrupt the reading frame, shortening the protein product. The affected cell proliferates, forming a growth that becomes a precancerous polyp when DNA loses protective methyl groups. Next, the *Ras* oncogene is activated. Loss of the *p53* tumor suppressor gene produces cancer, and other genes may contribute to the cancer's spread. Researchers continue to fill in the gaps in the genetic orchestration of this cancer.

toms suggests a chromosomal abnormality affecting several genes. Sure enough, the man's karyotype revealed a small deletion in the long arm of chromosome 5. This was the first piece to the puzzle of colon cancer.

Since 1985, researchers have discovered other genes that contribute in sequence to colon cancer, including *p53*. A gene on chromosome 5q, called *APC,* may start the process. A point mutation that changes a T to an A in the *APC* gene results in a stretch of eight consecutive A's, which destabilizes replication enzymes. The result is a shift in the reading frame and a shortened protein.

Key Concepts

Some cancers may be the culmination of a series of mutations in several genes. Determining which mutations are present in particular stages of a cancer can reveal the sequence of gene actions.

18.5 Cancer Prevention, Diagnosis, and Treatment

One way to lower the chance of developing cancer is to avoid certain high-risk environmental factors, such as cigarette smoking and excess sun exposure. A more active approach is chemoprevention, which is taking certain nutrients, plant extracts, or drugs to lower the risk of cancer. Promising "chemopreventatives" include folic acid, vitamins D and E, selenium, compounds from soybean, tomato, and green tea, and certain anti-inflammatory drugs.

Investigating Environmental Causes of Cancer

Diet affects the risk of developing some cancers, but determining precisely how a dietary intervention lowers the risk of—or actually prevents—cancer, can be complicated. Consider the cruciferous vegetables, such as broccoli and Brussels sprouts, which are associated with decreased risk of developing colon cancer. Experiments show that these vegetables release compounds called glucosinolates, which in turn activate "xenobiotic metabolizing enzymes" that detoxify carcinogenic products of cooked meat called heterocyclic aromatic amines. With a vegetable-poor, meaty diet, heterocyclic amines accumulate. They cross the lining of the digestive tract and circulate to the liver, where enzymes metabolize them into compounds that cause the mutations associated with colon cancer (**figure 18.12**).

Environmental exposures to carcinogens—in the workplace, home, or outdoors—can also raise cancer risk. Chemical carcinogens were recognized as long ago as 1775, when British physician Sir Percival Potts suggested that the high rate of skin cancer in the scrotums of chimney sweeps in London was due to their exposure to a chemical in soot. Since then, epidemiological studies have identified many chemicals as possibly causing cancer in certain popula- tions (**table 18.7**). However, most studies reveal correlations rather than cause-and-effect relationships. In the best cases, genetic or biochemical evidence explains the observed environmental connection.

Epidemiologists use different statistical tools to establish links between environmental exposures and cancer. Links are strengthened when different types of investigations yield consistent results. This is true, for example, of the association between eating whole grain cereals and reduced incidence of colorectal cancer.

A **population study** compares the incidence of a type of cancer among very different groups of people. If the incidence differs, then some difference between the populations may be responsible. For example, an oft-mentioned study from 1922 found that

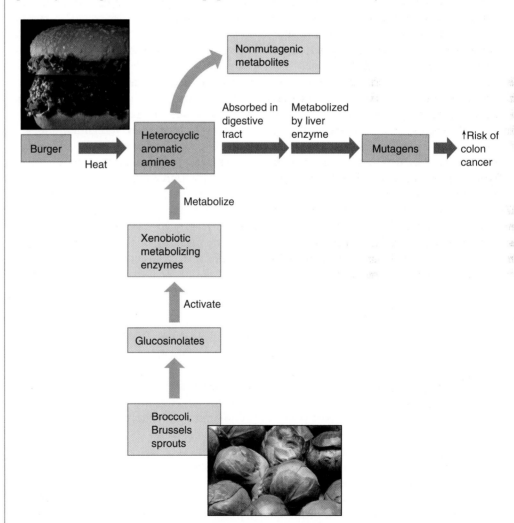

Figure 18.12 One way that cruciferous vegetables lower cancer risk.
Compounds called heterocyclic aromatic amines (HAs) form in cooking meat, are absorbed into the digestive tract, and are metabolized by a liver enzyme into mutagens, which may cause colon cancer. Broccoli and Brussels sprouts produce glucosinolates, which activate xenobiotic metabolizing enzymes that block part of the pathway that leads to production of the mutagens.

Table 18.7

Increase in Death Rates for Certain Cancers in Particular Geographical Areas in the United States

Cancer Type	Region	Possible Explanation
Breast	Northeast	*BRCA1* mutations, greater lifetime exposure to estrogens (early menstruation, late menopause, older age of first birth, exposure to pesticides)
Colon	Northeast	Dietary factors, medical screening
Lung	White men in south, white women in west, blacks in northern cities	Changes in regional trends in cigarette smoking
Lung	Men in southern coastal areas	Asbestos exposure while working in shipyards during World War II
Mouth, throat	Women in rural south	Smokeless tobacco
Esophagus	Washington, D.C., coastal South Carolina	Alcohol and tobacco, deficiencies of fruits and vegetables in diet

primitive societies have much lower rates of many cancers than more developed societies. The study attributed the lack of cancer to the high level of physical activity among the primitive peoples—but diet might also explain the difference.

Population studies often have too many variables to reveal cause and effect. Consider the very high incidence of breast cancer on Long Island, New York. One hypothesis attributes the mini-epidemic to pesticide exposure, but this population also has a high frequency of *BRCA1* mutations among its Ashkenazi citizens. Sociological factors come into play, too. In this population, women have frequent mammograms starting at a young age. As a result, the percentage of the population with recognized early stages of the disease may be higher than in other populations where women are less likely to have regular mammograms. All of these factors may contribute to the high breast cancer incidence in this area.

More informative is a **case-control study,** in which people with a type of cancer are matched with healthy individuals for age, sex, and other characteristics. Then researchers look for differences between the pairs. If, for example, the cancer patients had extensive dental X rays at a young age but the control group didn't, X-ray exposure may be a causal factor. The problem with this type of study is that much of the information is often based on recall, people make mistakes, and not all relevant factors are identified and taken into account.

The most informative type of epidemiological investigation is a **prospective study,** in which two or more groups of people follow a specified dietary regimen and are checked periodically for cancer. By looking ahead, the investigator has more control over the activities and can verify information. However, a limitation of this type of cancer study is that cancer usually takes many years to appear and progress.

The meaning of these epidemiological studies is far from certain. For a correlation to be elevated to the status of possible cause or preventative, a biological explanation is necessary. For example, certain vegetables contain antioxidant compounds, which deactivate the free radicals that can damage DNA, thereby preventing mutations. Still, on the basis of all of these types of studies, the National Cancer Institute advises consuming whole grains, fruits and vegetables, and limiting consumption of animal fat to lower cancer risk.

Diagnosing and Treating Cancer

Predicting that cancer will occur in a particular individual is only possible for a few disorders that are inherited in a Mendelian fashion through known genes. More often, discovery of cancer follows a screening test such as mammography or high levels of prostate specific antigen in the bloodstream, or after symptoms occur or a person feels a lump. Then treatments begin—and there are usually many options.

Cancer treatments focus on particular characteristics of cancer cells. The oldest treatment, surgery, is straightforward—it prevents invasiveness by removing the tumor. Radiation and chemotherapy use a different approach, killing all cells that divide rapidly. Unfortunately, this also affects healthy cells in the digestive tract, hair follicles, and bone marrow, causing nausea, hair loss, great fatigue, and susceptibility to infection. Patients receive several other drugs to help them tolerate the side effects, including colony stimulating factors to replenish bone marrow. These other drugs enable patients to withstand higher and more effective doses of chemotherapy. In the near future, pharmacogenomics will reveal gene variants and gene expression patterns that indicate which individuals will benefit the most from particular drugs.

Several new types of cancer drugs affect cancer cell characteristics or activities other than hiked division rate. Some treatments stimulate cells to regain specialized characteristics, such as drugs based on retinoic acid. Another approach is to inhibit telomerase, which prevents cancer cells from elongating their telomeres and continually dividing. In yet another approach, angiogenesis inhibitors rob a cancer of its blood supply. A drug called Avastin, for example, extends life in some people with colon cancer by inhibiting vascular endothelial growth factor (VEGF), which tumor cells secrete to attract and stimulate the extension of capillaries. Other anti-angiogenesis drugs shut off the signals in the cell that VEGF activates. Yet other treatment approaches induce apoptosis, which counters the runaway cell division of cancer.

The evolution of diagnosis and treatments for breast cancer illustrates how genetic and genomic information will increasingly refine how physicians manage these diseases. The earliest treatments simply removed or destroyed the affected tissue (**table 18.8**). Then physicians began to determine whether tumor cells have receptors for estrogen or progesterone, two hormones. Women with estrogen receptor-positive tumors typically begin a several-year course of a drug that

Table 18.8

Evolution of Treatments for Breast Cancer

Strategy	Examples
Remove or destroy cancerous tissue	Surgery, radiation, chemotherapy
Use phenotype to select drug	Estrogen receptor-positive women take a selective estrogen receptor modulator, followed by an aromatase inhibitor
Use genotype to select drug	Women with *Her-2/neu*-positive cancers take Herceptin (monoclonal antibody)
Genomic level	Gene expression profile on DNA microarray used to guide drug choice; 70-gene signature predicts metastasis

blocks these receptors from receiving signals to divide, and then another drug that inhibits an enzyme called aromatase.

Determining estrogen receptor status is subtyping by phenotype. With the discovery of single genes that cause cancer, diagnosis began to include genotyping, too; a woman might have *BRCA1* or *Her-2/neu* breast cancer. Increasingly, cancer diagnosis will be based on DNA microarrays that scan both genotype and gene expression patterns, enabling physicians to match a particular patient to the treatments most likely to work right from the start. Genomic analyses will also identify patients likely to suffer side effects from particular drugs. Some women with breast cancer, for example, develop gastrointestinal, bone marrow, and brain damage from the cancer drug 5-fluorouracil because they lack a liver enzyme that dismantles the drug. A gene test can spot this deficit.

The limitation of any cancer treatment, old or new, is defined by the strength of the enemy. Cancer cells are incredibly abundant and ever-changing. Surgery followed by a barrage of drugs and radiation can slow the course of the disease, but all it takes is a few escaped cancer cells—called micrometastases—to sow the seeds of a future tumor. The DNA of cancer cells mutates in ways that enable the cells to pump out any drug sent into them. In addition, cancer cells have redundancies, so that if a drug shuts down angiogenesis or invasiveness, the cell completes the task another way. Although cancer treatments can completely cure the illness, it is more likely that they kill enough cancer cells, and sufficiently slow the spread, that it takes the remainder of a lifetime for the tumors to grow back. In this way, cancer becomes a chronic, manageable condition.

Key Concepts

Lower cancer risk is associated with eating more fruits, vegetables, and whole grain cereals, and avoiding fats.
• Treatments for cancer target the characteristics of cancer cells. Surgery removes tumors. Chemotherapy and radiation nonselectively destroy rapidly dividing cells. Newer treatments target receptors on cancer cells, block telomerase, stimulate differentiation, or attack a tumor's blood supply. Diagnosis and treatment of cancer will increasingly consider genomic information.

Summary

18.1 Cancer as a Genetic Disorder

1. Cancer is a genetically dictated loss of cell cycle control, creating a population of highly proliferative cells that outgrows and overwhelms surrounding tissue.

2. Sporadic cancers result from mutations in somatic cells only. They are more common than germline cancers, which are caused by a **germline** mutation plus a somatic mutation in affected tissue. Cancer may also be polygenic. Changing gene expression patterns also contribute to cancer, and can be used to distinguish types.

3. Mutations in genes that encode or control transcription factors, cell cycle checkpoint proteins, growth factors, repair proteins, or telomerase may disrupt the cell cycle sufficiently to cause cancer.

18.2 Characteristics of Cancer Cells

4. A tumor cell divides more frequently or more times than cells surrounding it, has altered surface properties, loses the specializations of the cell type it arose from, and produces daughter cells like itself.

5. A malignant tumor infiltrates nearby tissues and can **metastasize** by attaching to basement membranes and secreting enzymes that penetrate tissues and open a route to the bloodstream. From there, a cancer cell can travel, establishing secondary tumors.

18.3 Genes That Cause Cancer

6. Cancer is often the result of a series of genetic changes involving the activation of **proto-oncogenes** to **oncogenes,** and the inactivation of **tumor suppressor** genes.

Mutations in DNA repair genes can cause cancer by increasing the mutation rate.

7. Proto-oncogenes normally promote controlled cell growth, but are overexpressed because of a point mutation, placement next to a highly expressed gene, or transcription and translation with another gene, producing a **fusion protein.** Oncogenes may also be overexpressed growth factor receptors.

8. A tumor suppressor is a gene that normally enables a cell to respond to factors that limit its division. Tumor suppressor genes include *RB, p53,* and *BRCA1.*

18.4 A Series of Genetic Changes Causes Some Cancers

9. Many cancers result from "two hits" or mutations, but some entail a longer series of genetic changes.

10. To decipher the gene action sequences that result in cancer, researchers examine the mutations in cells from patients at various stages of the same type of cancer. Those mutations present at all stages of the cancer are the first to occur.

11. Astrocytoma and FAP are two cancers that require several mutations to develop.

18.5 Cancer Prevention, Diagnosis, and Treatment

12. **Population, case-control,** and **prospective studies** can reveal correlations between environmental exposures and the development of certain cancers, but usually cannot establish cause and effect. Biochemical and/or genetic evidence is important to explain epidemiological observations.

13. Traditional cancer treatments consist of surgery, radiation, and chemotherapy. Newer approaches based on molecular biology include blocking hormone receptors, stimulating cell specialization, blocking telomerase, and inhibiting angiogenesis. A genomic approach identifies the differences in gene expression that define cancer subtypes and may correlate to the success of certain treatments.

Review Questions

1. How would mutations in genes that encode the following proteins lead to cancer?

   a. a transcription factor

   b. the p53 protein

   c. the retinoblastoma protein

   d. the *myl* oncogene's protein

   e. a repair enzyme

   f. the APC protein

   g. CHEK2 protein

2. How can the same cancer be associated with deletions as well as translocations of genetic material?

3. What would be the value of knowing whether a person's cancer is sporadic or inherited?

4. List four characteristics of cancer cells.

5. Cite three reasons why cancer may not follow a Mendelian pattern, but nevertheless involves abnormal gene function.

6. What is inaccurate about the statement that "cancer cells are the fastest dividing cells in the body?"

7. Distinguish among the following types of studies:

   a. population

   b. case-control

   c. prospective

8. Three percent of all cancer cells have chromosome rearrangements. What other type of genetic change might be present in a cancer cell?

9. List four new strategies for treating cancer, and explain how they work.

Applied Questions

1. An individual can develop breast cancer by inheriting a germline mutation, then undergoing a second mutation in a breast cell; or by undergoing two mutations in a breast cell, one in each copy of a tumor suppressor gene. Cite another type of cancer, discussed in the chapter, that can arise in these two ways.

2. For women under 55 with moderate-sized breast tumors that have not spread to the lymph nodes, treatment is surgery, then radiation and chemotherapy—but 60 percent of these women are cured with the surgery alone, and would not benefit further from the exhausting and painful follow-up treatment. Suggest how this treatment might be more targeted to individual women.

3. Humans missing both *p53* alleles in all cells are unknown. People with p53-related cancers either have a germline mutation and a somatic mutation in affected tissue, or two somatic mutations in the tissue. Experiments show that mice missing both

copies of their *p53* genes die as embryos, with massive brain abnormalities.

   a. Why don't we see people with two missing or mutant *p53* alleles in all cells?

   b. Under what circumstances might a human with two mutant *p53* alleles be conceived?

4. Von Hippel-Lindau disease is an inherited cancer syndrome. The responsible gene lifts control over the transcription of certain genes, which, when overexpressed, cause tumors to form in the kidneys, adrenal glands, and blood vessels. Would the von Hippel-Lindau gene be an oncogene or a tumor suppressor? Cite a reason for your answer.

5. A tumor is removed from a mouse and broken up into cells. Each cell is injected into a different mouse. Although all the mice used in the experiment are genetically identical and raised in the same environment, the animals develop cancers with different rates of metastasis. Some

mice die quickly, some linger, and others recover. What do these results indicate about the characteristics of the original tumor cells?

6. Colon, breast, and stomach cancers can be prevented by removing the affected organ. Why is this approach not possible for chronic myeloid leukemia?

7. A vegetarian develops pancreatic cancer and wants to sue the nutritionist who suggested she follow a vegetarian diet. Is her complaint justified? Why or why not?

8. Iron foundry workers in Finland and coke oven workers in Poland have high exposures to polycyclic aromatic hydrocarbons, and they tend to develop cancers caused by mutations in the *p53* gene. What information would help determine whether the chemical exposure causes the mutation and whether the mutation causes the cancers?

9. Elsie finds a small lump in her breast and goes to her physician, who takes a medical

and family history. She mentions that her father died of brain cancer, a cousin had leukemia, and her older sister was just diagnosed with a tumor of connective tissue. The doctor assures her that the family cancer history doesn't raise the risk that her breast lump is cancerous, because the other cancers were not in the breast. Is the doctor correct?

10. A project at the Sanger Centre in the United Kingdom is screening 1,500 types of cancer cells growing in culture to detect homozygous deletions. Will this approach identify oncogenes or tumor suppressor genes? Cite a reason for your answer.

11. How can a woman with breast cancer have an abnormally functioning BRCA1 or BRCA2 protein, yet not have a mutation in either of the genes?

12. A mutation in a gene called *FLT3*, which encodes a tyrosine kinase receptor, causes acute myelogenous leukemia, which has a dismal five-year survival rate of 20 percent. A new drug blocks the receptor on white blood cells. Explain how it works.

Web Activities

13. Go to http://www.cancerquest.org/ index.cfm?page=181 (for oncogenes) and the same website with 52 instead of 181 for tumor suppressors. Click on one oncogene and one tumor suppressor, and describe how, when mutant, they cause cancer.

Case Studies

14. Marcy goes to see a genetic counselor, terribly distressed. Her sister developed breast cancer at age 52, and her husband's sister at age 34. Marcy's mother was diagnosed with breast cancer at age 68. With these three cases in her family, she is convinced she has a mutant *BRCA1* gene and will suffer the same fate.

   a. What questions should the genetic counselor ask Marcy?

   b. Do you think she would benefit from a *BRCA1* gene test?

   c. What complications might arise from such testing?

Learn to apply the skills of genetic counselor with these additional cases found in the *Case Workbook in Human Genetics:*

   Li-Fraumeni family cancer syndrome

   Multiple endocrine neoplasia

   Thyroid cancer

Suggested Readings

Gibbs, W. Wayt. July 2003. Untangling the roots of cancer. *Scientific American,* 289(1):56–65. In cancer, the genome is shattered.

Levy-Lahad, Ephrat, and Sharon E. Plon. October 24, 2003. A risky business—assessing breast cancer risk. *Science* 302:574–75. It is difficult to estimate *BRCA1* and *BRCA2* penetrance when the environment intervenes.

Lewis, Ricki. February 10, 2003. Breast cancer: The big picture emerges. *The Scientist* 17(3):24–25. Many genes lead to breast cancer.

Lewis, Ricki. April 30, 2001. Herceptin earns recognition in breast cancer arsenal. *The Scientist* 15(9):10. A monoclonal antibody blocks extra growth factor receptors on the cells of some people with breast cancer, halting it.

McMurray, Cynthia T., and John A Tainer. July 2003. Cancer, cadmium, and genome integrity. *Nature* 411:366. The metal cadmium, found in paint, batteries, and metal coatings, disrupts mismatch DNA repair, causing cancer.

Page, Janice. August 7, 2001. Sometimes, it's the good news that makes the patient feel so bad. *The New York Times,* p. D7. A gene test that reveals absence of the *BRCA1* mutation causes another condition—survivor guilt.

Perou, Charles M., et al. August 17, 2000. Molecular portraits of human breast tumors. *Nature* 406:747–52. DNA microarrays reveal at a glance how tumor cells veer from normalcy.

Savage, David G., et al. February 28, 2002. Imatinib mesylate—A new oral targeted therapy. *The New England Journal of Medicine* 346(9):683–93. Gleevec is a wonder drug, but tumors can become resistant to it.

Sorlie, Therese, et al. September 11, 2001. Gene expression patterns of breast carcinomas distinguish tumor subclasses with clinical implications. *Proceedings of the National Academy of Sciences* 98(19):10869–74. Neural network algorithms are used to match patterns of gene expression to cancer subtypes.

Thilly, William G. July 2003. Have environmental mutagens caused oncomutations in people? *Nature Genetics* 34(3):255–59. Cancer is a genetic disease, but with varied environmental triggers.

"New Frontiers in Cancer," a supplement to *The Scientist* (September 22, 2003), has several articles by the author.

Weekly updates of current news related to human genetics are available through Power Web on your Online Learning Center.

Genetically Modified Organisms

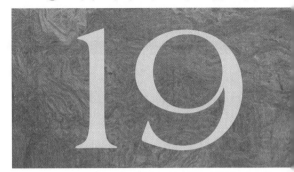

19

CHAPTER CONTENTS

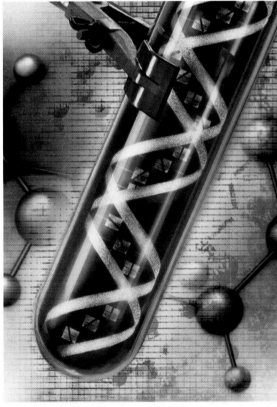

Biotechnology is possible because all organisms use DNA as the genetic material, and utilize the same genetic code.

Pig manure presents a serious environmental problem. The animals do not have an enzyme that would enable them to extract the mineral nutrient phosphorus from a compound called phytate in grain, so they are given dietary phosphorus supplements. As a result, their manure is full of phosphorus. The element washes into natural waters, contributing to fish kills, oxygen depletion in aquatic ecosystems, algal blooms, and even the greenhouse effect (**figure 19.1**). But biotechnology may have solved the "pig poop" problem.

19.1 Of Pigs and Patents

In the past, pig raisers have tried various approaches to keep their animals healthy and the environment cleaner. Efforts include feeding animal by-products from which the pigs can extract more phosphorus, and giving supplements of the enzyme phytase, which liberates phosphorus from phytate. But consuming animal by-products can introduce prion diseases, and giving phytase before each meal is costly. A "phytase transgenic pig," however, is genetically modified to secrete bacterial phytase in its saliva,

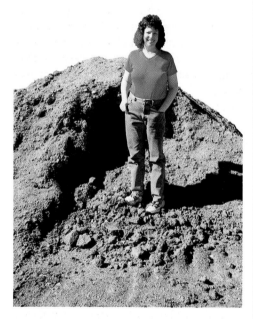

Figure 19.1 Genetically modified pig manure. Transgenic pigs given a bacterial digestive enzyme excrete less-polluting manure. The author poses amidst a pile of the nonmodified material, at the University of Georgia.

which enables it to excrete low-phosphorus manure.

A **transgenic** organism has a genetic change in each of its cells, often the addition of a gene from a different species. The transgenic pig has a phytase gene from the bacterium *E. coli*. Its manure has 75 percent less phosphorus than normal pig excrement. Says one researcher, "These pigs offer a unique biological approach to the management of phosphorus nutrition and environmental pollution in the pork industry."

The genetically modified pig, its genome manipulated so that its excrement is less polluting, is a product of **biotechnology,** which is the use or alteration of cells or biological molecules for specific applications. Biotechnology is, in a broad sense, hardly new. The ancient art of fermenting fruit with yeast to produce wine is a biotechnology, as is using yeast to make bread dough rise. Extracting biochemicals directly from organisms for various applications is also biotechnology.

The popular terms "genetic engineering" and "genetic modification" refer broadly to any biotechnology that manipulates genetic material. This includes altering the DNA of an organism to suppress or enhance the activities of its own genes as well as combining the genetic material of different species. The latter is possible because all life uses the same genetic code.

It is this mixing of DNA from different species that some people object to as unnatural. In fact, DNA does move and mix in nature—bacteria do it with abandon, and it is why we have viral DNA sequences nestled in our chromosomes. But genetic modification usually endows organisms with traits that they would probably not acquire naturally, such as pigs with low-phosphorus manure, tomatoes that grow in salt water, and bacteria that synthesize human insulin, discussed later in this chapter. **Figure 19.2** shows a dramatic example of a genetically modified organism—mice with a gene from a jellyfish that enables them to express green fluorescent protein.

Recombinant DNA technology, the first of the modern biotechnologies, adds genes from one type of organism to another. It was first done on bacteria. When bacteria bearing recombinant DNA divide, they yield many copies, or clones, of the foreign DNA and produce many copies of the protein the foreign DNA specifies.

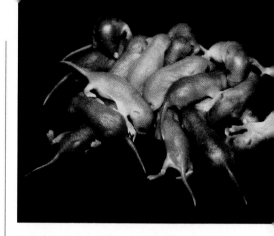

Figure 19.2 The universality of the genetic code makes biotechnology possible. Recombinant DNA technology is based on the fact that all organisms utilize the same DNA codons to specify the same amino acids. A striking illustration of the universality of the code appears in these transgenic mice that contain the gene encoding a jellyfish's green fluorescent protein (GFP). Researchers use GFP to mark genes of interest to follow their expression. The GFP mice glow less greenly as they mature and more hair covers the skin. The non-green mice are not genetically modified.

In the 1980s, researchers began to apply recombinant DNA technology to multicellular organisms. Researchers typically add foreign DNA at the one-cell stage: a gamete or fertilized ovum in animals, or to some cells of an early embryo, or to somatic (vegetative) cells in a plant. The transgenic organism that develops from the original altered cell carries the genetic change in every cell. Transgenic organisms have foreign DNA added to their genomes, and so the phenotype might be influenced by the organism's own version of the transgene. More precise is **gene targeting,** in which an introduced gene trades places with an existing gene, either removing and "knocking out" the gene's function, or replacing it, "knocking in" function.

The ability to combine genes from different types of organisms has raised legal questions—is a transgenic organism an invention, deserving of patent protection? By definition, to earn a patent an invention must be new, useful, and not obvious (see Technology Timeline).

Patent law has had to evolve in parallel to the unexpectedly accelerated pace of modern biotechnology. Early on, DNA sequences could be patented. In the mid-1990s, however, when the U.S. National Institutes of Health and biotech companies began seeking

Patenting Life and Genes

1790	U.S. patent act is enacted. An invention must be new, useful, and not obvious to earn a patent.
1873	Louis Pasteur is awarded first patent on a life form, for yeast used in industrial processes.
1930	New plant variants can be patented.
1980	First patent is awarded on a genetically modified organism, a bacterium given four plasmids (DNA rings) that enable it to metabolize components of crude oil. The plasmids are naturally occurring, but do not all occur naturally in a single type of bacterium.
1988	First patent is awarded for a transgenic organism, a mouse that manufactures human protein in its milk. Harvard University granted patent for "OncoMouse" transgenic for human cancer.
1992	Biotechnology company is awarded a broad patent covering all forms of transgenic cotton. Groups concerned that this will limit the rights of subsistence farmers contest the patent several times.
1996–1999	Companies patent partial gene sequences and certain disease-causing genes as the basis for developing specific medical tests.
2000	With gene and genome discoveries pouring into the Patent and Trademark Office, requirements tightened for showing utility of a DNA sequence.
2003	Attempts to enforce patents on nonprotein-encoding parts of the human genome anger researchers who support open access to the information.

Key Concepts

Biotechnology is the use or modification of cells or biological molecules for a specific application. Recombining DNA generates transgenic organisms. Gene targeting is a more precise modification that inactivates or replaces a gene. Patent law regarding DNA has evolved with the technology since the 1970s.

19.2 Recombinant DNA Technology

The origin of modern biotechnology dates to the 1970s, when researchers first began to ponder the potential uses and risks of mixing DNA from different species.

In February 1975, 140 molecular biologists convened at Asilomar, a seaside conference center on California's Monterey Peninsula, to discuss the safety and implications of a new type of experiment. Investigators had found a simple way to combine the genes of two species, and they were concerned about the safety of experiments requiring the use of a cancer-causing virus, and about where the field was headed. They discussed restricting the types of organisms used in recombinant DNA research and explored ways to prevent escape of a resulting organism from the laboratory. The guidelines drawn up at Asilomar outlined measures of "physical containment," such as using specialized hoods and airflow systems that would keep the organisms inside the laboratory, and "biological containment," ways to weaken organisms so that they could not survive outside the laboratory.

A decade after the Asilomar meeting, many members of the original group reconvened at the meeting site to assess progress in the field. Nearly all agreed on two points: Recombinant DNA technology was safer than expected, and the technology had spread to industry more swiftly and in more diverse ways than anyone had imagined. At a meeting twenty-five years after the event, attendees concluded that biotechnology had become so commercialized that the open atmosphere of the original gathering was no longer possible.

Recombinant DNA-based products have been slow to reach the marketplace because of the high cost of research and the long time it takes to develop any new drug. Today, several

patent protection for thousands of pieces of protein-encoding DNA sequences called expressed sequence tags (ESTs), the U.S. government's Patent and Trademark Office began to tighten the requirement for utility. Today, a DNA sequence alone is not patentable. It must be useful as a tool for research or as a novel and improved diagnostic test.

Despite the increasing stringency of patent requirements, problems still arise in patenting DNA sequences. A biotechnology company in the United States, for example, holds a patent on the *BRCA1* gene that includes any diagnostic tests based on the gene sequence. That company's tests, however, do not cover all mutations in the gene. A French physician working with a family that has a unique large deletion is challenging the patent, because to be tested, her patients must pay a high licensing fee to the U.S. company that "owns" the gene sequence. Bioethics: Choices for the Future on page 399 explores another case in which a gene patent adversely affected families with inherited disease.

Patenting genes may become even more complex as genome information floods the Patent and Trademark Office. One problem is redundancy. For the same gene, it is possible to patent:

- Genomic DNA (the protein-encoding sequence as well as noncoding regions)

- Expressed sequence tags

- cDNA (only the protein-encoding part of a gene)

- Mutations

- SNPs

A researcher or company wanting to develop a tool or test based on a protein thus might infringe upon five different patents, based on essentially the same information. Now, as genetics begins to shift from a single-gene focus to analyzing expression patterns of suites of interacting genes, and even entire genomes, the Patent and Trademark Office will have to cope with unprecedented change in the types of inventions submitted for protection from competition.

isolated from a genomic library. There are several ways to do this "needle in a haystack" type of search.

A synthetic piece of DNA that corresponds to the gene in question can be linked to a label, such as a radioactive or fluorescent molecule. This labeled gene fragment is called a **DNA probe.** It emits a signal when it binds to its complement in a cell that contains a recombinant plasmid. DNA probes can also be made using genes of similar sequence from other species. Using such a probe is a little like mistakenly using **hipropotamus** to search for **hippopotamus** on the Internet. You'd probably still come up with a hippo.

A genomic library contains too much information for a researcher seeking a particular protein-encoding gene—it may also contain introns, repeated sequences, the genes that encode rRNAs and tRNAs, and many repeated sequences. Another type of library, called a complementary DNA, or **cDNA library,** represents only protein-encoding genes. It is made from the mRNAs in a differentiated cell, which reflect the proteins manufactured there. For example, a muscle cell has abundant mRNA that encodes contractile proteins, whereas a fibroblast has many mRNAs that represent the connective tissue proteins collagen and elastin.

To make a cDNA library, researchers first extract the mRNAs from cells. Then, these RNAs are used to construct complementary or "c" DNA strands using reverse transcrip-tase, DNA nucleotide triphosphates, and DNA polymerase (**figure 19.6**). (Reverse transcriptase synthesizes DNA complementary to RNA.) DNA polymerase and the nucleotides then can synthesize the complementary strand to the single-stranded cDNA to form a double-stranded DNA. Different cell types yield different cDNA collections, or libraries, that reflect which genes are expressed. They do not, however, reveal protein abundance, because in a cell mRNA molecules are transcribed and degraded at different rates.

A specific cDNA can be taken from a cDNA library and used to isolate the original gene of interest from the genomic library. If the goal is to harness the gene and eventually collect its protein product, then the genomic version, and not the cDNA version, is required, because it includes control regions such as promoters. Once a gene of interest is transferred to a cell where it can be transcribed into mRNA and that RNA translated, the protein is collected. Such cells are typically grown in devices called bioreactors, with nutrients sent in and wastes removed. A researcher collects the desired product from the medium the cells are growing in.

Selecting Recombinant DNA Molecules

Much of the effort in recombinant DNA technology entails identifying and separating cells that contain the gene of interest, once the foreign DNA is inserted into the vector. Three types of recipient cells can result:

1. Cells that lack plasmids
2. Cells that contain plasmids that do not contain a foreign gene
3. Cells that contain plasmids that have picked up a foreign gene (the goal)

The procedure is cleverly set up so that recombinant plasmids are easily distinguished from plasmids that do not take up foreign DNA. In one strategy, a section of the foreign gene in the plasmid is detected by a color test (**figure 19.7**). The plasmid includes a gene conferring resistance to an antibiotic drug, as well as a gene called *lacZ* that produces blue colonies in the presence of a compound called x-gal. When the foreign DNA inserts into the plasmid, it does so at a restriction site that disables the *lacZ* gene. When bacteria are grown in the presence of the antibiotic, only those

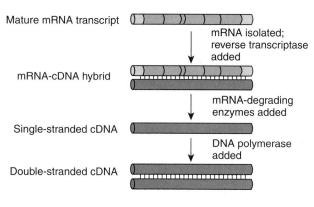

Figure 19.6 Copying DNA from RNA.
Researchers make cDNA from mRNA using reverse transcriptase, an enzyme from a retrovirus. A cDNA version of a gene includes the codons for a mature mRNA, but not sequences corresponding to promoters and introns. Labeled cDNAs are used as probes to locate genes in genomic libraries.

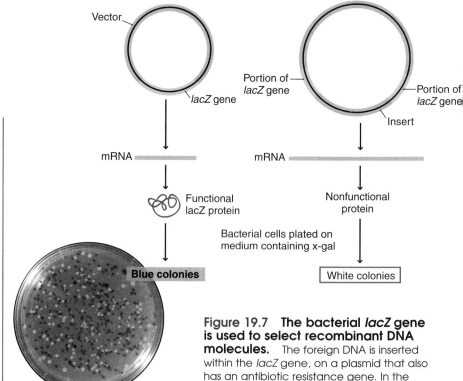

Figure 19.7 The bacterial *lacZ* gene is used to select recombinant DNA molecules. The foreign DNA is inserted within the *lacZ* gene, on a plasmid that also has an antibiotic resistance gene. In the presence of the antibiotic, and if *lacZ*'s substrate x-gal is introduced, white colonies represent cells and their descendants that have the recombinant plasmid.

cells that have incorporated plasmids can grow, because the plasmids include the antibiotic resistance gene. Secondly, bacterial cells containing plasmids that have taken up the foreign DNA do *not* turn the cell blue when x-gal is put into the medium. In contrast, cells with empty plasmids—and, therefore, a functional *lacZ* gene—turn blue.

When cells containing the recombinant plasmid divide, so does the plasmid. Within hours, the original cell gives rise to many harboring the recombinant plasmid. The enzymes, ribosomes, energy molecules, and factors necessary for protein synthesis transcribe and translate the plasmid DNA and its stowaway foreign gene, producing the desired protein.

Delivering DNA in Plants and Animals

When recombinant DNA technology is applied to multicellular organisms, they must be allowed to develop and bred to create homozygotes for recessive traits. The altered characteristic is apparent in the phenotype as a visible trait or an unusual secretion component. A transgenic plant can be derived from somatic cells. Different vectors and gene transfer techniques are sometimes used in plants because their cell walls, not present in animal cells, are difficult to penetrate. Some manipulations are done on plant cells that have had their cell walls removed. These denuded plant cells are called protoplasts.

Frequently used plant vectors include the **Ti plasmid** (for "tumor-inducing"), which occurs naturally in the bacterium *Agrobacterium tumefaciens,* and viruses found in plant cells (**figure 19.8**). A *Ti* plasmid normally causes a tumorlike growth to form, so researchers remove the genes controlling this process. For example, a gene from the bacterium *Bacillus thuringiensis* (*bt*) specifies a protein that destroys the stomach linings of certain insect larvae. The *bt* gene is introduced into corn cells via a *Ti* plasmid, and the cells are regenerated into plants that produce their own insecticide. More than two-thirds of the corn plants grown in the United States are transgenic for the *bt* insecticide gene, and organic farmers have been using its protein product for years.

Transgenic technology permits the rapid introduction of new traits. For example, a gene that confers an agriculturally useful

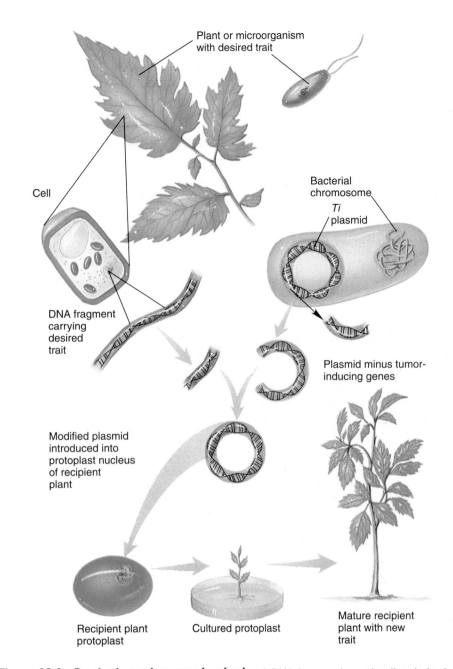

Figure 19.8 Producing a transgenic plant. A DNA fragment carrying the desired gene—conferring resistance to an herbicide, for example—is isolated from its natural source and spliced into a *Ti* plasmid with the tumor-inducing genes removed. The plasmid incorporating the foreign DNA is then allowed to invade a cell of the recipient plant, where it enters the nucleus and integrates into the plant's DNA. Finally, by means of cell culture, the cell is regenerated into a mature, transgenic plant that expresses the desired trait and passes it on to its progeny. A breeding step may be necessary to obtain plants homozygous for a recessive trait.

characteristic—such as the ability to withstand a particular pesticide—is isolated from one species and inserted into a vector; then the recombinant vector is placed into protoplasts. A whole plant regenerated from the genetically altered cell has the gene for the transferred trait in all of its cells. It is typically tested in the laboratory to see if the gene is expressed. Then the transgenic plant is grown in a greenhouse, and finally in experimental fields to see if the desired trait is present, and to assess effects of the transgenic plant on the ecosystem and beyond.

Researchers use several methods to insert DNA into animal cells (**table 19.2** and **figure 19.9**). Chemicals such as polyethylene glycol and calcium phosphate are used to open transient holes in plasma membranes, admitting DNA. **Liposomes** are fatty bubbles that can carry DNA into cells as plasma membranes envelop them. In **electroporation,** a brief jolt of electricity opens transient holes in plasma membranes that may permit foreign DNA to enter. DNA is also injected into cells using microscopic needles (see figure 19.9b). This is called **microinjection.**

Another way to introduce DNA into cells is **particle bombardment.** A gunlike device shoots tiny metal particles, usually gold or tungsten, coated with foreign DNA. When aimed at target cells, usually in plants, some of the projectiles enter. For example, gene guns shoot dividing cells in soybean seeds with an *E. coli* gene that stains cells expressing it a vibrant blue, allowing detection of the gene transfer.

Once foreign DNA is introduced into a target cell, it must enter the nucleus, replicate along with the cell's own DNA, and be transmitted when the cell divides. Finally, an organism must be regenerated from the altered cell. If the trait is dominant, the transgenic organism must express it in the appropriate tissues at the right time in development. If the trait is recessive, crosses between heterozygotes may be necessary to yield homozygotes that express the trait. Then the organisms must pass the characteristic on to the next generation.

Figure 19.10 illustrates transgenic silkworms that have been turned into a factory for a human protein, collagen. The silkworm *Bombyx mori* has been cultivated and its silk coveted for nearly five thousand years. About

Table 19.2
Gene Transfer Techniques

Approach	How It Works
Ti plasmid	Tumor-inducing genes are removed, gene of interest inserted, and modified plasmid sent into plant protoplasts.
Virus	A human gene is inserted into a virus, which infects a human cell, where it is expressed.
Retrovirus	An RNA virus carrying an RNA version of a human gene infects a somatic cell. The gene is reverse transcribed to DNA and inserts into a human chromosome. Here, it may produce a missing or abnormal protein.
Liposome transfer	A fatty bubble called a liposome carries a gene into a somatic cell. Here, the delivered gene may replace an abnormal one.
Chemical	Calcium phosphate or dextran sulfate opens transient holes in a plasma membrane, admitting replacement DNA.
Electroporation	An electrical current opens transient holes in a plasma membrane, admitting replacement DNA.
Microinjection	A tiny needle injects DNA into a cell lacking that DNA sequence.
Particle bombardment	Metal pellets coated with DNA are shot with explosive force or air pressure into recipient cells.

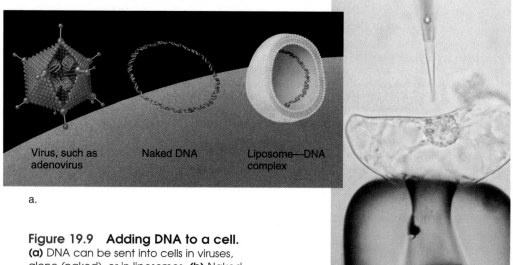

Figure 19.9 Adding DNA to a cell.
(a) DNA can be sent into cells in viruses, alone (naked), or in liposomes. **(b)** Naked DNA is injected into this plant cell.

Virus, such as adenovirus   Naked DNA   Liposome—DNA complex

a.

b.

Human procollagen gene
GFP gene
Silk protein promoter

Embryo

Larva with red fluorescent eye

Green fluorescent cocoon

Figure 19.10   Silk with human collagen, courtesy of transgenic silkworms. Early embryos receive injections of a human procollagen gene linked to a silk protein promoter, as well as to the green fluorescent protein (GFP) gene. The transgenic silkworms also have a red fluorescent protein gene linked to a promoter that causes it to be expressed in larval eyes. The affected larvae with red eyes indicate individuals that are homozygous for the transgenes, enabling their separation before they actually make their cocoons.

half of a larva's body is devoted to silk production. Two silk glands secrete threads consisting of linked proteins called fibroins. The insect pulls the strands out of its hindquarters in an elaborate figure-eight pattern, and once these strands hit the air, they harden into silk. Each cell in the silk glands has 400,000 copies of the genome, enabling the silkworm to build its cocoon rapidly.

To take advantage of the silkworm's mass-production capabilities, researchers placed recombinant DNA into a BAC vector, which they introduced in a transposon (a "jumping gene") naturally found in many insect cells. Then they injected the loaded vector into early embryo cells. The recombinant DNA included a promoter from a fibroin gene, so that when a larva got the hormonal urge to make silk, it would make silk and also human collagen. To mark the proteins, the investigators used GFP—from the same jellyfish gene that lights up the mice in figure 19.2. As an added guide, the recombinant DNA also included a gene for red fluorescent protein, but with a promoter that causes it to be expressed in the eye. The researchers simply selected red-eyed larvae for collagen-silk harvesting, then separated the collagen from the silk of the cocoons. Because the silk industry has been in place for centuries, the larvae may be a valuable resource for producing human proteins for varied uses. Collagen is used in cosmetics and in tissue engineering.

Key Concepts

In recombinant DNA technology, a cell receives a cloning vector that contains foreign DNA encoding a protein of interest. The universality of the genetic code and restriction enzymes, which cut DNA at specific sequences and create sticky ends, make recombinant DNA technology possible. • Genes are isolated from genomic DNA libraries or cDNA libraries. • Antibiotic sensitivity and resistance genes and gene variants that cause color changes to growth media are used to select single cells bearing plasmids containing recombinant DNA. • Recombinant DNA is introduced naked, in liposomes, or by electroporation, microinjection, or particle bombardment. The cell must transcribe and translate the foreign gene, and if the organism is multicellular, it must develop and be bred if the trait of interest is recessive. Homozygotes are necessary to express recessive alleles.

19.3 Applications of Recombinant DNA Technology

In basic research, recombinant DNA technology provides a way to isolate individual genes from complex organisms and observe their functions on the molecular level. Recombinant DNA has many practical uses, too.

Drugs

The first application of recombinant DNA technology was to mass produce protein-based drugs. The first such drug was human insulin.

Before 1982, people with type I diabetes mellitus got the insulin that they had to inject daily from pancreases removed from cattle in slaughterhouses. Cattle insulin is so similar to the human peptide, different in only 2 of its 51 amino acids, that most people with diabetes can use it. However, about 1 in 20 patients is allergic to cow insulin because of the slight chemical difference. Until recombinant DNA technology was possible, the allergic patients had to use expensive combinations of insulin from a variety of other animals or from human cadavers. A person with diabetes can now purchase "Humulin," the human protein made in *E. coli*, at a local drugstore. **Table 19.3** lists some drugs produced using recombinant DNA technology.

Table 19.3

Drugs Produced Using Recombinant DNA Technology

Drug	Use
Atrial natriuretic peptide	Dilates blood vessels, promotes urination
Colony stimulating factors	Help restore bone marrow after marrow transplant; restore blood cells following cancer chemotherapy
Deoxyribonuclease (DNase)	Thins pus in lungs of people with cystic fibrosis
Epidermal growth factor	Accelerates healing of wounds and burns; treats gastric ulcers
Erythropoietin (EPO)	Stimulates production of red blood cells in cancer patients
Factor VIII	Promotes blood clotting in treatment of hemophilia
Fertility hormones (follicle stimulating hormone, luteinizing hormone, human chorionic gonadotropin)	Treat infertility
Glucocerebrosidase	Treats Gaucher disease
Human growth hormone	Promotes growth of muscle and bone in people with very short stature due to hormone deficiency
Insulin	Allows cells to take up glucose in treatment of type I diabetes mellitus
Interferons	
Alpha	Treats genital warts, hairy cell leukemia, hepatitis C and B, Kaposi sarcoma
Beta	Treats multiple sclerosis
Gamma	Treats chronic granulomatous disease (a blood disorder)
Interleukin-2	Treats kidney cancer
Lung surfactant protein	Helps lung alveoli to inflate in infants with respiratory distress syndrome
Renin inhibitor	Lowers blood pressure
Somatostatin	Decreases growth in muscle and bone in pituitary giants
Superoxide dismutase	Prevents further damage to heart muscle after heart attack
Tissue plasminogen activator	Dissolves blood clots in treatment of heart attacks, stroke, and pulmonary embolism

Drugs developed using recombinant DNA technology must compete in the marketplace with conventional products. Deciding whether a drug produced this way is preferable to an existing, similar drug is often a matter of economics, marketing, and plain common sense. For example, interferon beta-1b helps some people with a certain type of multiple sclerosis, but it costs more than $20,000 per year per patient. British researchers calculated what it would cost to treat the nation's patients who would benefit from the drug, and then determined how else the funds could be spent. They concluded that more people would be served if the money were spent on improved supportive care for many rather than on a costly new treatment for a few.

A classic case of determining the value of a recombinant DNA-derived drug concerns tissue plasminogen activator (tPA), a clot-busting drug developed in the mid-1980s. If injected within four hours of a heart attack, tPA dramatically limits damage to the heart muscle by restoring blood flow, at a price of $2,200 a shot. However, an older drug, streptokinase, extracted from bacteria by conventional methods, is nearly as effective at $300 per injection. The recombinant drug is very valuable for patients who have already had streptokinase and could have an allergic reaction if they were to use it again. Bioethics: Choices for the Future considers another drug derived from recombinant DNA technology, erythropoietin (EPO).

Drugs may also be synthesized in transgenic plants. Seeds can serve as drug factories by harboring genes that encode proteins with therapeutic value, such as clotting factors. Seeds are abundant, easy to store, resistant to environmental extremes, and are alive. Soybeans are especially efficient miniprotein factories, because they are 40 to 45 percent protein. A plant's roots can also be tapped to produce proteins of interest, in a process called rhizosecretion (**figure 19.11**).

Textiles

In the textile industry, recombinant DNA technology has created a new source of indigo, the dye used to make blue jeans blue (**figure 19.12**). The dye originally came from mollusks and fermented leaves of the European woad plant or Asian indigo plant.

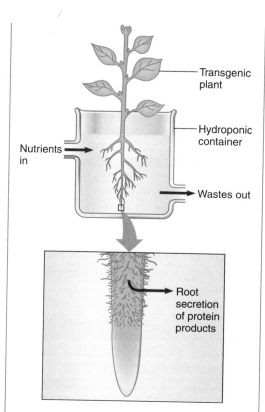

Figure 19.11   Rhizosecretion.
Transgenic plant technology has been problematic because of the difficulty of extracting protein products from plant cells. Rhizosecretion—enlisting roots to secrete—may solve the problem. A transgenic plant that expresses the gene for a desired protein in its roots can secrete the products directly into the surrounding medium.

The 1883 discovery of indigo's chemical structure led to the invention of a synthetic process to produce the dye using coal-tar. That method has dominated the industry, but it releases toxic by-products. In 1983, microbiologists discovered that E. coli, with a little help, can produce indigo. The bacterium converts glucose to the amino acid tryptophan, which then forms indole, a precursor to indigo. By learning the steps and offshoots of this biochemical pathway, researchers at a biotechnology company were able to alter bacteria to suppress the alternative pathways for metabolizing glucose, allowing the cells to synthesize much more tryptophan than they normally would. When the E. coli cells incorporate genes from another bacterial species, they extend the biochemical pathway all the way to produce indigo. The result: common bacteria that manufacture the blue dye of denim jeans from glucose, a simple sugar.

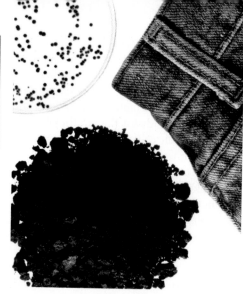

Figure 19.12   Genes for jeans. E. coli are genetically modified to produce indigo, the dye used in denim.

Cotton plants transgenic for bt toxins resist bollworm and budworm infections. The plants require little or no chemical insecticide, and yields are usually higher than with traditional crops.

Cotton can be improved in other ways. For example, two genes from a bacterium, Alcaligenes eutrophus, interact with a cotton gene to produce poly-hydroxybutyrate (PHB), a biodegradable plastic. A gene gun sends bacterial genes into cotton plant embryos. Plastic granules form within the cellulose strands of the fibers, so they are not noticeable in cotton fabric. This naturally plasticized cotton retains heat longer than unaltered cotton fibers and may be very useful in making outdoor clothing.

Paper and Wood Products

In the wood, pulp, and paper industries, the generation time of a tree can far exceed the lifespan of the researcher. For this reason, and because regenerating trees from altered cells is difficult, the development of transgenic trees has lagged behind other applications of recombinant DNA technology. However, several poplar species are emerging as valuable model systems for experimenting with transgenic trees. Researchers can evaluate new phenotypes on trees too young to reproduce, or incorporate sterility genes into experimental trees to control or contain the transmission of novel traits.

The Ethics of Using a Recombinant Drug: EPO

EPO is a hormone produced in the kidneys that consists of a 165-amino-acid protein portion plus four carbohydrate chains. When the oxygen level in the blood dips too low, cells in the kidneys produce EPO, which travels to the bone marrow and binds to receptors on cells that give rise to red blood cell progenitors. Soon, more red blood cells enter the circulation, carrying more oxygen to the tissues (**figure 1**).

The value of EPO as a drug became evident after the invention of hemodialysis to treat kidney failure in 1961. This otherwise highly successful treatment also causes severe anemia, because dialysis removes EPO from the blood. To counteract dialysis-induced anemia, it was necessary to boost patients' EPO levels. In 1970, the U.S. government sought ways to produce large amounts of the pure substance. But how?

Levels of EPO in human plasma are too low to make pooling from donors feasible. A more likely potential source was people suffering from disorders, such as aplastic anemia and hookworm infection, that cause them to secrete large amounts of EPO. The National Institute of Health set up a program to extract EPO from the urine of South American farmers with hookworm infections. Government planes transported the EPO in diplomatic pouches! Then, in 1976, the National Heart, Lung and Blood Institute began a grant program in search of ways to purify EPO. In 1977, supplies came in the form of 2,550 liters of urine from Japanese aplastic anemia patients.

Problems loomed for those trying to purify EPO from these sources. Was it ethical to obtain a scarce substance from the urine of sick, usually poor, people from one country to treat comparatively wealthy people from the United States? Then AIDS arose. Extracting any biochemical from human body fluids was no longer safe.

Recombinant DNA technology solved the EPO problem. The hormone is produced in hamster kidney cells, which can attach EPO's four carbohydrate groups. Today, EPO is sold under various names, including Epogen, Repotin, and Procrit. The Food and Drug Administration approved it to treat anemia in 1989 for dialysis patients, and in 1991 for AIDS patients. Today it is also widely used by people receiving chemotherapy, enabling them to avoid the need for transfusions.

Recombinant EPO found an unexpected market among Jehovah's Witnesses, whose religion forbids transfused blood, which they believe destroys the soul. They can, however, use EPO, because it has been declared a product of recent technology, rather than blood. Some Jehovah's Witnesses have used it before surgery to boost red blood cell supplies, or afterward to compensate for blood loss.

EPO's ability to increase the oxygen-carrying capacity of blood, and thereby to increase physical endurance, has attracted the attention of competitive athletes. Training at high altitudes increases endurance, and the reason is EPO. The scarcer oxygen in the air at high altitudes stimulates the kidneys to produce EPO, which in turn stimulates production of more red blood cells. Athletes have attempted to reproduce this effect by abusing EPO. A few Dutch bicyclists developed dangerous blood clots in their legs from taking

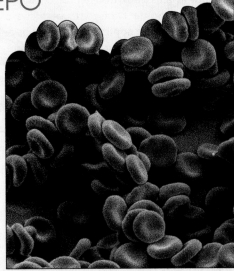

Figure 1 These red blood cells are mass-produced in a patient treated with erythropoietin (EPO).

overly high, and medically unnecessary, doses. It is now routine to screen Olympic athletes for EPO abuse.

One large Scandinavian family, however, gets its extra EPO quite naturally. They have an inherited condition, benign erythrocytosis, in which they overproduce the hormone. One of them won a gold medal for skiing in the Olympics. However, athletes who abuse EPO raise the issue of how to control the use of an otherwise valuable drug derived from biotechnology.

EPO is not the only abused biotech-derived drug. Body builders abuse a recombinant version of the hormone somatotropin, used to treat AIDS wasting syndrome, and the Internet is full of ads for recombinant human growth hormone.

Transgenic technology can protect trees from pests. For example, *B. thuringiensis* toxin renders larch, white spruce, pioneer elm, and American sweetgum trees resistant to attack by gypsy moth and forest tent caterpillars. Poplar trees transgenic for a gene from rice resist attack by the beetle *Chrysomella tremulae*, a major pest. The rice gene enables the trees to manufacture a polypeptide that blocks production of the insects' digestive enzymes.

Food

Products of recombinant DNA technology are also used in the food industry. The enzyme rennin, for example, normally produced in calves' stomachs, is used in cheese making. The gene that encodes the enzyme is inserted into plasmids and transferred to bacteria, which are mass cultured to produce large quantities of pure rennin.

Thanks to *Ti* plasmids and viral vectors, novel or easier-to-grow fruits and vegetables are available in countries that do not restrict the marketing of genetically modified foods. For example, *Ti* plasmids introduced a bacterial gene rendering sugar beets herbicide-resistant. This is an important trait because 37 percent of the world's sugar comes from this difficult-to-grow crop. Using a viral vector, another sweet crop, sugarcane, is given a gene encoding a corn protein that dismantles a bacterial toxin. The genetically modified sugarcane resists the corn pathogen, as well as a fungus known to decimate sugarcane crops. Some transgenic plants are strange. Macintosh apples given an antibacterial protein from a moth, for example, are resistant to a bacterial infection called fire blight.

Table 19.4 lists some useful transgenic plants, and table 19.5 describes some agricultural challenges that transgenic crops can address.

Bioremediation

In **bioremediation,** bacteria or plants with the ability to detoxify certain pollutants are released or grown in a particular area to cleanse the environment. Natural selection has sculpted such organisms, perhaps as adaptations that render them unpalatable to predators. Bioremediation uses genes that give an organism an appetite for some substance that, to another species, is a toxin. The technology uses unaltered organisms, and also transfers "detox" genes to other species so that the protein products can more easily penetrate a polluted area.

Nature offers many organisms with (to us) strange tastes. One type of tree that grows in a tropical rainforest on an island near Australia, for example, accumulates so much nickel from soil that slashing its bark releases a bright green latex ooze. Up to 20 percent of the tree's dry weight may be nickel. This tree can be used to clean up nickel-contaminated soil. Similarly, a microbe called *Citrobacter* absorbs the nuclear wastes plutonium and uranium from soils.

Bioremediation is helpful in environmental disasters. Ten weeks after a tanker drenched Alaska's Prince William Sound in oil in 1989, clean-up crews spread nitrogen and phosphorus fertilizer along the oil-slicked shore. The fertilizer stimulated an increase in native populations of bacteria that consume organic toxins in the oil. The pollutants disappeared, and the beaches whitened five times faster in treated areas.

Bioremediation that involves transgenesis usually taps the metabolisms of microbes, sending them into plants whose roots then

Table 19.4

Genetically Modified Crops

Altered Plant	Effect
Rice with beta carotene and extra iron	Added nutritional value
Canola with high-laurate oil	Can be grown domestically; less costly than importing palm and coconut oils
Delayed ripening tomato	Extended shelf life
Herbicide-resistant cotton	Herbicide kills weeds without harming crop
Minipeppers	Improved flavor, fewer seeds
Bananas resistant to fungal infection	Extended shelf life
Delayed-ripening bananas and pineapples	Extended shelf life
Elongated sweet pepper	Improved flavor, easier to slice
Altered cotton fiber	Easier fabric manufacturing
Altered paper pulp trees	Paper component (lignin) easier to process
High-starch potatoes	Absorb less oil when fried
Pest-resistant corn	Can resist European corn borer
Seedless minimelons	Single serving size
Sweet peas and peppers	Retain sweetness longer

Table 19.5

Transgenic Approaches to Agricultural Challenges

Challenge	Possible Solution
Frost damages crops	Spray crops with bacteria genetically altered to lack surface proteins that promote ice crystallization. Bacteria can also be manipulated to stimulate ice crystallization, then used to increase snow buildup in winter sports facilities.
Herbicides and pesticides damage crops	Isolate genes from an organism not affected by the chemical and insert it into the genome of a crop plant.
Crops need costly nitrogen fertilizer because atmospheric nitrogen is not biologically usable	Short-term: Genetically manipulate nitrogen-fixing *Rhizobium* bacteria to overproduce enzymes that convert atmospheric nitrogen to a biologically usable form in root nodules of legumes. Alter *Rhizobium* to colonize a wider variety of plants. Long-term: Transfer *Rhizobium* nitrogen-fixation genes into plant cells and regenerate transgenic plants.
A plant food is low in a particular amino acid	Transfer gene from another species that controls production of a protein rich in the amino acid the crop plant lacks.
A virus destroys a crop	Genetically alter crop plant to manufacture a protein on its cell surface normally found on the virus's surface. Plant becomes immune to virus.
Public concern about the safety of synthetic pesticides	Stimulate *Bacillus thuringiensis* to overproduce its natural pesticide, which destroys insects' stomach linings. Transfer *B. thuringiensis* bioinsecticide gene to crop plant.

distribute the detox proteins in the soil. For example, transgenic yellow poplar trees can thrive in mercury-tainted soil because they have a bacterial gene that encodes an enzyme, mercuric reductase, that converts a highly toxic form of mercury in soil to a less toxic gas. The tree's leaves then release the gas.

Bioremediation is used to clean up munitions dumps left over from wars past. One application uses bacteria that normally break down dinitrotoluene—better known as TNT, the major ingredient in dynamite and land mines. The enzyme that provides this capability is linked to the GFP gene (see figure 19.2) and when the bacteria are spread in a contaminated area, they glow where there are land mines, revealing the locations much more specifically than a metal detector could. Once the land mines are removed, the bacteria die because their food is gone. A related approach is to add the bacterial TNT-detecting gene and its GFP tag to various plants whose roots then glow to reveal the locations of buried explosives.

19.4 Gene Targeting

Transgenic technology is not very precise because it does not direct the introduced DNA to a particular chromosomal locus. The entry of the transgene can disrupt another gene's function, or the transgene can come under another gene's control sequence. Even if a transgene inserts into a chromosome and is expressed, the host's version of the same gene may overshadow the transgene's effect.

A more precise method of genetic modification, gene targeting, uses a natural process called **homologous recombination,** in which a DNA sequence displaces a similar or identical sequence in a host chromosome. The technique was developed in the late 1980s by introducing an inactivated gene into a mouse cell's nucleus, thereby "knocking out" function of the gene it replaced. By observing the effects of a gene's lack of function, researchers could deduce the gene's normal function as well as learn more about inherited disease. A variation on gene targeting swaps in genes that have an altered function, producing a "knock in."

Gene targeting in mammals entails genetic alteration plus complex developmental manipulations because it does not work on fertilized ova; instead, it is done in embryonic stem (ES) cells (see figure 2.24) later in development. Most gene targeting uses mice because their embryo cells are easiest to manipulate. The first attempts followed transmission of coat color genes, so that results would be easy to see. In one scheme, the knockout mice were white (**figure 19.13**). To begin, researchers used electroporation or microinjection to deliver an inactivated pigment gene into a pigmented mouse ES cell. Next, altered ES cells were injected into early embryos from colored mice. The embryos were implanted into surrogate mothers, where they continued development into individuals that had some cells bearing the targeted gene. The newborn mice were chimeras (mosaics), with patches of tissue whose cells contained the inactivated pigment gene. When the chimeric mice were mated to each other, some of the pups developed from a sperm and egg that each had the knocked-out gene. These rare homozygotes were easily distinguished because they were white, while their siblings were pigmented.

Gene-Targeted Mice as Models

Gene targeting is very useful in developing animal models of human genetic diseases. First, researchers identify the animal version of a human disease-causing allele. Then they transfer a corresponding human mutant

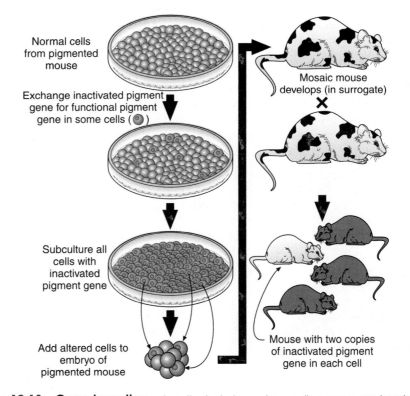

Figure 19.13 Gene targeting. Inactivated pigment-encoding genes are inserted into mouse embryonic stem (ES) cells, where they "knock out" functional pigment-encoding alleles. The modified ES cells are cultured and injected into early mouse embryos. Mosaic mice develop, with some cells heterozygous for the inactivated allele. These mice are bred to each other, and, if all goes well, yield some offspring homozygous for the knocked-out allele. It's easy to tell which mouse this is in the pigment gene example, but gene targeting is particularly valuable for revealing unknown gene functions by inactivating targeted alleles.

allele to mouse ES cells and follow the steps previously outlined to breed a homozygous animal. The mouse is a knockout if gene function is gone, and a knockin if it makes the human protein.

Knockout or knockin mice are valuable models of human disease because they provide a controllable test population. Consider severe combined immune deficiency (SCID) due to adenosine deaminase (ADA) deficiency, an immune disorder described in the next chapter (see figure 20.1). Phenotype varies, depending on a person's environment. A child raised in a protective bubble might be relatively healthy; a child out among others would suffer frequent infections. The disorder is so rare that it is difficult to study. This is where knockout SCID mice come in. Mice with knocked-out ADA genes can be raised under the same environmental conditions, bred to be genetically identical, and exposed to particular infectious agents or undergo treatments such as gene therapies.

Knockout mouse models of human disease can also reveal prenatal aspects of the condition. **Figure 19.14** compares a knockout mouse representing neurofibromatosis type 1 to a heterozygous sibling. In people, this disorder causes benign tumors beneath the skin and distinctive pigmented areas of skin. It is autosomal dominant, and affected individuals have one mutant allele and one normal one. For this condition and for most dominant genetic diseases, homozygous mutants are so severely affected that development ceases in the embryo, ending in spontaneous abortion. The mouse embryo on the left in figure 19.14 has two neurofibromin genes knocked out. The embryo has a severely abnormal heart and stopped developing in the middle of embryonic existence. The mouse embryo on the right has one knocked-out gene. It has some tumors, but is not nearly as severely affected as its homozygous sibling. Neurofibromin proteins in mice and humans share 98 percent of their amino acid sequences. In humans, a double dose of the mutant gene would cause a miscarriage.

Animals with knocked-out genes are also useful in studying polygenic disorders. For example, researchers are studying atherosclerosis by inactivating combinations of genes whose products oversee lipid metabolism. Similarly, scientists can study multiple genetic changes responsible for some cancers by targeting the genes in various combinations.

In a series of gene targeting experiments, two groups of researchers have developed mice that have human adult hemoglobin, fetal hemoglobin, or sickle cell hemoglobin. Recall from chapter 11 that the human globin genes occur in two clusters, on different chromosomes. One human research group knocked out the mouse's beta globin genes, and another knocked out the alpha genes— then each research team heard about the other. They joined forces, knocked out all the mouse globin genes, and knocked in their human counterparts. The mice with sickle cell hemoglobin have exactly the same symptoms as humans with sickle cell disease, and they are used to test new types of drugs and gene therapies.

When Knockouts Are Normal

The ability to knock out gene function has led to many surprises—especially when animals with supposedly vital genes knocked out are perfectly healthy, or much healthier than expected. This is the case for mice lacking a gene that encodes a type of collagen. Scientists thought that type X collagen promoted the normal growth and development of long bones in both mice and humans. Mutations in collagen genes cause a variety of syndromes in humans (see figure 12.3). Yet mice with knocked-out type X collagen genes have normal skeletons! How can this be?

A superhealthy knockout mouse forces researchers to rethink their assumptions about a gene's importance. Often these assumptions are based on knowing that the gene product has a vital function— such as contracting muscle or clotting blood. However, gene targeting experiments suggest that the importance of a gene's product must be considered in the context of the entire genome and organism. A broader view of interacting genes presents several possible explanations for healthy knockout mice:

1. Other genes that encode the same or similar proteins as the knocked-out gene may replace its function, so that disabling one gene does not affect the phenotype. The genome is redundant for important functions.

2. An absent protein in a knockout may not alter the phenotype, though an abnormal protein might.

3. The knocked-out gene may not do what we thought, and it may even have no function at all.

4. The knocked-out gene may function under different circumstances than the experiment provides. Various environmental challenges may be required to reveal the gene's function. For example, type X collagen, rather than being necessary for growth and development of a newborn's skeleton, may be called into action to repair fractures. It would therefore be unnecessary in embryonic and newborn mice.

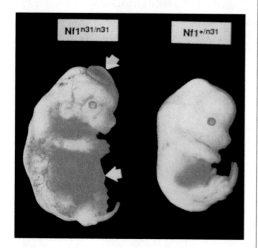

Figure 19.14 Knockout mouse embryos. Gene targeting can produce mice that are homozygous for disease-causing dominant alleles, such as those that cause neurofibromatosis type I (mouse embryo on the left). These effects are difficult to study in humans because they disrupt development very early. The arrows point to tumors.

Key Concepts

In gene targeting in mice, a gene of interest inserted into an embryonic stem cell recombines at the chromosomal site where it normally resides. The ES cell is then incorporated into a developing embryo from another individual, which is implanted into a surrogate. Animals with phenotypes indicating that they harbor cells with the targeted gene are bred to each other to yield homozygotes. Swapping an inactivated allele for a gene of interest produces a knockout mouse, and replacing a gene with another that has an altered function creates a knockin mouse. These animals can model human disease, but they sometimes reveal that a gene does not function as we thought.

19.5 Antisense Technology

Antisense technology selectively blocks expression of a gene —that is, it blocks synthesis of the gene's encoded protein. This is unlike transgenic technology or gene targeting, which add or replace a gene.

Antisense technology introduces part of a gene that already exists in the organism, but in reverse orientation. The mRNA transcribed from the inserted gene has a sequence complementary to the normal mRNA for that gene. The normal mRNA is called the "sense" sequence, and the complementary mRNA the "antisense" sequence. After transcription, the antisense sequence complementary base pairs to the sense sequence, preventing it from being translated into protein (**figure 19.15a**). This is a little like an intentional, single-stranded version of the recently discovered natural process of RNA interference (see section 11.3).

Antisense technology was conceived in the late 1980s and initially attracted great investor interest because it made so much sense. But as sometimes happens in biotechnology, experiments dashed initial hopes. Early apparent success in treating a variety of disorders turned out to reflect not the specific dampening of gene expression that lay at the heart of the idea, but instead a nonspecific alerting of the immune system. The short DNA sequences researchers used contained several dinucleotides consisting of CG. Because CGs are abundant in viruses and bacteria, their presence in the introduced antisense molecules looked like infection to the immune system.

Antisense drugs also proved difficult to deliver—they must be given intravenously, and they do not easily enter cells. Another roadblock was that an antisense sequence that theoretically would work by binding to its complement in an mRNA might not do so inside cells, where mRNA molecules tend to curl up with themselves, sometimes hiding the targeted sequences. Yet another limitation is that different exons may encode stretches of amino acids that become parts of different proteins. Therefore, an antisense treatment targeting one mRNA sequence might have unpredictable effects by silencing other genes.

Because of these limitations, only one drug derived from antisense technology is on the market. It is used to treat eye infections caused by cytomegalovirus in AIDS patients. Still, other antisense drugs are in clinical trials to treat diabetes, hepatitis C, cancers, psoriasis, Crohn disease, and rheumatoid arthritis.

Antisense technology has also had only limited success in plants. Best known was the doomed antisense "Flavrsavr" tomato, which squelched production of a ripening enzyme that normally breaks down pectin in cell walls, softening the fruit. The Flavrsavr tomatoes could stay on the vine longer, accumulating sugars and becoming redder (figure 19.15b). However, it failed to compete against tastier tomatoes already on the market, and once its origins were publicized, consumers' fear of genetically altered crops contributed to its failure.

Another application of antisense technology in plants is to reduce the amount of lignin, a component of the cell walls in wood that must be removed in the manufacture of pulp and paper. Lignin removal is costly and damaging to the environment. Researchers have used antisense technology to block production of a key enzyme in the lignin biosynthetic pathway of trembling aspen. The result is less lignin to remove from the wood, but other unexpected benefits also appeared. Blocking the enzyme leads to buildup of its substrate, which is then routed onto the biosynthetic pathway for cellulose. The extra cellulose, combined with less lignin, gives the trees a growth spurt.

The applications of biotechnology discussed in this chapter focused on generating products useful to humans. Genetic modification of ourselves, although based on the same techniques presented in this chapter, is an entirely distinct field, largely because of the bioethical implications. Gene therapy performed on somatic tissues is the topic of the next chapter—a natural follow-up to this one.

Sense mRNA •••UGACGCGAUUAGCCGAU•••

Antisense sequence —ACUGCGCUAAUCGGCUA

a.

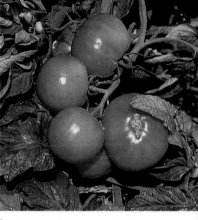

b.

Figure 19.15 Antisense RNA blocks protein synthesis and produces new crops. **(a)** The sense mRNA depicted on top cannot be translated into protein because an antisense sequence blocks it. **(b)** These tomatoes harbor an antisense gene that silences a ripening enzyme. This allows the fruit to remain longer on the vine, turning red but gaining a better flavor and texture, rather than becoming mushy. However, consumers rejected the tomatoes, which just didn't taste as good as older varieties.

Key Concepts

Antisense technology uses single-stranded RNA molecules to inhibit expression of a particular gene by binding to its mRNA. Limitations have slowed its progress, but products are still being tested.

Summary

19.1 Of Pigs and Patents

1. **Biotechnology** is the alteration of cells or biochemicals to provide a useful product. It includes extracting natural products, altering an organism's genetic material, and combining DNA from different species.

2. A **transgenic** organism has DNA from a different species in its genome. DNA from two sources is recombinant.

3. DNA can be patented in several guises, but it must be useful.

19.2 Recombinant DNA Technology

4. **Recombinant DNA technology** is possible because of the universality of the genetic code. It is used to mass-produce proteins in bacteria or other single cells. Begun hesitantly in 1975, the technology has matured into a valuable method to produce useful proteins.

5. Constructing a recombinant DNA molecule begins when **restriction enzymes** cut both the gene of interest and a **cloning vector** at a short palindromic sequence, creating complementary "sticky ends." The cut foreign DNA and vector DNA are mixed, and vectors that pick up foreign DNA are selected.

6. **Genomic libraries** consist of recombinant cells containing fragments of a foreign genome. **DNA probes** are used to select genes of interest from genomic libraries. DNA probes may be synthetic, taken from another species, or a **cDNA,** which is reverse transcribed from mRNA.

7. Genes conferring antibiotic sensitivity or resistance, and/or color change in growth medium, are used to select cells harboring recombinant DNA.

8. DNA is introduced into cells through liposomes, electroporation, microinjection, and particle bombardment.

9. For a multicellular transgenic organism, a single cell (a gamete in an animal or plant, or a somatic cell in a plant) or early embryo cells are genetically altered. The organism develops, including the change in each cell and passing it to the next generation. Heterozygotes for the transgene are then bred to yield homozygotes.

19.3 Applications of Recombinant DNA Technology

10. Single-celled organisms that have human genes manufacture proteins useful as drugs.

11. Novel or easier-to-manufacure textiles, wood products, and foods are possible using recombinant DNA technology.

12. Bioremediation uses natural detoxifying processes, sometimes expressing them in transgenic organisms.

19.4 Gene Targeting

13. **Gene targeting** uses the natural attraction of a DNA sequence for its complementary sequence, called **homologous recombination,** to swap one gene for another. It is more precise than transgenic technology.

14. Because homologous recombination will not occur in a gamete or fertilized ovum, the manipulation is done on an ES cell, which is then inserted into another embryo and transferred to a surrogate mother. Heterozygotes are bred to yield homozygotes.

15. Knockouts have the gene of interest inactivated. Knockins replace one gene with another allele with altered function.

16. Knockout mice with inactivated genes can model human disease. Sometimes, knockout mice reveal that a gene product is not vital to survival.

19.5 Antisense Technology

17. Antisense technology inserts a DNA sequence in reverse orientation so that the "antisense" mRNA transcribed from it complementary base pairs with the "sense" mRNA, squelching a gene's expression.

18. The technology was theoretically feasible, but presented various problems.

Review Questions

1. Define each of the following terms:
   a. biotechnology
   b. recombinant DNA technology
   c. a transgenic organism
   d. gene targeting
   e. homologous recombination

2. Describe the roles of each of the following tools in a biotechnology:
   a. restriction enzymes
   b. embryonic stem cells
   c. cloning vectors

3. How do researchers use antibiotics to select cells containing recombinant DNA?

4. List the components of an experiment to produce recombinant human insulin in *E. coli* cells.

5. Why would recombinant DNA technology be impossible if the genetic code was not universal?

6. Describe three ways to insert foreign DNA into cells.

7. Why isn't transgenic technology as precise as gene targeting?

8. How does Mendel's law of segregation for a monohybrid cross apply to carrying out transgenesis and gene targeting experiments?

9. How do gene targeting and antisense technology silence gene expression in different ways?

10. What is an advantage of a drug produced using recombinant DNA technology compared to one extracted from natural sources?

Applied Questions

1. Genetic modification can creatively combine parts of organisms. From the following three lists (choose one item from each list), devise an experiment to produce a particular protein, and suggest what it might be used for.

Organism	Biological Fluid	Protein Product
pig	milk	human beta globin chains
cow	semen	human collagen
goat	silk	human EPO
chicken	egg white	human tPA
aspen tree	sap	human interferon
silkworm	blood plasma	jellyfish GFP
rabbit	honey	human clotting factor
mouse	saliva	alpha-1-antitrypsin

2. Collagen is a connective tissue protein that is used in skincare products, shampoo, desserts, and in artificial skin. For many years it was obtained from the hooves and hides of cows collected from slaughterhouses. Human collagen can be manufactured in transgenic mice. Describe the advantages of the mouse system for obtaining collagen.

3. There was no public outcry over the development of Humulin, the human insulin produced in bacterial cells and used to treat diabetes. Yet many people object to mixing DNA from different species in agricultural biotechnology. Why do you think that the same general technique is perceived as beneficial in one situation, yet a threat in another?

4. A human oncogene called *ras* is inserted into mice, creating transgenic animals that develop a variety of tumors. Why are mouse cells able to transcribe and translate human genes?

5. A healthy knockout mouse cannot manufacture what was thought to be a vital enzyme. Suggest three possible explanations for this surprising finding.

6. In a mouse model of a human condition called "urge syndrome," in which the feeling of impending urination occurs frequently, researchers inactivate a gene encoding nitric oxide synthase, which produces nitric oxide (NO). NO is the neurotransmitter that controls muscle contraction in the bladder. What type of biotechnology could accomplish this?

7. Mouse models for cystic fibrosis have been developed by inserting a human transgene and by gene targeting to inactivate the mouse counterpart of the alleles that cause the disorder. How do these methods differ? Which method do you think produces a more accurate model of human cystic fibrosis, and why?

Web Activities

8. Use the web to identify three drugs made using recombinant DNA technology, and list the conditions they are used to treat.

Case Studies

9. Beginning in 1989 and continuing throughout the 1990s, Australian researcher Malcolm Simons filed many patent applications in many countries on the use of non-protein-encoding parts of the human genome to predict the risk of developing certain diseases. At the time the patents were filed, research interest largely focused on the protein-encoding parts of the genome—many researchers called the rest "junk." But towards the turn of the century, research correlating SNP (single nucleotide polymorphism) patterns in the "junk" to disease risk became a top priority at many biotech companies, and researchers seeking SNPs in noncoding portions of the genome encountered Simons's patents. He is now requesting that researchers pay a modest licensing fee to carry out their work. Many geneticists have publicly denounced Simons's actions as counter to the spirit of open access to information in the human genome. Do you support or object to Simons's restricting access to the DNA sequences he predicted would have clinical utility?

10. Nancy is a transgenic sheep who produces human alpha-1-antitrypsin (AAT) in her milk. This protein is normally found in blood serum and enables the microscopic air sacs in the lungs to inflate. Without it, inherited emphysema results—a severe illness that usually kills humans by early adulthood. Donated blood cannot yield enough AAT to help the thousands who need it. Describe the steps taken to enable Nancy to secrete this valuable drug in her milk.

Learn to apply the skills of a genetic counselor with additional cases found in the *Case Workbook of Human Genetics.*

Hemophilia A and B

Infertility drugs

Transgenic tobacco

Suggested Readings

Alvarez, Lizette. July 3, 2003. Europe acts to require labeling of genetically altered food. *The New York Times,* p. F1. The problem with labeling GM foods is that it implies a danger, which may not be scientifically accurate.

Bobrow, Martin, and Sandy Thomas. February 15, 2001. Patents in a genetic age. *Nature* 409:763–64. The Patent and Trademark Office can hardly keep up with single-gene applications. What will happen in this new age of genomics?

Dove, Alan. February 2002. Antisense and sensibility. *Nature Biotechnology,* 20:121–24. Antisense technology makes sense, but has hit many roadblocks.

Golovan, Serguei P., et al. August 2001. Pigs expressing salivary phytase produce low-phosphorus manure. *Nature Biotechnology* 19:741–42. Genetically modified pigs fight pollution.

Potrykus, I. March 2001. Golden rice and beyond. *Plant Physiology* 123:1157–61. Ingo Potrykus describes his invention of golden rice—and how both environmental activists and the media have misunderstood its status.

Roosevelt, Margot. May 26, 2003. Cures on the cob. *Time.* Transgenic plants can produce drugs.

Strauss, Steven H. April 4, 2003. Genomics, genetic engineering, and domestication of crops. *Science,* 300:61–62. Field test on transgenic plants will have to keep pace with plant genome projects.

Wurm, Florian M. January 2003. Human therapeutic proteins from silkworms. *Nature Biotechnology,* 21:34–35. Silkworms knit cocoons that include human collagen.

The October 2003 issue of *Nature Reviews Genetics,* 4(10), is devoted to genetically modified organisms.

Weekly updates of current news related to human genetics are available through Power Web on your Online Learning Center.

VISIT YOUR ONLINE LEARNING CENTER

Visit your online learning center for additional resources and tools to help you master this chapter. See us at

www.mhhe.com/lewisgenetics6.

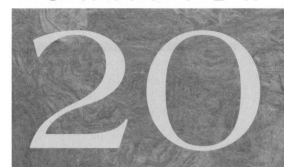

C H A P T E R

20

Gene Therapy and Genetic Counseling

CHAPTER CONTENTS

20.1   Gene Therapy Successes and Setbacks

The 1990s dawned with the first gene therapy experiments, which were partially successful and paved the way for improved methods. The decade closed, however, with the death of a young participant in a gene therapy trial, leading to a reexamination of the tools and approaches used in this still very promising technology. Gene therapy continues to yield some successes, but the challenges may be greater than anticipated.

20.2   The Mechanics of Gene Therapy

Designing a gene therapy requires the creative combining of genetic material. The gene of interest must be isolated and delivered to the tissue implicated in a particular illness, then coaxed to produce its encoded protein at the right time, in sufficient amounts (but not too much), and for long enough to improve symptoms. Gene therapies are being developed for a variety of illnesses.

20.3   A Closer Look: Treating Sickle Cell Disease

We know more about sickle cell disease than perhaps any other inherited illness. Several "traditional" gene therapies are being applied to this disorder, as well as the unique approach of "reawakening" genes that normally function only in the fetus.

20.4   Genetic Screening and Genetic Counseling

Genetic counselors combine scientific, medical, communication, and psychological skills to educate people facing the possibility of inherited illness, as well as other health care professionals. They guide individuals, couples, and families through the maze of decisions that accompanies testing for single gene disorders and, increasingly, susceptibilities for complex conditions such as cancers.

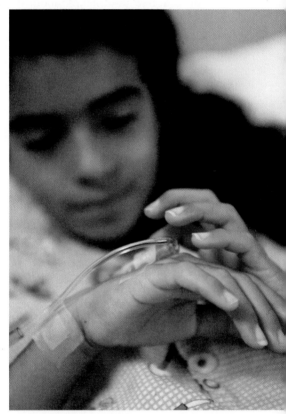

For a handful of inherited disorders, gene therapy offers hope.

Treatment for genetic diseases has evolved in three phases: (1) replacing missing proteins with material from donors, (2) obtaining pure proteins using recombinant DNA technology, and (3) delivering replacement genes to correct the problem at its source, called **gene therapy**. The Technology Timeline illustrates this evolution for hemophilia A, a disorder of blood clotting.

More than a thousand clinical trials of gene therapies have been conducted since 1990. This chapter introduces some of the patients who volunteered for the first gene therapies, then discusses the mechanics of the process. Researchers expected that the sequencing of the human genome would accelerate the pace of gene therapy development. Instead, new information about the complexity of how genes specify proteins, and a few cases where the experimental treatment harmed the patient, have led to a reevaluation of the idea that we can augment or replace a gene with predictable effects.

20.1 Gene Therapy Successes and Setbacks

Any new medical treatment or technology begins with creative minds and courageous volunteers. The first individuals to take new vaccines or to try new treatments know that they may give their lives, either directly or indirectly, in the process. Gene therapy, however, is unlike conventional drug therapy. It attempts to alter an individual's genotype in a part of the body that has malfunctioned. Because the potentially therapeutic gene must usually be delivered along with other DNA, and it may be taken up by cell types other than those that are affected in the disease, the body's reactions are unpredictable.

Adenosine Deaminase Deficiency—Early Success

For the first few years of her life, Laura Cay Boren didn't know what it was like to feel well (**figure 20.1a**). From her birth in July 1982, she fought infection after infection. Colds rapidly became pneumonia, and routine vaccines caused severe abscesses. In February 1983, doctors identified Laura's problem—severe combined immune deficiency (SCID) due to adenosine deaminase (ADA) deficiency. She had inherited the

autosomal recessive inborn error of metabolism from two carrier parents.

Lack of ADA blocks a biochemical pathway that normally breaks down a metabolic toxin into uric acid, which is then excreted (**figure 20.1b**). Without ADA, the substance that ADA normally acts upon builds up and destroys T cells. Without helper T cells to stimulate them, B cells cannot mature into the plasma cells that produce antibodies. Both branches of the adaptive immune system thus fail. The child becomes very prone to infections and cancer, and despite medical treatment, usually does not live beyond a year in the outside environment.

The Duke University Medical Center, where Laura celebrated her first and second birthdays, became her second home. In 1983 and again in 1984, she received bone marrow transplants from her father, which temporarily bolstered her immunity. Red blood cell transfusions also helped for a time. Still,

Laura was spending more time in the hospital than out. By the end of 1985, she was gravely ill. She had to be fed through a tube, and repeated infection had severely damaged her lungs. Laura's mother began to feel guilty for wishing that her child would die rather than suffer. Then, a medical miracle happened.

Laura was chosen to be the first recipient of a new treatment. She had been second in line to a boy who was even more ill, but he died just before beginning treatment. In the spring of 1986, Laura received her first injection of PEG-ADA. This is the missing enzyme, ADA, taken from a cow and stabilized by adding polyethylene glycol (PEG) chains to it. PEG is the major ingredient in antifreeze.

Previous enzyme replacement therapy hadn't worked, because what remained of the immune system rapidly destroyed the injected, unaltered enzyme. Patients needed frequent doses, which provoked the immune system further, causing allergic reactions too

---

Technology Timeline

Hemophilia A (Factor VIII Deficiency)

Hemophilia A is a bleeding disorder caused by a mutation in the gene on the X chromosome that encodes clotting factor VIII. It affects 1 in 10,000 newborns. Hemophilia A is an excellent candidate for gene therapy because it is a single-gene disorder, many cell types can secrete the clotting factor, it is well studied in animal models, and just modest increases in clotting factor production can improve health. The treatment of hemophilia A parallels the evolution of biotechnology, from enzyme replacement to recombinant DNA technology to gene therapy. Even though clinical trials are well under way, researchers are seeking improvements in gene delivery in mice using a variety of viruses—including disabled HIV.

1970s	Hemophilia A is treated with factor VIII pooled from donated plasma (cryoprecipitate). Recipients contract hepatitis.
Early 1980s	Up to 70 percent of patients receiving cryoprecipitate contract HIV infection.
1984	Factor VIII gene cloned, making prenatal diagnosis and carrier detection possible for some individuals.
1985	Invention of PCR allows detection of many more hemophilia A mutations, previously unknown because they occur in an intron.
1990	Recombinant factor VIII eliminates risk of infection from donated plasma while supplying missing gene product.
1999	First gene therapy experiment, using viral vector given intravenously, works (see In Their Own Words, chapter 1).
2001	In another gene therapy protocol, patients' skin fibroblasts are removed and cultured with cDNA for factor VIII, then reimplanted into abdominal fat. Four of six patients improve.
2002	Another gene therapy protocol injects cDNA for factor VIII carried in disabled mouse leukemia retrovirus.

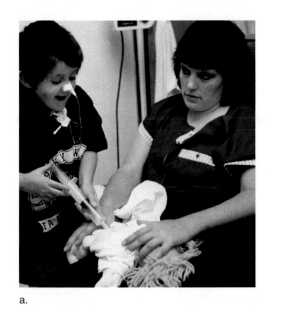

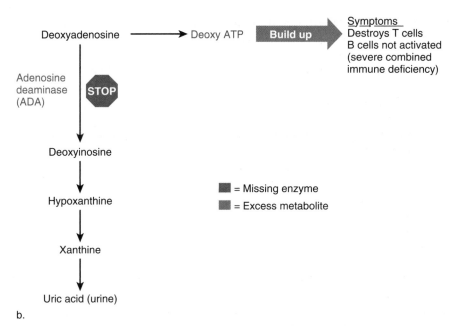

Deoxyadenosine → Deoxy ATP Build up → Symptoms
Destroys T cells
B cells not activated
(severe combined
immune deficiency)

Adenosine
deaminase
(ADA) STOP

Deoxyinosine

Hypoxanthine

Xanthine

Uric acid (urine)

■ = Missing enzyme
■ = Excess metabolite

a.

b.

Figure 20.1   Evolution of treatment for ADA deficiency.   **(a)** Laura Cay Boren spent much of her life in hospitals until she received the enzyme that her body lacks, adenosine deaminase (ADA). Here, she pretends to inject her doll as her mother looks on. Today, gene therapy is possible using cord blood stem cells. **(b)** ADA deficiency causes deoxy ATP to build up, destroying T cells, which therefore cannot stimulate B cells to secrete antibodies. The result is severe combined immune deficiency (SCID).

severe to continue treatment. Laura's physicians hoped that adding PEG would keep ADA in her blood long enough to work.

Laura began responding to PEG-ADA almost immediately. Within hours, her ADA level increased twentyfold. After three months, toxins no longer showed up in her blood, but her immunity was still suppressed. After six months, though, Laura's immune function neared normal for the first time ever—and stayed that way, with weekly doses of PEG-ADA. Her life changed drastically as she ventured beyond the hospital's germ-free rooms. By summer 1988, she could finally play with other children without fear of infection. She began first grade in fall 1989, but had to repeat the year—she had spent her time socializing!

PEG-ADA revolutionized treatment of this form of SCID, targeting the source of the disorder rather than trying to overcome the infections. But PEG-ADA therapy was only the opening chapter of the ongoing story of gene therapy, for it replaced the protein, not the gene.

The second chapter began on September 14, 1990, at 12:52 P.M. Four-year-old Ashanthi DeSilva sat up in bed at the National Institute of Health in Bethesda, Maryland, and began receiving her own white blood cells intravenously. Earlier, doctors had removed the cells and patched them with normal ADA

genes. This first gene therapy did not "heal" a sufficient percentage of cells, and treatment had to be repeated, or PEG-ADA given at intervals. But Ashanthi is now healthy, and she tells her story at scientific meetings (see In Their Own Words on page 394).

A longer-lasting treatment could result from altering progenitor cells (see figure 2.23). The progenitor of T cells accounts for one in several billion bone marrow cells—not a very promising ratio. Umbilical cord blood was a more plentiful source. If fetuses who had inherited ADA deficiency could be identified and their parents agreed to the treatment, then the appropriate stem cells could be extracted from the cord blood at birth, given ADA genes, and reinfused into the newborn. The third chapter in the ADA deficiency tale was about to begin.

Crystal and Leonard Gobea had already lost a five-month-old baby to ADA deficiency when amniocentesis revealed that their second fetus was affected. They and two other couples were asked to participate in the experiment. The May 31, 1993, issue of *Time* magazine featured newborn Andrew Gobea on the cover. He and the other two babies received their own bolstered blood cells on the fourth day after birth, and PEG-ADA to prevent symptoms in case the gene therapy did not work right away. The plan was to monitor the babies frequently to see if T cells carrying nor-

mal ADA genes would appear in their blood. The needed T cells accumulated slowly, but by the summer of 1995, the three toddlers each had about 3 in 100 T cells carrying the ADA gene, and they continued to improve.

A few years after the three children with ADA deficiency were treated, another gene therapy trial for a severe combined immune deficiency (SCID) began in France. Nine male infants with a type of X-linked SCID had T cell progenitors removed and given the gene they were missing, which encodes part of a cytokine receptor. The researchers hoped that restoring cells' ability to recognize cytokines would cure the immune deficiency. And it did, but there was a huge problem—in early 2003, two of the boys developed a rare leukemia. The retrovirus used to carry the healing gene had apparently inserted into a proto-oncogene. The boys have been treated for the leukemia, but this very unexpected side effect stalled many gene therapy trials, perhaps because it was not the first time such an experiment had a tragic outcome. First came Jesse Gelsinger.

Ornithine Transcarbamylase Deficiency—A Setback

The sad saga of Jesse Gelsinger stands in sharp contrast to the success stories of the children

The First Gene Therapy Patient

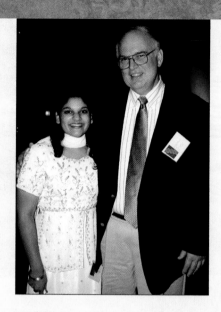

In the late 1980s, the DeSilva's did not think their little girl, Ashanthi ("Ashi"), would survive. She suffered near-continual coughs and colds, and was so fatigued that she could walk only a few steps before becoming winded, her father Raj recalls. "We took her to so many doctors that I stopped counting. One doctor after another would say it was asthma, an allergy, or bronchitis."

Raj's brother, an immunologist, suggested the blood tests that would eventually reveal Ashi's underlying problem—severe combined immune deficiency due to adenosine deaminase (ADA) deficiency. Although unlucky in inheriting a disease, Ashi was lucky in that it was a condition so well understood that it was first in line for gene therapy. Through a series of physician contacts, Ashi became the first recipient of gene therapy.

The medical team at the National Institute of Health—W. French Anderson, Kenneth Culver, and Michael Blaese—had spent years planning the gene therapy, and were fairly certain that it would work. Within weeks following the therapy, Ashi began to make her own, functional T cells. Although she required further treatments, today she is well and excited about her future, anticipating a career in the music industry after college.

Over the years, she has championed gene therapy at biomedical conferences. The photo shows her at a meeting when she was 17, where she introduced Dr. Blaese: "Our duty on Earth is to help others. I thank you from the bottom of my heart for all you have enabled me to do."

Gene therapy has hit snags in recent years, but overall has had an excellent track record. Says Dr. Blaese, "You have to consider the context. In the years since the first patient, there has been one death and two malignancies. Compare that to the first 100 heart transplants, where only one person lived more than a year. Gene therapy has had a remarkable safety record, yet there are still problems."

with ADA deficiency. In September 1999, the 18-year-old died, just days after receiving gene therapy. The cause of death was an overwhelming immune system reaction against the DNA used to introduce the healing gene.

Jesse had an inborn error of metabolism called ornithine transcarbamylase deficiency (OTC). In this X-linked recessive disorder, one of five enzymes required to break down amino acids liberated from dietary proteins is absent (**figure 20.2**). The nitrogen from the amino acids combines with hydrogens to form ammonia (NH_3), which rapidly accumulates in the bloodstream and travels to the brain, with devastating effects. The condition usually causes irreversible coma within 72 hours of birth. Half of affected babies die within a month, and another quarter by age five. The survivors can control their symptoms by following a special low-protein diet and taking drugs that bind ammonia.

Jesse wasn't diagnosed until he was two, because he was a mosaic—some of his cells could produce the enzyme, so his symptoms were milder. Still, when he went into a coma in December 1998 after missing a few days of his medications, he and his father began to consider whether he should volunteer for a gene therapy trial they had read about. The researchers would not accept Jesse until he turned 18, so the next summer, four days after his birthday, Jesse underwent testing at the University of Pennsylvania, where the gene therapy center is located, and was admitted to the trial. He was jubilant. He knew he would not directly benefit, at least not for awhile, but he had wanted to try to help the babies who die of the condition. A bioethics committee had advised that the experimental treatment could not be tried on newborns because the parents would be too distraught to give informed consent to an untried medical procedure. Instead, affected males and carrier females had volunteered. Said Jesse at the time, "What's the worst that can happen to me? I die, and it's for the babies."

The gene therapy consisted of an adenovirus—a type of virus that causes the common cold—with a functional human OTC gene stitched into it. This virus had already been used, apparently safely, in about a quarter of the gene therapy experiments done since 1990. It is a disabled virus, with the genes that enable it to replicate and cause disease removed. Three groups of six patients each were to receive three different doses, with the trial designed to identify the lowest dose that would fight the genetic disease without causing dangerous side effects.

Jesse entered the hospital on Monday, September 13, after the 17 others in the trial had already been treated and suffered nothing worse than a fever and aches and pains. Several billion altered viruses were introduced into an artery leading into his liver. That night, Jesse developed a high fever—still not unusual. But by morning, the whites of Jesse's eyes were yellow, indicating a high bilirubin level as his liver struggled to dismantle the hemoglobin released from burst red blood cells. A flood of hemoglobin meant a flood of protein, so the ammonia level in his liver soon skyrocketed, reaching 10 times normal levels by mid-afternoon. At the same time, his blood wasn't clotting well. Jesse became disoriented, then comatose. By Wednesday, doctors had controlled the ammonia buildup, but his lungs began to fail, and Jesse was placed on a ventilator. Thursday, Jesse's vital organs began to fail, and by Friday, he was brain dead. His dedicated and devastated medical team stood by as his father turned off life support, and Jesse died.

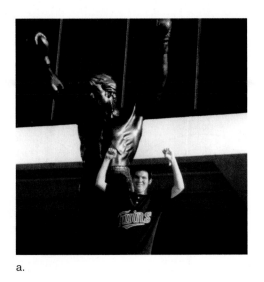

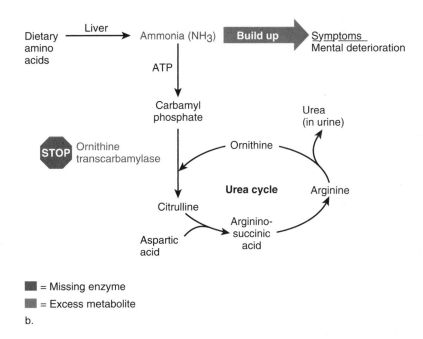

Figure 20.2   A brave example.   (a) Jesse Gelsinger received gene therapy for an inborn error of metabolism in September 1999. He died four days later from an overwhelming immune response. **(b)** Lack of ornithine transcarbamylase causes ammonia to accumulate, which is toxic to the brain.

At a public hearing in December, doctors explained that the autopsy showed that Jesse had had a parvovirus infection, which may have led his immune system to attack the adenovirus. In the liver, the adenovirus had traveled not to the targeted hepatocytes, but to a different cell type, the macrophages that function as sentries for the immune system. In response, interleukins flooded his body, and inflammation raged. Although parents of children with OTC who spoke at the hearing implored government officials to allow the research to continue, the death of Jesse Gelsinger led to suspension of several gene therapy trials. The death drew particular attention to safety because, unlike most other volunteers, Jesse was not very ill.

In the months following his death, representatives of the Food and Drug Administration and the National Institutes of Health (NIH) identified several procedural factors that may have contributed to the tragedy: failure to report all side effects in a timely fashion, failure to fill out the proper eligibility forms, and inadequately documented informed consent. Also, more careful attention should have been paid to screening potential participants for underlying medical conditions. When the NIH examined other gene therapy trials, the agency discovered extreme underreporting of adverse side effects. However, this appar-

ent oversight might reflect the fact that researchers attributed many adverse effects to the underlying disease, and not to the experimental treatment.

A Success in the Making— Canavan Disease

Jesse Gelsinger's death led to the halting or reevaluation of many gene therapy trials. However, efforts begun in 1995 to treat Canavan disease, which causes brain degeneration in children, continued. Canavan disease is an ideal candidate for gene therapy for several reasons: (1) the gene and protein are well known; (2) there is a window of time when affected children are healthy enough to be treated; (3) only the brain is affected; (4) brain scans can monitor response to treatment; and (5) there is no existing treatment.

Canavan disease disrupts the interaction between neurons and neighboring cells called oligodendrocytes, which produce the fatty myelin that coats neurons, enabling them to transmit impulses fast enough for the brain to function (**figure 20.3**). Specifically, neurons normally release N-acetylaspartate (NAA), which is broken down into harmless compounds by an enzyme, aspartoacylase, that the oligodendrocytes produce. In Canavan disease, the enzyme is missing, and the resulting NAA

buildup eventually destroys the oligodendrocytes. Without sufficient myelin, the neurons cease to function, and symptoms begin. The parents may first notice developmental delay—inability to sit and stand at ages when other children can. The children have poor vision, do not react much to their surroundings, may have seizures, require tube feeding, and may have muscle control so poor that they cannot even hold up their heads. In Their Own Words on page 397 and Bioethics: Choices for the Future on page 399 describe children with Canavan disease. Due to a powerful founder effect, Canavan disease is seen almost exclusively in the Ashkenazi Jewish population.

The first attempts at gene therapy for Canavan disease introduced the needed gene in a liposome, through holes bored into the skull. The first recipient, 18-month-old Lindsay Karlin, gained some skills for awhile. Previously, Lindsay could barely open her eyes and did not interact with anyone. But three months after the therapy, she looked around, moved, and vocalized. "It was as though she had awakened," wrote her mother. A magnetic resonance image of Lindsay's brain showed that myelination of neurons had begun in regions where it had vanished. Lindsay was not treated again until June 2001, when a viral vector replaced the liposomes. In the interim, while regulatory agencies argued

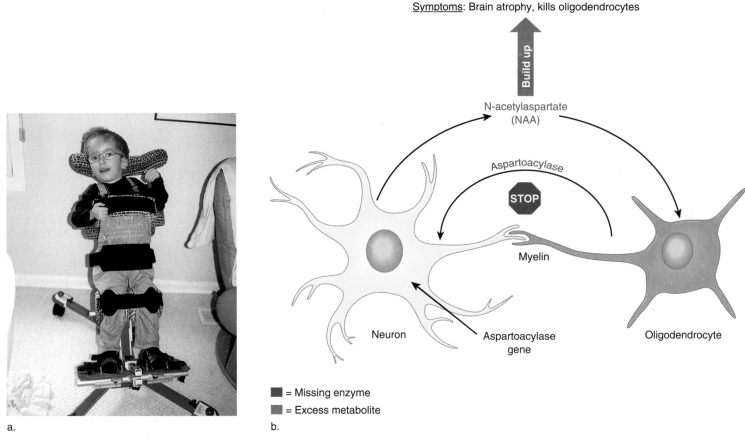

Symptoms: Brain atrophy, kills oligodendrocytes

Build up

N-acetylaspartate
(NAA)

Aspartoacylase

STOP

Myelin

Neuron

Aspartoacylase
gene

Oligodendrocyte

■ = Missing enzyme
■ = Excess metabolite

a.

b.

Figure 20.3 Canavan disease. (a) Max Randell, shown here at two-and-a-half years old, is battling Canavan disease. **(b)** In this condition, stripping of the lipid layer on brain neurons occurs because oligodendrocytes lack an enzyme that enables them to break down N-acetylaspartate, which neurons produce. Buildup of N-acetylaspartate eventually destroys the oligodendrocytes, so that the neurons lack myelin. Gene therapy enables the neurons to secrete the enzyme (rather than the oligodendrocytes), ultimately restoring the fatty covering that makes nerve transmission possible in the brain.

about the safety of this therapy for a disease that had no other treatment, Lindsay lost some of the gains from the first round, such as being able to hold her head up. But the gene therapy does appear to be working, in Lindsay and other children participating in current clinical trials.

Key Concepts

ADA deficiency was the first disorder treated with gene therapy. It began by replacing the missing enzyme, progressed to genetically altering mature white blood cells in ill children, and finally moved to infusing genetically modified umbilical cord stem cells into newborns. • Gene therapy for OTC deficiency led to a tragic death due to an unexpected severe immune reaction to the virus used to deliver the genes. • For Canavan disease, gene therapy may provide the only treatment.

20.2 The Mechanics of Gene Therapy

Altering genes to treat an inherited disorder theoretically can provide a longer-lasting effect than treating symptoms. The first gene therapy efforts focused on inherited disorders that researchers knew the most about, even though the conditions are very rare. With the increasing understanding of human genes and their functions made possible by knowing the human genome sequence, gene therapy efforts will be targeting more common illnesses, such as heart disease and cancer. **Tables 20.1** and **20.2** list some general requirements and concerns related to gene therapy.

Gene therapy approaches vary in invasiveness. The first gene therapy on Ashanthi DeSilva altered cells outside her body and then infused the corrected cells. This approach is called *ex vivo* **gene therapy.** In *in situ* **gene therapy,** the healthy gene plus the DNA that delivers it (the vector) is

injected into a very localized and accessible body part, such as a single melanoma skin cancer. In the most invasive approach, *in vivo* ("in the living body") **gene therapy,** the vector is introduced directly into the body, as it was into Jesse Gelsinger's liver.

Table 20.1
Requirements for Approval of Clinical Trials for Gene Therapy

1. Knowledge of defect and how it causes symptoms
2. An animal model
3. Success in human cells growing *in vitro*
4. Either no alternate therapies, or a group of patients for whom existing therapies are not possible or have not worked
5. Safe experiments

Gene Therapy for Canavan Disease

"On September 8, 1998, at 11 months old, little Max Randell became the youngest person in the world to receive gene therapy for a degenerative brain disease. He was one of four children, out of 14 total, in the safety trial to show an increase of myelin in his brain. His progress was amazing after the surgery, but unfortunately, was short-lived.

Finally, on June 19, 2001, Max received another injection of corrected genes using a new improved gene transfer system. Dr. Paola Leone, and her wonderful team at Thomas Jefferson University, worked tirelessly to develop this new system. They are truly lifesavers! This time, 90 billion viral particles carrying a corrected copy of the new gene were injected directly into Max's brain at six different sites. He was the second person in the world to receive a gene transfer using this experimental method.

The surgery was a success, and Max started to show signs of improvement after only ten days. After one month, the changes were being recorded by doctors, family, and all of Max's therapists. Previous data show that this time the new gene should stay active in Max's brain for at least two years, possibly even up to five years.

To see Max do things he hasn't done in the past one to two years is simply amazing! He is a very happy and well-adjusted child. His social, emotional, and cognitive skills are those of any normal three-and-a-half-year old. I cannot even begin to describe the joy we feel just seeing him regain even the slightest bit of functional mobility; he just beams with pride when his body does what he wants it to."

By Ilyce and Mike Randell

Table 20.2

Gene Therapy Concerns

Scientific	Bioethical
1. Which cells should be treated?	1. Does the participant in a gene therapy trial truly understand the risks?
2. What proportion of the targeted cell population must be corrected to alleviate or halt progression of symptoms?	2. If a gene therapy is effective, how will recipients be selected, assuming it is expensive at first?
3. Is overexpression of the therapeutic gene dangerous?	3. Should rare or more common disorders be the focus of gene therapy research and clinical trials?
4. Is it dangerous if the altered gene enters cells other than the intended ones?	4. What effect should deaths among volunteers have on research efforts?
5. How long will the affected cells function?	5. Should clinical trials be halted if the delivered gene enters the germline?
6. Will the immune system attack the introduced cells?	
7. Does the targeted DNA sequence occur in more than one gene?	

Treating the Phenotype

The phenotypes of some genetic disorders can be treated, often by replacing a missing protein. A child with cystic fibrosis sprinkles powdered cow digestive enzymes onto applesauce, which she eats before each meal to replace the enzymes her clogged pancreas cannot secrete. A boy with hemophilia receives a clotting factor. Even wearing eyeglasses is a way of altering the expression of one's inheritance. Today, newborns are routinely screened for certain inborn errors of metabolism whose symptoms can be prevented or alleviated by correcting the phenotype, such as by following a restrictive diet. Newborn screening is revisited at the chapter's end.

An inherited illness with an unusual phenotypic treatment is hereditary hemochromatosis (HH). Because HH results in "iron overload," the treatment is to periodically remove blood, because this action also removes iron, which is part of the hemoglobin molecule (see figure 11.3).

In the United States, 1.5 million people have this autosomal recessive condition, and 32 million people—1 in 8—carry a mutant allele for the HH gene. It is most common among those of Irish, Scottish, or British descent. In HH, cells in the small intestine absorb too much iron from food. Over many years, the excess iron is deposited throughout the body, causing various symptoms and secondary conditions. The liver develops cirrhosis (scarring) and sometimes cancer; the heart may fail or beat irregularly; an iron-loaded pancreas may cause diabetes; joints become arthritic; and the skin darkens. Early signs and symptoms include chronic fatigue, infection, hair loss, infertility, muscle pain, and feeling cold.

Diagnosis requires a blood test to detect the telltale blood-level increase in ferritin, a protein that carries iron, and a liver biopsy. Determining the genotype alone is not sufficient for diagnosis because the penetrance is very low. That is, although most people with iron overload have mutations in the HH gene, only a small percentage of people with a homozygous recessive genotype actually have symptoms. More men than women develop HH symptoms, because a woman loses some blood each month when she menstruates. Once women pass the age of menopause, the sex ratio equalizes. Donating blood every few months, however, is a simple way to keep the body's iron levels down. (The blood is discarded.)

Germline Versus Somatic Gene Therapy

Researchers distinguish two general types of gene therapy, depending upon whether it affects gametes or fertilized ova, or somatic tissue.

Germline gene therapy (also known as heritable gene therapy) alters the DNA of a gamete or fertilized ovum. As a result, all cells of the individual will have the change. Germline gene therapy is heritable—it passes to offspring. It is not being done in humans.

Correcting only the somatic cells that an illness affects is **somatic gene therapy.** This form of the technology is nonheritable, which means that a recipient does not pass the genetic correction to offspring. An example is clearing lungs congested from cystic fibrosis with a nasal spray containing functional CFTR genes. The treatment doesn't alter the gametes (sperm or oocytes), so a treated person could not pass a normal CFTR allele to offspring.

Many questions must be answered before somatic gene therapy can be applied. Which cells, in which tissues and organs, fail, and when in development do they do so? Which biochemical is abnormal or missing? What DNA sequence must be added to correct the defect? What percentage of cells in a tissue must be altered to alleviate symptoms? How long will the effects of the correction persist? Will it affect other cells in ways we can anticipate? Do other genes affect the function of the gene of interest? Even when we have much of this information, designing a gene therapy is challenging. Many early gene therapy experiments were disappointing because the correction wasn't sufficient to overcome symptoms or the immune system attacked the altered cells.

Sites of Somatic Gene Therapy

Current somatic gene therapy clinical trials, target several different tissues (**figure 20.4**). Delivery may be directly to the affected tissue, or via stem cells in bone marrow which can, under certain conditions, migrate to tissues other than blood—such as liver or muscle—where they either specialize into the needed cell types, or fuse with cells there, providing them with a functional copy of the gene.

Endothelium

One tissue that is very amenable to gene therapy is endothelium, which forms capillaries. Genetically altered endothelium can secrete a needed protein directly into the bloodstream. A person with diabetes, for example, might receive capillaries that secrete insulin; someone with hemophilia might receive an implant that manufactures a clotting factor. Endothelium is implanted with collagen to provide support and angiogenesis factors to stimulate capillary growth.

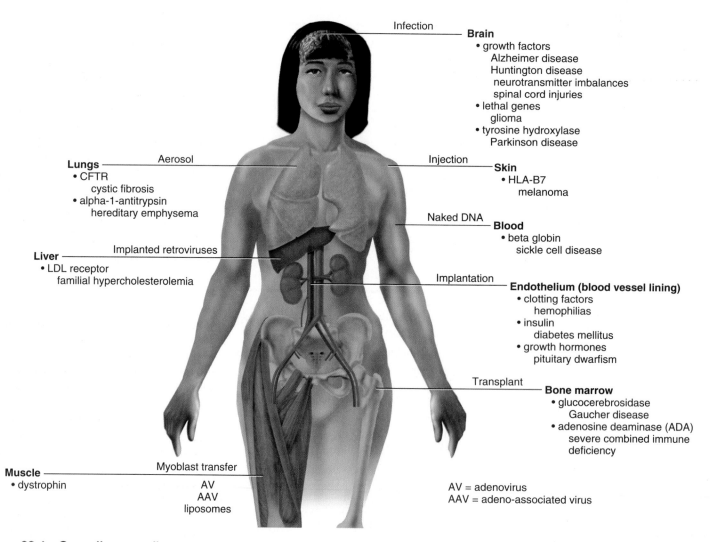

Figure 20.4 Gene therapy sites. Beneath the label for each site are listed the targeted protein (•) and then the disease.

Canavan Disease: Patients Versus Patents

When Debbie Greenberg gave birth to Jonathan in 1981, she and her husband Dan had no idea that they would one day be leading the first effort to challenge how a researcher and a hospital obtained a patent on a gene. Debbie and Dan first suspected all was not right with Jonathan when he was only three months old. The baby could not control his wobbly head, didn't seem able to maintain eye contact, and could not maneuver his fist into his mouth, a trademark of young babies. By six months of age, when he still was not progressing in attaining motor skills, the Greenbergs finally received a diagnosis for their son—Canavan disease. They were each carriers of the autosomal recessive condition. Although Jonathan would live 11 years, his brain never developed past infancy. The couple had an affected daughter, Amy, a few years after Jonathan was born, and three healthy children.

Shortly after Jonathan's diagnosis, the Greenbergs joined the National Tay-Sachs and Allied Diseases Association, Inc. Both disorders do not have treatments although gene therapy for Canavan disease has had temporary success in a few children. The Greenbergs started a patient support group, the Canavan Foundation, which established a tissue bank that stored blood, urine, and autopsy tissue from affected children. In 1987, the Greenbergs met Dr. Reuben Matalon at a Tay-Sachs screening event in Chicago, and convinced him to begin a search for the Canavan gene. The Greenbergs helped to collect tissue from families from all over the world, which was critical to Dr. Matalon's success in identifying the gene and the causative mutation in 1993, when he was working at Miami Children's Hospital.

Finding the gene made it possible to detect the mutation, which could be used to confirm diagnoses and detect carriers, and in prenatal diagnosis. By 1996, the Canavan Foundation was offering free testing. But unknown to the members of the organization who had donated their childrens' tissues for the gene search, Dr. Matalon and Miami Children's Hospital had filed for a patent on their discovery. The U.S. Patent and Trademark office granted invention number 5,679,635—the Canavan gene—in 1997. A year later, the American College of Obstetricians and Gynecologists advised their physician members to offer carrier testing for Canavan disease to Ashkenazi Jewish patients, because 1 in 40 such women is a carrier. Identifying couples in which both people are carriers would give them the option of avoiding giving birth to affected children, a strategy that has reduced the number of children born with the similar Tay-Sachs disease to nearly zero. That same year, Miami Children's Hospital began to exercise its patent rights by requiring that doctors and diagnostic laboratories charge for a Canavan test. Suddenly, families whose donations—both monetary and biological—had made the discovery of the gene possible had to pay for carrier and prenatal tests. They were outraged.

On November 30, 2000, a group of parents and three nonprofit organizations filed suit in Chicago against Dr. Reuben Matalon and Miami Children's Hospital. The suit does not challenge the patent, but does challenge the way in which it was obtained—in secret, they claim. They wish to recover earnings from the gene test to be turned over to the families who had to pay to offset licensing fees.

The Greenbergs' fight against a disease gene patent not only is a legal precedent, but also sounded a warning bell to other patient groups. As a direct result of the Canavan case, Sharon and Patrick Terry, of Sharon, Massachusetts, started a support group and tissue bank for the disorder their child has—pseudoxanthoma elasticum (PXE), which causes connective tissue to calcify. Like the Greenbergs, the PXE parents supplied their childrens' tissue, but they stipulated that their group be listed as a coinventor on any gene patents. By doing this, the families hope they will be able to retain control over the fate of the gene that they helped discover.

Skin

Like endothelium, skin cells also grow well in the laboratory. A person can donate a patch of skin the size of a letter on this page; after a genetic manipulation, the sample can grow to the size of a bathmat within just three weeks, and the skin can then be grafted back onto the person. Skin grafts can be genetically modified to secrete therapeutic proteins, which may provide a new drug delivery route.

Muscle

Muscle tissue is a good target for gene therapy for several reasons. It comprises about half of the body's mass, is easily accessible, and is near a blood supply. However, it is a challenge to correct enough muscle cells to alleviate symptoms. Consider gene therapy for Duchenne muscular dystrophy (DMD) (see figure 2.1a). An early milestone was to cut the dystrophin gene—about 3 million bases—down to a size small enough to deliver to cells. This was eventually accomplished, and the gene sent into immature muscle cells (myoblasts), but this approach worked only on small sections of muscle. An alternative strategy is to direct stem cells from bone marrow that can naturally migrate to muscle, where they differentiate and produce dystrophin.

Liver

This largest organ in the body is an important candidate for gene therapy because it has many functions and can regenerate. An implant of corrected cells can take over liver function. For the inborn error of metabolism tyrosinemia, for example, effective gene therapy would have to "fix" only about 5 percent of the liver's 10 trillion cells.

Gene therapy to deliver the gene that encodes the LDL receptor can treat familial hypercholesterolemia, discussed in figure 5.2. Recall that when liver cells lack LDL receptors, cholesterol accumulates on artery interiors. Heterozygotes have half the normal number of LDL receptors and suffer heart attacks in early or mid-adulthood. Homozygotes die in childhood. Genetically altering liver cells to produce more LDL receptors can reverse the effects of FH. One young woman who is heterozygous for FH had 15 percent of her liver removed. The cells were isolated and given functional LDL receptor genes, and then redelivered into the body through a major liver vein. Eighteen months later, the grafted liver cells bore more LDL receptors, and the woman's serum cholesterol levels had improved.

Lungs

The respiratory tract is easily accessed with an aerosol spray, eliminating the need to remove, treat, and reimplant cells. Several aerosols to treat cystic fibrosis attempt to replace the defective gene, but so far the correction is short-lived and localized. Another lung disorder that may be treatable with gene therapy is alpha-1-antitrypsin (AAT) deficiency, which causes hereditary emphysema. Absence of the enzyme AAT enables levels of another enzyme, elastase, to accumulate and destroy lung tissue. White blood cells in the lungs normally produce elastase to destroy infecting bacteria, but in AAT deficiency, elastase levels rise too high. Delivering the AAT gene may normalize levels of both enzymes.

Nervous Tissue

Many common illnesses and injuries affect the nervous system, including seizures, strokes, spinal cord injuries, and degenerative disorders such as Alzheimer disease, Parkinson disease, Huntington disease, and amyotrophic lateral sclerosis. Gene therapy on nervous tissue therefore isn't restricted to correcting inherited diseases. If a protein could be used to correct an abnormal situation, then cell implants or gene delivery can possibly heal. However, neurons are difficult targets for gene therapy because they do not divide. Gene therapy efforts can alter other cell types, such as fibroblasts (connective tissue cells), to secrete nerve growth factors or manufacture the enzymes necessary to produce certain neurotransmitters. Then the altered cells can be implanted.

Cancer

About half of current gene therapy trials target cancer. Two promising strategies are **suicide gene therapy** and manipulation of the immune response to create **cancer vaccines.**

Viruses are used to treat a type of brain tumor, called a glioma, that affects a type of neuroglial cell that supports and interacts with neurons. Unlike neurons, neuroglia can divide. Cancerous neuroglia divide very fast, usually causing death within a year. Researchers reasoned that an agent directed against only the dividing cells might halt the cancer. One candidate was a "suicide" gene from the herpes simplex virus. In the presence of a certain drug, activation of the gene kills the cell that contains it. Would cancer cells infected with a virus carrying this gene self-destruct?

Figure 20.5 illustrates the herpes suicide gene therapy system. First, mouse fibroblasts are infected with a retrovirus or adenovirus vector that contains a herpes gene that encodes an enzyme called thymidine kinase. Any cell that produces thymidine kinase is susceptible to the anti-herpes drug ganciclovir. Because a retrovirus can only infect dividing cells, it does not harm nondividing, healthy brain neurons, but does enter cancerous neuroglia. The modified mouse fibroblasts are injected into a person's brain tumor through a hole drilled in the skull. The implanted cells release viruses, which infect neighboring tumor cells, which then produce thymidine kinase. When the patient takes ganciclovir, the drug is changed into a toxin that kills the cancer cells as well as nearby cells in what is called a "bystander effect." A few people have improved with this treatment, but studies on animal cells reveal a chronic immune response to the vectors.

Cancer vaccines enable tumor cells to produce immune system biochemicals or mark tumor cells so that the immune system recognizes them more easily. In one approach, a patient's cancer cells are removed, altered in a way that attracts an immune response, then reimplanted. The tumor cells are altered to overproduce cytokines or HLA cell surface molecules.

Melanoma, a skin cancer, is amenable to cancer vaccine treatment because it is on the body's surface and therefore easily accessible. In one group of experiments, melanoma cells were removed, given genes encoding interleukins, and reimplanted. The genes were then expressed, evoking an immune response. The tumors shrank. In another strategy, researchers inject liposomes bearing genes encoding HLA proteins directly into tumors. **Figure 20.6** describes this approach for an HLA protein called HLA-B7. This protein, when displayed on tumor cell surfaces, stimulates the immune system to respond to the tumor as if it were foreign tissue.

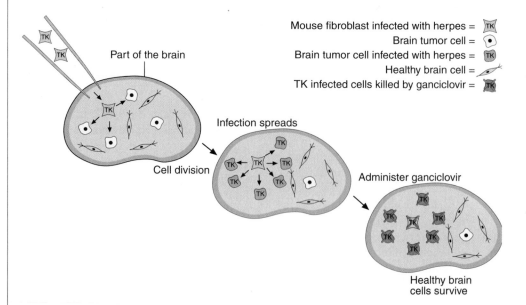

Figure 20.5 A herpes virus attacks cancer. Mouse fibroblasts harboring a thymidine kinase gene from the herpes simplex virus, in a retrovirus vector, are implanted near the site of a brain tumor. The altered viruses infect the rapidly dividing tumor cells. When the patient takes the antiviral drug ganciclovir, the cells producing thymidine kinase are selectively killed, providing a gene-based cancer treatment from within.

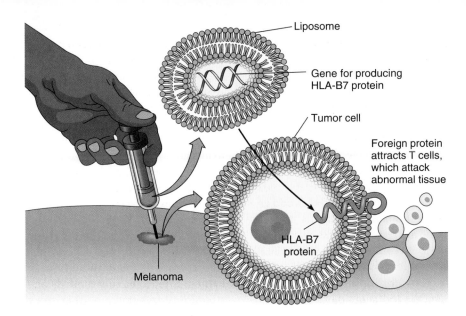

Figure 20.6 Gene therapy for skin cancer. A gene that encodes a cell surface protein that attracts the immune system's tumor-killing T cells is injected directly into a melanoma tumor. (The size of the liposome relative to the tumor cell is greatly exaggerated.)

Gene Delivery

Researchers send foreign DNA into cells in several ways (see table 19.2). Physical methods include electroporation, microinjection, and particle bombardment. Chemical methods include liposomes that enclose the gene cargo and lipid molecules that carry DNA across the plasma membrane. The lipid carrier can penetrate the plasma membrane that DNA alone cannot cross. However, lipid-based methods often fail to deliver a sufficient payload, and gene expression is transient.

One way to improve upon lipid-mediated gene delivery is to link the lipid to a peptide that carries the gene of interest and also binds it to a specific integrin on the target cell. (Recall from chapter 2 that an integrin is a cellular adhesion molecule.) So far this approach has restored enzyme production in the cells of patients with certain lysosomal storage diseases. Another strategy is to alter liposome surfaces so that they resemble viruses that can enter particular cell types.

Biological approaches to gene transfer utilize a vector, which often is a viral genome. Researchers remove the viral genes that cause symptoms or alert the immune system and add the corrective gene. Different viral vectors are useful for different types of experiments. A certain virus may transfer its cargo with great efficiency but carry only a short DNA sequence. Another virus might carry a large piece of DNA but send it to many cell types, causing side effects. Still another virus may not infect enough cells to alleviate symptoms.

Some retroviruses have limited use because they infect only dividing cells. Adenovirus as a vector has been replaced in many clinical trials because of Jesse Gelsinger's reaction to it. **Table 20.3** lists the characteristics of viral vectors used in gene therapy clinical trials.

Researchers choose some viral vectors to suit the cells that are normally infected. For example, adenoviruses used to transport CFTR genes to the airway passages of people with cystic fibrosis normally infect lung tissue. By adding portions of other viruses, researchers can redirect a virus to infect a certain cell type. Adeno-associated virus (AAV), for example, infects many cell types, but adding a promoter from a parvovirus B19 gene restricts infectivity to red blood cell progenitors in bone marrow. Add a human gene that encodes a protein normally found in red blood cells, and the entire vector can treat an inherited disorder of blood, such as sickle cell disease (**figure 20.7**).

Table 20.3

Vectors Used in Gene Therapy

Vector	Characteristics	Applications
Adeno-associated virus (AAV)	Integrates into specific chromosomal site Long-term expression Nontoxic Infects dividing and nondividing cells Carries small genes	Cystic fibrosis Sickle cell disease Thalassemias
Adenovirus (AV)	Large virus, carries large genes Transient expression Evokes immune response Infects dividing and nondividing cells, particularly in respiratory system	Cystic fibrosis Hereditary emphysema
Herpes	Long-term expression Infects neuroglia	Brain tumors
Retrovirus	Stable but imprecise integration Long-term expression Most types infect only dividing cells Nontoxic Most established in clinical experience	Gaucher disease HIV infection Several cancers Severe combined immune deficiency

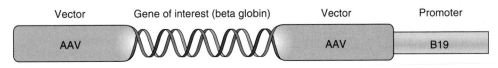

Figure 20.7 Correcting defects in red blood cells. A promoter from a parvovirus B19 gene directs the adeno-associated virus (AAV) genome harboring a human beta globin gene to erythroid progenitor cells, which give rise to cells that mature into red blood cells.

20.3 A Closer Look: Treating Sickle Cell Disease

Sickle cell disease is perhaps the best-studied inherited illness. The molecular defect was identified in 1949. We also understand the precise mutation that causes the disease, how the phenotype arises, and how the globin genes are regulated in the embryo, fetus, and newborn (see figure 11.2). Knowledge of this developmental regulation has led to a unique type of treatment.

Recall from chapter 12 that sickle cell disease is caused by a missense mutation in the beta globin gene that replaces a glutamic acid with valine at the sixth amino acid position (see figure 12.2). The valine protrudes from the otherwise globular molecule, causing it to latch onto other beta globin molecules and form sheets that bend the red blood cell. Then the red blood cell's plasma membrane changes, exposing receptors that glue it to blood vessel linings, rather than deforming and moving along in the circulation. The sickle-shaped, sticky cells lodge in the small passageways of the circulatory system. But all of these changes occur only when the blood is low in oxygen. Blocked circulation causes the acute pain of a sickle cell crisis, affecting different body parts. Impeded circulation in the brain can cause stroke; in the retina, blindness; in the lungs, a painful condition called "acute chest syndrome"; kidney damage; and a persistent state of penile erection called priapism. One boy described the pain of a part of the disease called "hand-foot syndrome" as similar to having his hand crushed in a closing door.

Sickled red blood cells live only 20 days, compared to the normal 120-day lifespan, and as they die, anemia develops. The spleen works overtime to handle the onslaught of dying cells, abandoning its immune functions. Infections ensue. Newborn screening tests detect babies who have inherited sickle cell disease, and prophylactic antibiotic treatment from then on can prevent infections.

Treatments for sickle cell disease have extended the average survival from 14 years in 1973 to more than 50 years today. Transfusions that replace sickled blood and pain medications help patients through crises. Bone marrow transplants are risky, but they have led to complete cures (**figure 20.8**). Experimental gene therapy uses AAV.

A drug, hydroxyurea, prevents sickling by altering the regulation of the globin protein chains. The story began with the observation that people who have "hereditary persistence of fetal hemoglobin" (HPFH) are healthy or have very mild anemia, indicating that fetal hemoglobin does no harm in an adult. Could "turning on" fetal hemoglobin cure sickle cell disease by replacing

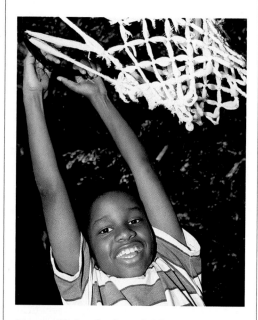

Figure 20.8 Curing sickle cell disease.   Seye Arise was born with sickle cell disease. At a year of age, his hands and feet swelled due to blocked circulation, and he needed frequent transfusions to dilute his sickled red blood cells with normal ones. At age four, he began limping from a stroke. He had a bone marrow transplant, with brother Mayo donating the marrow. Four months later, Seye ran and played for the first time. Bone marrow transplant is 80 percent effective, but carries a 10 percent fatality rate.

the mutant beta chains with normal gamma (fetal) globin chains?

In adults, the gamma genes are normally silenced with methyl groups. A drug that removes the methyl groups might expose the gamma genes, enabling their expression. In 1982, researchers found that a drug called 5-azacytidine indeed removed the methyl groups and raised the proportion of fetal hemoglobin in the blood. But this drug causes cancer. Then, researchers discovered that 5-azacytidine not only removes methyl groups, but is also toxic to (or "stresses") red blood cells. Which effect actually stimulates production of fetal hemoglobin, removing methyls or adding stress? Researchers found that an existing, safer drug, hydroxyurea, stresses red blood cell progenitors. Could it also turn on fetal globin genes?

From 1984 until 1992, experiments in monkeys, healthy people, and sickle cell disease patients showed that hydroxyurea raises fetal hemoglobin levels. A trial began on 299 adults with sickle cell disease to see if this effect improved symptoms—half of the group received the drug, half received a placebo. By 1995, researchers called off the study. The participants receiving the drug were doing so much better than the others that it was unethical to deny the placebo group treatment. The patients receiving hydroxyurea had half the number of crises and needed fewer transfusions than the others. By 2003, mortality among those who had received hydroxyurea was down by 40 percent, presumably because they suffered fewer sickle cell crises.

The way hydroxyurea works involves biology, chemistry, and physics. First, the drug increases the proportion of gamma globin molecules in the blood. Some of the gamma globins bind to mutant beta globins, preventing them from forming the circulation-strangling sheets. This prolongs the time it takes for the mutant beta globin chains to join, simply because gamma chains are now in the mix (**figure 20.9**). The delay is long enough for a red blood cell to return to the lungs. Once the cell picks up oxygen, sickling cannot occur. By slowing the sickling process, hydroxyurea corrects a devastating phenotype.

Teaming hydroxyurea with the kidney hormone erythropoietin (EPO) might work even better because EPO stimulates

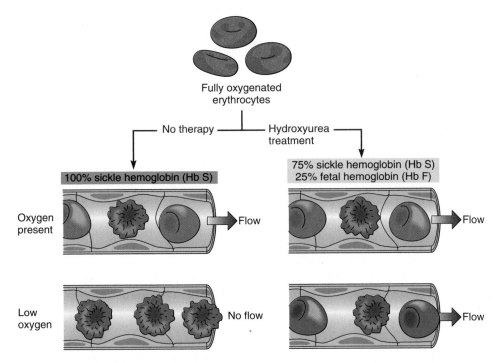

Fully oxygenated
erythrocytes

No therapy ———— Hydroxyurea
treatment

100% sickle hemoglobin (Hb S)

75% sickle hemoglobin (Hb S)
25% fetal hemoglobin (Hb F)

Oxygen
present

Flow

Flow

Low
oxygen

No flow

Flow

Figure 20.9 Reactivating globin genes. Hydroxyurea stimulates production of fetal hemoglobin (Hb F), which dilutes sickled hemoglobin (Hb S). With fewer polymerized hemoglobin molecules, the red blood cells do not bend out of shape as much and can reach the lungs. Oxygen restores the cells' shapes, averting a sickling crisis.

bone marrow to produce more red blood cells (see p. 383, Bioethics: Choices for the Future). Other compounds are also being tested for their ability to reactivate dormant fetal globin genes.

Key Concepts

The more we know about a genetic disease, the more different treatment options we can develop. Conventional gene therapy protocols, as well as a unique approach that reactivates fetal hemoglobin genes, are being applied to treat sickle cell disease.

20.4 Genetic Screening and Genetic Counseling

Despite setbacks in gene therapy experiments, thousands of people have already participated in clinical trials. Given the wealth of information from the sequencing of the human genome, gene therapies are likely to become more common. Until recently, however, most medical professionals received very limited training in genetics. Bridging the gap as human genetics becomes increasingly clinical is a small group of health care professionals, **genetic counselors.** In the United States, about 2,200 genetic counselors have masters degrees in the field. Physicians, nurses, social workers, and PhD geneticists also provide genetic counseling.

Since the 1970s, genetic counselors have led the way in explaining single gene disease inheritance patterns and recurrence risks to patients, with the goal of reducing anxiety through knowledge. Their role is expanding to embrace multifactorial disorders, such as cancer and cardiovascular disease. Genetic counselors work in medical centers, clinics, hospitals, biotechnology companies, pharmaceutical companies, research and diagnostic testing laboratories, and medical practices. Other healthcare workers incorporate genetics into their practices. One survey of hospitals, clinics, geriatric facilities, and schools found that 70 percent of dietitians, social workers, physical therapists, psychologists, occupational therapists, audiologists, and speech-language pathologists regularly discuss genetic principles with their patients.

Genetic Counselors Provide Diverse Services

The knowledge that genetic counselors share with their patients reflects what you have read so far in this book, but counselors present this information in a personalized manner. A genetic counselor might explain Mendel's laws, but substitute the particular family's situation for the pea plant experiments.

A genetic counseling session begins with a discussion of the family's health history. Using a computer program or pencil and paper, the counselor derives a pedigree, then explains the risks of recurrence for particular family members for their particular inherited illness (**figure 20.10**). The counselor provides detailed information on the condition and refers the family to support groups. If a couple wants to have a biological child who does not have the illness, a discussion of assisted reproductive technologies (see chapter 21) might be in order.

A large part of the genetic counselor's job is to determine when specific biochemical, gene, or chromosome tests are appropriate, and to arrange for people to take the tests (**table 20.4**). In addition, certain tests for newborns, mandated by law, are conducted on a small blood sample taken from the heels of newborns (**table 20.5**). The counselor interprets test results and helps the patient or

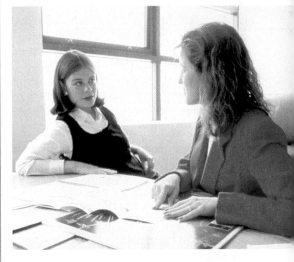

Figure 20.10 Genetic counselors provide genetic information. A genetic counseling session may include an analysis of the family's health history, calculations of the risk of recurrence of an inherited disease, and explanation of appropriate genetic tests and assisted reproductive technologies.

Table 20.4

Types of Genetic Screening Tests

Type	Examples
Prenatal	Amniocentesis, chorionic villus sampling, maternal serum markers, ultrasound for detection of increased risk for certain trisomies and neural tube defects
Newborn screening	Sickle cell disease, PKU, maple syrup urine disease
Carrier screening	Heterozygote tests for cystic fibrosis, sickle cell disease, Tay-Sachs disease, thalassemia
Inherited predisposition	Breast and ovarian cancer genes *BRCA1* and *BRCA2*
Characterizing tumor type	Breast cancer variant *Her-2/neu* indicating patient may respond to monoclonal antibody-based drug Herceptin
Diagnosis of genetic disease to confirm physical exam	Inborn errors of metabolism, muscular dystrophies, DNA repair disorders, inherited anemias, neurofibromatosis, Prader-Willi syndrome, Tay-Sachs disease, movement disorders
Predictive testing for adult-onset Mendelian disorder	Huntington disease
Identity	Paternity testing, forensics to identify bodies

family choose among medical options. Genetic counselors are also often asked to provide information on drugs that can cause birth defects, although this really is related to development, not genetics.

Counseling prospective parents on genetic issues is different from working with families dealing with a specific inherited disease. Prenatal genetic counseling is typically a straightforward analysis of population (empiric) and family-based risks, an explanation of tests, and a determination of whether or not the benefits of testing outweigh the risks. The family decides how to proceed, and, happily, most of the time, amniocentesis, chorionic villus sampling, or maternal serum screening indicates no detectable problem or increased risk. A genetic counselor must explain that tests do not guarantee a healthy baby. For example, many people assume that amniocentesis checks every gene, when it actually is limited to detecting large-scale chromosome aberrations. Single-gene tests must be requested separately. If a test reveals that the fetus has a serious medical condition, the counselor discusses possible outcomes, treatment plans, and the options of ending the pregnancy or treating an ill newborn.

Counseling when there is an inherited disease in a family is another matter. For recessive disorders, the affected individual is usually a child, whose condition often came as quite a surprise. Counseling for subsequent pregnancies requires great sensitivity and sometimes a little bit of mind reading. Many people will not terminate a pregnancy when the fetus has a condition that already affects their living child. Genetic counselors must respect these feelings, and tailor the options discussed accordingly. Counseling for adult-onset disorders may include helping a patient decide whether to take a predictive test, such as that for Huntington disease. Predictive tests are introducing a new type of patient, the "genetically unwell"—those with mutant genes but no symptoms.

Until recently, genetic counseling was "nondirective," meaning that the practitioner did not offer an opinion or suggest a course of action, but only presented options. That approach is changing as the field moves from analyzing single-gene disorders, to considering inherited susceptibilities to more common illnesses that are more likely to have treatments. A recent definition of the role of the genetic counselor is "shared deliberation and decision-making between the counselor and the client." Although genetic counselors educate physicians on genomic medicine, some are concerned that their expertise is being ignored in other situations, such as web sites that offer direct-to-consumer genetic

tests, and diagnostic testing companies that use nurses with limited training in genetics to counsel patients who take the tests, such as for cancer-predisposing mutations.

Scene from a Sickle Cell Disease Clinic

To get an idea of the diversity of skills a genetic counselor must develop, imagine a family with a newborn child who has sickle cell disease. The family might first meet the counselor a few days after the child's birth, when the state-mandated newborn screening test detects the mutation. The counselor talks about the switch from fetal to adult hemoglobin, explaining why the newborn will be healthy for about six months. This might help the family to understand why the child will be started on antibiotics to prevent infection several weeks before the six-month mark. The counselor refers the family to support groups and provides as much information as the family seeks.

After explaining autosomal recessive inheritance, the counselor draws a pedigree, indicating which other individuals might be carriers and suggesting that the parent's siblings be tested. Often the hardest information to communicate is the risk to subsequent children. Many people assume that if one child has sickle cell disease, the next three will be healthy. Probability doesn't work this way. Each conception is a separate event.

The genetic counselor will probably meet with the family during future pregnancies to review the mode of inheritance and recurrence risk. Parents may want to test the fetus, to see if it has inherited the disease. Perhaps the affected child will be a candidate for a bone marrow or cord blood stem cell transplant if a sibling is healthy and compatible as a donor—the counselor can explain these risky procedures and help make plans. The counselor becomes a source of information and a liaison between the growing family and the staff of the medical center.

Genetic Counseling Quandaries and Challenges

Because genetic counseling is based on communication, misunderstandings and tough situations involving confidentiality can arise. Because genetic counselors are human, they

Table 20.5

Newborn Screening Tests

Disease	Incidence	Symptoms	Treatment
Biotinidase deficiency	1/70,000 Rare in blacks or Asians	Convulsions, hair loss, hearing loss, vision loss, developmental abnormalities, coma, sometimes death	Most physical symptoms reversed by oral biotin
Maple syrup urine disease	1/250,000–300,000 More common in blacks and Asians	Lethargy, mental retardation, urine smells sweet, irritable, vomiting, coma, death by age one month	Diet very low in overproduced amino acids
Congenital adrenal hyperplasia	1/12,000 whites 1/15,000 Jews 1/680 Yupik eskimos	Masculinized female genitalia, dehydration, precocious puberty in males, accelerated growth, short stature, ambiguous sex characteristics	Hormone replacement, surgery
Congenital hypothyroidism	1/3,600–5,000 whites Rare in blacks, more common in Hispanics	Mental retardation, growth failure, hearing loss, underactive thyroid, neurological impairment	Hormone replacement
Galactosemia	1/60,000–80,000	Muscle weakness, cerebral palsy, seizures, mental retardation, cataracts, liver disease	Galactose-free diet
Homocystinuria	1/50,000–150,000	Blood clots, thin bones, mental retardation, seizures, muscle weakness, mental disturbances	Low-methionine, high-cysteine diet, drugs
Phenylketonuria (PKU)	1/10,000–25,000	Mental retardation	Low phenylalanine diet
Sickle cell and other hemoglobinopathies	1/400 U.S. blacks	Joint pain, severe infection, leg ulcers, delayed maturation	Prophylactic antibiotics

risk revealing their opinions or feelings. Consider the following true examples:

- A couple has suffered several miscarriages, then have a child with multiple problems. A chromosome check finds that the father carries a translocation. The man's siblings may also carry the translocated chromosome, but the couple does not want to tell anyone the test result.

- A man and woman have the same autosomal recessive form of blindness but want to have children, even though they know that the children will be blind because they, too, will be homozygous recessive. A genetic counselor suggests adoption or intrauterine insemination by a donor. The couple considers this suggestion a value judgment on their choice to have a child.

- Mr. and Mrs. Gold know that their mildly retarded son has a chromosomal deletion. A questionnaire from the special education department in their school district asks if he's ever had a chromosome test. If the parents answer yes, their child may be stigmatized. If they answer no, he may not get appropriate support. They do not know what to do.

- A couple has a child with PKU. It costs $8,000 a year to supply the special diet that prevents her from becoming mentally retarded. The woman becomes pregnant again. A prenatal test to detect PKU costs $1,200. Insurance will not cover the cost of the test, nor will it pay to feed a second child with PKU. The couple elect not to have more children.

- A subway driver has familial hypercholesterolemia. Although he has chest pains and high blood pressure and serum cholesterol, he has never had a heart attack. He knows that he may suddenly die, but he won't tell the transportation department because he is retiring in a few months. The genetic counselor knows the diagnosis.

Perspective: A Slow Start, New Complications, But Great Promise

Medical genetics is no longer just the realm of a few physician specialists, genetic counselors, and the families that have conditions so rare that they are called "orphan" diseases. As we begin to understand precisely how genes control the functioning of the human body, genetic testing, counseling, and therapy will likely become routinely applied to common as well as rare disorders. But it has been a long time in coming.

When the age of gene therapy dawned in the 1990s, expectations were high—and for good reason. Work in the 1980s had clearly shown abundant, pure, human biochemicals, useful as drugs, could come from transgenic organisms. It was merely a matter of time, researchers speculated, before genetic altering of our own somatic tissue would treat a variety of ills.

In reality, gene therapy progress has been painstakingly slow. Boys with Duchenne muscular dystrophy who receive myoblasts with healthy dystrophin genes do not walk again. Instead, they might be able to wiggle a toe for a time. People with cystic fibrosis who sniff viruses bearing the CFTR gene do not permanently breathe easier, but might feel relief for a few weeks. Jesse Gelsinger, and the two boys whose SCID gene therapy caused leukemia, demonstrate that delivered genes do not always go where intended.

The sequencing of the human genome has not provided a list of new gene defects to correct—many of the disease-causing genes were already known—but instead has revealed a complexity to genome structure and function that will impact gene therapy. Consider the fact that copies of the same exon can be parts of different genes. Targeting an exon because it is part of one gene may affect others, healing one set of symptoms while unexpectedly causing some other problems. As researchers continue to identify gene functions, this risk should lessen.

Discovery of RNA interference, discussed in chapter 11, may also throw a wrench into the basic idea of gene therapy. That is, correcting a genetic mistake in the nucleus may not counter a disease phenotype because of what may happen in the cytoplasm—the mRNA transcribed from the delivered gene may be silenced before the needed protein is even synthesized. Yet another area of uncertainty is the issue of somatic versus germline gene therapy. It is remotely possible for a corrected gene targeted to a particular tissue to find its way, in the circulation, to the reproductive tract, enter a gamete, and thereby affect the next generation.

Despite these drawbacks—real and theoretical—at a molecular and cellular level, gene therapy *is* working. The patients with muscular dystrophy, cystic fibrosis, and SCID have cells that have accepted and expressed therapeutic genes. The challenge now is to find just the right vector to deliver a sustained, targeted, and safe genetic correction without alerting the immune system.

Key Concepts

A genetic counselor provides information to individuals, couples, and families on modes of inheritance, recurrence risks, genetic tests, and treatments. The counselor helps make decisions while being sensitive to individual choices. Gene therapy has been in development for many years.

Summary

20.1 Gene Therapy Successes and Setbacks

1. Protein supplementation, from donors and then from recombinant DNA technology, preceded gene therapy.

2. **Gene therapy** replaces malfunctioning genes.

3. Gene therapy for ADA deficiency began with enzyme replacement, then gene therapy in white blood cells, then gene therapy in progenitor cells that could better replace affected cells.

4. Two children developed leukemia from gene therapy to treat SCID. A death in a gene therapy trial for OTC deficiency was due to an immune system response to the viral genome used to introduce the gene.

5. Gene therapy for Canavan disease enables brain neurons to produce a missing enzyme.

20.2 The Mechanics of Gene Therapy

6. *Ex vivo* **gene therapy** is applied to cells outside the body that are then reimplanted or reinfused into the patient. *In situ* **gene therapy** occurs directly on accessible body parts. *In vivo* **gene therapy** is applied in the body.

7. Hereditary hemochromatosis is treated by having blood removed.

8. **Germline gene therapy** affects gametes or fertilized ova, affects all cells of an individual, and is transmitted to future generations. It is not performed in humans.

9. **Somatic gene therapy** affects somatic tissue and is not passed to offspring.

10. Gene therapy delivers new genes and encourages production of a needed substance at appropriate times and in therapeutic (not toxic) amounts.

11. Several types of vectors are used in gene therapy, including liposomes and viral genomes.

20.3 A Closer Look: Treating Sickle Cell Disease

12. We know the mutation that causes sickle cell disease, how the phenotype arises, and how the globin genes are developmentally regulated.

13. In addition to genes delivered on vectors, drugs to reactivate fetal globin genes can treat sickle cell disease.

20.4 Genetic Screening and Genetic Counseling

14. **Genetic counselors** provide information on inheritance patterns, disease risks and symptoms, and available tests and treatments.

15. Prenatal counseling and counseling a family coping with a particular disease pose different challenges.

Review Questions

1. What are the three stages of the evolution of treatments for single-gene disorders?

2. Describe how a gene therapy works to treat
   a. ADA deficiency.
   b. ornithine transcarbamylase deficiency.
   c. Canavan disease.
   d. sickle cell disease.

3. What are two challenges in providing gene therapy for Duchenne muscular dystrophy?

4. Explain the differences among *ex vivo, in situ,* and *in vivo* gene therapies. Give an example of each.

5. Would somatic gene therapy or germline gene therapy have the potential to affect evolution? Explain your answer.

6. What factors would a researcher consider in selecting a viral vector for gene therapy?

7. Why is a bone marrow transplant from a healthy child to a sibling with sickle cell disease technically not gene therapy, while removing an affected child's bone marrow and replacing the mutant gene with a normal one in particular cells is gene therapy?

8. Why is it easier to "fix" a liver with gene therapy than to treat a muscle disease?

9. Gene therapies for Duchenne muscular dystrophy have used AV, AAV, and liposomes. Explain how each approach works.

Applied Questions

1. Magazine articles sometimes portray gene therapy as if it were a brand new idea. How inaccurate is this view?

2. A lentivirus is a rare type of retrovirus that can infect nondividing cells, therefore widening its applicability as a gene therapy vector. HIV is a lentivirus that is being evaluated in a disabled form as a vector for gene therapy. What would have to be done to it to make this feasible?

3. Researchers have discovered that red blood cells from people with sickle cell disease hold oxygen longer when exposed to nitric oxide in a test tube. How can this observation be used to develop a new treatment for sickle cell disease?

4. Parkinson disease is a movement disorder in which neurons in a part of the brain called the substantia nigra can no longer produce the neurotransmitter dopamine. This neurotransmitter is not a protein. What are two difficulties in developing gene therapy for Parkinson disease?

5. Create a gene therapy by combining items from the three lists below. Describe the condition to be treated, and how a gene therapy might correct the symptoms.

Cell Type	Vector	Disease Target
fibroblast	AV	Duchenne muscular dystrophy
skin cell	AAV	Alzheimer disease
neuroglial cell	retrovirus	sickle cell disease
red blood cell progenitor	liposome	cystic fibrosis
myoblast	herpes virus naked DNA	glioma melanoma

6. Genes can be transferred into the cells that form hair follicles. Would gene therapy to treat baldness most likely be *ex vivo, in situ,* or *in vivo*? Cite a reason for your answer.

7. Suggest three specific ways to use protein or gene therapy to treat sickle cell disease.

8. Why might a gene therapy for Canavan disease be more likely to pass requirements of a bioethics review board than the trial that Jesse Gelsinger took part in?

Web Activities

9. Use OMIM to identify a disease that might be treated with gene therapy, and describe how the therapy would work.

10. How would you, as a genetic counselor, handle the following situations (all real)? (You might have to consult past chapters for specific information.)

    a. A couple in their early forties is expecting their first child. Amniocentesis indicates that the fetus is XXX, which might never have been noticed without the test. When they learn of the abnormality, the couple asks to terminate the pregnancy.

    b. A couple's two sons have Duchenne muscular dystrophy. They want to have a third child, but would like it to be a girl, so that she could not inherit this illness.

    c. A 25-year-old woman gives birth to a baby with trisomy 21 Down syndrome. She and her husband are shocked—they thought that this could only happen to a woman over the age of 35.

    d. Two people of normal height have a child with achondroplastic dwarfism, an autosomal dominant trait. They are concerned that subsequent children will also have the condition.

    e. A newborn has a medical condition not associated with any known gene mutation or chromosomal aberration. The parents want to sue the genetics department of the medical center because the amniocentesis did not indicate a problem.

Case Studies

11. Two women are in the hospital suffering from emphysema. Linda, 20 years old, does not smoke. She has battled the condition all her life—she has an inherited form of emphysema called alpha-1-antitrypsin deficiency. She knows that she is unlikely to survive to see her thirtieth birthday. Linda's roommate in the hospital, Bernice, is also struggling to breathe with emphysema. She is 58 years old and developed the condition from smoking since age 16. A pair of lungs becomes available for transplant, and they match the tissue types of both Linda and Bernice. If Linda has the transplant, the new lungs will eventually become diseased, because her underlying enzyme deficiency is still present. Still, she could gain a decade of life. If the lungs go to Bernice, they would likely stay healthy, as long as she does not smoke —which she is not certain she can do. What criteria should the transplant and bioethics teams consider to decide who receives the lungs?

12. Three-year-old Tawny Fitzgerald has been to the emergency department four times in her short life, for broken bones. At the last visit, a nurse questioned Tawny's parents, Donald and Rebecca, about possible child abuse. No charges were filed—the child just appeared to be clumsy. Then Tawny's brother Winston was born. When he was six months old, Donald found him screaming in pain one morning. A trip to the hospital revealed a broken arm. This time, a social worker was sent to the Fitzgerald home. Donald and Rebecca were interviewed in great depth and advised to find a lawyer. A relative in medical school suggested that they have the children examined for osteogenesis imperfecta, also known as "brittle bone disease."

    Consult OMIM and list the facts about a form of this condition that could affect both sexes, with carrier parents. If you were the genetic counselor hired to help this couple, what would you ask them, and tell them, to help them deal with the legal and social services authorities who might need a biology lesson?

Learn to apply the skills of a genetic counselor with these additional cases found in the *Case Workbook in Human Genetics:*

Gene doping

Hemophilia B

Newborn screening

Suggested Readings

Bennett, Robin L., et al. November 2003. Genetic counselors: translating genomic science into clinical practice. *The Journal of Clinical Investigation* 112(9):1274–79. Genetic counselors help physicians and patients apply knowledge about the human genome.

Claster, Susan and Elliott P. Vichinsky. November 15, 2003. Managing sickle cell disease. *The British Medical Journal* 327:1151–55. Treatments have greatly extended the lives of people with sickle cell disease.

Check, Erika. December 19/26, 2002. Shining hopes dented—but not dashed. *Nature* 420:735. Cancer is a rare side effect of gene therapy.

Cohen, Hal. October 14, 2002. Gene therapy marches forward. *The Scientist* 16(20):24. Despite setbacks, many gene therapy trials have continued.

Holtzman, Neil A. November 19, 2003. Expanding newborn screening—how good is the evidence? *The Journal of the American Medical Association* 290:2606–08. Expansion of newborn screening may increase parental anxiety.

Juengst, Eric T. June 28, 2003. What next for human gene therapy? *The British Medical Journal* 326:1410–11. Human genome sequence information reveals a complexity that will impact how likely gene therapy is to work.

Lewis, Ricki. October 20, 2003. Genetic testing timeline. *The Scientist* 17(18):23. Population screening for Tay-Sachs and sickle cell diseases paved the way for testing for cystic fibrosis and Huntington disease today.

Lewis, Ricki. October 20, 2003. A genetic checkup: Lessons from Huntington disease and cystic fibrosis. *The Scientist* 17(18):24–26. Screening for single-gene disorders is helping researchers plan future screens for complex conditions.

Lewis, Ricki. April 11, 2002. Hereditary hemochromatosis: Too soon for genetic testing? *The Scientist* 16(8):22. Many people who inherit the genotype for this disorder do not develop the phenotype.

Mannucci, Pier M., and Edward G. D. Tuddenham. June 7, 2001. The hemophilias—From royal genes to gene therapy. *The New England Journal of Medicine* 344 (23):1773–79.

Steinberg, Douglas. September 17, 2001. Gene therapy targets Canavan disease. *The Scientist* 15(18):20–21. Sending genes into the brain aboard a virus may seem like an extreme treatment, but for children with this disease, it is the only option.

Weiner, Debra L., and Carlo Brugnara. April 2, 2003. Hydroxyurea and sickle cell disease: A chance for every patient. *The Journal of the American Medical Association* 289:1692–94. Treatment for an inherited disease need not be complex.

Weekly updates of current news related to human genetics are available through Power Web on your Online Learning Center.

VISIT YOUR ONLINE LEARNING CENTER

Visit your online learning center for additional resources and tools to help you master this chapter. See us at

www.mhhe.com/lewisgenetics6.

Reproductive Technologies

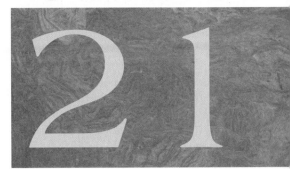

CHAPTER CONTENTS

21.1 Infertility and Subfertility
The male and female reproductive systems are each a series of tubes and associated structures. Blockages, abnormalities, and incompatibilities can disrupt the precise interactions necessary for sperm to approach, meet, and merge with an oocyte, kickstarting development. For one in six couples, something goes wrong, but most problems can be treated.

21.2 Assisted Reproductive Technologies
Technology and generous people can help others to have children. Gametes and embryos can be donated, uteruses borrowed, and early embryos screened for chromosomal problems.

21.3 On the Subject of "Spares"
In vitro fertilization usually generates extra fertilized ova or early embryos that couples must elect to implant, discard, donate to infertile couples, store, or designate for research. Although studying these embryos is revealing new facts about early human development, many people object to using human embryos in research.

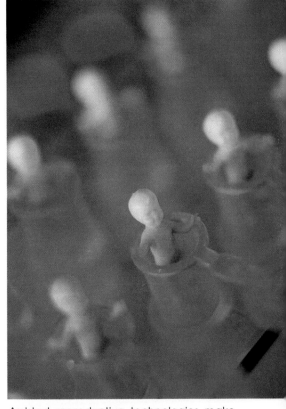

Assisted reproductive technologies make headlines and may seem more like science fiction when they are new, but they produce normal children—more than a million have been born following *in vitro* fertilization, for example.

A couple in search of an oocyte donor places an ad in a college newspaper seeking an attractive woman under age 30 from an athletic family. A cancer patient has her oocytes stored before undergoing treatment. Two years later, she has several of them fertilized in a laboratory dish with her partner's sperm, and has a cleavage embryo implanted in her uterus. She survives the cancer and becomes a mother. A man paralyzed from the waist down has sperm removed and injected into his partner's oocyte. He, too, becomes a parent when he never thought he would.

Lisa and Jack Nash sought to have a child for a different reason. Their daughter Molly, born on July 4, 1994, had Fanconi anemia, an autosomal recessive condition that would destroy her bone marrow, severely impairing her immunity. An umbilical cord stem cell transplant from a sibling could likely cure her, but Molly had no siblings. Nor did her parents wish to conceive a child with a 1 in 4 chance of also inheriting the disorder, as Mendel's first law dictates. Technology offered another solution.

In late 1999, researchers at the Reproductive Genetics Institute at Illinois Medical Center mixed Jack's sperm with Lisa's oocytes in a laboratory dish. After allowing 15 of the fertilized ova to develop to the 8-cell stage, researchers then separated and applied DNA probes to one cell from each embryo. A cell that had a normal Fanconi anemia allele and that matched Molly's human leukocyte antigen (HLA) type was identified and its 7-celled counterpart implanted into Lisa's uterus. Adam was born in late summer, and a month later, physicians infused his umbilical cord stem cells into his sister, saving her life (**figure 21.1**). The Nash's journey wasn't easy—they began treatment in 1995, suffered several miscarriages, then faced media scrutiny for their action. Other similar cases have followed.

Increased knowledge of how the genomes of two individuals come together and interact has spawned several novel ways to have children. **Assisted reproductive technologies** replace the source of a male or female gamete, aid fertilization, or provide a uterus. These procedures, developed to treat infertility, are becoming a part of genetic screening, a role that will likely increase with the influx of human genome information.

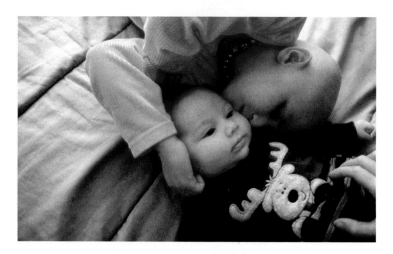

Figure 21.1 Special siblings. Adam Nash was conceived and selected to save his sister's life. But he is also a much-loved sibling and son. Several other families have followed the Nash's example in conceiving one child to help another. Criticism has faded.

21.1 Infertility and Subfertility

Infertility is the inability to conceive a child after a year of frequent intercourse without the use of contraceptives. Some specialists use the term *subfertility* to distinguish those individuals and couples who can conceive unaided, but for whom this may take longer than usual. On a more personal level, infertility is a seemingly endless monthly cycle of raised hopes and crushing despair. In addition, as a woman ages, the incidence of pregnancy-related problems rises, including chromosomal anomalies, fetal deaths, premature births, and low-birthweight babies. For most conditions, the man's age does not raise the risk of pregnancy complications.

Physicians who specialize in infertility treatment can identify a physical cause in 90 percent of cases. Of these, 30 percent of the time the problem is primarily in the male, and 60 percent of the time it is primarily in the female. However, for cases in which a physical problem is not obvious, the cause is usually a mutation or chromosomal aberration that impairs fertility in the male. The statistics are somewhat unclear, because in 20 percent of the 90 percent, both partners have a medical condition that could contribute to infertility or subfertility. A common combination, for example, is a woman with an irregular menstrual cycle and a man with a low sperm count.

One in six couples has difficulty in conceiving or giving birth to children. **Table 21.1** summarizes causes of subfertility and infertility.

Male Infertility

Infertility in the male is easier to detect but sometimes harder to treat than female infertility. One in 25 men is infertile. Some men have difficulty fathering a child because they produce fewer than the average 120 million sperm cells per milliliter of ejaculate, a condition called oligospermia that has several causes. If a low sperm count is due to a hormonal imbalance, administering the appropriate hormones may boost sperm output. Sometimes a man's immune system produces IgA antibodies that cover the sperm and prevent them from binding to oocytes. Male infertility can also be due to a varicose vein in the scrotum. This enlarged vein produces too much heat near developing sperm, and they cannot mature. Surgery can remove a scrotal varicose vein.

Until recently, no cause could be identified for 30 to 40 percent of cases of male infertility. Researchers then discovered that many of these men have small deletions of the Y chromosome that remove the only copies of key genes whose products control spermatogenesis. Clues to this cause of male infertility came from men who cannot make any sperm, and who also have very large Y chromosome deletions. If a deletion is very small, the man may still make some sperm. Other genetic causes of male infertility include mutations in genes that encode androgen receptors or protein fertility hormones, or that regulate sperm development or motility. Overall, most cases of male infertility are genetic.

For many men with low sperm counts, fatherhood is just a matter of time: They are

Table 21.1

Causes of Subfertility and Infertility

Men

Problem	Possible Causes	Treatment
Low sperm count	Hormone imbalance, varicose vein in scrotum, possibly environmental pollutants	Hormone therapy, surgery, avoiding excessive heat
	Drugs (cocaine, marijuana, lead, arsenic, some steroids and antibiotics, chemotherapy)	
	Oxidative damage	
	Y chromosome gene deletions	
Immobile sperm	Abnormal sperm shape	Intracytoplasmic sperm injection
	Infection	
	Malfunctioning prostate	Antibiotics
	Deficient apoptosis	Hormones
Antibodies against sperm	Problem in immune system	Drugs

Women

Problem	Possible Causes	Treatment
Ovulation problems	Pituitary or ovarian tumor	Surgery
	Underactive thyroid	Drugs
	Polycystic ovary syndrome	
Antisperm secretions	Unknown	Acid or alkaline douche, estrogen therapy
Blocked fallopian tubes	Infection caused by IUD, abortion, or by sexually transmitted disease	Laparotomy, oocyte removed from ovary and placed in uterus
Endometriosis	Delayed parenthood until the thirties	Hormones, laparotomy

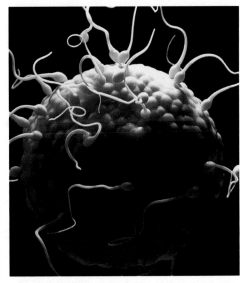

a.

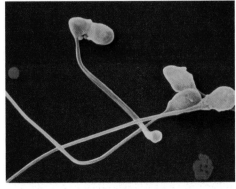

b.

Figure 21.2 Sperm shape and motility are important. **(a)** Healthy sperm in action. **(b)** A misshapen sperm cannot fertilize an oocyte.

subfertile, not infertile. If an ejaculate contains at least 60 million sperm cells, fertilization is likely eventually. To speed conception, a man with a low sperm count can donate several semen samples over a period of weeks at a fertility clinic. The samples are kept in cold storage, then pooled. Some of the seminal fluid is withdrawn to leave a sperm cell concentrate, which is then placed in the woman's reproductive tract. It isn't very romantic, but it is highly effective at achieving pregnancy.

Sperm quality is more important than quantity. Sperm cells that are unable to move—a common problem—cannot reach an oocyte. If the lack of motility is structural, such as sperm tails that are misshapen or missing, or bumps near the sperm head, no treatment is available (**figure 21.2**). If the cause is hormonal, however, replacing the absent hormones can sometimes restore sperm motility.

Hampered sperm motility is also associated with the presence of white blood cells in semen. The blood cells produce toxic compounds called reactive oxygen species, which bind sperm cell plasma membranes and destroy enzymes essential for the reactions within the sperm cell that generate ATP. With too little ATP to supply energy, sperm cannot move effectively. Fertility declines. Clinical trials are underway to test antioxidants to treat this form of male infertility.

Faulty apoptosis (programmed cell death) can also cause male infertility. Apoptosis selectively kills abnormally shaped sperm. Studies show that men with high percentages of abnormally shaped sperm often have cell surface molecules that indicate impaired apoptosis.

Female Infertility

Female infertility can be caused by abnormalities in any part of the reproductive system (**figure 21.3**). Many women with subfertility or infertility have irregular menstrual cycles, making it difficult to pinpoint when conception is most likely. In an average menstrual cycle of 28 days, ovulation usually occurs around the 14th day after menstruation begins, and this is when a woman is most likely to conceive.

For a woman with regular menstrual cycles who is under 30 years old and not using birth control, pregnancy typically happens within three or four months. A woman with irregular menstrual periods can use an ovulation predictor test, which detects a peak in the level of a certain hormone that precedes ovulation by a few hours, or record her

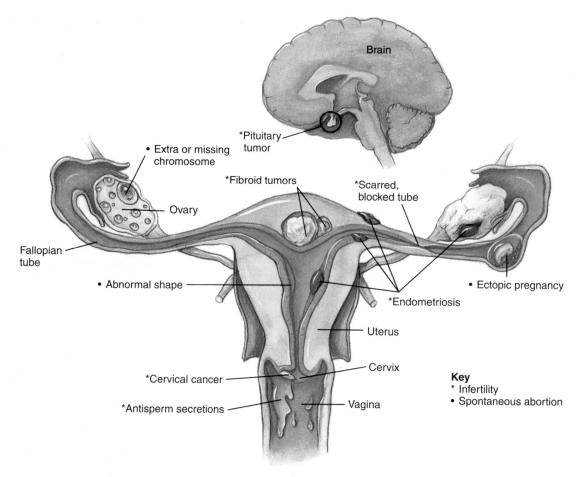

Figure 21.3   Sites of reproductive problems in the human female.

body temperature each morning using a special thermometer with very fine subdivisions. She can then time intercourse for when she is most likely to conceive. Sperm can fertilize oocytes if they have been in the woman's body for up to five days before ovulation, but can fertilize for only a short time after ovulation.

The hormonal imbalance that usually underlies irregular ovulation has various causes—a tumor in the ovary or in the pituitary gland in the brain that hormonally controls the reproductive system, an underactive thyroid gland, or use of steroid-based drugs such as cortisone. Sometimes a woman produces too much prolactin, the hormone that normally promotes milk production and suppresses ovulation in new mothers. If prolactin is abundant in a nonpregnant woman, she will not ovulate and therefore cannot conceive.

Fertility drugs can stimulate ovulation, but they can also cause women to "superovulate," producing more than one oocyte each month. A commonly used drug, clomiphene, raises the chance of having twins from 1 to 2 percent to 4 to 6 percent. If a woman's ovaries

are completely inactive or absent (due to a birth defect or surgery), she can become pregnant only if she uses a donor oocyte. Ovary transplants have succeeded only between identical twins, or in the same woman if she has ovarian tissue removed before cancer treatment and implanted after.

A common cause of female infertility is blocked fallopian tubes. Fertilization usually occurs in open tubes. Blockage can prevent sperm from reaching the oocyte, or entrap a fertilized ovum, keeping it from descending into the uterus. The embryo begins developing in the tube and if it is not removed and continues to enlarge, the woman can die. This "tubal pregnancy" is called an **ectopic pregnancy.**

Fallopian tubes can also be blocked due to a birth defect or, more likely, from an infection such as pelvic inflammatory disease. A woman may not know she has blocked fallopian tubes until she has difficulty conceiving and medical tests uncover the problem. Surgery can sometimes open blocked fallopian tubes.

Excess tissue growing in the uterine lining may make it inhospitable to an embryo. This tissue can include benign tumors, called **fibroids,** or a condition called **endometriosis,** in which tissue builds up inside and sometimes outside of the uterus. In response to the hormonal cues to menstruate, the tissue bleeds, causing cramps. Endometriosis can make conception difficult, but curiously, once a woman with endometriosis has been pregnant, the cramps and bleeding usually subside.

Sometimes secretions in the vagina and cervix are hostile to sperm. If cervical mucus is unusually thick or sticky, as can happen during infection, sperm become entrapped and cannot move far enough to encounter an oocyte. Vaginal secretions may be so acidic or alkaline that they weaken or kill sperm. For example, some women with cystic fibrosis are unable to secrete bicarbonate from the cells lining their reproductive tracts, which is normally required to activate sperm. Douching daily with an acidic solution such as acetic acid (vinegar) or an alkaline solution, such as bicarbonate, can alter the pH of the vagina so that in some cases it is more receptive to sperm cells. Too little mucus is treated with low daily doses of oral estrogen. Sometimes mucus in a woman's body harbors antibodies that attack sperm. Infertility may also result if the oocyte fails to release sperm-attracting biochemicals.

One reason female infertility increases with age is that older women are more likely to produce oocytes with an abnormal chromosome number, which often causes spontaneous abortion. Losing very early embryos may appear to be infertility because the bleeding accompanying the aborted embryo resembles a heavy menstrual flow. The higher incidence of meiotic errors in older women may occur because their oocytes have been exposed longer to harmful chemicals, viruses, and radiation. In other cases, women are simply prone to producing oocytes with abnormal numbers of chromosomes.

Infertility Tests

A number of medical tests can identify the cause or causes of infertility. The man is checked first, because it is easier, less costly, and certainly less painful to obtain sperm than oocytes.

Sperm are checked for number (sperm count), motility, and morphology (shape). An ejaculate containing up to 40 percent unusual forms is still considered normal, but many more than this can impair fertility. A urologist performs sperm tests. A genetic counselor may also be of help in identifying the cause of male infertility. He or she can interpret the results of a PCR analysis of the Y chromosome to detect deletions associated with lack of sperm. If a male cause of infertility is not apparent, the next step is for the woman to consult a gynecologist, who checks to see that the structures of the woman's reproductive system are present and functioning.

Some cases of subfertility or infertility have no clear explanation. Psychological factors may be at play, or it may be that inability to conceive results from consistently poor timing. Sometimes a subfertile couple adopts a child, only to conceive one of their own shortly thereafter; at other times, the couple's infertility remains a lifelong mystery.

Key Concepts

Male infertility is due to a low sperm count or sperm that cannot swim or are abnormal in structure. • Female infertility can be due to an irregular menstrual cycle or blocked fallopian tubes. Fibroid tumors, endometriosis, or a misshapen uterus may prevent implantation of a fertilized ovum, and secretions in the vagina and cervix may inactivate or immobilize sperm. Oocytes may fail to release a sperm-attracting biochemical. Early pregnancy loss due to abnormal chromosome number may be mistaken for infertility; this is more common among older women. • A variety of medical tests can pinpoint some causes of infertility.

21.2 Assisted Reproductive Technologies

A growing number of couples with fertility problems are turning to alternative ways to achieve pregnancy, many of which were perfected in nonhuman animals. The Technology Timeline on reproductive technologies depicts the chronology for these assisted reproductive technologies.

Donated Sperm— Intrauterine Insemination

The oldest assisted reproductive technology is **intrauterine insemination,** in which a doctor places donated sperm into a woman's reproductive tract, typically the cervix or uterus. The sperm are washed free of seminal fluid, which can inflame female tissues. Her partner may be infertile or carry a gene for an inherited illness that the couple wishes to avoid passing to their child, or a woman may undergo intrauterine insemination if she desires to be a single parent without having sex.

The first intrauterine insemination in humans was done in 1790. For many years, physicians donated sperm, and this became a way for male medical students to earn a few extra dollars. By 1953, sperm could be frozen and stored and intrauterine insemination became much more commonplace. Today, donated sperm is frozen and stored in sperm banks, which provide the cells to obstetricians who perform the procedure.

A couple who chooses intrauterine insemination can select sperm from a catalog that lists the personal characteristics of donors, such as blood type, hair and eye color, skin color, build, and even educational level and interests. Of course, not all of these traits are inherited. If a couple desires a child of one sex—such as a daughter to avoid passing on an X-linked disorder—sperm can be separated by weight into fractions enriched for X-bearing or Y-bearing sperm.

Problems can arise in intrauterine insemination, as they can in any pregnancy. For example, a man who donated sperm years ago developed a late-onset genetic disease, cerebellar ataxia. Eighteen children conceived using his sperm now face a 1 in 2 risk of having inherited the mutant gene. In 1983, the Sperm Bank of California became the first to ask donors if they wished to be contacted by their children years later. In 2002, the first such meeting occurred, evidently quite successfully.

A male's role in reproductive technologies is simpler than a woman's. A man can be a genetic parent, contributing half of his genetic self in his sperm, but a woman can be both a genetic parent (donating an oocyte) and a gestational parent (donating the uterus). Problems can crop up when a second female assists in conception and/or gestation.

A Donated Uterus— Surrogate Motherhood

If a man produces healthy sperm but his partner's uterus is absent or cannot maintain a pregnancy, a **surrogate mother** may help by being inseminated with the man's sperm. When the child is born, the surrogate mother gives the baby to the couple. In this variation of the technology, the surrogate is both the genetic and the gestational mother. Attorneys usually arrange surrogate relationships. The surrogate mother signs a statement signifying her intent to give up the baby, and she is paid for her nine-month job.

The problem with surrogate motherhood is that a woman may not be able to predict her responses to pregnancy and childbirth in the cold setting of a lawyer's office. When a surrogate mother changes her mind about giving up the baby, the

Landmarks in Reproductive Technology

	In Animals	In Humans
1782	Intrauterine insemination in dogs	
1790		Pregnancy reported from intrauterine insemination
1890s	Birth from embryo transplantation in rabbits	Intrauterine insemination by donor
1949	Cryoprotectant successfully freezes animal sperm	
1951	First calf born after embryo transplantation	
1952	Live calf born after insemination with frozen sperm	
1953		First reported pregnancy after insemination with frozen sperm
1959	Live rabbit offspring produced from *in vitro* ("test tube") fertilization (IVF)	
1972	Live offspring from frozen mouse embryos	
1976		First reported commercial surrogate motherhood arrangement in the United States
1978	Transplantation of ovaries from one cow to another	Baby born after IVF in United Kingdom
1980		Baby born after IVF in Australia
1981	Calf born after IVF	Baby born after IVF in United States
1982	Sexing of embryos in rabbits	
	Cattle embryos split to produce genetically identical twins	
1983		Embryo transfer after uterine lavage
1984		Baby born in Australia from frozen and thawed embryo
1985		Baby born after gamete intrafallopian transfer (GIFT)
		First reported gestational surrogacy arrangement in the United States
1986		Baby born in the United States from frozen and thawed embryo
1989		First preimplantation genetic diagnosis (PGD)
1992		First pregnancies from sperm injected into oocytes
1994	Intracytoplasmic sperm injection (ICSI) in mouse and rabbit	62-year-old woman gives birth from donated oocyte
1995	Sheep cloned from embryo cell nuclei	Babies born following ICSI
1996	Sheep cloned from adult cell nucleus	
1998	Mice cloned from adult cell nuclei	Baby born 7 years after his twin
1999	Cattle cloned from adult cell nuclei	
2000	Pigs cloned from adult cell nuclei	
2001		Sibling born following PGD to treat sister for genetic disease
		Human preimplantation embryo cloned, survives to 6 cells
2003		3000^{+} preimplantation genetic diagnoses performed to date

results are wrenching for all. A prominent early case involved Mary Beth Whitehead, who carried the child of a married man for a fee and then changed her mind about relinquishing the baby. Whitehead's ties to "Baby M" were perhaps stronger because she was both the genetic and the gestational mother.

Another type of surrogate mother lends only her uterus, receiving a fertilized ovum conceived from a man and a woman who has healthy ovaries but lacks a functional uterus. The gestational-only surrogate mother turns the child over to the donors of the genetic material.

In Vitro Fertilization

In *in vitro* fertilization (IVF), which means "fertilization in glass," sperm and oocyte join in a laboratory dish. Then the embryo is placed in the oocyte donor's uterus (or another woman's uterus), and, if all goes well, implants into the uterine lining.

Louise Joy Brown, the first "test-tube baby," was born in 1978. Initial media attention was great, with cartoons depicting a newborn with the word "Pyrex," a test-tube and glassware manufacturer, branded on her thigh. Yet Louise was, despite her unusual beginnings, a rather ordinary child. The technology has since led to the births of more than a million children.

A woman might undergo IVF if her ovaries and uterus work but her fallopian tubes are blocked. Using a laparoscope, a physician removes several of the largest oocytes and transfers them to a dish. Just before ovulation, 15 to 20 or so oocytes enlarge, and can be cultured in a dish. If left in the body, only one oocyte would pop out of the ovary, but in a culture, many of them can mature sufficiently to be fertilized *in vitro*. In the past, women took drugs to make them "superovulate" and produce many mature oocytes at once, but this is being phased out. Chemicals that mimic those in the female reproductive tract are added to the culture, and sperm are applied to the oocytes.

If the sperm cannot readily penetrate the oocyte, they may be sucked up into a tiny syringe and microinjected into the female cell. This is called **intracytoplasmic sperm injection** (ICSI), and it is more effective than IVF alone **(figure 21.4)**. ICSI is very helpful for men who have low sperm counts or high percentages of abnormal sperm. The procedure even works with immature sperm, making fatherhood possible for men who cannot ejaculate, such as those who have suffered spinal cord injuries. ICSI has been very successful, performed on thousands of men with about a 30 percent success rate. The Bioethics: Choices for the Future on page 416 considers an unexpected problem with ICSI—transmitting infertility.

A day or so after sperm wash over the oocytes in the dish, or are injected into them, some of the embryos—balls of 8 or 16 cells—are transferred to the woman's uterus. If the hormone human chorionic gonadotropin appears in her blood a few days later, and its level rises, she is pregnant.

IVF costs from $8,000 to $15,000 per attempt, and the success rate is up to 30 percent. (The cover of a celebrity magazine featured a well-known actress who had finally had a baby after seven IVF attempts—a cost that clearly very few people can afford.) By contrast, two-thirds of embryos conceived through sexual intercourse implant. The lower success rate of IVF is due both to the difficulty of the procedure and to the fact that couples who choose it have a higher incidence of subfertility or infertility than the general population. Children born following IVF have twice the rate of birth defects (about 9 percent) compared to children conceived naturally, which may also reflect the underlying medical problems of parents. In the past, several embryos were implanted to increase the success rate, but this led to many multiple births. In many cases, embryos had to be removed to make room for others to survive. Section 21.3 considers what to do with extra embryos.

Measures to improve the chance that IVF will culminate in a birth include:

1. Transferring embryos slightly later in development, at the blastocyst stage.

2. Culturing fertilized ova and early embryos with other cells that normally surround the oocyte in the ovary. These "helper" cells provide extra growth factors.

3. Screening early embryos for chromosome abnormalities, and implanting only those with apparently normal karyotypes.

Embryos resulting from IVF that are not soon implanted in the woman are frozen in liquid nitrogen, with cryoprotectant chemicals added to prevent salts from building up or ice crystals from damaging delicate cell parts. Freezing takes a few hours; thawing about a half hour. The longest an embryo has been frozen and then successfully revived is 13 years; the "oldest" pregnancy using a frozen embryo occurred 9 years after the freezing!

Gamete Intrafallopian Transfer

As the world marveled at the miracle of "test-tube" babies, disillusioned couples were learning that IVF is costly, time-consuming, and for years rarely worked. IVF may fail because of the artificial environment for fertilization. A procedure called GIFT, which stands for **gamete intrafallopian transfer,** improves the setting. Fertilization is assisted in GIFT, but it occurs in the woman's body rather than in glassware. Certain religions approve of GIFT, but not IVF, because GIFT preserves more natural reproductive function.

In GIFT, a woman has several of her largest oocytes removed. The man submits a sperm sample, and the most active cells

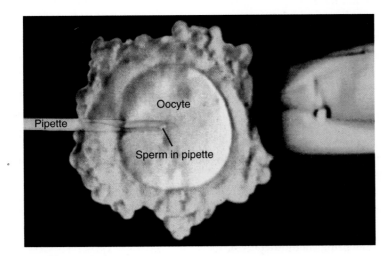

Figure 21.4 ICSI. Intracytoplasmic sperm injection (ICSI) enables some infertile men, men with spinal cord injuries, or men with certain illnesses to become fathers. A single sperm cell is injected into the cytoplasm of an oocyte.

Technology Too Soon? The Case of ICSI

Intracytoplasmic sperm injection (ICSI), available since 1995, has been extremely successful in enabling men with AIDS, paralysis, very low sperm counts, or abnormal sperm to become fathers. The birth defect rate is the same as for normal conceptions, although abnormal embryos and sex chromosome aberrations are slightly more common. But as more ICSI procedures are performed and tests on nonhuman animals continue, potential problems are emerging, based on the fact that ICSI bypasses what one researcher calls "natural sperm selection barriers."

ICSI is now commonly used on men who have azoospermia—lack of sperm—or oligospermia—very few sperm. The rare sperm are sampled from an ejaculate or taken from the testes with a needle, then injected into an oocyte. Sometimes these men produce spermatids but not mature sperm, and spermatids that have already elongated can also successfully fertilize oocytes using ICSI. However, a complication has developed that involves not science, but logic. About 10 percent of infertile men have microdeletions in the Y chromosome. When their sperm cells are used in ICSI, they pass on the infertility to their sons. This is true for other causes of infertility and subfertility, too. For example, if a man's above-average proportion of abnormally shaped sperm is due to abnormal apoptosis, he could pass a susceptibility to cancer to his offspring.

Bioethicists are debating whether it is right to intentionally conceive a male who is genetically destined to be infertile. On the positive side is the opportunity ICSI is providing to study that infertility. It is possible that adolescents with microdeleted Y chromosomes can produce viable sperm or spermatids, and if so, these cells can be sampled and stored for later use. In the past, these men would not have suspected that they had Y chromosome abnormalities until they had difficulty fathering children. Alternatives to transmitting deletions and other mutations include selecting and using only X-bearing sperm in ICSI, or selecting and implanting only female fertilized ova. Because of the transmission of Y-linked infertility with ICSI, men undergoing fertility testing and considering the procedure now have their Y chromosomes screened for deletions, and genetic counseling is provided.

Meanwhile, experiments on rhesus monkeys are pinpointing the sources of damage to those ICSI embryos that do not continue to develop:

- Injecting sperm at the site of the polar body on the oocyte can disrupt the meiotic spindle, leading to nondisjunction (an extra or missing chromosome).

- Injected sperm DNA does not always condense properly, also leading to nondisjunction.

- Spermatids that have not yet elongated are often unable to fertilize an oocyte. Culturing them in the laboratory until

they mature may help improve the odds of success.

- Spermatids may not be completely imprinted, leading to problems in gene expression.

- Mitotic cell cycle checkpoints are altered at the first division following ICSI.

- Injected sperm sometimes lack a protein that normally associates with the sex chromosomes. This may explain the elevation in sex chromosome anomalies.

- Injected sperm can include surface proteins normally left outside the oocyte, producing unanticipated effects. They may also include mitochondria from the male.

Despite these largely theoretical concerns, parents of children conceived with ICSI do not have any cause to worry, researchers insist. Tests on these children so far have not revealed any problems. Says one researcher, "In spite of its potential risks, ICSI still seems to be remarkably safe." Still, it would be comforting to some to have more research to back up this new way to start development. Ongoing studies are following the children of ICSI for longer times, and investigating any correlations between health problems in offspring and the cause of subfertility or infertility in the fathers.

---

are separated from it. The collected oocytes and sperm are deposited together in the woman's fallopian tube, at a site past any obstruction that might otherwise block fertilization. GIFT is about 26 percent successful, and costs about half as much as IVF.

A variation of GIFT is ZIFT, which stands for **zygote intrafallopian transfer.** In this procedure, an IVF ovum is introduced into the woman's fallopian tube. Allowing the fertilized ovum to make its own way to the uterus seems to increase the chance that it will implant. ZIFT is 23 percent successful.

Oocyte Banking and Donation

Oocytes can be stored, as sperm are, but the procedure may introduce problems. Candidates for preserving oocytes for later use include:

- Women wishing to have children later in life

- Women undergoing chemotherapy or other toxic or teratogenic treatments

- Women who work with toxins or teratogens

Oocytes are frozen in liquid nitrogen at −30 to −40 degrees Celsius, when they are at metaphase of the second meiotic division. At this time, the chromosomes are aligned along the spindle, which is sensitive to temperature extremes. If the spindle comes apart as the cell freezes, the oocyte may lose a chromosome, which would devastate development. Another problem with freezing oocytes is retention of a polar body, leading to a diploid oocyte.

Alternative approaches try to overcome the difficulty of freezing oocytes. Researchers are developing ways to nurture in the laboratory 1-millimeter-square ovary sections that are packed with oocytes. Laboratory culture of oocytes appears to require a high level of oxygen and a complex combination of biochemicals. One approach that helps women undergoing radiation treatments to the abdomen for cancer is to implant a strip of ovarian tissue beneath the skin of their arms. The oocytes there are easy to retrieve later and are not exposed to the radiation.

Women can also obtain oocytes from donors, typically younger women. Often these women are undergoing IVF and have "extra" harvested oocytes. The potential father's sperm and donor's oocytes are placed in the recipient's uterus or fallopian tube, or fertilization occurs in the laboratory, and an 8- or 16-celled embryo is transferred to the woman's uterus.

The first baby to result from oocyte donation was born in 1984 (**figure 21.5**). The success rate ranges from 20 to 50 percent, and the procedure costs at least $10,000. The technique is useful for the reasons cited for freezing oocytes, as well as to avoid transmitting a disease-causing gene.

Embryo adoption is a variation on oocyte donation. A woman with malfunctioning ovaries but a healthy uterus carries an embryo that results when her partner's sperm is used in intrauterine insemination of a woman who produces healthy oocytes. If the woman conceives, the embryo is gently flushed out of her uterus a week later and inserted through the cervix and into the uterus of the woman with malfunctioning ovaries. The child is genetically that of the man and the woman who carries it for the first week, but is born from the woman who cannot produce healthy oocytes. "Embryo adoption" is also the term used to describe use of IVF "leftovers."

In another technology, **cytoplasmic donation,** older women have their oocytes injected with cytoplasm from the oocytes of younger women to "rejuvenate" the cells. Although resulting children conceived through IVF appear to be healthy, they are being monitored for a potential problem—heteroplasmy, or two sources of mitochondria in one cell. Researchers do not yet know the health consequences of having mitochondria from the donor cytoplasm plus mitochondria from the recipient's oocyte. These conceptions also have an elevated incidence of XO syndrome, which often causes spontaneous abortion. After the birth of the first child from this technique in 2001,

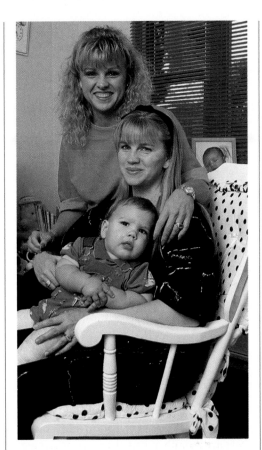

Figure 21.5 Oocyte donation.
Anthony Miceli was born from Vicki Miceli's uterus, but he was conceived when Jerry Miceli's sperm fertilized an oocyte donated by Bonny De Irueste, Vicki's sister (in pink). Says Bonny, "I'm his aunt, that's it." Not all reproductive technologies have such joyous outcomes.

the media made much of the unnatural situation of having three parents—the father, the mother, and the ooplasm donor. The U.S. government has banned this procedure unless it is part of a clinical trial.

Because oocytes are harder to obtain than sperm, oocyte donation technology has lagged behind that of sperm banks, but is catching up. One IVF facility that has run a donor oocyte program since 1988 has a patient brochure that describes 120 oocyte donors of various ethnic backgrounds, like a catalog of sperm donors. The oocyte donors are young and have undergone extensive medical and genetic tests. Recipients may be up to 55 years of age.

Preimplantation Genetic Screening and Diagnosis

Prenatal diagnostic tests such as amniocentesis, chorionic villus sampling, and fetal

cell sorting can be used in pregnancies achieved with assisted reproductive technologies. A test called **preimplantation genetic diagnosis** (PGD) detects genetic and chromosomal abnormalities *before* pregnancy starts. The couple selects a very early embryo—termed a "preimplantation embryo" because it would not normally have yet arrived at the uterus for implantation—that is free of a certain detectable genetic condition. This was the technology used to select Adam Nash, whose umbilical cord stem cells cured his sister's Fanconi anemia (see figure 21.1). PGD has about a 29 percent success rate.

PGD is possible because one cell, or blastomere, can be removed for testing from an 8-celled embryo, and the remaining 7 cells can complete development normally in a uterus. Before the remaining embryo is implanted into the woman, the single cell is karyotyped, or its DNA amplified and probed for particular genes that the parents carry. (Soon it will be possible to quickly scan the entire genome.) Healthy embryos are selected. At first, researchers implanted the remaining seven cells, but they have found that letting the embryo continue developing in the laboratory until day 5, when it is 80 to 120 cells, more often leads to success. Obtaining the cell to be tested is called "blastomere biopsy" (**figure 21.6**). Accuracy is about 97 percent. Errors are generally due to mosaics—when a somatic mutation occurs in a blastomere—or during amplification of blastomere DNA.

The first children who had PGD were born in 1989. In these cases, probes for Y chromosome-specific DNA sequences were used to select female preimplantation embryos, which developed into girls not affected by the X-linked conditions their mothers carried. The conditions avoided included Lesch-Nyhan syndrome (profound mental retardation with self-mutilative behavior) and adrenoleukodystrophy, in which seizures and nervous system deterioration end in sudden death in early childhood. The alternative would have been to risk Mendel's ratios and face the 25 percent chance of conceiving an affected male.

In March 1992, the first child was born who underwent PGD to avoid a specific inherited disease in the family. Chloe O'Brien was checked as an 8-celled preimplantation embryo to see if she had escaped inheriting the cystic fibrosis that affected

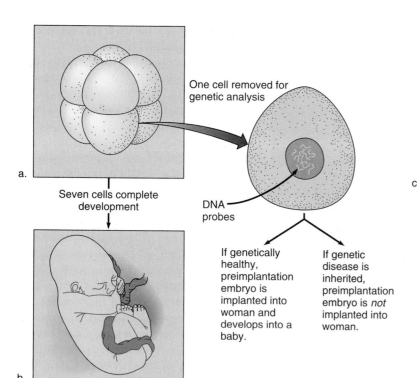

a.

Seven cells complete development

One cell removed for genetic analysis

DNA probes

If genetically healthy, preimplantation embryo is implanted into woman and develops into a baby.

If genetic disease is inherited, preimplantation embryo is *not* implanted into woman.

b.

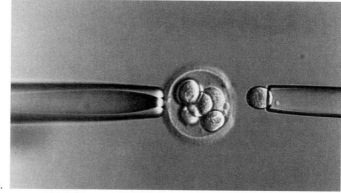

c.

Figure 21.6   Preimplantation genetic diagnosis.
A blastomere biopsy provides material for assessing the health of an embryo. Preimplantation genetic diagnosis probes disease-causing genes or chromosome aberrations in an 8-celled preimplantation embryo. **(a)** A single cell is separated from the ball of cells and tested to see if it contains a disease-causing gene combination or chromosome imbalance. **(b)** If it doesn't, the remaining seven cells, or the embryo after a few more cell divisions, is transferred to the oocyte donor to complete development. **(c)** This preimplantation embryo is held still by suction applied on the left. On the right, a pipette draws up a single blastomere. Fertilization took place 45 hours previously, *in vitro.*

her brother. Since then, PGD has helped to select thousands of children free of several dozen types of inherited illnesses. It has been used for the better-known single-gene disorders as well as for many rare ones. For example, a couple who had lost two children to familial holoprosencephaly used PGD to have a healthy daughter. This condition blocks the separation of the two sides of the brain in the embryo. If the fetus survives to be born, the child may have one giant eye (a cyclops), and usually also has a severe cleft lip and palate and a very small head.

Today, preimplantation genetic diagnosis is increasingly being used to screen fertilized ova and early embryos derived from IVF for chromosome abnormalities before implanting them into women. This quality control of sorts ensures that the implanted embryos will not be spontaneously aborted due to chromosomal abnormalities, increasing the likelihood of success. PGD with IVF is primarily used for older women who have suffered several spontaneous abortions, because they are at higher risk of having oocytes with abnormal numbers of chromosomes. One woman who had undergone several failed IVF attempts had five preimplantation embryos karyotyped. Four were abnormal, yet in different ways. One embryo lacked chromosome 14; one lacked chromosome 4 but had an extra

chromosome 16; a third embryo lacked a chromosome 8 and 9 but had an extra chromosome 1; another had three chromosomes missing and three extra! The couple's remaining embryo became their daughter. Obviously, one parent had very defective meiosis.

Like many technologies, preimplantation genetic diagnosis can introduce a bioethical "slippery slope" when it is used for reasons other than ensuring that a child is free of a certain disease, such as for gender selection. A couple with five sons might, for example, use PGD to select a daughter. But this use of technology might just be a new expression of age-old human nature, according to one physician who performs PGD. "From the dawn of time, people have tried to control the sex of offspring, whether that means making love with one partner wearing army boots, or using a fluorescence-activated cell sorter to separate X and Y bearing sperm. PGD represents a quantum leap in that ability—all you have to do is read the X and Y chromosome paints," he says.

While PGD used solely for family planning is certainly more civilized than placing baby girls outside the gates of ancient cities to perish, the American Society for Reproductive Medicine endorses the use of PGD for sex selection only to avoid passing on an X-linked disease. Yet even PGD to

avoid disease can be controversial. A woman with early-onset familial Alzheimer disease used PGD to select a daughter free of the dominant mutant gene—but that child will have to experience life with her mother's illness. **Table 21.2** summarizes the assisted reproductive technologies.

Key Concepts

In intrauterine insemination, donor sperm is placed in a woman's reproductive tract. • A genetic and gestational surrogate mother is intrauterinally inseminated, becomes pregnant, then gives the baby to the father and his partner. A gestational surrogate mother gestates a baby conceived *in vitro* with gametes from a man and a woman who cannot carry a fetus. • In IVF, sperm and oocyte unite outside the body, and the resulting embryo is transferred to the uterus. Early embryos can also be frozen and used later. • In GIFT, sperm and oocytes are placed in a fallopian tube at a site past a blockage. • In ZIFT, an IVF embryo is placed in a fallopian tube. • Oocytes can be donated. In embryo adoption, an artificially inseminated woman has an early embryo washed out of her uterus and transferred to a woman who lacks oocytes. • PGD removes cells from early embryos and screens them for genetic or chromosomal abnormalities.

Table 21.2

Assisted Reproductive Technologies

Technology	Procedures
Blastomere biopsy	Samples cell from 8-celled embryo and performs genetic or chromosomal test on it.
Embryo adoption	Allows woman to carry embryo of her partner, after his sperm is used for intrauterine insemination of oocyte donor.
Gamete intrafallopian transfer (GIFT)	Deposits collected oocytes and sperm in fallopian tube.
In vitro fertilization	Mixes sperm and oocytes in a laboratory dish, with chemicals to simulate intrauterine environment to encourage fertilization.
Intrauterine insemination	Places or injects washed sperm into the cervix or uterus.
Intracytoplasmic sperm injection	Injects immature or rare sperm into oocyte, before IVF.
Polar body biopsy	Indicates wild type allele in oocyte when specific mutant allele is present in first polar body attached to oocyte from carrier female. IVF can proceed using that oocyte.
Preimplantation genetic diagnosis	Searches for specific mutant allele in sampled cell of 8-celled embryo. Its absence indicates remaining 7-celled embryo can be nurtured and implanted in woman, and child will be free of genetic condition.
Surrogate mother	Allows woman to undergo pregnancy for a female who cannot become or stay pregnant.
Zygote intrafallopian transfer (ZIFT)	Places IVF ovum in fallopian tube.

21.3 On the Subject of "Spares"

In the United States, federal funds cannot be used for research that uses human embryos, and efforts are underway to criminalize such work. As a consequence, most strides in human reproductive research have been funded by patients or companies, or have occurred outside the United States. Nearly half a million embryos derived from IVF have been in U.S. deep freezers for years. These embryos are an obvious source of material for basic research on stem cells. The donors must decide whether to use the embryos, donate them to an infertile couple, allow them to be used in research, or, after a certain time has elapsed, allow them to be discarded.

As government bioethics committees debate manipulating human embryos, privately funded researchers are gleaning information from "spares," the fertilized ova and early embryos that couples choose to discard, donate, or freeze. These glimpses into early human prenatal development sometimes challenge long-held ideas, indicating that we still have much to learn about early human prenatal development. This was the case for a study from Royal Victoria Hospital at McGill University in Montreal. Researchers examined the chromosomes of sperm from a man with Klinefelter (XXY) syndrome. Many of the sperm would be expected to have an extra X chromosome, due to nondisjunction (see figure 13.12), which could lead to a preponderance of XXX and XXY offspring. Surprisingly, only 3.9 percent of the man's sperm had extra chromosomes, but five out of ten of his spare embryos had an abnormal X, Y, or chromosome 18. That is, even though most of the man's sperm were normal, his embryos weren't. The source of reproductive problems in Klinefelter disease, therefore, might not be in the sperm, but in early embryos—a finding that was previously unknown and not expected.

In another study, Australian researchers followed the fates of single blastomeres that had too many or too few chromosomes. They wanted to see whether the abnormal cells preferentially ended up in the inner cell mass, which develops into the embryo, or the trophectoderm, which becomes extraembryonic membranes. The study showed that cells with extra or missing chromosomes become part of the inner cell mass much more frequently than one would expect by chance. This finding indicates that a prediction of a healthy offspring based on preimplantation genetic diagnosis can go awry if a mutation occurs in a cell of the inner cell mass, a case of chromosomal mosaicism that arises after PGD.

Not everyone agrees that fertilized ova or embryos designated for discard should be used in research. With regulations not extending to privately funded research, ethically questionable experiments can happen. For example, researchers reported at a conference that they had mixed human cells from male embryos with cells from female embryos, to see if the normal male cells could "save" the female cells with a mutation. Sex was chosen as a marker because the Y chromosome is easy to detect. But the idea of human embryos with mixed sex parts caused a public outcry.

The major source of fertilized ova and early embryos for research—IVF—will diminish if yet another artificial reproductive technology becomes commonplace. **Polar body biopsy** is based on Mendel's first law, the segregation of alleles. In the technique, if a polar body resulting from the first meiotic division in a woman who is a carrier of an X-linked disorder has the mutant allele, then it is inferred that the oocyte to which it clings lacks that allele. Oocytes that pass this test can then be fertilized in vitro and the resulting embryo implanted in the woman. Polar body biopsy is possible because the polar body is attached to the much larger oocyte. A large pipette is used to hold the two cells in place, and a smaller pipette is used to pluck off the polar body. Then, DNA probes and FISH are used to look at genes and chromosomes in the polar body and infer the genotype of the oocyte (**figure 21.7**). Polar body biopsy followed by PGD is quite effective in avoiding

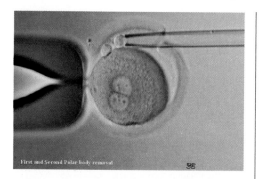

First and Second Polar body removal

Figure 21.7 Polar body biopsy.
The fact that an oocyte shares a woman's divided genetic material with a much smaller companion, the polar body, allows physicians to screen oocytes for use in IVF. If a woman is a known carrier of a genetic disorder and the polar body contains the disease-causing gene variant, it is inferred that the oocyte has received the wild type allele. A polar body biopsy is possible because the polar body remains attached to the oocyte. In the procedure, a large pipette holds the oocyte still, and then a smaller pipette draws up the attached polar body. Genetic tests are then performed on the polar body.

conceptions with chromosome abnormalities or single-gene disorders.

The area of assisted reproductive technology introduces a hotbed of bioethical issues. **Table 21.3** lists some complicated cases. Human genome information is providing more traits to track and perhaps control in coming generations. Already preimplantation genetic diagnosis is being used to screen out embryos destined to face a high risk of developing a particular disorder later in life, such as Huntington disease or cancer. It is easy to envision, instead of a quick Y chromosome FISH test, or a probe for a single gene that is mutant in a particular family, whole human genome DNA microarrays widely applied to gametes, fertilized ova, or preimplantation embryos. Who will decide which traits are worth living with, and which aren't? This coming genomic fortunetelling could spiral out of control.

Assisted reproductive technologies operate on molecules and cells, but with repercussions for individuals and families. Ultimately, if it becomes widespread enough, it will affect the gene pool. Let us hope that regulations will evolve along with the technologies to assure that they are applied sensibly and humanely.

Table 21.3

Assisted Reproductive Disasters

1. A physician in California used his own sperm to perform intrauterine insemination on 15 patients, telling them that he had used sperm from anonymous donors.
2. A plane crash killed the wealthy parents of two early embryos stored at –320°F (–195°C) in a hospital in Melbourne, Australia. Adult children of the couple were asked to share their estate with two 8-celled siblings-to-be.
3. Several couples in Chicago planning to marry discovered that they were half-siblings. Their mothers had been inseminated with sperm from the same donor.
4. Two Rhode Island couples sued a fertility clinic for misplacing several embryos.
5. Several couples in California sued a fertility clinic for implanting their oocytes or embryos in other women without donor consent. One woman requested partial custody of the resulting children if her oocytes were taken, and full custody if her embryos were used, even though the children were of school age and she had never met them.
6. A man sued his ex-wife for possession of their frozen fertilized ova. He won, and donated them for research. She had wanted to be pregnant.

Key Concepts

IVF produces extra fertilized ova and early embryos. They may be used, frozen, donated, or discarded. Used in basic research, such embryos are adding to our knowledge of early human development. Polar body biopsy enables physicians to identify and select out defective oocytes.

Summary

21.1 Infertility and Subfertility

1. **Infertility** is the inability to conceive a child after a year of unprotected intercourse. Subfertility refers to individuals or couples who manufacture gametes, but may take longer than usual to conceive.

2. Causes of infertility in the male include low sperm count, a malfunctioning immune system, a varicose vein in the scrotum, structural sperm defects, drug exposure, and abnormal hormone levels. In cases not associated with an obvious physical problem, a mutation is often the cause of the subfertility or infertility.

3. Female infertility can be caused by absent or irregular ovulation, blocked fallopian tubes, an inhospitable or malshaped uterus, antisperm secretions, or lack of sperm-attracting biochemicals. Early pregnancy loss due to abnormal chromosome number is more common in older women and may appear to be infertility.

21.2 Assisted Reproductive Technologies

4. In **intrauterine insemination,** sperm are obtained from a donor and introduced into a woman's reproductive tract in a clinical setting.

5. A gestational and genetic **surrogate mother** provides her oocyte. Then intrauterine insemination is performed from a man whose partner cannot conceive or carry a fetus. The surrogate also provides her uterus for nine months. A gestational surrogate mother receives an *in vitro fertilized* ovum that belongs genetically to the couple who ask her to carry it.

6. In IVF, oocytes and sperm meet in a dish, fertilized ova divide a few times, and the resulting embryos are placed in the woman's body, circumventing blocked tubes or the inability of the sperm to penetrate the oocyte.

7. Embryos can be frozen and thawed and then complete development when placed in a woman's uterus.

8. **GIFT** introduces oocytes and sperm into a fallopian tube past a blockage; fertilization occurs in the woman's body. **ZIFT** places an early embryo in a fallopian tube.

9. Oocytes can be frozen and stored. In **embryo adoption,** a woman undergoes intrauterine insemination. A week later, the embryo is washed out of her uterus and introduced into the reproductive tract of the woman whose partner donated the sperm.

10. Seven-celled embryos can develop normally if a blastomere is removed at the 8-cell stage and examined for abnormal chromosomes or genes. This is **preimplantation genetic diagnosis.**

21.3 On the Subject of "Spares"

11. In the United States, funding for assisted reproductive technologies can only come from private sources.

12. Extra fertilized ova and early embryos generated in IVF are used, donated to couples, stored, donated for research, or discarded. They enable researchers to study aspects of early human development that they could not investigate in other ways.

13. **Polar body biopsy** enables physicians to perform genetic tests on polar bodies and to infer the genotype of the accompanying oocyte, eliminating the problem of having to decide the fate of extra fertilized ova or early embryos.

Review Questions

1. Which assisted reproductive technologies might help the following couples? (More than one answer may fit some situations.)

   a. A woman who is born without a uterus, but who manufactures healthy oocytes.

   b. A man whose cancer treatments greatly damage his sperm.

   c. A woman who undergoes a genetic test that reveals she will develop Huntington disease. She wants to have a child, but she does not want to pass on this presently untreatable illness.

   d. Two women who wish to have and raise a child together.

   e. A man and woman are each carriers of sickle cell disease. They do not want to have an affected child, but they also do not want to terminate a pregnancy.

   f. A woman's fallopian tubes are scarred and blocked, so an oocyte cannot reach the uterus.

   g. A young woman must undergo abdominal radiation to treat ovarian cancer, but wishes to have a child in the future.

2. Why are men typically tested for infertility before women?

3. A man reads his medical chart and discovers that the results of his sperm analysis indicate that 22 percent of his sperm are shaped abnormally. He wonders why the physician said he had normal fertility if so many sperm are abnormally shaped. Has the doctor made an error?

4. Cite a situation in which both man and woman contribute to subfertility.

5. How does ZIFT differ from GIFT? How does it differ from IVF?

6. A Tennessee lower court, in ruling on the fate of seven frozen embryos in a divorce case, called them "children *in vitro.*" In what sense is this label incorrect?

7. Explain how preimplantation genetic diagnosis is similar to and different from CVS and amniocentesis.

8. What are some of the causes of infertility among older women?

9. How do each of the following assisted reproductive technologies deviate from the normal biological process?

   a. *in vitro* fertilization

   b. GIFT

   c. embryo adoption

   d. gestational surrogacy

   e. intrauterine insemination

   f. cytoplasmic donation

Applied Questions

1. At the same time that 62- and 63-year-old women gave birth, actors Tony Randall and Anthony Quinn became fathers at ages 77 and 78—and didn't receive nearly as much criticism as the women. Do you think this is an unfair double standard, or a fair criticism based on valid biological information?

2. Many people spend thousands of dollars pursuing pregnancy. What might be an alternative solution to their quest for parenthood?

3. An Oregon man anonymously donated sperm that were used to conceive a child. The man later claimed, and won, rights to visit his child. Is this situation for the man more analogous to a genetic and gestational surrogate mother, or an oocyte donor who wishes to see the child she helped to bring into existence?

4. Big Tom is a bull with valuable genetic traits. His sperm are used to conceive 1,000 calves. Mist, a dairy cow with exceptional milk output, has many oocytes removed, fertilized *in vitro,* and implanted into surrogate mothers. With their help, Mist becomes the genetic mother of 100 calves—far more than she could give birth to naturally. Which two reproductive technologies performed on humans are based on these two agricultural examples?

5. State who the genetic parents are and who the gestational mother is in each of the following cases:

   a. A man was exposed to unknown burning chemicals and received several vaccines during the first Gulf war, and abused drugs for several years before and after that. Now he wants to become a father, but he is concerned that past exposures to toxins have damaged his sperm. His wife undergoes intrauterine insemination with sperm from the husband's brother, who has led a calmer and healthier life.

   b. A 26-year-old woman has her uterus removed because of cancer. However, her ovaries are intact and her oocytes are healthy. She has oocytes removed and fertilized *in vitro* with her husband's sperm. Two resulting embryos are implanted into the uterus of the woman's best friend.

c. Max and Tina had a child by IVF in 1986. At that time, they had three extra embryos frozen. Two are thawed years later and implanted into the uterus of Tina's sister, Karen. Karen's uterus is healthy, but she has ovarian cysts that often prevent her from ovulating.

d. Forty-year-old Christensen von Wormer wanted children, but not a mate. He donated sperm, which were used for intrauterine insemination of an Indiana mother of one. The woman carried the reulting fetus to term for a fee. On September 5, 1990, von Wormer held his newborn daughter, Kelsey, for the first time.

e. Two men who live together want to raise a child. They go to a fertility clinic, have their sperm collected and mixed, and used to inseminate a friend, who nine months later turns the baby over to them.

6. Delaying childbirth until a woman is over age 35 is associated with certain physical risks, yet an older woman is often more mature and financially secure. Many women delay childbirth so that they can establish careers. Can you suggest societal changes, perhaps using a reproductive technology, that would allow women to more easily have both children and careers?

7. An IVF attempt yields 12 more embryos than the couple who conceived them can use. What could they do with the extras?

8. What do you think children born of an assisted reproductive technology should be told about their origins?

9. Wealthy couples could hire poor women as surrogates or oocyte donors simply because the adoptive mother does not want to be pregnant. Would you object to this practice? Why or why not?

10. Cloning could potentially help people who cannot make gametes. Madeline is fertile, but her partner Cliff had his testicles removed to treat cancer when he was a teenager. He did not bank testicular tissue. To have a child that is genetically theirs, the couple wishes to use a nucleus from one of Cliff's somatic cells, which would be transferred to an oocyte of Madeline's that has had its nucleus removed. The resulting fertilized ovum would be cultured in the laboratory and then transferred to Madeline's uterus via standard IVF. Is the couple correct in assuming that the child would be genetically theirs? Cite a reason for your answer.

11. An IVF program in Bombay, India offers preimplantation genetic diagnosis to help couples who already have a daughter to conceive a son. The reasoning is that because having a male heir is of such great importance in this society, offering PGD can enable couples to avoid aborting second and subsequent female pregnancies. Do you agree or disagree that PGD should be used for sex selection in this sociological context?

Web Activities

12. Go to http://www.cdc.gov/nccdphp/drh/art.htm. Click on ART Trends, and use the information to answer the following questions.

a. Since 1996, to what extent has the use of assisted reproductive technologies (ART) in the U.S. increased?

b. Which is more successfully implanted into the infertile woman's uterus, a fresh or frozen donor oocyte?

c. Which is more successfully implanted into the infertile woman's uterus, a donated oocyte or one of her own?

d. What are two factors that could complicate data collection on ART success rates?

Case Studies

13. Natallie Evans had to have her ovaries removed at a young age because they were precancerous, so she and her partner had IVF and froze their embryos for use at a later time. Under British law, both partners must consent for the continued storage of frozen embryos. Evans and her partner split, and he revoked his consent. She sued for the right to use the embryos. She told the court, "I am pleased to have the opportunity to ask the court to save my embryos and let me use them to have the child I so desperately want."

What information should the court consider in deciding this case? Whose rights do you think should be paramount?

Learn to apply the skills of a genetic counselor with these additional cases found in the *Case Workbook in Human Genetics:*

Charcot-Marie-Tooth disease

Male infertility

Suggested Readings

Boyle, Robert J., and Julian Savulescu. November 22, 2001. Ethics of using preimplantation genetic diagnosis to select a stem cell donor for an existing person. *British Medical Journal* 323:1240–43. An analysis of the Nash case.

Ford, W. C. L. April 21, 2001. Biological mechanisms of male infertility. *The Lancet* 357:1223–24. Deranged apoptosis can lead to sperm with an excess of abnormal forms.

Gottlieb, Scott. June 23, 2001. Scientists screen embryo for genetic predisposition to cancer. *The British Medical Journal* 322:1505. A

couple used PGD to ensure that their child did not inherit Li-Fraumeni family cancer syndrome. The father had been diagnosed at age two.

Hall, Judith G. July 2001. Neonatal outcome after preimplantation genetic diagnosis by analysis of the polar bodies. *Growth, Genetics, and Hormones* 17, no. 2:30–31. A mutant allele in a polar body may mean that the oocyte has been spared.

Hansen, Michéle. March 7, 2002. The risk of major birth defects after intracytoplasmic sperm injection and *in vitro* fertilization.

The New England Journal of Medicine 346:725–30. Children born following IVF or ICSI face twice the risk of birth defects—but this may reflect the reason for a parent's infertility.

Hughes, Edward G., and Mita Giacomini. September 2001. Funding in *in vitro* fertilization treatment for persistent subfertility: The pain and the politics. *Fertility and Sterility* 76, no. 3:431–42. Assisted reproductive technologies remain prohibitively expensive.

Josefson, D. October 14, 2000. Couple select healthy embryo to provide stem cells for sister. *The British Medical Journal* 321:917. The Nash family used PGD to save their daughter from an inherited disease.

Lewis, Ricki. November 13, 2000. Preimplantation genetic diagnosis—the next big thing? *The Scientist* 14(22):16. PGD "leftovers" reveal details of the basic mechanisms of early human development.

Magli, M. C., et al. August 2000. Chromosome mosaicism in day three aneuploid embryos that develop to morphologically normal blastocysts *in vitro*. *Human Reproduction* 15:1781–86. Mutations that occur in the early embryo can confound the predictions of preimplantation genetic diagnosis.

Powell, Kendall. April 17, 2003. Seeds of doubt. *Nature* 422:656–58. Do children conceived with ARTs have higher rates of birth defects because of the procedures, or because their parents are more likely to have reproductive problems?

Robertson, J. A. March 2003. Extending preimplantation genetic diagnosis: The ethical debate. *Human Reproduction* 18(3):465–71. Who should determine for which conditions PGD should be used?

Sheldon, Tony. March 16, 2002. Children at risk after sperm donor develops late-onset genetic disease. *The British Medical Journal* 324:631. Eighteen English children conceived by intrauterine insemination face a 1 in 2 chance of developing cerebellar ataxia because their biological father did not know he would develop it.

Weekly updates of current news related to human genetics are available through Power Web on your Online Learning Center.

VISIT YOUR ONLINE LEARNING CENTER

Visit your online learning center for additional resources and tools to help you master this chapter. See us at

www.mhhe.com/lewisgenetics6.

C H A P T E R

The Age of Genomics

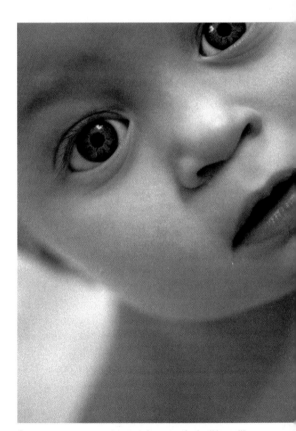

22

Soon, genome sequencing early in life will provide individualized backdrops of inherited disease risks, against which people can attempt environmental interventions.

As sciences go, genetics is young, genomics younger still. The milestones along the way, as one field evolved into the other, have come at oddly regular intervals. A century after Gregor Mendel announced and published his findings, the genetic code was deciphered; a century after his laws were rediscovered, the human genome was sequenced, beginning the age of genomics. This chapter chronicles the rise of this new science, and glimpses the future.

The completion of the first draft human genome sequence was a huge accomplishment (**figure 22.1**). The information will affect us in many ways. This chapter is the story of how the human genome came to be sequenced.

22.1 Genome Sequencing: A Continuation of Genetics

The term *genome* was coined in 1920 by geneticist H. Winkler. A hybrid of "gene" and "chromosome", genome denotes a complete set of chromosomes and its genes. The term *genomics* is credited to T. H. Roderick, coined in 1986 to indicate the study of genomes. A year later, a journal was founded by that name.

Thoughts about genomes in general, and the human genome in particular, lay in the background throughout the twentieth century, as researchers defined and described the units of inheritance from various perspectives. Francis Crick, writing in his 1966 book *Of Molecules and Men,* described the size of a human genome in terms of the amount of DNA in a single sperm cell. "This comes to about 500 large books, all different—a fair-sized private library." Just as you wouldn't read every word on every page of every book to locate a particular volume, but would scan the book titles, the human genome project began with deciphering signposts and discovering shortcuts. Many of the initial steps and tools grew from existing technology.

The linkage maps from as long ago as the 1950s, and the many studies of families that associated chromosomal aberrations with syndromes, provided a wealth of mapping data, assigning a handful of genes to their chromosomes. Then a technological revolution, in the form of automated DNA sequencing, enabled researchers to go from mapping genes to sequencing them, determining the actual order of A, C, T, and G that make up the chromosomes. **Figure 22.2** schematically illustrates the refinement and increasing resolution of different types of genetic maps, from the chromosomal (cytogenetic) and linkage maps generated by family data, to the physical maps derived from restriction fragment length polymorphisms and overlapping large pieces of DNA cloned into vectors.

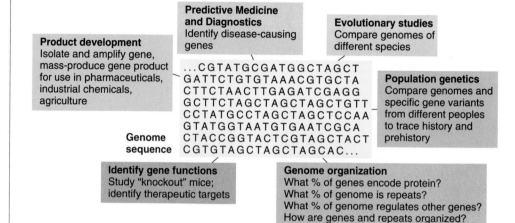

Figure 22.1 Some applications of human genome information.

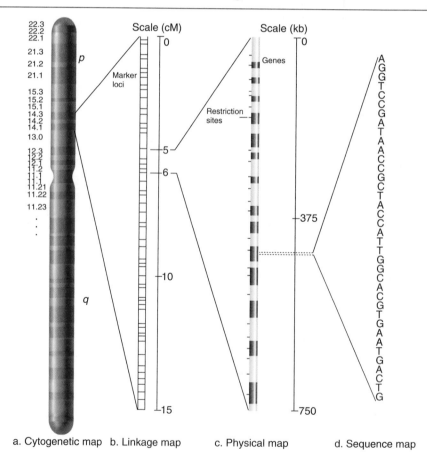

a. Cytogenetic map b. Linkage map c. Physical map d. Sequence map

Figure 22.2 Different levels of genetic maps. **(a)** A cytogenetic map, based on associations between chromosome aberrations and syndromes, can distinguish DNA sequences that are at least 5,000 kilobases (kb) apart. **(b)** A linkage map derived from recombination data distinguishes genes hundreds of kb apart. **(c)** A physical map constructed from DNA pieces cloned in vectors and then overlapped distinguishes genes tens of kb apart. **(d)** A sequence map is the ultimate genetic map, consisting of all the nucleotide bases ordered as they are on the chromosomes, including protein-encoding genes and other sequences.

The human genome project examined hundreds or thousands of pieces of DNA at a time, cataloguing their sequences in a public database called GenBank maintained by the National Library of Medicine, and at some companies. **Figure 22.3** depicts schematically the two approaches used to determine the first draft sequence, unveiled officially in 2000 and 2001, but posted, little by little, in GenBank all along. One research group, The International Consortium, unofficially headed by Francis Collins, divided the genome into "BAC clones." Recall from table 19.1 that a BAC is a bacterial artificial chromosome. The ones used in the human genome project each housed about 100,000 bases of inserted human DNA. The BAC contents were known to correspond to specific places among the chromosomes called sequence tagged sites (STSs). Several copies of each BAC were cut, or "shotgunned," into up to 80 overlapping pieces, and the pieces sequenced. A powerful computer program then assembled the overlaps to derive the overall sequence for each chromosome. Finally, teams of researchers filled in gaps and analyzed sequences, "annotating" each chromosome with functional descriptions of protein-encoding genes. More detailed views of the chromosomes continue to be published.

The second group to obtain the first draft sequence of the human genome, who actually came in first if one looks at the accomplishment as a race, was Celera Genomics Corporation, of Rockville, Maryland, headed by J. Craig Venter. The Celera team skipped the BAC stage, instead shotgunning multiple copies of the entire genome into small pieces, and using a computer program to assemble the overlaps into larger pieces called scaffolds. They then also used STSs to anchor the resulting 119,000 scaffolds to the chromosomes.

In parallel to the human genome project, many individual laboratories continued to investigate specific genes that cause specific diseases. This approach, called **positional cloning,** began with examining a particular phenotype corresponding to a Mendelian disorder, then gradually following clues to find a chromosomal locus or position for the responsible gene.

In contrast to the genome project's "sequence now—interpret later" strategy, the positional cloning experiments that had dominated medical genetics pinpointed particular genes. It was a time-consuming approach, yet yielded a steady stream of discoveries of disease-causing genes throughout the 1980s and 1990s. For example, mapping, identifying, and finally sequencing the gene that causes Huntington disease took a multicenter team from 1983 until 1993. Today, given the availability of the entire human genome sequence and the tools to analyze it, a graduate student can find a gene in weeks.

The entire way we look at gene discovery has changed in this new age of genomics. Today, gene discovery is largely an

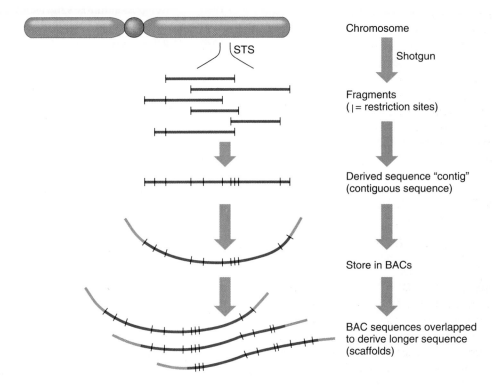

a. International Human Genome Mapping Consortium "BAC by BAC"
(BAC = bacterial artificial chromosome)

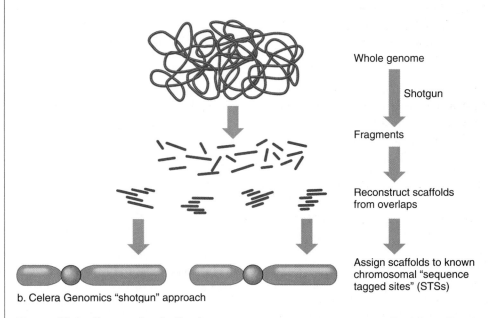

b. Celera Genomics "shotgun" approach

Figure 22.3 Two routes to the human genome sequence. (a) The International Consortium began with known chromosomal sites and overlapped large pieces, called contigs, that in turn were reconstructed from many small, overlapping pieces. **(b)** Celera Genomics shotgunned several copies of a genome into small pieces, overlapped them to form scaffolds, and then assigned scaffolds to known chromosomal sites. They used some Consortium data.

informational science, where researchers mine genome databases for DNA sequence similarities. Each time a new species has its genome sequenced, researchers can go back to those that came before and identify gene functions to fill in many blanks. At first, nearly half of the genes uncovered in genomes were mysteries. The field is also no longer focused on single genes. DNA microarrays can reveal the simultaneous functions of thousands of genes.

Key Concepts

Sequencing the human genome built upon linkage and cytogenetic information gained from decades of work. Genome sequencing handles many pieces of DNA at once, with analysis later. The International Consortium pinned sequences in BACs to known chromosomal sites; Celera Genomics used a whole-genome shotgunning approach. In contrast, positional cloning, which contributed much genetic information in the 1980s and 1990s, sought specific genes based on the disorders that they cause when mutant.

22.2 The Origin of the Idea

The idea of sequencing an entire genome probably occurred to many researchers as soon as Watson and Crick determined the structure of DNA. In 1966, Francis Crick proposed sequencing all genes in *E. coli,* to reveal how the organism works, writing that "this particular problem will keep very many scientists busy for a long time to come." Jacques Monod, who described the first genetic control system in bacteria, wrote at about the same time, "What is true for *Escherichia coli* is true for the elephant," meaning that to know genomes is to understand all life. It was a gross oversimplification.

For sequencing genomes to evolve from science fiction to science required the development of key tools and technologies (see Technology Timeline). First was the need to obtain the nucleotide base sequence of pieces of DNA. Then, computer programs would have to align and detect overlaps in sequence in pieces cut from multiple copies of a genome, and assemble them to reconstruct each chromosome.

Technology Timeline

Evolution of the Human Genome Project

1985–1988	Idea to sequence human genome is suggested at several scientific meetings.
1988	Congress authorizes the Department of Energy and the National Institutes of Health to fund the human genome project.
1989	Researchers at Stanford and Duke Universities invent DNA chip (microarray) technology.
1990	Human genome project officially begins.
1991	Expressed sequence tag (EST) technology identifies protein-encoding sequences.
1992	First DNA microarrays become available.
1993	Need to automate DNA sequencing is recognized.
1994	U.S. and French researchers publish preliminary map of 6,000 genetic markers, one every 1 million bases along the chromosomes.
1995	Emphasis shifts from gene mapping to sequencing.
1996	Resolution passed at Second International Strategy Meeting on Human Genome Sequencing to make all data public and update it daily at GenBank (www.ncbi.nlm.nih.gov).
1998	Public Consortium releases preliminary map of pieces covering 98 percent of human genome. Millions of sequences are listed in GenBank. Directions for developing DNA microarrays are posted on the Internet.
1999	Rate of filing of new sequences in GenBank triples.
	A full 30 percent of human genome is sequenced by year's end.
	Public Consortium and two private companies race to complete sequencing.
2000	Ninety-nine percent of the human genome is sequenced privately.
	Microarray technology explodes as researchers investigate gene functions and interactions.
2001	Two versions of human genome sequence are published in mid-February issues of *Science* and *Nature.*
2003	Finished version of human genome sequence announced to coincide with fiftieth anniversary of discovery of DNA structure.
	Entire protein-encoding part of human genome becomes available on DNA microarrays.
	U.S. National Human Genome Research Institute publishes "A Vision of the Future of Genomics Research."
2004 and beyond	Annotation continues as genomics gradually impacts health care.

The Sanger Method of DNA Sequencing

Modern DNA sequencing instruments utilize a basic technique that Frederick Sanger developed in 1977. The goal is to generate a series of DNA fragments of identical sequence that are complementary to the sequence of interest. These fragments differ in length from each other by one end base (see figure to right).

Sequence of interest: T A C G C A G T A C
Complementary sequence:
Series of fragments:

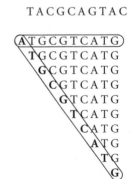

Note that the entire complementary sequence appears in the sequence of end bases of each fragment. If the complement of the gene of interest can be cut into a collection of such pieces, and the end bases distinguished with a radioactive or fluorescent label, then polyacrylamide gel electrophoresis (see figure 14.5) can be used to separate the fragments by size. Then, once the areas of overlap are aligned, reading the labeled end bases in size order reveals the sequence of the complement. Replacing A with T, G with C, T with A, and C with G establishes the sequence of the DNA in question.

Sanger invented a way to generate the DNA pieces. In a test tube, he included the unknown sequence and all of the biochemicals needed to replicate it, including supplies of the nucleotide bases. Some of each of the four types of bases were chemically modified at a specific location on the base sugar to contain no oxygen atoms instead of one—in the language of chemistry, they were *di*deoxyribonucleotides rather than deoxyribonucleotides. A radioactive nucleotide, usually C, was also included. DNA synthesis

halted when DNA polymerase encountered a "dideoxy" base, leaving only a piece of the newly replicated strand.

Sanger repeated the experiment four times, each time using a dideoxy version of A, T, C, then G. The four experiments were run in four lanes of a gel (**figure 22.4**). Today, fluorescent labels are used, one for each of the four base types, to reveal the sequence in a single experiment. The four types of pieces, ending in any of the four types of labeled bases, are collected in thin glass tubes called capillaries, rather than on cumbersome slabs of gel. The data appear as a sequential readout of the wavelengths of the fluorescence from the labels (**figures 22.5** and **22.6**). In the mid-1980s, Leroy Hood automated Sanger's method of DNA sequencing, which was essential to the ability to analyze entire genomes.

DNA sequencing occurs on a vast scale today. Many individual laboratories or academic departments have one or more automated DNA sequencers, while companies devoted to genome sequencing may have hundreds. But the automated Sanger method

of DNA sequencing, although the workhorse of the human genome project, is now considered too slow to handle the routine genome sequencing that will be part of clinical medicine and perhaps such fields as forensics and agriculture. Today's version of the human genome race is to find a way to sequence one for under $1,000.

Several companies are pursuing a new, fast and inexpensive route to DNA sequencing called single-molecule detection. This technique unwinds a long DNA molecule by passing it through a microfluidics environment, which is a small, fluid-filled chamber containing intricate nooks and crannies. Imagine a large group of children walking through a tight maze—navigating the twists and turns would gradually draw them into a single-file line. In one variation on this theme, the DNA is initially labeled with four fluorescent dyes. After passing through the nooks and crannies, the unwound DNA encounters a multi-laser scanner that "reads" 10 to 30 million base pairs per second. Researchers caution, however, that the new devices must undergo rigorous testing on

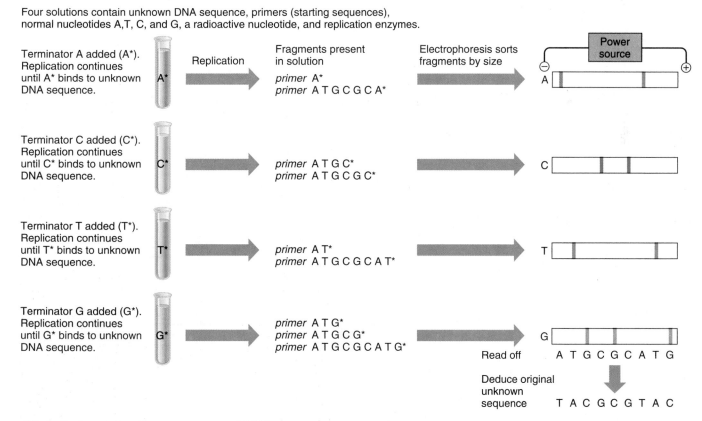

Figure 22.4 **Determining the sequence of DNA.** In the Sanger method of DNA sequencing, complementary copies of an unknown DNA sequence are terminated early because of the incorporation of dideoxynucleotide "terminators." A computer deduces the sequence by placing the fragments in size order. Radioactive or fluorescent labels are used to visualize the sparse quantities of each fragment.

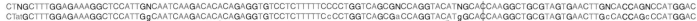

```
CTNGCTTTGGAGAAAGGCTCCATTGNCAATCAAGACACACAGAGGTGTCCTCTTTTTCCCCTGGTCAGCGNCCAGGTACATNGCACCAAGGCTGCGTAGTGAACTTGNCACCAGNCCATGGAC
CTatGCTTTGGAGAAAGGCTCCATTGgCAATCAAGACACACAGAGGTGTCCTCTTTTTCcCCTGGTCAGCGaCCAGGTACATgGCACCAAGGCTGCGTAGTGAACTTGcCACCAGcCCATGGAC
```

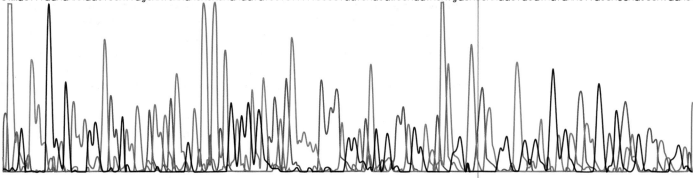

Figure 22.5 DNA sequence data. In automated DNA sequencing, a readout of sequenced DNA is a series of wavelengths that represent the terminally labeled DNA base.

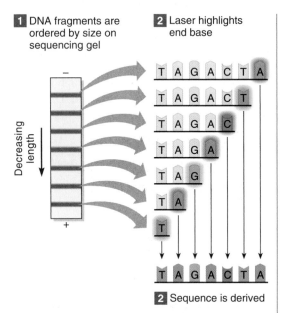

1 DNA fragments are ordered by size on sequencing gel

2 Laser highlights end base

Decreasing length

2 Sequence is derived

Figure 22.6 Reading a DNA sequence. A computer algorithm detects and records the end base from a series of size-ordered DNA fragments.

actual DNA samples before sequencing your genome becomes as simple as taking your blood pressure at the supermarket! As of early 2004, single molecule detection was still far from the marketplace, with the cost of sequencing the protein-encoding portion of the human genome still about $400,000.

The Project Starts

During the 1980s, the idea to sequence the human genome evolved for several reasons. It surfaced at a meeting held by the Department of Energy in 1984 to discuss the long-term population genetic effects of exposure to low-level radiation. In 1985, at another gathering, Robert Sinsheimer, chancellor of the University of California, Santa Cruz, called for an institute to sequence the human genome, basically because it could be done. The next year, virologist Renato Dulbecco proposed that the key to understanding the origin of cancer lay in knowing the human genome sequence. In the summer of 1986, many of the major players in genetics and molecular biology convened at the Cold Spring Harbor Laboratory on New York's Long Island to discuss the feasibility of a human genome project. Worldwide planning soon began.

The idea to systematically sequence the human genome shifted the goals of life science research. A furious debate ensued, with detractors claiming that the project would be more gruntwork than a creative intellectual endeavor, comparing it to conquering Mt. Everest just because it is there. Some researchers feared that such an unprecedented "big science" project would divert government funds from basic research and the AIDS budget. Finally, the National Academy of Sciences convened a committee composed of both detractors and supporters to debate the feasibility, risks, and benefits of the project. The naysayers were swayed to the other side. So in 1988, Congress authorized the National Institutes of Health (NIH) and the Department of Energy (DOE) to fund the $3 billion, 15-year human genome project. For the first few years, it appeared that the NIH was still unconvinced—DOE was the more active participant.

The government-sponsored human genome project officially began in 1990 with James Watson at the helm. Recognizing the profound effect that genetic information would have on public policy and on peoples' lives, the project set aside 3 percent of its budget for the ELSI program, which stands for ethical, legal, and social issues. ELSI helps ensure that genetic information is not misused to discriminate against people with particular genotypes.

The human genome project expanded both in scope and in number of participants. In addition to ten major sequencing centers, the largest in England, France, Germany, and Japan, many hundreds of other basic research laboratories and biotechnology companies contributed DNA sequence data. The project also, from the start, sequenced the genomes of several different species to investigate how life forms on earth are related.

Key Concepts

DNA sequencing and computer software to align DNA pieces were essential technological developments necessary for genome projects to proceed. In the Sanger method of DNA sequencing, complementary copies of an unknown DNA sequence are terminated early by incorporating dideoxynucleotides. A researcher or automated DNA sequencer deduces the sequence by labeling the end bases and placing fragments in size order. • Single-molecule detection uses microfluidics to unwind DNA, which is sequenced as it passes a laser scanner. This method is much faster and cheaper than Sanger sequencing. • The idea to sequence the human genome emerged in the mid-1980s, with several goals. The project officially began in 1990.

22.3 Technology Drives the Sequencing Effort

The human genome project progressed in stages as sequencing technology and computer capability to align and derive continuous sequence improved. At first the project focused on developing tools and technologies to divide the genome into pieces small enough to sequence, and to improve the efficiency of sequencing techniques. **Table 22.1** summarizes the overall steps in genome sequencing.

In 1991, two key inventions entered the picture. Venter, then a government researcher at the NIH, introduced a very powerful shortcut called **expressed sequence tag** (EST) technology. ESTs are cDNAs that are pieces of the genes expressed in a particular cell type. Identifying ESTs enabled researchers to quickly pick out genes most likely to be implicated in disease, because they encode protein, and are expressed in the cell types affected in a particular illness. Venter left the NIH to develop ESTs at The Institute for Genomic Research (TIGR), which he founded. TIGR has sequenced the genomes of many organisms, especially microbes.

Also in 1991, Patrick Brown at Stanford University developed a way to embed DNA pieces of known sequence into tiny glass squares, then use this array to pull out complementary sequences from a sample of unknown DNA pieces. These devices were first called DNA chips, then DNA microarrays. The idea grew out of a whimsical suggestion in 1989 that genes, like transistors, be placed on chips.

Sequencing and mapping techniques improved greatly from 1993 to 1998. At the start of the project, researchers cut the genome into overlapping pieces of about 40,000 bases (40 kilobases), then randomly cut the pieces into small fragments. Researchers would cut up several genomes in a single experiment, so that many of the resulting fragments overlapped. By finding the overlaps, the pieces could be assembled to reveal the overall sequence. The greater the number of overlaps, the more likely that the final assembled sequence would not omit anything. Today, computers recognize the overlaps and align and derive the sequences, either beginning with larger sections or using many small pieces. It is important that the sites of overlap be unique sequences, found in only one place in the genome. Overlaps of repeated sequences present in several places could lead to more than one derived overall sequence. This requirement is why the Y chromosome, with its many repeats, was extremely difficult to sequence, and had to be cut into very small pieces. Another problem is to determine which side of the double helix to sequence for each piece. **Figure 22.7** illustrates the strategy of overlapping sequences using a sentence from the English language, and **figure 22.8** depicts how a DNA sequence might be reconstructed from overlapping pieces.

By many people's accounts, 1995 was a turning point in the human genome project, as "proteomics" entered the growing vocabulary of genome jargon, referring to all the proteins that an organism can

Table 22.1

Steps in Genome Sequencing and Analysis

1. Obtain chromosome maps with landmarks from classical linkage or cytogenetic studies, or RFLP sites.
2. Obtain chromosome pieces maintained in gene libraries, or shotgun entire sequence.
3. Sequence the pieces.
4. Overlap aligned sequences to extend the known sequence.
5. Compare the sequence to those in other species.

```
                    FEELING WE'RE NOT
       TOTO, I HAVE A FEE
                         ELING WE'RE NOT IN KANSAS ANYMORE
                    A FEELING
         AVE A FEELING WE'RE NOT IN KANSAS A
                 ING WE'R
                        'RE NOT IN KANSAS ANYMORE
              ELING WE'RE NOT IN KANS
       I HAVE A FEELING WE
              FEELING WE'R
                    NG WE'RE NOT IN KANSAS ANYMO
       TOTO, I HAVE A FEELING WE'RE NOT IN KANSAS ANYMORE
```

Figure 22.7 Overlapping sequences. Deriving a DNA sequence requires overlapping a number of fragments according to where their sequences match. This English sentence provides a model.

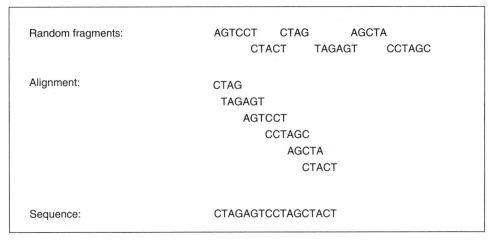

Figure 22.8 Deriving a DNA sequence. Automated DNA sequencers first determine the sequences of short pieces of DNA, or sometimes of just the ends of short pieces. Then algorithms search for overlaps. By overlapping the pieces, the software derives the overall DNA sequences.

synthesize, as well as how the proteins are distributed among different cell types. Researchers began to see that proteomics would present an even greater challenge than sequencing the genome.

The year 1995 was also when efforts shifted from mapping genes to chromosomes, to DNA sequencing. For the first time, the number of gene sequences deposited in GenBank outnumbered the number of papers in the scientific literature introducing disease genes identified by positional cloning. The reason: the automation of DNA sequencing. Although similar to their 1980s prototypes in concept, devices could now produce lines of A, T, C, and G ten times as fast as in the early days.

The deadline for completion of the human genome project inched forward as optimism soared. In 1995, Venter's company, TIGR, developed computer software that could rapidly locate the unique sequence overlaps among many small pieces of DNA and assemble them into a continuous sequence, eliminating the preliminary step of gathering large guidepost pieces. Using this software, TIGR obtained the first complete genome sequence for an organism, in under a year! Many more would follow.

The distinction of being the first organism to have its genome sequenced went to *Haemophilus influenzae,* a bacterium that causes meningitis and ear infections. The researchers cut the bacterium's 1,830,137 bases into 24,000 fragments, sequenced them, and the software assembled the overlaps of several genomes worth of pieces. The human genome is 1,500 times larger than that of *H. influenzae.*

Meanwhile, the partners of the International Consortium met in Bermuda, establishing the "Bermuda rules." These guidelines bound researchers to release new DNA sequences to the public database within 24 hours of determination. By 1998, Venter had founded Celera Genomics, with the goal of sequencing the human genome faster and at less cost than the consortium, a feat possible because of the company's powerful assembler software. Unlike the consortium's public posting of data, Celera planned to sell access to its sequence, even though they had to use some of the public data to get that sequence. And so began the fierce bioethical battle over public access to human genome information that continues today.

In 1999, the human genome project became intensely competitive, with Venter and Collins, director of the U.S. arm of the International Consortium since 1993, racing to finish and sacrificing a degree of accuracy for speed. The first map of an entire human chromosome, number 22, was published near year's end. In March 2000, Celera Genomics completed the sequence of the genome of the fruit fly, *Drosophila melanogaster,* in collaboration with a public consortium. It was considered a "trial run" for the human genome.

Venter claimed privately to have reached the first draft goal for the human genome by March 2000, while the consortium's sequence was completed June 22, following a month of frantic work by University of California at Santa Cruz graduate student James Kent. His invention of the GigAssembler program immediately catapulted him to cult hero status in the genome project. The task that GigAssembler tackles has been compared to putting together a million-piece puzzle

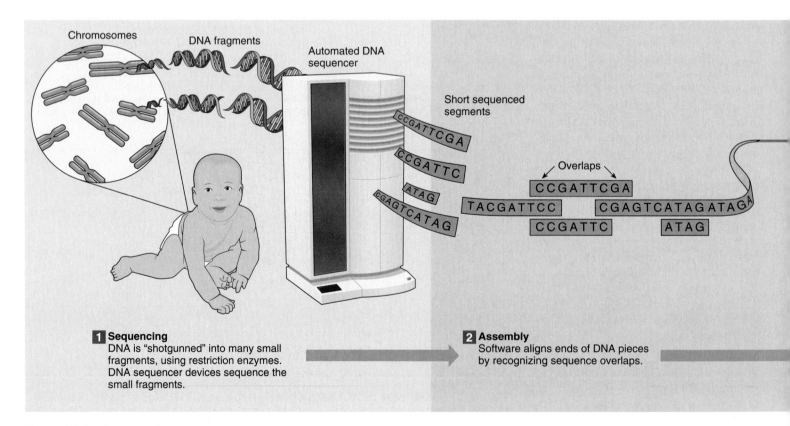

1 Sequencing
DNA is "shotgunned" into many small fragments, using restriction enzymes. DNA sequencer devices sequence the small fragments.

2 Assembly
Software aligns ends of DNA pieces by recognizing sequence overlaps.

Figure 22.9   Sequencing genomes.   Determining the DNA sequence of a genome is just a first step—albeit a huge one. After pieces are assembled into a whole, protein-encoding genes are identified, and then patterns of gene expression in different tissues are assessed.

using thousands of preassembled pieces. The program looks for the connections between the pieces to present the final view of the human genome.

In the end, the battling factions called a truce. On June 26, 2000, Venter and Collins flanked President Clinton in the White House rose garden to announce the shared accomplishment of obtaining a "first draft" of the human genome sequence. To those unfamiliar with genetics, the news must have seemed to have come out of nowhere, and perhaps to have been the work of just these two men. In actuality, the milestone capped a decade-long project involving thousands of researchers, which in turn was the culmination of a century of discovery. The historic date of June 26 came about because it was the only opening in the White House calendar! In other words, the work was monumental; its announcement, staged.

Figure 22.9 is an overview of genome sequencing and one application—gene expression profiling using DNA microarrays, discussed in chapter 11. Reading 22.1 considers the human genome sequence in a broader context.

Key Concepts

The human genome project switched from mapping to sequencing in 1995. EST technology enabled researchers to focus on protein-encoding genes, and microarray technology considered many expressed genes at a time. In the second half of the 1990s, the race intensified. The first draft sequence was announced in June 2000.

22.4 Into the Future

During the frantic final months of the race to sequence the human genome, thoughts turned to what would happen afterwards. Meanwhile, the public became confused by the intermittent media coverage. The announcement of the first draft in June 2000, then publication of the initial annotated sequence eight months later, followed by the unveiling of the completed draft to coincide with the fifty-year anniversary of the discovery of DNA's structure in 2003, made it seem that scientists were claiming the same coup over and over. However, also timed to the fifty-year mark, but not as prominently reported, was publication of a paper that finally put the entire project into a practical perspective that would guide the future.

A Multilevel House

In the paper, "A Vision for the Future of Genomics Research," the leaders of the U.S. National Human Genome Research Institute explained applications of the sequence information using a metaphor of a building with three stories—representing basic biological research, health, and society—resting on the foundation of the human genome project (**figure 22. 10**). The three "floors" do not have to occur in any sequence, although the impact will often flow from research to health to society. For example, comparison of a human DNA sequence to those of other organisms (floor 1, biology) can lead to identification of a disease-causing gene (floor 2, health), which in turn spawns discussion of the repercussions of testing for that gene (floor 3, society). The approaches represented in the three floors overlap as physicians read genetics journals and imagine new therapies, and bioethicists and lawyers consider the impact of new tests and technologies.

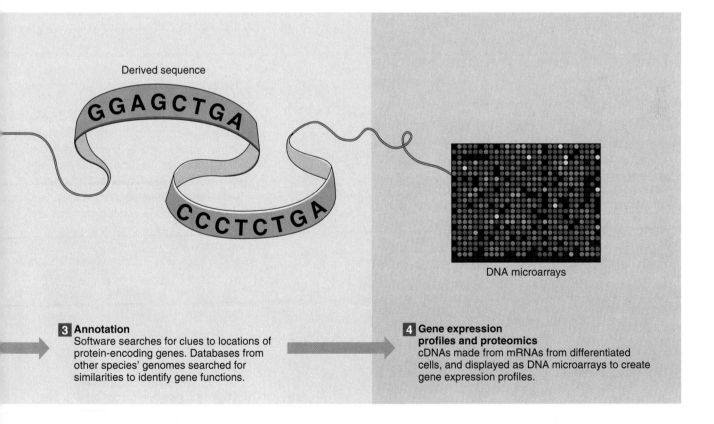

Derived sequence

GGAGCTGA
CCCTCTGA

DNA microarrays

3 Annotation
Software searches for clues to locations of protein-encoding genes. Databases from other species' genomes searched for similarities to identify gene functions.

4 Gene expression profiles and proteomics
cDNAs made from mRNAs from differentiated cells, and displayed as DNA microarrays to create gene expression profiles.

The Human Genome Among Others: Comparative Genomics

Sequencing the human genome is important because it is *us*, the information that reveals how our bodies work and how they malfunction. From a broader perspective, the human genome represents just one species among many thousand living today. Comparative genomics is the field that searches for similarities and differences among genomes. A limited way to do this is through targeted comparative sequencing, which aligns corresponding sequences in different organisms, discussed in chapter 16. A way to ask more profound questions is to compare genomes of organisms that lie at the boundaries of great evolutionary leaps, when life changed drastically. Following are some examples.

The minimum gene set required for life. The smallest cell known to be able to reproduce is *Mycoplasma genitalium*. It infects cabbage, citrus fruit, corn, broccoli, honeybees, and spiders, and causes respiratory illness in chickens, pigs, cows, and humans. Researchers call its tiny genome the "near-minimal set of genes for independent life." Of 480 protein-encoding genes, researchers

think that 265 to 350 are essential for life. Considering how *Mycoplasma* uses its genes reveals the fundamental challenges of being alive (**table 1**). When the organism's genome was sequenced, nearly a quarter of the genes had no known counterpart in other organisms. Taking cues from the tiny mycoplasma genome, Venter's current research group is attempting to build a synthetic genome, starting with simple, harmless viral genomes.

Fundamental distinctions among the three domains of life. *Methanococcus jannaschii* is a microorganism that lives at the bottom of a 2,600-meter-tall "white smoker" chimney in the Pacific Ocean, at high temperature and pressure and without oxygen. It is a member of the Archaea, cells that lack nuclei, yet that replicate DNA and synthesize proteins in ways similar to those of multicellular organisms. The genome sequence confirms that this organism represents a third form of life. Fewer than half of its 1,738 genes had known counterparts among the bacteria, other archaea, or eukaryotes when the genome was sequenced. Even the genome of *E. coli*, the

Table 1

The Minimal Functional Gene Set for Life (Distribution of Gene Function in *Mycoplasma genitalium*)

Percentage of Genome	Function
30.0%	Maintaining plasma membrane
24.0%	Protein synthesis
22.0%	Unknown (doesn't match any known gene)
9.0%	DNA replication
8.0%	Acquiring energy
4.5%	Evading immune attack by host cell
4.0%	Synthesizing and recycling nucleic acids

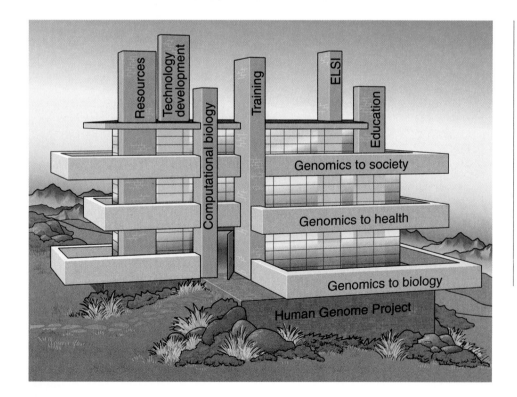

Each floor also intersects six other areas that can be looked at as subdivisions. They are resources (such as databases), technology development, computational biology, training, ELSI (ethics, legal, and social issues), and education. Training can refer to that of health professionals and others who impart information about genetics and genomics, such as teachers, lawyers, and bioethicists; education refers to the public. The paper describes "grand challenges" for each floor, posed as questions in **table 22.2**.

Figure 22.10 An architectural metaphor. The human genome project serves as a foundation for biological, health, and societal applications of the human genome sequence.

organism that geneticists supposedly knew the best, held surprises. The functions of more than a third of *E. coli*'s 4,288 genes remain a mystery.

The simplest organism with a nucleus. The paper in *Science* magazine that introduced the genome of the yeast *Saccharomyces cerevisiae* was entitled "Life with 6,000 Genes." But the unicellular yeast is more complex than this title implies. About a third of its 5,885 genes have counterparts among mammals, including those implicated in more than 70 human diseases. Understanding what a gene (such as one that controls the cell cycle) does in yeast can provide clues to how it affects human health.

The basic blueprints of an animal. The genome of the tiny, transparent, 959-celled nematode worm *Caenorhabditis elegans* is packed with information on what it takes to be an animal. Thanks to researchers who, in the 1960s, meticulously tracked the movements of each cell as the animal developed, much of the biology of this organism was already known before its 97 million DNA bases were revealed late in 1998. The worm's signal transduction pathways, cytoskeleton, immune system, apoptotic pathways, and even brain proteins are very similar to our own.

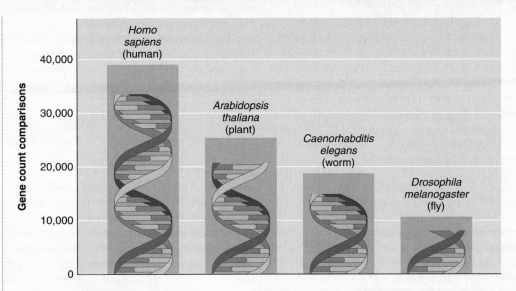

Figure 1 Comparative genomics. The human genome is not much larger than that of other organisms and shares much of the DNA sequence. At a genome-size level, we are actually similar to pufferfish and brussels sprouts! Clearly, genome organization as well as DNA sequence are important in establishing the many differences among Earth's inhabitants.

The sequencing of the fruit fly genome held a big surprise—it has 13,601 genes, fewer than the 18,425 in the much simpler *C. elegans* worm (**figure 1**). Apparently the way that genes control the development and functioning of an organism is more complex than studying single genes suggested. Also, of 289 human disease-causing genes, the fly sequencers identified 177—about 60 percent—in *Drosophila*. The fly might therefore serve as a model for humans in testing new treatments.

Table 22. 2

"Grand Challenges" from the U.S. National Human Genome Research Institute

Genomics to Biology	Genomics to Health	Genomics to Society
1. What are the structural and functional components of the human genome—our "parts list?"	1. Which genes cause or contribute to which diseases and to our responses to the drugs used to treat them?	1. How can we develop policies to balance the benefits of personalized medicine with risk of discrimination based on knowledge of genetic information?
2. What are the pathways and networks through which genes and their protein products interact in different cell types, under different conditions?	2. Which gene variants promote health or provide resistance to particular diseases?	2. How are genes and genomes related to population subgroups, such as races?
3. How greatly do we vary at the DNA sequence level?	3. How can genome information be used to predict disease susceptibility and drug response, diagnose illness early, and subclassify diseases based on a new "molecular taxonomy?"	3. How do genes and genomes influence our behavior and other human traits?
4. How does DNA sequence variation among species reflect evolution?	4. How can identification of genes be used to develop new drugs?	4. What are the ethical limits to the applications of genomics and genome information?
5. How can we keep genome information freely available to basic and clinical researchers?	5. How do healthcare consumers receive and use genetic risk information, and what is its impact?	
	6. How can new tools based on genome information help everyone?	

New Types of Studies

The applications of this new biology are diverse, and some have probably not even occurred to us yet. Past chapters have examined several of them, from more powerful DNA profiling, to new types of foods, to tracing the origins and migrations of early humans, to predictive medicine.

Human genome information will fuel an approach that is opposite that of classical genetics—focusing on the healthy many, rather than the ill few, to better understand disease. For example, researchers are assembling a "healthy cohort"—a group of exceptionally disease-free and vigorous people whose genomes can be searched to reveal shared gene variants that presumably help to keep them well. This project is not an attempt to define a "perfect" genetic blueprint, but one that might suggest new types of treatments based on how particular gene variants optimally function and interact. It is a broader version of the centenarian genome project, discussed in Reading 3.1. Comparing the lucky healthy cohort to groups of people who share the same molecularly defined disorder will help to pinpoint the exact deviations that underlie the pathology.

Another type of study made feasible by the sequencing of the human genome will scrutinize the genomes of people at high risk for an illness, but who do not have it—much as researchers study healthy people repeatedly exposed to HIV who never become infected to identify protective gene variants. Why does one 40-year, two-pack-a-day smoker *not* develop lung cancer, while another does? Why does an 85-year-old man who has eaten three eggs a day all his life have low cholesterol—a real case reported years ago in a medical journal. Why do only some people who inherit *BRCA1* mutations develop cancer?

At the same time that human genome information reveals the underpinnings of health, the identification of disease-causing genes that has proceeded for half a century will continue, but with unprecedented precision. Breast cancer will no longer be considered "a" disease, but several distinct errors in cell cycling—sharing a phenotype, but not a genotype, and hence requiring different treatments. Each genetically influenced disease in an individual will be considered in the context of the entire genome.

Future treatments based on genome information will not be limited to correcting or circumventing genetic flaws, or supplying missing proteins. Discovering which gene variants contribute to which diseases, and how they do so, will enable us to identify risk factors that are easier to control—those from the environment. (This has, of course, been obvious for years for diseases such as lung cancer that have clear environmental triggers.) With the entire protein-encoding part of the human genome already available on a tiny chip, and fast, economical genome sequencing coming, the testing that Laurel and Mackenzie undergo in chapter 1 may soon represent a small and primitive fraction of what is possible.

Key Concepts

Genome researchers use a multistory building metaphor to describe the applications of genome information. The three floors represent biological research, health care, and society, and they are each intersected by six categories: resources (such as databases); technology development; computational biology; training; ELSI (ethics, legal, and social issues); and education. Studies of genome sequence information in groups of individuals can reveal how healthy people stay that way, how disease arises, and how and why individuals experience the same disorders differently.

Epilogue: Genome Information Will Affect You

Since the dawn of humanity, people have probably noted inherited traits, from height and body build, to hair and eye color, to talents, to behavioral quirks, to illnesses. Genetics provides the variety that makes life interesting.

The science of genetics grew out of questions surrounding plant and animal breeding, then became human-oriented in the mid-twentieth century with the recognition that certain characteristics and conditions run in families, sometimes recurring with predictable frequencies. Today, genetics and genomics are often in the news, and are beginning to impact many areas of clinical medicine. Once covered only in obscure scientific journals, genetic and genomic analyses of diseases are regularly featured in the top medical journals, as physicians embrace a field that was not so long ago barely touched upon in medical school.

You will likely encounter many of the genetic technologies discussed in this book. In the near future, you might

- be offered a DNA microarray test to diagnose or treat a medical condition.

- serve on a jury and be asked to evaluate DNA profiling evidence.

- undergo a panel of genetic tests before trying to have a child.

- seek preimplantation genetic diagnosis to ensure that your child does not inherit a particular gene.

- help a parent or other loved one through chemotherapy, with some assurance, thanks to DNA testing, that the most effective drugs will be tried first.

- eat a genetically modified fruit or vegetable (you likely have already done this).

- receive a body part from a pig, with cell surfaces matched to your own.

- take medicine manufactured in a transgenic organism.

The list of applications of genetic technology is long and ever-expanding. I hope that this book has offered you glimpses of the future and prepared you to deal personally with the choices that genetic technology will present to you. Let me know your thoughts!

Ricki Lewis
rickilewis@nasw.org

Summary

22.1 Genome Sequencing: A Continuation of Genetics

1. Genetic maps have increased in detail and resolution, from cytogenetic and linkage maps to physical and sequence maps.

2. The International Consortium used BAC clones pinned to sequence tagged sites on chromosomes. Celera Genomics used a whole genome shotgun strategy.

3. **Positional cloning** discovered individual genes by beginning with a phenotype and gradually identifying a causative gene, localizing it to a particular part of a chromosome.

22.2 The Origin of the Idea

4. Automated DNA sequencing and the ability of computers to align and derive long base sequences were vital to sequencing the human genome.

5. In the Sanger method of DNA sequencing, DNA fragments differing in size and with one labeled end base are aligned, and the sequence read off from the end bases.

6. Single-molecule detection quickly and economically unwinds DNA through a microfluidics environment, then a laser scanner reads off fluorescently tagged bases as they pass by.

7. Many people thought of sequencing the human genome, for different reasons. The project officially began in 1990 under the direction of the DOE and NIH.

22.3 Technology Drives the Sequencing Effort

8. **Expressed sequenced tags** enable researchers to find protein-encoding genes. DNA microarrays reveal gene expression. Both were developed in the early 1990s.

9. In 1995, with better technology, the focus shifted from mapping to sequencing. Interest in proteomics began.

10. By 1999, competition had intensified. The first draft of the genome sequence was announced in 2000.

22.4 Into the Future

11. Three main areas that human genome sequence information will impact are basic biological research, health care, and society. Each also has six subdivisions: resources, technology development, computational biology, training, ELSI, and education.

12. Comparing the genomes of a healthy cohort to groups of people with certain diseases may reveal how gene combinations maintain health. Clues to health also lie in the genome sequences of people at high risk for certain disorders who do not become ill.

13. Understanding how genes contribute to disease will reveal more controllable risk factors.

Review Questions

1. How did the following technologies contribute to sequencing the human genome, or to the start of genomics?
   a. expressed sequence tags
   b. positional cloning
   c. DNA microarray technology
   d. automated DNA sequencing
   e. assembler computer programs

2. Why is a cytogenetic map less precise than a sequence map?

3. In 1966, Francis Crick suggested that knowing the genome of a simple bacterial cell would reveal how life works. Why was he mistaken?

4. Two difficulties in sequencing the human genome were the large number of repeat sequences, and the fact that DNA is double-stranded. Explain how these characteristics complicated sequencing efforts.

5. If a researcher wanted to attempt to create a genome of a free-living life form, which organism could serve as a model? Cite a reason for your answer.

6. What has comparative genomics revealed about our relationships to yeast, worms, and flies?

7. Why did the Sanger method of DNA sequencing suffice for the human genome project, but is now considered to be too slow?

Applied Questions

1. Why must several copies of a genome be cut up to sequence it?

2. Celera Genomics actually sequenced several different genomes (one of which was J. Craig Venter's). Why would the sequences not be identical?

3. How could DNA microarray technology grow before human genome sequencing was completed?

4. Axenfeld-Rieger anomaly is an autosomal dominant condition whose symptoms include absent eye muscles, flattened leg bones and associated abnormal gait, mild hearing loss, a flattened midface, prominent forehead, large nose, and bulging eyes. How might a researcher use DNA microarray technology and human genome information to identify the gene that causes this condition?

5. Restriction enzymes break a sequence of DNA bases into the following pieces:

   T T A A T A T C G

   C G T T A A T A T C G C T A G

   G C T T C G T T

   A A T A T C G C T A G C T G C A

   C T T C G T

   T A G C T G C A

   G T T A A T A T C G C T A G C T G C A

   How long is the original sequence? Reconstruct it.

6. One newly identified human gene has counterparts (homologs) in bacteria, yeast, roundworms, mustard weed, fruit flies, mice, and chimpanzees. A second gene has homologs in fruit flies, mice, and chimpanzees only. What does this information reveal about the functions of these two human genes with respect to each other?

7. Many physicians do not have much training in genetics, but these are the professionals to whom most people turn for genetic information. Genetic counselors convey information, but Ph.D. scientists are the ones who are pioneering genomics. Suggest a way for physicians to attain new expertise that will assist them in translating research discoveries into clinical applications.

8. Do you think the human genome sequence should be in the public domain, available to all researchers, or should companies own the information and make it available for a fee? How might the amount of such a fee be determined?

9. It is possible now to measure your blood pressure using a machine available in a supermarket, or mail a blood sample to a laboratory to test for HIV infection or hereditary hemochromatosis. Do you think it would ever be useful, or safe, to be able to mail a plucked hair or cheek scraping to a laboratory and receive an analysis of your genome?

10. Write out the three-story building metaphor for the future of human genome information, including the six areas, in outline form, and provide an example of each of the eighteen intersecting areas.

11. Suggest a study design to reveal why siblings with the same genetic disorder may experience different severities of the family's illness.

12. Consult figure 22.10 and table 22.2.

   a. Suggest a project that could encompass all three "floors" of the human genome building metaphor at one time.

   b. A researcher wishes to identify all the proteins in a contracting human muscle cell. Which building level would this project fit into?

   c. Can you think of any questions that are not addressed in table 22.2, or of a different way to organize ideas about how we should proceed in using human genome information?

13. Headlines about sequencing genomes of such unusual organisms as sea squirts and pufferfish often serve as material for comedians. Why, scientifically, is it important to sequence the genomes of a variety of organisms?

14. If the "$1,000 genome" can be achieved, how should we decide who should have their genomes sequenced, under what conditions, and who should have access to the resulting information?

Web Activities

15. Go to the ELSI web pages at: http://www.ornl.gov/TechResources/Human_Genome/elsi/elsi.html.

   Discuss one societal concern arising from genomics, and how it might affect you.

Case Studies

16. Reread chapter 1, look through this book again, and devise a plan for yourself. Which genes would you like to know about, and when? What will you do with the information? Will you tell anyone what you find out? Who?

Learn to apply the skills of a genetic counselor with these additional cases found in the *Case Workbook in Human Genetics.*

   Diffuse large B cell lymphoma

   Muscle cell DNA microarray

Suggested Readings

Baltimore, David. February 15, 2001. Our genome unveiled. *Nature* 409:814–16. A summary of the human genome project, including a great glossary of jargon and acronyms.

Collins, Francis S., et al. April 24, 2003. A vision for the future of genomics research. *Nature* 422:835–47. A plan for responsible utilization of human genome information based on an architectural metaphor.

Constans, Aileen. June 30, 2003. Beyond Sanger: Toward the $1000 genome. *The Scientist*, 17(13):36–38. The time and cost to sequence a human genome are falling fast.

International Human Genome Mapping Consortium. February 15, 2001. A physical map of the human genome. *Nature* 409:934–41. The public first-draft human genome sequence. Other articles in this issue discuss specific chromosomes.

Lewis, Ricki. July 24, 2000. Keeping up: Genetics to genomics in four editions. *The Scientist* 14(15):46. A look at the coevolution of this textbook and genomics.

Lewis, Ricki. January 5, 1998. Comparative genomics reveals the interrelatedness of life. *The Scientist* 12(1):5. Probing genomes shows that species are more alike than different.

Maher, Brendan. February 4, 2002. The human genome—one year later. *The Scientist* 16(5):29. A look back at the human genome annotation.

Olson, Maynard. February 15, 2001. Clone by clone by clone. *Nature* 490:816–18. How the International Consortium sequenced the human genome.

Pevzner, Pavel A. September 2001. Assembling puzzles from preassembled blocks. *Genome Research* 11(9):1–2. A clear explanation of how a DNA genome sequence assembler program works.

Roberts, Leslie. February 16, 2001. Controversial from the start. *Science* 291:1182–88. The first draft human genome project got off to a rocky start, and ended with a fight.

Singer, Peter A., and Abdallah S. Daar. October 5, 2001. Harnessing genomics and biotechnology to improve global health equity. *Science* 294:87–89. Researchers hope that genomic technologies will improve health care in all nations.

Venter, J. C., et al. February 16, 2001. The sequence of the human genome. *Science* 291:1304–51. Celera Genomics's first-draft human genome sequence and annotation.

Wade, Nicholas. February 13, 2001. Grad student becomes gene effort's unlikely hero. *The New York Times*, p. F1. How a graduate student compressed the work of six months into four weeks to save the public human genome project.

Weekly updates of current news related to human genetics are available through Power Web on your Online Learning Center.

Answers

to End-of-Chapter Questions

Chapter 1 Overview of Genetics

Answers to Review Questions

1. Gene pool, genome, chromosome, gene, DNA

2. a. An autosome does not carry genes that determine sex. A sex chromosome does.

   b. Genotype is the allele constitution in an individual for a particular gene. Phenotype is the physical expression of an allele combination.

   c. DNA is a double-stranded nucleic acid that includes deoxyribose and the nitrogenous bases adenine, guanine, cytosine, and thymine. DNA carries the genetic information. RNA is a single-stranded nucleic acid that includes ribose and the nitrogenous bases adenine, guanine, cytosine, and uracil. RNA carries out gene expression.

   d. A recessive allele determines phenotype in two copies. A dominant allele determines phenotype in one copy.

   e. Absolute risk refers to an individual's personal risk. Relative risk is in comparison to another group, and is less precise.

   f. A pedigree is a chart of family relationships and traits. A karyotype is a chart of chromosomes.

   g. A gene is a sequence of DNA that encodes a protein. A genome is all the DNA in a cell.

3. Inherited disease differs from other types of diseases in that recurrence risk is predictable for particular individuals in families; predictive testing detection is possible; and different populations have different characteristic frequencies of traits or disorders.

4. CF is caused by one malfunctioning gene. Height reflects the actions of several genes and environmental influences, such as diet.

5. A mutant is a variant, usually uncommon, but not necessarily harmful.

6. A genetic test can predict symptoms.

Answers to Applied Questions

1. 16

2. An individual shares more genes with a sibling (1/2) than with a first cousin (1/8).

3. The benefits: more convictions and exonerations would be obtained at the risk of invading the privacy of many people. Use of a population database is not foolproof. An adopted person might have an identical twin who is a suspect in a crime, and not know it. The database would implicate both twins. To be effective, DNA data should not be the only evidence considered.

4. Genetic engineering could mean any intentional change to DNA, whereas a transgenic organism has DNA from a member of a different species. A transgenic organism is created using a type of genetic engineering.

5. Restricting publication of pathogen genome sequences might or might not prevent development of bioweapons, but would hamper research. An answer might balance the gains possible from microbiological research—such as new vaccines and treatments—against the possibility of abuse of that information.

6. "ATCG" on the http://gnn.tigr.org/articles/art_gallery.shtml website depicts James Watson's DNA.

7. Many cartoons state that the genetic code is human and was recently cracked, that geneticists are evil or rich or both, and that genetically modified foods are known to be dangerous.

8. Oxidative stress profile for skin health and aging; obesity susceptibility profile; osteopenia
   Pro: If you have one, you can change your behavior to lower the risk.
   Con: If you think the problem is genetic, you may stop efforts to follow a healthy lifestyle. The tests are SNP based. Treat skin aging before wrinkles appear. Dangers unknown.

9. The wife

10. More likely than general population: coronary artery disease, kidney cancer, lung cancer, depression.
    Less likely than general population: addictive behaviors, diabetes.

11. Multiple sclerosis is multifactorial, and because of interacting, multiple causes, precise recurrence risks are not possible.

12. a. It is crucial to know what percentage of people with the carpal tunnel gene variant actually develop the condition, and whether an individual's job assignment would overwork the wrists.

    b. The test is not scientifically sound because a predisposition indicates increased probability of a future event, not an absolute prediction.

    c. Do not compel a person to take a genetic test, such as threatening job loss.

Chapter 2 Cells

Answers to Review Questions

1. a. In signal transduction, an outside stimulus triggers a chain reaction among membrane proteins that causes production or activation of a second messenger, which activates the genes that directly provide the cell's response.

   b. In cell adhesion, cell surface molecules direct how cells attach and move.

   c. In the cell cycle, a cell proceeds through an interphase consisting of two gap phases, when proteins and lipids are synthesized, and a synthesis phase when DNA is replicated, then mitosis, when the DNA divides, followed by cytokinesis, when other cellular constituents are distributed between the resulting two daughter cells.

   d. In apoptosis, a death receptor receives a death signal, then activates caspases that destroy the cell in a series of steps. Membranes surround the pieces, preventing inflammation.

e. In mitosis, the replicated DNA condenses, the nucleolus temporarily breaks down, and the centromeres part and two sets of chromosomes move to opposite ends of the cell. Then the cell physically divides in two.

f. In secretion, proteins produced in the rough ER join carbohydrates and lipids in the Golgi apparatus, and exit the cell encased in lipid vesicles.

2. a. Tubulin forms microtubules and actin forms microfilaments, which comprise the cytoskeleton.

b. Caspases carry out apoptosis.

c. Changing levels of cyclins and kinases regulate the cell cycle.

d. Checkpoint proteins provide choices during the cell cycle.

e. Cellular adhesion molecules allow certain cell types to stick to each other.

3. Hormones, growth factors, cyclins, and kinases.

4. Specialized cells express different subsets of all the genes that are present in all cell types, except for red blood cells.

5. a. A bacterial cell is usually small and lacks a nucleus and other organelles. A eukaryotic cell contains membrane-bounded organelles, including a nucleus, that compartmentalize biochemical reactions.

b. During interphase, cellular components are replicated. During mitosis, the cell divides, distributing its contents into two daughter cells.

c. Mitosis increases cell number. Apoptosis eliminates cells.

d. Rough ER is a labyrinth of membranous tubules, studded with ribosomes that synthesize proteins. Smooth ER is the site of lipid synthesis and lacks ribosomes.

e. Microtubules are tubules of tubulin and microfilaments are rods of actin. Both form the cytoskeleton.

f. A stem cell has greater developmental potential than a progenitor cell.

g. A totipotent cell can differentiate as any cell type; a pluripotent cell's fate is more restricted.

6. a. Mitochondria extract energy from nutrients to fuel cellular activities.

b. Lysosomes are sacs of enzymes that break down debris.

c. Peroxisomes break down certain lipids and rare biochemicals, synthesize bile acids and detoxify compounds that result from excess oxygen exposure.

d. Smooth ER is the site of lipid synthesis.

e. Rough ER is the site of protein synthesis.

f. The Golgi apparatus is the site of carbohydrate addition to proteins to form secretions.

g. The nucleus houses the genetic material.

7. Compartmentalization separates biochemicals that could harm certain cell constituents. It also organizes the cell so it can function more efficiently.

8. The plasma membrane is the backdrop that holds many of the molecules that intercept incoming signals. These molecules contort in ways that amplify and spread the message.

9. The genome from a stem cell derived from an IVF embryo is that of the fertilized ovum; the genome in a stem cell obtained with SCNT is that of the nucleus donor, typically a patient.

Answers to Applied Questions

1. a. Lack of cell adhesion can speed the migration of cancer cells.

b. Impaired signal transduction can block a message to cease dividing.

c. Blocking apoptosis can cause excess mitosis, and an abnormal growth.

d. Lack of cell cycle control can lead to too many mitoses.

e. If telomerase is abnormal, a cell might not cease to divide when it normally would.

2. Because enzymes are proteins, genes encode them.

3. Nucleus and lysosomes

4. Stem cells maintain their populations because each mitosis produces a daughter cell that differentiates, as well as one that remains a stem cell.

5. Too frequent mitosis leads to an abnormal growth. Too little mitosis can limit growth or repair of damaged tissues. Too much apoptosis

can kill healthy tissue. Too little apoptosis can lead to abnormal growths.

6. A cell in an embryo would not be in G_o because it has to divide frequently to support the high growth rate.

7. Mitochondria

8. Disrupting microtubules can prevent the spindle apparatus from either forming or breaking down, either of which would halt mitosis. A drug that disables telomerase might enable chromosomes to shrink, which might stop mitosis. A drug can intercept an extracellular signal to divide.

9. Signals from outside the cell interact with receptors embedded in the plasma membrane, and the plasma membrane's interior face contacts the cytoskeleton.

10. a. Abnormal chloride channels in cell membranes of lung lining cells and pancreas.

b. Lack of a transport protein in peroxisomes leads to build up of long-chain fatty acids.

c. Abnormal growth factors and signal transduction cause nerve overgrowth under skin.

d. Lack of CAMs impairs wound healing.

e. Syndactyly is a failure of apoptosis to fully separate digits.

11. Stem cells in the body may sense and respond to signals that indicate injury or a crisis. They may home to the affected site and divide to form cells that can heal the injury.

12. AIDS patient donates a cell with a nucleus, such as a skin fibroblast. Donor oocyte has its nucleus removed or destroyed. Patient's nucleus injected into oocyte. Oocyte with donor nucleus allowed to develop to blastocyst stage. Inner cell mass cells removed and cultured to become ES cells, then appropriate biochemicals applied to stimulate development to form a thymus gland. Tissue grafted into AIDS patient.

13. Senate bill 245 and House of Representatives bill 234 prohibit and criminalize reproductive cloning and SCNT to treat patients and in research. S303 and HR801 ban reproductive cloning but allow SCNT for research.

14. U.S., Germany, Norway = neither

U.K., Israel, China = both

Canada, France = IVF ok, no SCNT

Belgium, Sweden = no IVF, SCNT ok

15. **a.** Anthony was more likely to have it, because his abnormal cells were not replaced immediately, as were Julia's.

   b. The stem cells came from an umbilical cord, not an embryo.

   c. Julia might have relapsed because not all of her affected cells were obliterated prior to the cord blood stem cell transplant.

Chapter 3 Development

Answers to Review Questions

1. **a.** 2 **b.** 2 **c.** 1 **d.** 2 **e.** 1 **f.** 1 **g.** 1

2. Male: Sperm are manufactured in seminiferous tubules packed into the testes, and mature and are stored in the epididymis. The epididymis is continuous with the vas deferens, which carries sperm to the urethra, which sends them out through the penis. The prostate gland and the seminal vesicles secrete into the vas deferens, and the bulbourethral glands secrete into the urethra, forming seminal fluid.
   Female: Oocytes develop within the ovaries and are released into the fallopian tubes, which carry them to the uterus, which narrows to form the cervix, which opens to the vagina.

3. 2^{39}. This is an underestimate because it does not account for crossing over.

4. Mitosis divides somatic cells into two daughter cells with the same number of chromosomes as the diploid parent cell. Meiosis forms gametes, in which the 4 daughter cells have half the number of chromosomes of the parent cell. Recombination occurs in meiosis.

5. Both produce gametes, but oogenesis takes years and spermatogenesis takes months.

6. In female gamete maturation, most of the cytoplasm concentrates in one huge cell. In male gamete maturation, 4 same-size sperm derive from an original cell undergoing meiosis.

7. Hundreds of millions of sperm are deposited in the vagina during intercourse. There, the sperm are chemically activated and the oocyte secretes a sperm attractant. Sperm tail movement and contraction of the woman's muscles aid sperm movement. When sperm contact follicle cells, their acrosomes release enzymes that penetrate the oocyte. When the plasma membranes of sperm and oocyte meet, a wave of electricity spreads physical and chemical changes over the oocyte surface, blocking other sperm. The nuclei approach, merge, and the chromosomes of the two cells meet. The fertilized ovum is a zygote.

8. Teratogens are more dangerous to an embryo than they are to a fetus because structures form in the first eight weeks.

9. Teratogens include thalidomide, alcohol, excess nutrients, cocaine, cigarettes, and infections. Exposure to teratogens during critical periods can have drastic effects.

10. Accelerated aging disorders and studies on adopted individuals indicate an inherited component to longevity.

Answers to Applied Questions

1. Answers may vary. A commonly used cutoff point for experimentation is after the second week, when primary germ layers begin to form.

2. The chromosomes in a polar body resulting from the first meiotic division would be replicated, unlike those from the second meiotic division.

3. yes

4. Stem or progenitor cells

5. A polar body does not have enough cytoplasm and organelles to support an embryo.

6. Some people believe that a pregnant woman should be held legally responsible for knowingly exposing an embryo or fetus to a teratogen.

7. opinion

8. Prenatal environmental stress, such as lack of nutrients, can alter gene expression in ways that enhance utilization of nutrients, which is adaptive for the fetus but may set the stage for future diabetes or heart disease. Evidence is epidemiological and based on animal studies.

9. Don't: smoke, eat nitrites in cured meats, eat charred meats, eat a lot of fat, drink excess alcohol, breathe polluted air, drink excess coffee. Avoid excess sun, calories and risky behavior. Exercise.

10. Pigment patterns of cloned calves differ.

11. **a.** The basis of these tests is that the cells whose DNA is tested descend from the fertilized ovum, and should therefore be genetically identical to it.

   b. Cleavage embryo

   c. The structures in Diana and Max's fetus are more detailed than those in Anna and Peter's, but organs are present in both.

Chapter 4 Mendelian Inheritance

Answers to Review Questions

1. The law of segregation derives from the fact that during meiosis, alleles separate into different gametes. The law of independent assortment is based on the fact that distribution of alleles of two unlinked genes into gametes occurs at random.

2. The two laws of inheritance were derived from pea crosses. Without knowing about chromosomes, Mendel observed offspring phenotypes and predicted results of crosses.

3. **a.** An autosomal recessive trait is inherited from carriers and affects both sexes. An autosomal dominant trait can be inherited from one parent, who is affected. Autosomal recessive inheritance can skip generations; autosomal dominant inheritance cannot.

   b. Mendel's first law concerns inheritance of one trait. The second law follows inheritance of two genes on different chromosomes.

   c. A homozygote has identical alleles for a particular gene, and a heterozygote has different alleles.

   d. The parents of a monohybrid cross are heterozygotes for a single gene. Parents of a dihybrid cross are heterozygous for a pair of genes.

   e. A Punnett square tracks the distribution of alleles of genes on different chromosomes from parents to offspring. A pedigree depicts family members and their inherited traits.

4. If Mendel had chosen two traits on the same chromosome, he would have observed a higher percentage of offspring inheriting two alleles together rather than independently.

5. Blood relatives share alleles inherited from common ancestors.

6. The Egyptian pedigree only traces genealogy and not inheritance of traits. The pedigree a genetic counselor would use today would trace inherited traits too.

7. The parents of a person who is homozygous dominant for HD must be heterozygotes.

8. 100 percent

Answers to Applied Questions

1. Autosomal dominant—it affects both sexes, and occurs every generation.

2. Pedigree

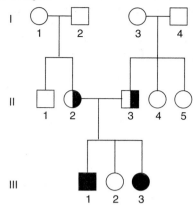

3. Carriers are I-3, I-4, II-4, III-3, III-4.

4. One in 2 chance the child has double eyelashes.

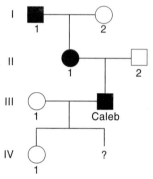

5. Consanguinity

6. Genotypic ratios:

4/32 = BbHhEe	2/32 = bbHhee
4/32 = bbHhEe	1/32 = BbHHEE
2/32 = BbHhEE	1/32 = BbhhEE
2/32 = BbJJEe	1/32 = BbHHee
2/32 = BbhhEe	1/32 = Bbhhee
2/32 = BbHhee	1/32 = bbHHEE
2/32 = bbHhEE	1/32 = bbhhEE
2/32 = bbHHEe	1/32 = bbHHee
2/32 = bbhhEe	1/32 = bbhhee

Phenotypic ratios:

9/32 = yellow urine, colored eyelids, short fingers

9/32 = red urine, colored eyelids, short fingers

3/32 = yellow urine, normal eyelids, short fingers

3/32 = red urine, normal eyelids, short fingers

3/32 = yellow urine, colored eyelids, long fingers

3/32 = red urine, colored eyelids, long fingers

1/32 = yellow urine, normal eyelids, long fingers

1/32 = red urine, colored eyelids, long fingers

7. II-1 and II-2 must be carriers. All of the individuals in generation 1 could be carriers.

8. $.10 \times .002 = .0002 = 2$ in 10,000

9. a. Uncles and nieces having children together.

   b. Carriers = III-5, III-6, III-9, IV-1 and niece, IV-6, IV-11, V-4, V-5, V-6, V-9, V-10

10. No

11. First cousins

12. His normal allele enables enough of the enzyme to be produced so that his nervous system can function normally.

13. Glycogen storage disease type VII is autosomal recessive and causes muscle cramps with exercise. Edna and Murray Schwartz are in their 70s, and neither has experienced muscle pain with exercise, although they are both sedentary, so would not know. Their son, Zeppo, is a distance runner, as is his wife, Marsha. They are surprised when their daughter Kelly wants to try out for the gymnastics team, but becomes paralyzed with cramps upon exertion.

Macroglossia is autosomal dominant, and causes a large tongue, feeding problems, and snoring. The McDoofis family has a long history of babies with feeding problems, and loud snorers. In each generation, at least one individual has a very large tongue.

14. The retinoblastoma gene on chromosome 20 and the cystic fibrosis gene on chromosome 7 independently assort. The genes for xeroderma pigmentosum and brachydactyly type B1, each on chromosome 9, do not.

15. a. Autosomal recessive

   b. Both sexes are affected, and it skips generations

   c. Pedigree

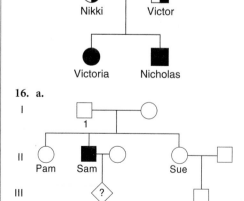

16. a.

b. 1/2

c. 1/4

d. She is incorrect because each family member is an independent event.

Chapter 5 Extensions and Exceptions to Mendel's Laws

Answers to Review Questions

1. a. Lethal alleles eliminate a progeny class that Mendel's laws predict should exist.

   b. Multiple alleles create the possibility of more than two phenotypic classes.

   c. Incomplete dominance introduces a third phenotype for a gene with two alleles.

   d. Codominance introduces a third phenotype for a gene with two alleles.

   e. Epistasis eliminates a progeny class when a gene masks another's expression.

   f. Incomplete penetrance produces a phenotype that does not reveal the genotype.

   g. Variable expressivity can make the same genotype appear to different degrees.

   h. Pleiotropy can make the same genotype appear as more than one phenotype because subsets of effects are expressed.

   i. A phenocopy mimics inheritance, but is an environmental effect.

   j. Conditions with the same symptoms but caused by different genes (genetic heterogeneity) will not recur with the frequency that they would if there was only one causative gene.

2. Dominant and recessive alleles are of the same gene, whereas epistasis is an interaction of alleles of different genes.

3. It can skip generations in terms of phenotype.

4. The I^A allele is codominant with the I^B allele; both are completely dominant to i.

5. Knowing the human genome sequence has revealed genetic heterogeneity, which reflects redundant function. It has identified many new alleles of already known genes. Gene interactions explain penetrance and expressivity—these were once thought to be characteristic of individual genes. DNA microarrays reveal which genes contribute to pleiotropy. Epistasis is more common than once thought.

6. Maternal inheritance describes transmission of mitochondrial genes, which sperm do not usually contribute to oocytes and therefore these traits are always passed from mothers only. Linked genes are transmitted on the same chromosome. Mendel's second law applies to genes transmitted on different chromosomes.

7. Only females transmit maternally inherited traits. All of a woman's children inherit a mitochondrial trait, but a male does not pass the trait to his children.

8. Additional genes may affect expression of a particular gene, and therefore the same genotype for that gene may be associated with a different phenotype in different individuals.

9. Twenty-four linkage groups, including 22 pairs of autosomes, and the X and the Y.

Answers to Applied Questions

1. **a.** D **b.** A **c.** E **d.** C **e.** H **f.** F **g.** G **h.** G **i.** E

2. Haplotypes can reveal if people without symptoms have the haplotype associated with the condition. These people are non-penetrant. If the genotype is lethal, individuals with the haplotype containing the lethal allele should not exist.

3. **a.** 1/2 **b.** 1/2 **c.** 0 **d.** 0

4. 1/4

5. **a.** This alters the phenotype.

   b. Bombay phenotype

6. It would be Mendelian because the gene that causes the condition when mutated is in the nucleus.

7. $.45 \times .05 = .0225$

8. The sperm are all of genotype *hh se se*. The oocytes are of genotype *Hh Se se*, with the alleles in cis:

$$H \underline{\quad\quad} Se$$
$$h \underline{\quad\quad} se$$

All sperm are *h se*.

Oocytes: *H Se* 49.5% *h se* 49.5%
          H se 0.5% *h Se* 0.5%

Chance offspring like father =
   1 (*h se*) × 49.5 (*h se*) = 49.5

9. **a.** Male: *RrHhTt*
   Female: *rrhhtt*

   b. Parental progeny classes: Round eyeballs, hairy tail, 9 toes; square eyeballs, smooth tail, 11 toes

   Recombinant progeny classes: Round eyeballs, hairy tail, 11 toes; square eyeballs, smooth tail, 9 toes; round eyeballs, smooth tail, 11 toes; square eyeballs, hairy tail, 9 toes

   c. Crossover frequency between eyeball shape (*R*) and toe number (*T*): Round eyeballs, 11 toes = 6 + 4; square eyeballs, 9 toes = 6 + 4; crossover frequency = $20/100 = 20\%$

10. Ehlers-Danlos syndrome, FG syndrome, Kabuki syndrome, VATER association

11. Kearn-Sayre syndrome, heart failure, infections, anemia, hearing loss, pancreatic failure, visual loss

12. chromosome 3: genes for sodium channel, voltage-gated, type V, alpha and contactin 3 and chondroitin sulfate proteoglycan 5

13. **a.** a, b, c, d

    b. People with one copy have abnormalities so mild that they are not noticeable without a test. People with two copies can be severely affected.

    c. The parents are heterozygotes, so each of their offspring has a 1 in 4 probability of inheriting two wild type alleles, like Tina.

    d. Phenotype

Chapter 6 Matters of Sex

Answers to Review Questions

1. Sex is expressed at the chromosomal level as inheriting XX or XY; at the gonadal level by developing ovaries or testes; at the phenotypic level by developing male or female internal and external structures; and at the gender identity level by feelings.

2. Genes in the pseudoautosomal region are the same as certain X-linked genes, but X-Y genes share only sequence similarities.

3. **a.** Female **b.** Female **c.** Female

4. Sustentacular cells secrete anti-Müllerian hormone, which stops development of female reproductive structures. Interstitial cells secrete testosterone, which promotes development of male reproductive structures.

5. Absence of the *SRY* gene product causes the Müllerian ducts to develop into ovaries. The ovaries produce female hormones, which influence the development of external and internal reproductive structures.

6. Feelings of very young children; twin studies in which identical twins are more likely to both be homosexual than are fraternal twins; fruit fly behavior; genes on the X chromosome that segregate with homosexuality.

7. A female homozygous dominant for an X-linked dominant allele would probably be so severely affected that she would not be alive or healthy enough to reproduce.

8. Coat color in cats is X-linked. In females, one X chromosome in each cell is inactivated, and the pattern of a calico cat's coat depends on which cells express which coat color allele. A male cat, with only one coat color allele, would have to inherit an extra X chromosome to be tortoiseshell or calico.

9. Inactivation of the gene in some cells but not others results in a patchy phenotype.

10. Each cell in a female's body contains only one active X chromosome, which makes females genetically equivalent (in terms of X-linked genes) to males.

11. An X-linked trait appears usually in males and may affect structures or functions not distinct to one sex. A sex-limited trait affects a structure or function distinct to one sex. A sex-influenced trait is inherited as a recessive in one sex and dominant in the other.

12. Mouse zygotes with two female pronuclei or two male pronuclei are abnormal. In humans, two male and one female genome in the same embryo yields placental tissue, while two female and one male genome yields a normal embryo with an abnormal placenta.

Answers to Applied Questions

1. **a.** 1/2 **b.** 1/2 **c.** 1/2 **d.** A carrier might have symptoms if the mutated gene is expressed in tissues affected by the condition.

2. Girls may have milder cases because X inactivation might inactivate a more severe allele in some cells, and because hormonal differences from males may affect the phenotype.

3. The unevenness of the teeth of affected females may reflect expression of the defect in only some cells as the result of X inactivation.

4. XXX female

5. Genomic imprinting

6. Rett syndrome, OMIM 312750: autism, dementia, loss of hand use, jerky movements, seizures, poor growth

7. Cornelia de Lange syndrome, which causes growth retardation, characteristic facial features, and mental retardation, comes from the mother. Wolf-Hirschhorn syndrome, with severe growth retardation, microcephaly, "Greek helmet face," heart defects, and cleft lip or palate, comes from the father.

8. 1/4

9.

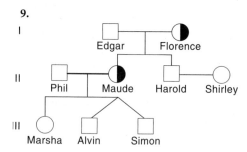

10. a. Because the phenotype is not severe.

   b. 1 in 2, because she is a carrier.

   c. 1 in 1

11. 1/2

12. a. Carriers = I-4, II-3, III-2, III-5 **b.** 1/2 **c.** 1/2 **d.** Women would have to inherit kinky hair disease from an affected father and a carrier mother; affected males would not live long enough to have children.

Chapter 7 Multifactorial Traits

Answers to Review Questions

1. Body weight is more likely to be multifactorial than eye color, because eating and exercise habits greatly influence weight. We can't change eye color.

2. FH, leptin deficiency, lipodystrophy, melanocortin-4 receptor deficiency

3. A Mendelian multifactorial trait is caused by one gene and environmental influences, whereas a polygenic multifactorial trait is caused by more than one gene and environmental influences.

4. Eye color has a greater heritability because the environment has a greater influence on height than on eye color.

5. Heritability for skin color changes because the duration and intensity of sun exposure contribute to skin color.

6. The environment determines which infections a person with CF contracts.

7. a. Empiric risk is based on observations of trait prevalence in a particular population or group of individuals.

   b. Twin studies approximate the degree of heritability by comparing trait prevalence among pairs of MZ twins to DZ twins. The greater the difference, the higher the heritability.

   c. Inherited traits may stand out in an adoptee's family where each member lives in the same environment, but the adopted individual has different genes.

   d. Association studies establish correlations between particular gene variants or sections of chromosomes (haplotypes) and inheritance of certain traits or susceptibilities.

8. Many people must be surveyed to determine whether a certain haplotype (and its SNPs) is exclusively associated with a particular phenotype. Enough DNA must be considered so that several SNPs are analyzed, and a case-control strategy must be employed to ensure that the same SNPs are not found among affected individuals as well as unaffected ones. Finally, if many SNPs are considered, many combinations must be correlated to phenotypes.

9. Cardiovascular: apolipoproteins, lipoprotein lipase and proteins that regulate blood pressure or homocysteine metabolism

Body weight: neuropeptide Y, genes that control leptin, melanocortin-4 receptor

10. More genotypes specify a medium brown skin color than other colors.

Answers to Applied Questions

1. a. The different affected sibs results and heritabilities from two populations suggest ADHD has a large environmental component. Increased relative risk among sibs and in adoptees of affected individuals also suggests a large environmental component.

   b. Differences in classroom restrictiveness.

   c. Attempt to identify specific genes and determine effects their protein products would have to exert to cause symptoms of ADHD.

   d. Drugs for ADHD are overprescribed, because diagnosis is based on symptoms, which might not always reflect illness. Knowing genetic

susceptibility could avoid prescribing drugs to people in whom they would not work.

   e. A genetic test for ADHD might also identify highly creative, talented people! If there is a gene for ADHD, it is likely affected by other genes in ways that make the overall phenotype a talent, not a disorder.

2. A drug for obesity would block neuropeptide Y or stimulate production of the melanocortin-4 receptor.

3. A genetic change in a population would not occur in so short a time. Therefore, the cause for the increase in obesity is largely environmental, perhaps acting on inherited susceptibilities.

4. It is important to publish negative results so that the findings can be duplicated, and research stopped or misinformation that could affect health care choices corrected.

5. Heritability, 0.54, suggests the influence of genes and the environment is about equal.

6. Broad

7. a. .5 **b.** .5 **c.** Selfishness is difficult to assess, and is a normal part of childhood.

8. http://www.bovineengineering.com/ Heritability_Table.html traits with heritability <.5 in cattle: carcass loin eye area; efficiency of gain in feed lot; yearling weight; carcass tenderness; length of teats

9. 3 causes of death with high heritability: Alzheimer disease, cancer, asthma. These are multifactorial. 3 causes of death with low heritability: HIV infection, firearms injury, accidents. These are largely environmentally caused.

10. a. Topography of back of iris intensifies the color, or Tanya inherited dark pigment alleles from each parent

   b. Different allele combinations

   c. Height

   d. Height is genetically determined as evidenced by Jamal and Tanya's above average height since early childhood. Effect of diet is seen in their greater height compared to the parents, who did not eat as well.

   e. Eye color

11. During starvation, shrinking fat cells release less leptin, which stimulates neuropeptide Y and inhibits production of melanocortin-4 receptors. Appetite increases.

Chapter 8 The Genetics of Behavior

Answers to Review Questions

1. Proteins whose products are involved in neurotransmission or signal transduction can affect behavior.

2. The older techniques of empiric risk and adoptee and twin studies estimate the proportion of the contribution of genetics to a trait. Linkage, SNP association studies, and genome-wide scans seek to identify particular genes that contribute to a particular behavior.

3. ADHD has a very distinctive phenotype; it is common; and linkage studies point to a candidate gene. In contrast, autism is rare, and linkage points to several candidate genes, suggesting genetic heterogeneity (different ways to inherit the same condition).

4. **a.** sleep disorders **b.** addiction **c.** addiction

5. We must understand how a gene variant affects behavior, and how other genes and the environment affect its expression.

6. **a.** N-CAM

   b. dopamine D(2) receptor

   c. ADH

   d. serotonin receptor or transporter

   e. dopamine or glutamine transporter

7. Genetic heterogeneity; when a behavior is part of several disorders; behaviors that fall within the range of normal, although they are extreme; ability to imitate a behavior.

8. A trait that is polygenic has varying degrees of expression. A trait that is genetically heterogeneic is the same even though caused by mutations in different genes.

9. With age, the environment has had longer to affect gene expression.

Answers to Applied Questions

1. **a.** The same neurotransmitter controls different behaviors. The differences arise from which neurons are involved.

   b. Dopamine

2. Instead of demonstrating the existence and extent of inherited influences, DNA microarrays implicate specific genes, revealing clues to the biological basis of a behavior or behavioral disorder.

3. For all choices—drug addiction, eating disorder, and depression—a SNP profile indicating increased risk could be helpful if the person can take action to lower the risk of developing the condition, but can be harmful if the person just gives up, thinking that fate cannot be avoided. SNP profiling might also be used to discriminate.

4. This is an opinion question. If drugs are outlawed based on their addiction potential, then alcohol and nicotine should be included with other drugs that are illegal. An alternate approach would be to outlaw drugs that impair one's ability to function. Such an approach might outlaw alcohol and cocaine, yet permit tobacco or possibly marijuana use.

5. Yes—a criminal cannot alter his or her inherited behavior. No—the environment can override inherited criminal tendencies.

6. Depression and bipolar disorder each might actually be several conditions that have similar symptoms.

7. Identify what is abnormal in the Utah family, develop a drug to treat the condition, and then try the drug on elderly people who are having difficulty sleeping.

8. The IQ test could be flawed or measure intelligence in a way that does not compensate for differences in educational opportunities.

9. Environmental component about equals genetic susceptibility

10. Research can isolate a chromosomal region where the DNA sequence is common to people with Wolfram syndrome, and eventually discover and describe the causative gene. The specific nature of the corresponding protein product may explain how a half normal gene dose causes the behavioral problems of relatives.

11. These data suggest a large inherited component to alcoholism.

12. Schizophrenia, bipolar disorder, unipolar depression

13. Advantages of genetic testing for an eating disorder: Alleviates guilt and can warn people at high risk so that they can take preventive action in themselves or in their children. Disadvantages: Genetic testing will not change the phenotype and may even discourage someone from trying to control the condition and stigmatization. Does not address underlying societal problem of pressure to be thin.

Chapter 9 DNA Structure and Replication

Answers to Review Questions

1. DNA is replicated so that it is not used up in directing the cell to manufacture protein.

2. 1 E   2 C   3 D   4 B   5 A

3. The nucleotide base sequence encodes information.

4. One end of a strand of nucleotides has a phosphate group attached to the 5′ carbon of deoxyribose. The other end has a hydroxyl group attached to the 3′ carbon. The opposite (complementary) strand has the reverse orientation.

5. Helicases, primase, DNA polymerase, ligase, photolyases

6. **a.**   A G C T C T T A G A G C T A A

   b.   G G C A T A T C G G C C A T G

   c.   T A G C C T A G C G A T G A C

7. Histone protein, nucleosome, chromatin

8. **a.** Opposite orientations of the two DNA chains of a double helix

   b. The fact that a new DNA double helix retains a parental strand

   c. Hydrogen bonding of A with T, T with A, G with C, and C with G in the DNA double helix

9. Hershey and Chase showed that DNA is the genetic material and protein is not. Meselson and Stahl showed that DNA replication is semiconservative, but not conservative or dispersive.

10. Strands separate and are held apart. Primase makes RNA primer. DNA polymerase adds DNA bases to RNA primer. Proofreading, repair. Continuous on one strand only. RNA primers removed. Ligase seals sugar-phosphate backbone.

11. PCR wouldn't work because if DNA replication is conservative, the daughter strand would not be complementary.

Answers to Applied Questions

1. The sugar-phosphate backbone of replicating DNA cannot attach.

2. Primase, DNA polymerase, helicase, binding proteins, and ligase are required for DNA replication.

3. 20 cycles × 2 minutes/cycle = 40 minutes

4. Such a molecule would bulge where purines paired with each other, yet be narrow where pyrimidines pair.

5. Lacking DNA polymerase makes life impossible, because cells cannot divide.

6. PCR can directly detect HIV RNA, rather than a sign that the human body is responding to the presence of the virus.

7. Determining the structure of DNA led to discoveries of the mechanism of heredity, whereas sequencing the human genome provided information.

8. CCACCCTTGGAGTTCACTCA
GGTGGGAACCTCAAGTGAGT

9. Hans and Eva
CGTGCCGCTCG
CGTGCTGCTCG

Peter
CGTGCCGCTCG
CGTGCCGCTCG

Anna
CGTGCTGCTCG
CGTGCTGCTCG

Chapter 10 Gene Action and Expression

Answers to Review Questions

1. a. H bonds between A and T and G and C join the strands of the double helix.

b. In DNA replication, a new strand is synthesized semiconservatively, with new bases inserted opposite their complementary bases to form a new strand.

c. An mRNA is transcribed by aligning RNA nucleotides against their complements in one strand of the DNA.

d. The sequence preceding the protein-encoding sequence of the mRNA base pairs with rRNA in the ribosome.

e. A tRNA binds to mRNA by base pairing between the three bases of its anticodon and the three mRNA bases of a codon.

f. The characteristic cloverleaf of tRNA is a consequence of H bonding between complementary bases.

2. The direction of the flow of genetic information in retroviruses is opposite that of the central dogma.

3. a. The start of a gene

b. tRNA

c. A pseudogene

d. rRNA

e. mRNA

4. a. Proteins with an incorrect sequence of amino acids may not function.

b. If the initial amino acid is released, additional amino acids cannot add on.

c. If rRNA cannot bind to the ribosome, then mRNAs cannot be translated into protein.

d. If ribosomes cannot move, then a protein would not exceed two amino acids in length.

e. If a tRNA picks up the wrong amino acid, the protein's amino acid sequence will be abnormal.

5. Both respond to environmental conditions.

6. RNA contains ribose and uracil and is single-stranded. DNA contains deoxyribose and thymine and is double-stranded. DNA preserves and transmits genetic information; RNA expresses genetic information.

7. DNA replication occurs in the nucleus of eukaryotes. Prokaryotes have no nucleus so replication occurs in the cytoplasm. The same is true of transcription. In eukaryotes, translation occurs in the nucleus and cytoplasm, and some ribosomes are attached to the ER.

8. Transcription controls cell specialization by turning different sets of genes on and off in different cell types.

9. The same mRNA codon can be at the A site and the P site because the ribosome moves.

10. In transcription initiation, the DNA double helix unwinds locally, transcription factors bind near the promoter, and RNA polymerase binds to the promoter.

11. mRNA is the intermediate between DNA and protein, carrying the genetic information to ribosomes. tRNA connects mRNA and amino acids, and transfers amino acids to ribosomes for incorporation into protein. rRNA associates with proteins to form ribosomes.

12. Post-transcriptional changes to RNA include adding a cap and poly A tail, and removing introns.

13. Ribosomes consist of several types of proteins and rRNAs in two subunits of unequal size.

14. An overlapping code constrains protein structure because certain amino acids would always be followed by the same amino acids in every protein.

15. Transcription and translation recycle tRNAs and ribosomes.

16. Proinsulin is shortened to insulin after translation. RNA editing shortens apolipoprotein B post-transcriptionally.

17. Each of these types of abnormalities could affect more than one protein.

18. The amino acid sequence determines a protein's conformation by causing attractions and repulsions between different parts of the molecule.

19. A two-nucleotide genetic code would only specify 17 types of amino acids. There are 20 amino acids in biological proteins.

20. To create a mature mRNA for translation, snurps (small RNAs and proteins) excise introns in pre-mRNAs. Ribozymes assist in peptide bond formation. Proteins make up part of the structure of ribosomes, and enzymes are involved in protein synthesis.

Answers to Applied Questions

1. a. 46

b. 44

2. a. AAUGUGAACGAACUCUCAG

b. UGAACCCGAUACGAGUAAT

c. CCGACGUUAUCGGCAUCUA

d. CCUUAUGCAGAUCGAUCGU

3. a. CGATAGACAGTATTTCTC CT

b. CACCGCATAAGAAAAGGCC CATCC

c. CTCCCTTAAGAAAGAGTTC GTTCA

d. TCCTTTTGGGGAGAATAAT ATCTA

4. Many answers are possible, using combinations of *his* (CAU or CAC), *ala* (CGU, GCC, GCA, GCG), *arg* (CGU, CGC, CGA, CGG), *ser* (AGU, AGC, AGA, AGG), *leu* (CUU, CUC, CUA, CUG), *val* (GUC, GUG), and *cys* (UGU, UGC).

5. Several answers are possible because of the redundancy of the genetic code. One answer is: C A T A C C T T T G G G A A A T G G.

6. There is only one genetic code.

7. Use ACA with any triplet other than CAA, and see whether threonine or histidine occurs. Whichever occurs, ACA encodes.

8. 26,927

9. 125, but this doesn't account for degenerate codons.

10. 1

11. 3,777 DNA bases (plus promoter sequence)

12. a. *Candida cylindrical* (fungus) CTG = serine, normal CUG = leucine

   b. *Mycoplasma* (microorganism) CGG is not used, normal = arginine

   c. Acetabularia (alga) UAA = glutamine, normal = STOP

13. http://medweb.bham.ac.uk/http/depts/clin_neuro/teaching/tutorials/parkinsons1.html Parkinson disease and Lewy body dementia brains accumulate neurofilaments that ubiquitin binds, indicating they are destined for proteasomes.

http://www.lougehrigsdisease.net/als_causes_of_als.htm
"The aggregates may be a byproduct from overwhelmed cells attempting to repair incorrectly folded proteins."

http://www.the-scientist.com/yr2003/may/hot_030519.html
Huntingtin protein plugs up proteasomes.

14. a. Shortens **b.** No change **c.** Shortens **d.** Lengthens **e.** No protein made

Chapter 11 Gene Expression

Answers to Review Questions

1. Transcription and translation must be controlled so that the appropriate amounts of proteins are present for specific cell types.

2. After the genetic code was elucidated, the steps of transcription and translation needed to be determined. After sequencing the genome, genes and their functions had to be identified, and the functions of non-protein encoding sequences discovered.

3. Oxygen level

4. Progenitor cells in the pancreas divide to give rise to daughter cells that differentiate as either exocrine or endocrine cells.

5. A genetic change is a change to DNA. An epigenetic change is not to DNA, but to something that affects it.

6. Histones are proteins, so genes encode them. Yet histones control which genes are transcribed, and under what conditions.

7. Methylation, RNA interference

8. siRNAs dismantle certain mRNAs; proteasomes dismantle misfolded proteins

9. Genes come in pieces. Genes can move. The same sequence of DNA can encode more than one protein because of exon shuffling.

10. Introns interrupt genes. Exons from different genes can contribute to the same protein. An intron on one strand may be an exon on the other.

11. a. Add or remove acetyl groups to lysines on histones

   b. Cuts long double-stranded RNAs into 21- or 22-base-long pieces

   c. Binds and unwinds RNA pieces cut by dicer

   d. Attracts acetylase to add lysines to certain histones

   e. Controls hemoglobin chain switching

   f. Controls fate of progenitor cells in pancreas

12. One protein is degraded faster than the other.

13. Exon shuffling

14. Encoding rRNA and tRNA; introns; repeats; promoters and other control sequences

Answers to Applied Questions

1. In drug development, targeting the product of a gene that shares exons with other genes could lead to side effects.

2. Dermatomics = genes that affect the skin; musculomics = genes that affect muscle; imaginomics = genes that affect creativity

3. Acetylase

4. Parts of the protein-encoding genes mix and match. The genes contain many large introns.

5. Exon shuffling; pseudogenes; exons are part of different genes.

6. Transcription factors are most needed before birth.

7. SARS inhibition

8. The promoter for the adjacent gene activates the aromatase gene.

9. Gene expression patterns and the alleles differ. The man has mutations in oncogenes or tumor suppressor genes and those that control blood pressure. The woman has wild type alleles of these genes.

Chapter 12 Gene Mutation
Answers to Review Questions

1. A germinal mutation occurs in a gamete or a fertilized ovum, and therefore affects all the cells of an individual and is more serious than a somatic mutation, which affects only some tissues and is not transmitted to future generations.

2. The gene for collagen is prone to mutation because it is very symmetrical.

3. A spontaneous mutation can arise if a DNA base is in its rare tautomeric form at the instant when the replication fork arrives. A wrong base inserts opposite the rare one.

4. Mutational hot spots are direct repeats or symmetrical regions of DNA.

5. Gaucher disease is caused by an insertion, a missense mutation, or a crossover with a pseudogene.

6. Mutations in the third codon position can be silent. Mutations in the second position may replace an amino acid with a similarly shaped one. 61 codons specify 20 amino acids.

7. (1) A degenerate codon, (2) a mutation that replaces an amino acid with a structurally similar one, (3) a mutation that replaces an amino acid in a nonessential part of the protein, and (4) a mutation in an intron

8. A conditional mutation is only expressed under certain conditions, such as increased temperature or exposure to particular drugs or chemicals.

9. Frameshift, deletion, duplication, insertion, transposable element

10. Retention of an intron and expanding triplet repeats may provide a new function for a gene, which may cause disease.

11. A jumping gene can disrupt gene function by altering the reading frame or shutting off transcription.

12. A new recessive mutation will not become obvious until two heterozygotes produce a homozygous recessive individual with a phenotype.

13. The gene is expanding.

14. Short repeats can cause mispairing during meiosis. Long triplet repeats add amino acids, which can disrupt the encoded protein's function, often adding a function. Repeated genes can cause mispairing in meiosis and have dosage-related effects.

15. Whether the symptoms differ in type rather than severity.

16. Excision repair corrects ultraviolet-induced pyrimidine dimers. Mismatch repair corrects replication errors. They use different enzymes.

Answers to Applied Questions

1. Glycine to arginine: GGU to CGU, GGC to CGC, GGA to AGA, GGG to AGG

2. The frameshift mutation can create a stop codon, leading to a shortened polypeptide.

3. Any change that produces UAA, UAG, or UGA.

4. A transcription factor controls the expression of several genes, in a time and tissue-specific manner. Therefore a mutation in it affects several genes, producing multiple symptoms.

5. GAU to AAU or GAC to AAC

6. The second boy's second mutation, further in the gene, restores the reading frame so that part of the dystrophin protein has a normal structure, providing some function.

7. *asn* to *lys*: AAU to AAA AAC to AAG
ile to *thr*: AUU to ACU AUC to ACC AUA to ACA

8. Nonsense

9. *Arg* to *his*: CGU to CAU CGC to CAC

10. GAU to GUU or GAC to GUU

11. Nonsense

12. The repair enzymes could correct UV-induced pyrimidine dimers.

13. a. *de novo,* because not in parents

b. The mutation creates an intron splice site.

c. Emery-Dreifuss muscular dystrophy, dilated cardiomyopathy, Dunnigan-type familial partial lipodystrophy, limb girdle muscular dystrophy, obesity, Charcot-Marie-Tooth disease

14. Marcia's case is more severe because she lacks CFTR protein, whereas Jan is missing part of the protein.

15. They shouldn't be concerned, because they have mutations in two different genes.

Chapter 13 Chromosomes

Answers to Review Questions

1. Essential parts of a chromosome are telomeres, the centromere, and origin of replication sites. A centromere includes repeats of alpha satellites; centromere-associated proteins; and centromere protein A.

2. Protein-encoding genes become denser from the telomeres inward toward the centromere.

3. Centromeres and telomeres contribute to chromosome stability and have many repeats.

4. a. Homologs do not separate in meiosis I or II, leading to a gamete with an extra or missing chromosome.

b. DNA replicates, but is not apportioned into daughter cells, forming a diploid gamete.

c. Increased tendency for nondisjunction in the chromosome 21 pair.

d. Crossing over in the male yields unbalanced gametes, which can fertilize oocytes, but too much or too little genetic material halts development.

e. A gamete including just one translocated chromosome will have too much of part of the chromosome, and too little of other parts. Excess chromosome 21 material causes Down syndrome.

5. Patches of octaploid cells in liver tissue may arise as a result of abnormal mitosis in a few liver cells early in development.

6. a. A XXX individual has no symptoms, but she may conceive sons with Klinefelter syndrome by producing XX oocytes.

b. A female with XO Turner syndrome has wide-set nipples, flaps of skin on the neck, and no secondary sexual development.

c. A female with trisomy 2 Down syndrome. Phenotype includes short, sparse, straight hair, wide-set eyes with epicanthal folds, a broad nose, protruding tongue, mental retardation, and increased risk of a heart defect, suppressed immunity, and leukemia.

7. Basketball players may have an extra Y chromosome that makes them tall.

8. Triploids are very severely abnormal. Trisomy 21 is the least severe trisomy, and involves the smallest chromosome. Klinefelter syndrome symptoms are worse if there is more than one extra X chromosome.

9. A balanced translocation causes duplications or deletions when a gamete contains one translocated chromosome, plus has extra or is missing genes from one of the chromosomes involved in the translocation. A paracentric or pericentric inversion can cause duplications or deletions if a crossover occurs between the inverted chromosome and its homolog. Isochromosomes result from centromere splitting in the wrong plane, duplicating one chromosome arm but deleting the other.

10. Chromosomes would not contort during meiosis because their genes are aligned.

11. a. High resolution chromosome banding: Cells in culture are synchronized in early mitosis, then the chromosomes are spread and stained.

b. FISH: Fluorescently-labeled DNA probes bind homologous regions on chromosomes.

c. Amniocentesis: Fetal cells and fluid are removed from around a fetus. Cells are cultured and their chromosomes stained or exposed to DNA probes, and karyotyped.

d. Chorionic villus sampling: Chromosomes in chorionic villus cells are directly karyotyped.

e. Fetal cell sorting: A fluorescence activated cell sorter separates fetal from maternal cells, and fetal chromosomes are karyotyped.

f. Maternal serum markers: Abnormal levels of proteins such as AFP and hCG in a pregnant woman's blood indicate increased risk of certain disorders.

g. Quantitative PCR amplifies sequences that are unique to specific chromosomes that are most often part of trisomies.

h. Human artificial chromosomes are created by synthesizing and attaching the minimal requirements of chromosome components.

12. Trisomies 13 and 18 are highly represented in spontaneous abortions, therefore they are often lethal before birth. Chromosomes 5 and 16 are less often part of trisomies because they have high gene densities.

13. 48

14. A female cannot have Klinefelter syndrome because she does not have a Y chromosome, and a male cannot have Turner syndrome because he has a Y chromosome.

15. Nondisjunction in oocyte. Nondisjunction in sperm. Large deletion in X chromosome.

Answers to Applied Questions

1. a. 35

   b. Karen Martini

   c. The risks in the right hand column are higher because they include many conditions.

   d. One in 66 is greater than 1 percent.

   e. Age 40 trisomy 21 risk = 1/106. Age 45 risk = 1/30. Her risk approximately triples in the five years.

2. The person is a girl missing part of the short arm of chromosome 5. This is cri du chat syndrome, and she will be mentally retarded with a catlike cry.

3. FISH

4. a. Reciprocal translocation

   b. She doesn't have extra or missing genes.

   c. She might have a child with translocation Down syndrome.

5. At the second mitotic division, replicated chromosomes failed to separate, yielding one of four cells with an extra two sets of chromosomes.

6. Down syndrome caused by aneuploidy produces an extra chromosome 21 in each cell. In mosaic Down syndrome, the extra chromosome is only in some cells. In translocation Down syndrome, unbalanced gametes lead to an individual with extra chromosome 21 material in each cell.

7. The XXY son could have gotten two X chromosomes from his mother, or an XY-bearing sperm from his father.

8. a. A translocation carrier can produce an unbalanced gamete that lacks chromosome 22 material.

   b. The microdeletion may be more extensive than the deleted region in the translocation individuals.

   c. Translocation family members might be infertile or have offspring with birth defects.

9. a. 4 + 5, 9 + 10, 11 + 12   The lower chromosome # should have more bases.

   b. 19

   c. Y

   d. 6.2 times

10. Student should create a karyotype.

11. Chromosome 13:
   cataract-clouded lens   OMIM   601885
   deafness   220290
   leukemia/lymphoma—blood cancer 602221
   ectodermal dysplasia—no hair   129500
   or nails, dark skin

12. a. Uniparental disomy

   b. The first condition might arise from an oocyte that has two copies of the long arm of chromosome 14 being fertilized by a sperm that lacks this segment. The situation would be the reverse for the second condition.

   c. A deletion mutation could remove the copy of the gene that is expressed.

13. One of the Watkins probably has a balanced translocation, because there is more than one Down syndrome case. The two spontaneous abortions were the result of unbalanced gametes. Their problems are likely to repeat with a predictable and high frequency, because the translocated chromosome is in half of the carrier parents' gametes. In contrast, the Phelps' child with Down syndrome is more likely the result of nondisjunction, which is unlikely to repeat. The Phelps child has trisomy Down syndrome; the Watkins' child may only have a partial extra copy of chromosome 21.

Chapter 14 When Allele Frequencies Stay Constant

Answers to Review Questions

1. A gene pool refers to a population.

2. Evolution is not occurring.

3. Knowing the incidence of the homozygous recessive class makes it possible to derive the "q" part of the Hardy-Weinberg equation.

4. The possibility of two unrelated Caucasians without a family history of CF having an affected child is $1/4 \times 1/23 \times 1/23 = 1/2,116$. If one person knows he or she is a carrier, the risk is $1/4 \times 1/23 = 1/92$.

5. Natural selection does not act on STRs.

6. Population databases are necessary to interpret DNA fingerprints because alleles occur with different frequencies in different populations.

7. For females use the standard formula. For males, gene frequency equals phenotypic frequency.

Answers to Applied Questions

1. $q^2 = .25$ $q = .5$ Carrier percentage = $2pq = (2)(.5)(.5) = .5$

2. $q^2 = .001$ $q = .0316$ $p = .968$
   $2pq$ = carrier frequency = $(2)(.0316)(.968) = .061$

3. a. $q^2 = 1/190 = 0.005$. Square root of 0.005 = 0.071 = frequency of mutant allele q

   b. Frequency of wild type allele = $p = 1 - 0.071 = 0.929$

   c. Carriers = $2pq = 2 \times 0.071 \times 0.929 = 0.132$

   d. Nonrandom mating

4. $0.1 \times 0.1 = 0.01$ = chance both are carriers. If both are carriers, $0.25 \times 0.01 = 0.0025 = 0.25\%$ chance child will be affected.

5. $q^2 = 1/8,000 = 0.000125$ $q = 0.011$ $p = 1 - 0.011 = 0.989$

   Carrier frequency = $2pq = 2 \times 0.011 \times 0.989 = 0.022$

6. $4/177 = 0.0225 = 2.25\%$ are carriers

7. Students genotypes: 6 TT 4 Tt 10 tt

   Parents genotypes:
      of 6 TT students = 9 TT 2 Tt 1 tt
      of 4 Tt students = 2 TT 4 Tt 2 tt
      of 10 tt students = 8 Tt 12 tt

   Students allele frequencies: $T = p = 1/2Tt + TT = 1/2 (4) + 6 = 8/20$ students = .4

   $t = q = .6$

   Parents allele frequencies: $T = p = 1/2Tt + TT = 1/2 (14) + 11 = 18/40$ parents = .45

   $t = q = .55$

   The gene is evolving because the allele frequencies change between generations.

8. a. In 1990, DNA profiling did not consider as many sites in the genome as it does now, and juries and judges did not understand the outlandish statistics.

   b. Sperm cells in victim, any somatic cells of suspects and victim

   c. Their ethnic/population group

d. It is unfair to convict and punish suspects without using an available technology to evaluate their guilt or innocence (opinion).

e. Eddie Joe Lloyd was exonerated in 2002, after serving 17 years in prison for a rape and murder of a 16-year-old girl in Detroit in 1984. Police tricked him into confessing by feeding him details, then using his repeating the details as evidence of knowledge of the crime. Semen stain on underwear used to strangle her was used as evidence, but not tested for DNA.

9. Autosomal recessive class = $900/10,000 = .09 = q^2$ $q = .3$ $p = .7$

   Normal lashes = $p^2 + 2pq = .49 + .42$

   Homozygote with normal lashes = $.49/.49 + .42 = .538$

10. **a.** Genes 2 and 4 have 2 alleles because they generate 2 bands on the gel

    b. $(.2)^2 + (2)(.3)(.7) + (.10)^2 + (2)(.4)(.2)$ $= .04 \times .42 \times .01 \times .16 = .0000268$

    c. The man might have close male relatives who cannot be ruled out as suspects.

    d. It makes his guilt even more likely.

Chapter 15 Changing Allele Frequencies

Answers to Review Questions

1. **a.** Agriculture

   b. Cities, as groups of immigrants arrive and mix in

   c. Endangered species, survivors of massacres or natural disasters and their descendants

   d. Introducing an inherited disease into a population

2. **a.** Highly virulent TB bacteria are selected against because they kill hosts quickly. Resistant hosts are selected for because they survive infection and live to reproduce. In this way, TB evolved from an acute systemic infection into a chronic lung infection. In the 1980s, antibiotic-resistant TB strains led to re-emergence of the disease.

   b. Bacteria that become resistant to antibiotics by mutation or by acquiring resistance factors from other bacteria selectively survive in the presence of antibiotics.

   c. Viral diversity is low at the start of infection because the immune system is vulnerable—viral variants aren't necessary. As symptoms ebb, viral diversity increases, then it decreases again as the immune system becomes overwhelmed.

   d. CF may be maintained in populations where heterozygosity protects against diarrheal disease.

3. Increasing homozygosity increases the chance that homozygous recessives will arise, who may be too unhealthy to reproduce. The population may decline.

4. Misuse of antibiotics provides a selective pressure that benefits and maintains populations of drug-resistant bacteria.

5. Recessive alleles persist in heterozygotes.

6. Sickle cell disease protects against malaria.

7. The incidence of the phenotype is less than that predicted by the genotype and mode of inheritance.

8. Historical records, geographical information, and linguistics

9. Decreased variation in mitochondrial and Y chromosome DNA sequences indicate the genetic uniformity of a population bottleneck.

10. In the Dunker population, the frequencies of blood type genotypes are quite different from those of the surrounding U.S. population and the ancestral population in Europe.

11. The most common CF allele is more common in France (70 percent) than in Finland (45 percent). Therefore the test would be more likely to detect a carrier in France than in Finland.

12. The same mutation in a population group and linkage disequilibrium (shared haplotypes) suggest a founder effect.

13. The causes of founder effects and population bottlenecks differ. A founder effect reflects a small group moving to start a new population, whereas a population bottleneck results from removal of individuals with certain genotypes from the population.

14. A gradual cline might reflect migration over many years. An abrupt cline could be due to a cataclysmic geological event that separates two populations, such as an earthquake or flood.

15. Genetic drift is the chance sampling of some genotypes from a population, and this may lead to nonrandom mating, in which the most fit individuals reproduce more successfully. Environmental conditions help determine which genotypes reproduce and are thus selected for.

16. **a.** A founder effect is a type of genetic drift that occurs when a few individuals found a settlement and their alleles constitute a new gene pool, amplifying the alleles they introduce and eliminating others.

    b. Linkage disequilibrium is the inheritance of certain combinations of alleles of different genes at a higher frequency than can be accounted for by their individual frequencies.

    c. Balanced polymorphism is the persistence of a disease-causing allele in a population because the heterozygote enjoys a health or reproductive advantage.

    d. Genetic load is the proportion of deleterious alleles in a population.

17. Shifts in allele frequency should parallel people's movements, which are often described in historical records, and explained by sociology and anthropology.

Answers to Applied Questions

1. Not balanced polymorphism because being homozygous recessive for glycophorin C deficiency does not cause symptoms.

2. Tasting bitter is harmful—see whether people who can taste bitter substances are overrepresented among people with cancer, because they may have avoided protective vegetables.

   Tasting bitter is protective—see whether people who cannot taste bitter are overrepresented among those who have been poisoned.

3. Microevolution refers to changes in allele frequencies in populations. Examples: changing virulence of infectious diseases, antibiotic resistance, infectious diseases that jump species.

4. Balanced polymorphism as an explanation requires 12 rare events; drift requires one, the sequestering of the population.

5. **a.** All modern Afrikaners with porphyria variegata descend from the same person in whom the disorder originated.

   b. One person, who had the dental disorder, contributed disproportionately to future generations.

ANSWERS TO END-OF-CHAPTER QUESTIONS

c. Heterozygotes for cystic fibrosis and sickle cell disease resist certain infectious diseases, maintaining the disease-causing allele in populations.

d. The Pima Indian population has a high incidence of an allele that predisposes to develop type I diabetes mellitus, but it wasn't expressed until certain dietary and lifestyle changes became popular.

e. The Amish and Pakistani groups have high incidences of certain inherited diseases because of consanguinity.

f. Migration patterns are responsible for the different frequencies of the galactokinase deficiency allele across Europe.

g. The same haplotype for CJD in different populations reflects descent from a shared ancestor followed by migration.

h. Varying mtDNA sequences along the Nile river valley are due to migration.

i. The alleles responsible for BRCA1 breast cancer originated in different ancestors for Ashkenazim and African-Americans.

6. a. Founder effect

b. Geographical barriers and natural selection, acting over time, make two populations have different variants of inherited characteristics.

c. Nonrandom mating

d. Natural selection

7. Treating PKU has increased the proportion of mutant alleles in the population because without treatment, affected individuals would not have been able to reproduce.

8. The mutations arose independently.

9. The high incidence is due to extreme consanguinity—nearly everyone is related to nearly everyone else. Tracking the incidence of this condition is difficult because the symptoms exist independently, and may be caused by environmental factors rather than genes.

10. Natural selection

11. Balanced polymorphism

12. a. Balanced polymorphism b. Founder effect c. Migration

13. West Nile virus-associated illness is evolving. It arrived in the U.S. in New York City in 1999 and has since spread nearly everywhere in the nation.

14. European males settled in India. Later, Asian immigrants arrived. The male European Indians had children with Asian Indian women.

Chapter 16 Human Origins and Evolution

Answers to Review Questions

1. Hominoids are ancestral to apes and humans, whereas hominids are ancestral to humans only. Therefore, hominoids are more ancient.

2. Physically, chimpanzees are not as similar to us as were the australopithecines, yet the australopithecines are in a different genus from us.

3. A single gene can control the rates of development of specific structures, causing enormous differences in the relative sizes of organs in two species.

4. The hunting behavior of *A. garhi* and the time and place where it lived suggests that it could have been a bridge between *Australopithecus* and *Homo*.

5. Fossil evidence and mtDNA evidence support an "out of Africa" emergence of modern humans. Anthropological evidence indicates three waves of migration of native Americans from Siberia, but molecular evidence suggests one migration.

6. Y chromosome and mitochondrial DNA sequences enable researchers to trace the genetic contributions of fathers and mothers, respectively.

7. Bipedalism, larger brain, improved fine coordination

8. Exons are highly conserved because they affect the phenotype by encoding protein and are therefore subject to natural selection.

9. Small insertions and deletions might alter the regulation of the same protein in chimps and humans, but not introduce a new structure or function or drastically alter an existing one.

10. Estimating passage of time requires a steady interval, such as a minute. Mutation rates vary.

11. a. Differences in genes that control rates of development of particular structures

b. Variants of single genes with obvious effects, such as body hair

In general, differences in gene expression can account for phenotypic distinctions between humans and chimps despite similarity in genome sequence.

12. Gene sequences are more specific because different codons can encode the same amino acids.

13. Mutation rates are not the same across genomes. Genes mutate at different rates.

14. One gene encodes one polypeptide, and so comparing the evolution of a gene tracks a tiny part of the biology of the organism. DNA hybridization assesses relationships among many genes, and thus means more. Also, much of the genome does not encode protein.

15. A chromosome band may contain many genes, and so comparing them is not specific.

16. Knowledge of a DNA, RNA, or polypeptide sequence and the mutation rate is necessary to construct an evolutionary tree diagram. An assumption is that mutation rate is constant. A limitation is that only one biochemical is considered, and not large scale characteristics such as behavior and anatomy.

17. Sterilizing people with mental retardation
Encouraging poor people to limit family size
Avoiding marriage to a person who carries a disease-causing allele

18. European men were among the first settlers, and contributed to the higher castes. Asian women arrived later and contributed to lower castes.

Answers to Applied Questions

1. a. A small duplication occurred in human chromosome 11 to give rise to the Betazoid karyotype. The Klingon and Romulan karyotypes could have arisen from fusion of human chromosomes 15 and 17.

b. The Betazoids are our closest relatives because of greater similarity in chromosome bands and chromosome arrangement. Cytochrome *c* sequences and intron pattern in the collagen gene are identical between humans and Betazoids.

c. They are not distinct species because they can interbreed.

d. (3)

2. Negative eugenics:
—sterilizing people who are mentally retarded
—restricting certain groups from immigrating
—encouraging people with inherited disease or carriers not to reproduce

Positive eugenics:

—a sperm bank where Nobel prizewinners make deposits

—people seeking very smart people as mates

— governments paying people with the best jobs and education to have larger families

3. People in third world nations might be alarmed by white-coated strangers wielding hypodermic needles seeking blood samples. A compromise would be to collect hair instead of blood, and use PCR to amplify the genes. Another compromise is to offer vaccines in exchange for tissue samples.

4. The action was eugenic because it indirectly selected against nonwhite students. It was not eugenic in that, superficially, all applicants were evaluated using the same criteria.

5. The child would be a modern human.

6. A law can be passed stating that no laws can be passed or restrictions imposed based upon genetic data.

7. **a.** *K. platyops* had facial characteristics of more than one type of australopithecine.

b. Skeletal remains are incomplete.

8. Ease of cultivation might not be a biologically sound way to select a model organism, because that species might not suffer the same inherited disorders as humans, or have the same mutant phenotypes.

9. The *BAZ1B* gene encodes a bromodomain next to a zinc finger domain. It is deleted in Williams-Beuren syndrome, which is a developmental disorder, OMIM 605681. Chimp and baboon have similar sequences.

10. Most similar to humans is Otzi, then Neanderthal, *H. sapiens idalta, H. habilis, A. afarensis,* baboon.

11. **a.** Forced sterilization

b. If a trait in one family is deemed inherited, it might be assumed to be inherited in another family, when that might not be the case.

c. Wealthy people seeking partners among other wealthy people

d. How common the negative traits were in the general population. Whether the family members were really related biologically. Environmental influences on the traits considered. Evidence of family members without the negative traits who have beneficial ones.

Chapter 17 Genetics of Immunity

Answers to Review Questions

1. 1. d   2. e, g   3. a   4. b   5. h   6. b

2. Blood type is determined by specific glycoprotein antigens on red blood cell surfaces. Incompatibility results when a person's immune system manufactures antibodies that attack red blood cells bearing antigens of other blood types.

3. **a.** Collapse of entire immune system

b. Increase in viral infections and cancer

c. Increase in bacterial infections

d. Total collapse of immune system

4. **a.** Destruction of bacteria and viruses, stimulation of inflammation

b. Destruction of bacteria, yeasts, some viruses

c. Bind to and stimulate destruction of bacteria

d. Cause changes in body that are inhospitable to pathogens

5. HIV mutates rapidly, replicates rapidly, the site where it binds to T cells is shielded, and resistance alleles are very rare.

6. Thymocytes are selected as others die, rather than undergoing an "education."

7. Allergens stimulate production of IgE antibodies that bind mast cells, causing them to release allergy mediators. In an autoimmune disorder, antibodies attack the body's cells and tissues.

8. **a.** Transplanted bone marrow cells (the graft) recognize cells in the recipient (the host) as foreign. The donor's cells attack the host's cells.

b. ADA deficiency may result in severe combined immune deficiency, in which a lack of ADA poisons T cells, which then cannot activate B cells.

c. Autoantibodies attack cells that line joints.

d. In AIDS, HIV infects helper T cells and reproduces, eventually killing enough T cells to overcome cellular immunity. Opportunistic infections occur.

e. Grass antigens (allergens) induce production of IgE that causes mast cells to release histamines, causing allergy symptoms.

9. T cells control B cell function.

10. Memory and plasma B cells respond specifically to one antigen following a cytokine cue from a T cell. Plasma B cells secrete antigen-specific antibodies and are in the circulation for only a few days. Memory B cells remain, providing a fast response the next time the antigen is encountered.

11. A polyclonal antibody response attacks an invader at several points simultaneously, hastening recovery. MAbs are useful as a diagnostic tool because of their specificity.

12. Memory cells alert the immune system of the first exposure, and ensure that a secondary immune response occurs on subsequent exposure to the Coxsackie virus.

Answers to Applied Questions

1. O negative blood lacks ABO cell surface antigens and the Rh antigens, so it is less likely to evoke a rejection reaction than other types of blood.

2. Autoimmune, because of presence of autoantibodies

3. It is working. Lowered IgE signifies less of an allergic reaction, and increased levels of IgG and IgA indicate protection.

4. Antibiotics treat the bacterial infection, but not the inflammation in the joints, which is an autoimmune response.

5. Innate antibodies. A mutation in the host that prevents the pathogen from infecting.

6. Colony stimulating factor

7. The bonobo's cells would bear antigens specific to a particular human.

8. Stockpile antibiotics locally, but control their use. Better vaccine coverage. Publicize what people should look out for, and how to disinfect themselves or suspicious materials.

9. SCID heritability is higher because it is caused by a mutation that usually removes a gene's function. An allergy in contrast, reflects an overactive, misdirected immune response, which is more acquired than inherited.

10. http://allonhealth.com/human-immune-system-booster.htm
This website claims that "Barleygreen" ingredients "give your body the nutrients it needs to rebuild your immune system." Assumes your immune system is broken down. Product claims to prevent immune system diseases, slow aging, fight bacteria and viruses, destroy cancer cells, and distinguish "live" and "dead" nutrients. A

nutrient is a chemical and cannot be alive. This product is vitamins, minerals, and enzymes. The enzymes are digested by the stomach and small intestine, before they can function. Taking a multivitamin, or eating a balanced diet, would have the same effect as this bogus product.

11. a. Allograft **b.** Isograft **c.** Xenograft **d.** Autograft

12. There will not be an Rh incompatibility because the female would have to be Rh⁻.

Chapter 18 The Genetics of Cancer

Answers to Review Questions

1. a. An overexpressed transcription factor could function as an oncogene, causing too frequent cell division.

b. Mutations in the *p53* gene lift tumor suppression, allowing too many cell divisions.

c. Mutations in the retinoblastoma gene lift tumor suppression.

d. The *myc* oncogene allows too frequent cell division.

e. DNA repair fixes errors that would otherwise lead to cancer (turning on an oncogene or turning off a tumor suppressor).

f. Mutations in the *APC* gene lift tumor suppression by making the DNA more prone to replication errors.

g. *CHEK2* controls *BRCA1,* so a mutation in it would lift tumor suppression, causing cancer.

2. Cancer is a consequence of disruption of the cell cycle. Deletion of a tumor suppressor gene and translocation of an oncogene next to a highly active gene would have the same effect of uncontrolled division.

3. Only an inherited cancer susceptibility can pass to future generations.

4. Cancer cells divide continuously and indefinitely; they are heritable, transplantable, dedifferentiated, and lack contact inhibition.

5. One inherits a susceptibility to cancer, not the cancer itself. Cancer may affect only somatic tissue. Many mutations may be necessary for cancer to develop.

6. Cancer cells divide faster than cells from which they derive. Some normal cells divide faster than cancer cells.

7. a. A population study examines disease incidence in different populations, at any time.

b. A case-control study analyzes pairs of people who differ only in the characteristic of interest.

c. A prospective study is any study that evaluates results as they occur, rather than relying on recall.

8. A cancer cell could have a point mutation.

9. Inducing apoptosis halts runaway cell division. Inducing differentiation enables cancer cells to specialize, which would slow down their division rate. Blocking hormone receptors prevents cancer cells from receiving signals to divide. Inhibiting angiogenesis prevents tumors from building a blood supply. Blocking telomerase stops cell division.

Answers to Applied Questions

1. Retinoblastoma

2. DNA expression microarrays could predict which women would respond to chemotherapy and/or radiation and which would not.

3. a. Missing both *p53* alleles is lethal.

b. A person with two mutant *p53* alleles could be conceived if both parents have one mutant allele.

4. It is an oncogene because it caused overexpression of a transcription factor.

5. The cells from the original tumor are not genetically identical.

6. Treatment for leukemia is more complex than removal of a solid organ because bone marrow must be replaced.

7. No diet can guarantee that an individual will not develop cancer.

8. Are certain *p53* mutations more prevalent among exposed workers, compared to people not exposed to PAHs? If so, the PAHs may cause the mutation.

9. The woman could have a familial cancer syndrome.

10. Tumor suppressors. These genes cause cancer when inactivated or removed.

11. She could have a mutation in a gene that controls the expression of *BRCA1* or *BRCA2.*

12. If the receptor is blocked, the cell cannot receive the signal to divide.

13. a. *hTERT* keeps telomeres long by encoding telomerase. When overexpressed it is an oncogene.

b. *p53* is a tumor suppressor gene that when underexpressed due to a germinal mutation and a somatic mutation causes Li-Fraumeni family cancer syndrome.

14. a. The counselor should ask about ethnic background, and other types of cancer in the family.

b. This woman would probably not benefit from a BRCA1 test, because her two affected blood relatives were older when affected.

c. A complication of BRCA1 testing is that if no mutation is found, a person might assume that she cannot develop breast cancer. We do not know all of the ways that this disease can develop, and in fact it may be several different disorders.

Chapter 19 Genetically Modified Organisms

Answers to Review Questions

1. a. Biotechnology—Specific uses of altered cells or biochemicals.

b. Recombinant DNA technology—Inserting foreign genes into bacteria or other single cells, which express them.

c. Transgenic technology—A genetic alteration of a gamete or fertilized ovum, perpetuating the change in every cell of the individual that develops.

d. Gene targeting—An introduced gene exchanges places with its counterpart in a chromosome.

e. Homologous recombination—A gene introduced into a cell exchanging places with a gene on a chromosome.

2. a. Restriction enzymes cut DNA at specific sequences. They can be used to create DNA fragments for constructing recombinant DNA molecules.

b. In gene targeting, genes of interest are added to embryonic stem cells where they exchange places with a homologous gene. After construction of chimeric embryos and crosses of mosaic animals, heterozygotes are bred to yield homozygous transgenic animals with a particular gene knocked out.

c. Cloning vectors carry DNA molecules into cells.

3. Antibiotics are used to set up a system where only cells that have taken up foreign DNA can survive.

4. Human insulin DNA cut with a restriction enzyme, vector DNA cut with the same restriction enzyme, *E. coli*, DNA ligase, selection mechanism (such as antibiotic)

5. Bacteria couldn't manufacture human proteins if the genetic code was not universal.

6. Foreign DNA can be inserted on a virus, carried across plasma membranes in liposomes, microinjected, electroporated, or sent in with particle bombardment.

7. Transgenic technology is not precise because introduced DNA is not directed to a particular chromosomal locus, as it is in gene targeting.

8. When a transgene or knocked out gene is present in one copy in animals, the animals must be bred to obtain homozygous individuals that express the phenotype. This is a monohybrid cross.

9. Gene targeting exchanges a gene that is expressed for a copy that is not. Antisense technology blocks an mRNA by binding it to its complementary sequence.

10. A drug obtained using recombinant DNA technology does not contain contaminants found in proteins extracted from organisms.

Answers to Applied Questions

1. A goat produces human EPO in its semen.

A mouse produces jellyfish GFP in its plasma.

A chicken produces human clotting factor in its egg whites.

2. Human collagen produced in transgenic mice is less likely to include infectious agents than collagen obtained from hooves and hides. It is also the human protein, which is less likely to stimulate an immune response than the cow type.

3. Perhaps people do not object to genetic modification of bacteria because bacteria are not easily visible and the drug is used to treat an illness. GM foods are more familiar, and do not improve upon an existing product, as Humulin does.

4. Mice can express human genes because they use the same genetic code.

5. Another gene specifies the same enzyme; another gene specifies a different enzyme with the same or a similar function; the enzyme isn't vital.

6. Gene targeting

7. Gene targeting shows the result of no CFTR protein. A transgenic model shows effects of an abnormal CFTR protein. Gene targeting models the most extreme expression of CF.

8.

Insulin	type 1 diabetes mellitus
Beta interferon	multiple sclerosis
EPO	kidney failure, anemia
TPA	stroke, coronary heart disease
CSF	restores white blood cell count

9. Object: A novel idea in 1989 is now obvious.

Support: He thought of using the noncoding DNA first.

10. Give a ewe hormones to make her superovulate. Apply ram sperm to ewe's reproductive tract. Flush out fertilized ova, and inject them with human *AAT* gene linked to sheep gene promoter that will control its expression. Place GM fertilized ova into sheep surrogate mothers. Select heterozygous offspring, breed them to obtain homozygotes. Milk female homozygotes and extract human drug.

Chapter 20 Gene Therapy and Genetic Counseling

Answers to Review Questions

1. (a) Replace protein; (b) use recombinant DNA technology to obtain pure, human protein; (c) gene therapy.

2. a. ADA gene in cord blood cells.

b. OTC gene delivered to liver.

c. Implant gene in brain.

d. Activate fetal hemoglobin production.

3. Fitting the huge dystrophin gene into a vector, and getting gene expression in enough muscle cells to affect symptoms.

4. *Ex vivo* gene therapy alters cells outside the body, then injects or implants them. SCID is treated this way. *In situ* gene therapy is a localized procedure on accessible tissue, such as treating melanoma. *In vivo* gene therapy occurs inside the body, such as a nasal spray to deliver the CFTR gene to a person with cystic fibrosis.

5. Germline gene therapy can affect evolution because the changes are heritable.

6. Researchers should consider the amount of DNA the virus can carry, the types of cells the virus normally infects, how stable the incorporated vector is in the human genome, if toxic effects are associated with use of the virus, and whether or not the virus stimulates a strong immune response.

7. A bone marrow transplant is a cell implant; genes are not altered. Removing bone marrow and adding a functional gene is gene therapy because the DNA is altered.

8. A liver is in only one place in the body. Muscle is more difficult to treat because it comprises much of the body's bulk. It is nearly everywhere.

9. AV and AAV are viral vectors, and the dystrophin gene is stitched into them using recombinant DNA technology. A liposome is a fatty bubble that can encase the gene and introduce it into a cell across the lipid-rich plasma membrane.

Answers to Applied Questions

1. The first gene therapy experiments in humans took place in 1990—it isn't new.

2. HIV would have to have the genes that make it destroy the immune system deleted.

3. Small amounts of nitric oxide could be used to prevent sickling. The cells sickle only in a low-oxygen environment.

4. There is no dopamine gene to manipulate—a gene therapy would be applied to an enzyme necessary to synthesize dopamine. It is difficult to deliver a gene therapy to the brain, because of the blood-brain barrier.

5. To treat Duchenne muscular dystrophy, the gene for dystrophin is delivered via a retrovirus into immature muscle cells.

To treat sickle cell disease, the beta globin gene is delivered as naked DNA into immature red blood cells.

To treat glioma, mouse fibroblasts are given retroviruses with a herpes gene that encodes thymidine kinase. The fibroblasts are implanted into the tumor, and an anti-herpes drug given, which selectively destroys dividing cells, including the cancer cells.

6. *In situ,* because only the scalp need be treated.

7. (a) A viral vector (AAV) to add globin genes to red blood cell precursor cells, (b) a bone marrow transplant, (c) hydroxyurea to stimulate production of fetal hemoglobin.

8. Jesse Gelsinger was relatively healthy. Children with Canavan disease have no other treatment options.

9. Any disease where the affected tissue can be reached and an overexpressed gene silenced or a deficient gene's activity boosted or replaced. RNA interference to squelch mRNA for huntingtin in Huntington disease. For cystic fibrosis, a viral vector to introduce *CFTR* gene into airway lining cells.

10. a. The counselor should explain to the couple that even though the fetus has an extra X chromosome, the individual will most likely not have any related symptoms other than perhaps great height.

 b. The counselor might suggest a technique to separate X-bearing sperm, to increase the chances of conceiving a female. Or, the couple could test the fetus for the muscular dystrophy gene and terminate an affected fetus.

 c. Explain that risk increases with age, but a young woman can still conceive a child with trisomy 21—it is just rare.

 d. If the parents are of normal height, then their child with achondroplasia is a new mutation, and there should be no elevated risk to other children.

 e. Genetic counselors tell patients that amniocentesis can rule out certain chromosomal and biochemical disorders, but it cannot guarantee a healthy child.

11. Which patient is sicker, closer to death, more likely to be cured, did not contribute to her condition by smoking, or has more to contribute to society.

12. OMIM 259420 describes osteogenesis imperfecta type III, which, unlike the other forms, is recessive. It is autosomal. In addition to easily broken bones, the whites of the eyes may appear bluish and the teeth rotted. The genetic counselor should take a family history to determine the mode of inheritance. One or both parents may be affected if the disorder is dominant. The counselor should point out symptoms other than broken bones, describe how collagen contributes to bone structure and integrity (the phenotype), and how the disorder is transmitted (the genotype).

Chapter 21 Reproductive Technologies

Answers to Review Questions

1. a. Surrogate mother

 b. Intrauterine insemination

 c. Oocyte donation, preimplantation genetic diagnosis

 d. Intrauterine insemination

 e. Preimplantation genetic diagnosis or intrauterine insemination

 f. IVF, ZIFT, or GIFT

 g. Preservation of her ovarian tissue in her arm

2. It is easier, less costly, and less painful to detect infertility in men than in women.

3. A man can have up to 40 percent abnormally shaped sperm and still be considered fertile.

4. A man with a low sperm count and a woman with an irregular menstrual cycle.

5. ZIFT and GIFT occur in the fallopian tube, whereas IVF takes place in the uterus. ZIFT and IVF transfer a zygote, whereas GIFT transfers gametes. In IVF, fertilization occurs outside the body.

6. They are "embryos *in vitro*" because a uterus is required for the embryos to develop—and there is no guarantee that this will happen.

7. Preimplantation genetic diagnosis is similar to amniocentesis and CVS in that it allows prenatal detection of disease-causing genes. It is different in that it takes place much earlier in gestation.

8. Endometriosis, scarred fallopian tubes, irregular ovulation, nondisjunction

9. a. Fertilization occurs outside of the body.

 b. Oocytes and sperm are collected and placed in the fallopian tubes.

 c. Conception occurs in a woman other than the one who gives birth.

 d. Conception occurs outside the body, and a woman other than the genetic mother carries the fetus.

 e. Conception does not occur as a result of sexual intercourse, but in a Petri dish.

 f. The nucleus and cytoplasm in a cell come from different individuals.

Answers to Applied Questions

1. An older man fathering a child does not have to alter his physiology the way a postmenopausal woman must to conceive.

2. Adoption

3. Oocyte donor

4. Big Tom illustrates intrauterine insemination. Mist illustrates surrogate motherhood.

5. a. The genetic parents are the sperm donor and the woman, who is also the gestational mother.

 b. The genetic parents are the woman whose uterus is gone, and her husband. The gestational mother is the woman's friend.

 c. The genetic parents are Max and Tina; the gestational mother is Karen.

 d. The genetic parents are von Wormer and the Indiana woman, who was also the gestational mother.

 e. The genetic and gestational mother is the woman who is the friend of the men. The genetic father can be determined if DNA profiles of the child are compared to those of the sperm donors.

6. Younger women can freeze oocytes or early embryos, to be fertilized or implanted years later.

7. Extra preimplantation embryos can be donated to infertile couples.

8. People will vary in when they think children born from assisted reproductive technologies should be told of their origins.

9. Paying for reproductive services because one is lazy is not the same as seeking assistance because one has a fertility problem.

10. The child would be a clone of Cliff.

11. Agree: it prevents abortion

 Disagree: sex selection is abhorrent

12. a. For year 2000 data, use of ART has increased 54% since 1996.

 b. Fresh

 c. Her own

 d. If she becomes naturally pregnant; couple who have had ART more than once: couple who have had more than one type of ART; several causes of infertility

13. The court might investigate why the man revoked his consent, and whether he has children. One might argue that the woman's rights should be paramount, because she is the one who would be pregnant.

Chapter 22 The Age of Genomics

Answers to Review Questions

1. a. Expressed sequence tags sped the discovery of protein-encoding genes by working with cDNAs reverse transcribed from mRNAs.

   b. Positional cloning identified many important disease-causing genes.

   c. DNA microarray technology enables researchers to analyze gene expression.

   d. Automated DNA sequencing sped determination of the base sequence of the genome.

   e. Assembler computer programs overlapped genome pieces.

2. A cytogenetic map provides only a few landmarks per chromosome, whereas a sequence map consists of the DNA bases.

3. No

4. Repeated sequences could be mapped to several chromosomal sites. Not knowing which strand a sequence comes from could lead to duplicating some parts of the genome sequence and missing others.

5. *Mycoplasma genitalium,* because it is the smallest genome sequenced.

6. We share a great deal, genetically speaking, with yeast and worms.

7. The Sanger method sufficed for sequencing a few genomes, but is not fast enough to support genome sequencing as a routine medical test.

Answers to Applied Questions

1. The pieces must be overlapped to derive the sequence, so several genome copies must be used.

2. SNPs differ among individuals.

3. DNA microarrays detect expression of selected genes. Many genes had been well-studied before the draft human genome sequence was unveiled.

4. DNA microarrays could be used to identify a particular gene variant that is expressed in the affected tissues of affected individuals, but not in other tissues.

5. G C T T C G T T A A T A T C G C T A G C T G C A

6. The first gene is more ancient than the second.

7. MDs should be required to take continuing education courses in genetics.

8. Most people think human genetic/genomic information should be free. If there is a fee, it could reflect intent—that is, whether the user will make money.

9. A genome analysis without someone to interpret the results could lead to decisions or actions based on erroneous information. Genes interact with each other and the environment, and many are not fully penetrant, so that genotype does not reflect phenotype. This isn't so for a blood pressure reading or cholesterol measurement, which is accurate when taken.

10. I. Genomics to Biology
    1. Determining percentage of genome that encodes protein
    2. How is the cell cycle controlled in a normal cell lining a milk duct compared to a cancer cell?
    3. How do people's SNP patterns differ?
    4. Targeted comparative sequencing to compare the same genome region in several species
    5. A company charging for access to human genome information

    II. Genomics to Health
    1. Detecting genes that cause cancer, and genes and gene expression patterns that predict an individual's response to a particular drug
    2. What do people who are exposed to an infectious disease (such as SARS or WNV), but who do not get sick, share at the genome sequence level?
    3. Breast cancer is about 20 distinct diseases, depending on which genes are implicated. Response to treatment might be predicted by considering type.
    4. Genes reveal components of biochemical pathways, some of which might be new drug targets.
    5. A *BRCA1* mutation that confers a very high cancer risk in an Ashkenazi family with several cases would not do so in a non-Jewish family that has several cases by chance.
    6. Integration of new genetics tests into health care practices, used before illness to reveal individual risks

    III. Genomics to Society
    1. Pass legislation to outlaw genetic discrimination. Educate public that genotype does not indicate present symptoms.
    2. Race as defined by skin color is a social, not a biological concept, but certain gene variants are more common in some groups due to culture and geography and our choices in partners.
    3. Genes affect neurotransmission.
    4. Application of genetic/genomic information should not harm anyone, in terms of discrimination or limited opportunities.

11. List all of the symptoms of the family's illness, and devise tests for other genes that may cause them directly, or by interacting with the product of the recognized causative gene. Also investigate different environmental exposures of the family members that might account for different symptoms or symptom severity.

12. A study to identify all of the genes that cause breast and prostate cancer would reveal the biological bases of these cancers and provide information on subtypes that might be associated with prognosis or response to specific treatments. At the societal level, a study might compare workplace/employer/insurer responses to knowledge that an individual has breast cancer to the same for prostate cancer, to identify gender bias.

13. Comparative genomics reveals evolutionary relatedness and may identify useful model organisms. For example, a sea squirt's primitive kidney is used to test new drugs.

14. If genome sequencing remains costly, access might be decided in a way similar to distribution of organs for transplant—by who could benefit most in terms of survival.

15. Psychological impact and stigma: learning that you have a high risk of developing a certain disease, or that your child-to-be has inherited an illness.

16. Personal

Glossary

A

absolute risk The probability that an individual will develop a particular condition, based on family history and/or test results.

acrocentric chromosome A chromosome in which the centromere is located close to one end.

acrosome A protrusion at the front end of a sperm cell containing enzymes that help cut through an oocyte's plasma membrane.

adaptive immunity A slow, specific immune response that develops after exposure to a foreign antigen.

adenine One of two purine nitrogenous bases in DNA and RNA.

allantois A membrane surrounding the fetus that gives rise to umbilical blood vessels.

allele An alternate form of a gene.

allergen A substance that elicits an allergic response.

allograft A transplant in which donor and recipient are the same species.

alpha satellite A repeated 171-base sequence that is an essential part of a centromere.

alternate splicing Building different proteins by combining the information encoded in exons of different genes, or only transcribing and translating some of the exons of a gene.

amino acid A small organic molecule that is a protein building block. Contiguous triplets of DNA nucleotide bases encode the 20 types of amino acids that polymerize to form biological proteins.

amniocentesis A prenatal diagnostic procedure in which a physician inserts a needle into the uterus to remove a small sample of amniotic fluid, which contains fetal cells and biochemicals. A chromosome chart is constructed from cultured fetal cells, and tests for certain inborn errors of metabolism are conducted on fetal biochemicals.

amniotic cavity The space between the inner cell mass and the outer cells anchored to the uterine lining.

anaphase The stage of mitosis when the centromeres of replicated chromosomes part.

aneuploid A cell with one or more extra or missing chromosomes.

angiogenesis Growth of new blood vessels.

antibody A multisubunit protein, produced by B cells, that binds a specific foreign antigen at one end, alerting other components of the immune system or directly destroying the antigen.

anticodon A three-base sequence on one loop of a transfer RNA molecule that is complementary to an mRNA codon, and that therefore brings together the appropriate amino acid and its mRNA instructions.

antigen A molecule that elicits an immune response.

antigen binding site The region of an antibody molecule that includes the idiotype, where foreign antigens bind.

antigen-presenting cell A cell displaying a foreign antigen.

antigen processing A macrophage's display of a foreign antigen on its surface, next to an HLA self antigen. This alerts the immune system.

antiparallel The head-to-tail arrangement of the two entwined chains of the DNA double helix.

antisense technology Using a piece of RNA that is complementary in sequence to a sense RNA to stop expression of a particular gene.

apoptosis A form of cell death that is a normal part of growth and development.

A site Part of ribosome that holds incoming amino acid in growing peptide chain.

assisted reproductive technologies Procedures that replace a gamete or the uterus to help people with fertility problems have children.

association study A case-control study in which genetic variation, often measured as SNPs that form haplotypes, is compared between people with a particular condition and unaffected individuals.

autoantibodies Antibodies that attack the body's own cells.

autograft A transplant of tissue from one part of a person's body to another.

autoimmunity An immune attack against one's own body.

autosomal dominant The inheritance pattern of a dominant allele on an autosome. The phenotype can affect males and females and does not skip generations.

autosomal recessive The inheritance pattern of a recessive allele on an autosome. The phenotype can affect males and females and can skip generations.

autosome A non-sex-determining chromosome. A human cell has 22 pairs of autosomes.

B

bacteriophage A virus that infects bacterial cells; used as a vector to introduce foreign DNA into cells.

balanced polymorphism Maintenance of a harmful recessive allele in a population because the heterozygote has a survival or reproductive advantage.

Barr body A dark-staining, inactivated X chromosome in a cell.

base excision repair Removal of five or fewer bases to correct damage due to reactive oxygen species.

B cell A type of lymphocyte that secretes antibody proteins in response to nonself antigens displayed on other immune system cells.

bioethics A field of study that analyzes personal issues that arise from the application of biological information.

bioinformatics Comparison and analysis of DNA sequences.

bioremediation Use of an organism's natural or modified metabolic abilities to remove toxins from the environment.

biotechnology The alteration of cells or biochemicals with a specific application.

bipedalism Walking upright.

bipolar affective disorder A mood disorder in which periods of depression alternate with periods of mania.

blastocyst A hollow ball of cells descended from a fertilized ovum.

blastomere A cell in a blastocyst.

bulbourethral glands Glands joined to the male urethra that contribute mucus to the seminal fluid, easing sperm release.

C

cancer A group of disorders resulting from loss of cell cycle control.

capacitation Activation of sperm in a woman's body.

carbohydrate A type of macromolecule; sugars and starches.

carcinogen A substance that induces cancerous changes in a cell.

case-control study An epidemiological method in which people with a particular condition are considered against individuals as much like them as possible, but without the disease.

cell The fundamental unit of life.

cell cycle A cycle of events describing a cell's preparation for division and division itself.

cellular adhesion molecules (CAMs) Proteins that join certain cells.

cellular immune response T cells release cytokines to stimulate and coordinate an immune response.

centromere The largest constriction in a chromosome, located at a specific site in each chromosome type.

centromere-associated proteins Various types of proteins that appear at the centromeres in interphase.

cervix The opening between the vagina and the uterus.

chaperone protein A protein that binds a polypeptide as it begins to fold, directing the folding.

checkpoint A part of the cell cycle where a protein controls the process.

chorionic villi Fingerlike growths that extend from an embryo where it implants in the uterine wall.

chorionic villus sampling (CVS) A prenatal diagnostic technique that analyzes chromosomes in chorionic villus cells, which, like the fetus, descend from the fertilized ovum.

chromatid A single, very long DNA molecule and its associated proteins, forming half of a replicated chromosome.

chromatin DNA and its associated histone proteins.

chromatin remodeling Adding or removing chemical groups to or from histones, which can alter gene expression.

chromosome A structure within a cell's nucleus that carries genes. A chromosome consists of a continuous molecule of DNA and proteins wrapped around it.

cleavage A series of rapid mitotic cell divisions after fertilization.

clines Allele frequencies that change from one area to another.

cloning vector A piece of DNA used to transfer DNA from a cell of one organism into that of another.

coding strand The side of the double helix for a particular gene from which RNA is not transcribed.

codominant A heterozygote in which both alleles are fully expressed.

codon A continuous triplet of mRNA that specifies a particular amino acid.

collectins Proteins that protect against bacteria, yeasts, and some viruses.

colony stimulating factors A class of cytokines that stimulate bone marrow to produce lymphocytes.

complement A set of biochemicals that destroy microbes and attack transplanted tissue.

complementary base pairs The pairs of DNA bases that hydrogen bond together; adenine hydrogen bonds to thymine and guanine to cytosine in the DNA double helix.

complementary DNA (cDNA) A DNA molecule that is the complement of an mRNA, copied using reverse transcriptase.

concordance A measure indicating the degree to which a trait is inherited, calculated by determining the percentage of twin pairs in which both members express a particular trait. High concordance among monozygotic (identical) twins indicates a considerable genetic component.

conditional mutation A genotype that is expressed only under certain environmental conditions.

conformation The three-dimensional shape of a molecule.

constant regions The lower portions of an antibody amino acid chain, which are similar in different species.

contact inhibition Tendency of noncancer cells to cease dividing once they touch each other.

correlation coefficient Comparison of the actual incidence of a trait among related individuals to the expected incidence. Used to calculate heritability.

critical period The time during prenatal development when a structure is sensitive to damage from an abnormal gene or an environmental intervention.

crossing over An event during prophase I when homologs exchange parts, adding to genetic variability.

cytogenetics A discipline that matches phenotypes to detectable chromosomal abnormalities.

cytokine A biochemical that a T cell secretes that controls immune function.

cytokinesis Division of cellular parts other than DNA at the end of mitosis.

cytoplasm Cellular contents other than organelles.

cytosine One of the two pyrimidine nitrogenous bases in DNA and RNA.

cytoskeleton A framework composed of protein tubules and rods that supports the cell and gives it a distinctive form.

cytotoxic T cells Lymphocytes that attack nonself cells by binding them and releasing chemicals that attack the cell.

D

dedifferentiated A cell less specialized than the cell it descends from, such as a cancer cell.

deletion mutation A missing sequence of DNA or part of a chromosome.

density shift experiment Experiments in which bacterial cultures labeled with radioactive isotopes were centrifuged to separate those that incorporated the "heavier" isotopes into their DNA. This allowed researchers to study DNA replication.

deoxyribonucleic acid (DNA) The genetic material; the biochemical that forms genes.

deoxyribose The 5-carbon sugar in a DNA nucleotide.

dicentric A chromosome that has two centromeres.

differentiation The process by which cells develop distinctive characteristics, reflecting the expression of particular subsets of genes.

dihybrid cross A cross of individuals who are heterozygous for two traits.

diploid cell A cell containing two sets of chromosomes.

dizygotic (DZ) twins Twins that originate as two different fertilized ova and that are thus not identical. (Commonly known as fraternal twins.)

DNA *See* deoxyribonucleic acid.

DNA microarray Also called a DNA chip. A set of target genes embedded in a glass chip, to which labeled cDNAs from a sample bind and fluoresce. Microarrays show patterns of gene expression.

DNA polymerase An enzyme that inserts into replicating DNA and corrects mismatched base pairs.

DNA probe A labeled short sequence of DNA that corresponds to a specific gene. When applied to a biological sample, the probe base pairs with its complementary sequence, and the label reveals its locus.

DNA replication Construction of a new DNA double helix using the information in parental strands as a template.

dominant A gene variant expressed when present in even one copy.

duplication An extra copy of a gene or DNA sequence, usually caused by misaligned pairing in meiosis; a chromosome containing repeats of part of its genetic material.

dynein A protein necessary for microtubule movement.

E

ectoderm The outermost primary germ layer.

ectopic pregnancy An embryo that grows outside of the uterus, usually in a fallopian tube.

electroporation Using a brief jolt of electricity to open transient holes in a plasma membrane, allowing foreign DNA to enter.

elongation The stage of protein synthesis in which ribosomes bind to the initiation complex and amino acids join.

embryo In humans, prenatal existence until the end of the eighth week of development. The cells in an embryo can be distinguished from each other, but all basic structures are not yet present.

embryo adoption A woman carries an embryo conceived with her partner's sperm and a donor oocyte.

embryonic stem (ES) cell A cell from a preimplantation embryo that is manipulated in gene targeting, and may be useful in regenerative medicine because it can give rise to all differentiated cell types.

empiric risk Probability that a trait will recur based upon its incidence in a particular population.

endoderm The innermost primary germ layer.

endometriosis Abnormal buildup of uterine tissue in and on the uterus, causing cramps and impairing fertility.

endoplasmic reticulum (ER) A labyrinth of membranous tubules on which proteins, lipids, and sugars are synthesized.

enzyme A type of protein that speeds the rate of a specific biochemical reaction, making it fast enough to be compatible with life.

epididymis A tightly coiled tube in the male reproductive tract where sperm cells mature and are stored.

epigenetic A layer of information placed on a gene that is a modification other than a change in DNA sequence.

epistasis One gene masking expression of another.

epitope Parts of an antibody that antigen binds.

equational division The second meiotic division, producing four cells from two.

euchromatin Parts of chromosomes that do not stain and that contain active genes.

eugenics The control of individual reproductive choices to achieve a societal goal.

eukaryotic cell A complex cell containing organelles, including a nucleus.

euploid (cell) A somatic cell with the normal number of chromosomes for that species.

excision repair Enzyme-catalyzed removal of pyrimidine dimers in DNA, which corrects errors in DNA replication.

exon The DNA base sequences of a gene that encode amino acids.

expanding triplet repeat A type of mutation in which a gene grows with each generation by adding copies of a specific 3-base sequence.

expressed sequence tags (ESTs) Short pieces of cDNAs used to locate and isolate protein-encoding genes.

expressivity Severity or degree of a phenotype.

***ex vivo* gene therapy** Genetic alteration of cells removed from a patient, then reinfused or implanted back into the patient.

F

fallopian tubes Tubes leading from the ovaries to the uterus.

fertilized ovum An oocyte that a sperm has penetrated.

fetus The prenatal human after the eighth week of development, when structures grow and specialize.

fibroids Noncancerous tumors in the uterus.

fluorescence *in situ* hybridization (FISH) A technique that binds a DNA probe and an attached fluorescent molecule to its complementary sequence on a chromosome.

follicle cells Nourishing cells surrounding a developing oocyte.

founder effect A type of genetic drift in populations in which a few members leave to found a new settlement, perpetuating a subset of the alleles from the original population.

frameshift mutation A mutation that alters a gene's reading frame.

fusion protein A protein that forms from transcription of two genes as a unit and then translation. Can cause cancer.

G

gamete   A sex cell.

gamete intrafallopian transfer (GIFT)   An infertility treatment in which sperm and oocytes are placed in a woman's fallopian tube.

gap 1(G₁) phase   The stage of interphase when proteins, carbohydrates, and lipids are synthesized in preparation for impending mitosis.

gap 2(G₂) phase   The stage of interphase when additional proteins are synthesized in preparation for impending mitosis.

gastrula   A three-layered embryo.

gene   A sequence of DNA that instructs a cell to produce a particular protein.

gene expression   Transcription of a gene and translation of the mRNA transcript into protein. On a genome level, the pattern of transcribed genes in a cell.

gene flow   Movement of alleles between populations.

gene pool   All the genes in a population.

gene targeting   A biotechnology in which an introduced gene exchanges places with its counterpart on a host cell's chromosome by homologous recombination.

gene therapy   Replacing a malfunctioning gene to alleviate symptoms.

genetic code   The correspondence between specific RNA triplets and the amino acids they specify.

genetic counseling   A medical specialty in which a counselor calculates the risk of recurrence of inherited disorders in families, applying the laws of inheritance to pedigrees.

genetic determinism   The idea that the environment cannot modify expression of an inherited trait.

genetic drift   Changes in gene frequencies that occur when small groups of individuals are separated from a larger population.

genetic heterogeneity   A phenotype that can be caused by variants of any of several genes.

genetic load   The collection of deleterious recessive alleles in a population.

genetics   The study of inherited variation.

genome   All the genetic material in the cells of a particular type of organism.

genomic imprinting   A process in which the phenotype differs depending upon which parent transmits a particular allele.

genomics   The study of the functions and interactions of many genes at a time.

genotype   The allele combinations in an individual that cause particular traits or disorders.

genotypic ratio   The ratio of genotype classes expected in the progeny of a particular cross.

germline gene therapy   Genetic alterations of gametes or fertilized ova, which perpetuate the change throughout the organism and transmit it to future generations.

germline mutation   A mutation that occurs in every cell in an individual.

glycolipid   A molecule that consists of a sugar bonded to a lipid.

glycoprotein   A molecule that consists of a sugar bonded to a protein.

Golgi apparatus   An organelle, consisting of flattened, membranous sacs, where secretion components are packaged.

gonads   Paired structures in the reproductive system where sperm or oocytes are manufactured.

growth factor   A protein that stimulates mitosis.

guanine   One of the two purine nitrogenous bases in DNA and RNA.

H

haploid (cell)   A cell containing one set of chromosomes (half the number of chromosomes of a somatic cell).

haplotype   A series of known DNA sequences or single nucleotide polymorphisms linked on a chromosome.

Hardy-Weinberg equilibrium   An idealized state in which gene frequencies in a population do not change from generation to generation.

heavy chain   Either of the two longer amino acid chains of the four that comprise an antibody subunit.

helicase   A type of enzyme that unwinds and holds apart strands of replicating DNA.

helper T cells   Lymphocytes that recognize foreign antigens on macrophages, activate B cells and cytotoxic T cells, and secrete cytokines.

hemizygous   The sex that has half as many X-linked genes as the other; a human male.

heritability   An estimate of the proportion of phenotypic variation in a group due to genes.

heterochromatin   Dark-staining genetic material that is inactive but that maintains the chromosome's structural integrity.

heterogametic sex   The sex with two different sex chromosomes; a human male.

heteroplasmy   The phenomenon of mitochondria within the same cell having different alleles of a particular gene.

heterozygous   Having two different alleles of a gene.

highly conserved   Genes or proteins whose sequences are very similar in different species.

histamine   A biochemical that mast cells release that causes allergy symptoms.

histone   A type of protein around which DNA entwines.

hominids   Animals ancestral to humans only.

hominoids   Animals ancestral to apes and humans only.

homogametic sex   The sex with identical types of sex chromosomes; the human female.

homologous pairs   Chromosomes with the same gene sequence.

homologous recombination   A naturally occurring process in which a piece of DNA exchanges places with its counterpart on a chromosome.

homozygous   Having two identical alleles of a gene.

hormone   A biochemical secreted in one part of the body that travels in the bloodstream to another part, where it exerts an effect.

human chorionic gonadotropin (hCG)   The hormone that prevents menstruation and indicates that a woman is pregnant.

human leukocyte antigen (HLA) **complex**   Polymorphic genes closely linked on the short arm of chromosome 6 that encode cell surface proteins important in immune system function.

humoral immune response   Process in which B cells secrete antibodies into the bloodstream.

I

ideogram   A diagram of a chromosome showing bands and locations of known genes. An ideogram combines cytogenetic and molecular information.

idiotype The part of an antibody's antigen binding site that fits around a particular foreign antigen.

inborn error of metabolism An inherited disorder resulting from a malfunctioning or absent enzyme.

incomplete dominance A heterozygote intermediate in phenotype between either homozygote.

independent assortment The random arrangement of homologous chromosome pairs, in terms of maternal or paternal origin, down the center of a cell in metaphase I. Inheritance of a gene on one chromosome does not influence inheritance of a gene on a different chromosome. Mendel's second law.

infertility The inability to conceive a child after a year of unprotected intercourse.

inflammation Part of the innate immune response that causes an infected or injured area to swell with fluid, turn red, and attract phagocytes.

initiation complex Aggregation of the components of the protein synthetic apparatus formed before mRNA is translated.

initiation site The site where DNA replication begins on a chromosome.

innate immunity Components of immune response that are present at birth and do not require exposure to an environmental stimulus.

inner cell mass A clump of cells on the inside of the blastocyst that will continue developing into an embryo.

insertion mutation A mutation that adds DNA bases.

in situ gene therapy Localized gene therapy in an easily accessible body part.

interferons A class of cytokines that fight viral infections and cancers.

interleukins A class of cytokines that control lymphocyte differentiation and growth.

intermediate filament A type of cytoskeletal component made of different proteins in different cell types.

interphase The stage of the cell cycle when a cell is not dividing.

intracytoplasmic sperm injection (ICSI) Injection of a sperm cell nucleus into an oocyte, to overcome lack of sperm motility.

intrauterine insemination An infertility treatment in which donor sperm is placed in the cervix or uterus.

introns Base sequences within a gene that are transcribed but are excised from the mRNA before translation into protein.

invasiveness The ability of cancer cells to squeeze into tight places and break through basement membranes.

in vitro fertilization (IVF) Placing oocytes and sperm in a laboratory dish with appropriate biochemicals so that fertilization occurs, then, after a few cell divisions, transferring the embryos to a woman's uterus.

in vitro gene therapy Direct genetic manipulation of cells in the body.

isochromosome A chromosome with identical arms, which forms when the centromere splits in the wrong plane.

isograft A transplant in which the donor and recipient are identical twins.

K

karyotype A chart that displays chromosome pairs in size order.

kinetochore A structure built of centromere-associated proteins that extends from the centromere during mitosis and meiosis and contacts spindle fibers.

L

lethal allele An allele that causes death before reproductive maturity or a ceasing of prenatal development.

ligand A molecule that binds to a receptor.

ligase An enzyme that catalyzes the formation of covalent bonds in the sugar-phosphate backbone of DNA.

light chain Either of the two shorter polypeptide chains of the four that comprise an antibody subunit.

linkage The relationship between genes on the same chromosome.

linkage disequilibrium Extremely tight linkage between DNA sequences.

linkage maps Maps that show how genes are ordered on chromosomes, determined from crossover frequencies between pairs of genes.

lipid A type of organic molecule that has more carbon and hydrogen atoms than oxygen atoms. Includes fats and oils.

liposomes Fatty bubbles that can enclose and transport DNA into cells.

LOD score A statistical measurement that indicates whether DNA sequences are usually inherited together due to linkage or chance.

lymphocytes Types of white blood cells that provide immunity; they include B cells and T cells.

lysosome A saclike organelle containing enzymes that degrade debris.

M

macroevolution Genetic change sufficient to form a new species.

macrophage A large, wandering scavenger cell that alerts the immune system by binding foreign antigens.

major depressive disorder A mood disorder characterized by prolonged, inexplicable sadness.

major histocompatibility complex (MHC) A gene cluster, on chromosome 6 in humans, that includes many genes that encode components of the immune system.

manifesting heterozygote A female carrier of an X-linked recessive gene who expresses the phenotype because the normal allele is inactivated in some affected tissues.

mast cells Circulating cells that have IgE receptors. They release allergy mediators when IgE binds to receptors on their surfaces. This causes allergy symptoms.

meiosis A type of cell division that halves the usual number of chromosomes to form haploid gametes.

memory cells Descendants of activated B cells that participate in a secondary immune response.

Mendelian trait A trait that a single gene specifies.

mesoderm The middle primary germ layer.

messenger RNA (mRNA) A molecule of RNA complementary in sequence to the coding strand of a gene. Messenger RNA carries the information that specifies a particular protein product.

metacentric chromosome A chromosome with the centromere located approximately in the center.

metaphase The stage of mitosis when chromosomes align along the center of the cell.

metastasis Spread of cancer from its site of origin to other parts of the body.

microevolution   Change of allele frequency in a population.

microfilament   A solid rod of actin protein that forms part of the cytoskeleton.

microtubule   A hollow structure built of tubulin protein that forms part of the cytoskeleton.

mismatch repair   Proofreading of DNA for misalignment of short, repeated segments (microsatellites).

missense   A single base change mutation that alters an amino acid in the gene product.

mitochondrion   An organelle consisting of a double membrane that houses enzymes responsible for catalyzing reactions that extract energy from nutrients.

mitosis   Division of somatic (nonsex) cells.

mode of inheritance   The pattern in which a gene variant passes from generation to generation, determined by whether it is dominant or recessive and is part of an autosome or a sex chromosome.

molecular clock   A tool for estimating the time elapsed since two species diverged from a shared ancestor, based on DNA or protein sequence differences and mutation rates for individual genes.

molecular evolution   Changes in protein and DNA sequences over time used to estimate how recently species diverged from a common ancestor.

monoclonal antibody (MAb)   A single antibody type, produced from a B cell fused to a cancer cell (a hybridoma).

monohybrid cross   A cross of two individuals who are heterozygous for a single trait.

monosomy   A human cell with 45 (one missing) chromosomes.

monozygotic (MZ) twins   Twins that originate as a single fertilized ovum and are thus identical.

morula   The very early prenatal stage that resembles a mulberry.

multifactorial trait   A trait or illness determined by several genes and the environment.

mutagen   A substance that changes, adds, or deletes a DNA base.

mutant   An allele that differs from the normal or most common allele, altering the phenotype.

mutation   A change in a protein-encoding gene that has an effect on the phenotype.

N

natural selection   Differential survival and reproduction of individuals with particular phenotypes in particular environments, which may alter allele frequencies in subsequent generations.

neural tube   A structure in the embryo that develops into the brain and spinal cord.

nitrogenous base   A nitrogen-containing base that is part of a nucleotide.

nondisjunction   The unequal partitioning of chromosomes into gametes during meiosis.

nonsense mutation   A point mutation that changes an amino-acid-coding codon into a stop codon, prematurely terminating synthesis of the encoded protein.

notochord   An embryonic structure that forms the framework of the skeleton and induces formation of the neural tube.

nucleic acid   DNA or RNA.

nucleolus   A structure within the nucleus where ribosomes are assembled from ribosomal RNA and protein.

nucleosome   A unit of chromatin structure.

nucleotide   The building block of a nucleic acid, consisting of a phosphate group, a nitrogenous base, and a 5-carbon sugar.

nucleotide excision repair   Replacement of up to 30 nucleotides to correct damage of several types.

nucleus   A large, membrane-bounded region of a eukaryotic cell that houses the genetic material.

O

oncogene   A dominant gene that promotes cell division. An oncogene normally controls the cell cycle, but causes cancer when overexpressed.

oocyte   The female gamete (sex cell).

oogenesis   Oocyte development.

oogonium   The diploid cell that begins oogenesis.

organelle   A specialized structure in a eukaryotic cell that carries out a specific function.

organogenesis   Development of organs from a three-layered embryo.

orgasm   Pleasurable sensations associated with sperm release or rubbing of the clitoris.

ovaries   Paired structures in the female reproductive tract where oocytes mature.

ovulation   Release of an oocyte from an ovary.

P

p53   A tumor-suppressor gene whose loss of function is implicated in a number of different types of cancer. The functional allele enables a cell to repair damaged DNA or cease dividing.

paracentric inversion   An inverted chromosome that does not include the centromere.

parsimony analysis   A statistical method used to identify the most realistic evolutionary tree that can be derived from a given data set.

PCR   See polymerase chain reaction.

pedigree   A chart consisting of symbols for individuals connected by lines that depict genetic relationships and transmission of inherited traits.

penetrance   Percentage of individuals with a particular genotype who have an associated phenotype.

pericentric inversion   An inverted chromosome that includes the centromere.

peroxisome   An organelle consisting of a double membrane that houses enzymes with various functions.

phagocytes   Cells that surround a smaller cell or particle and destroy it.

phenocopy   An environmentally caused trait that occurs in a familial pattern, mimicking inheritance.

phenotype   The expression of a gene in traits or symptoms.

phenotypic ratio   The ratio of phenotypic classes expected in the progeny of a particular cross.

plasma cells   Descendants of activated B cells that produce large amounts of a single antibody type.

plasma membrane   The selective barrier around a cell, consisting of proteins, glycolipids, glycoproteins, and lipid rafts on or in a phospholipid bilayer.

plasmid   A small circle of double-stranded DNA found in some bacteria in addition to their DNA. Plasmids are used as vectors for recombinant DNA technology.

pleiotropic   A Mendelian disorder with several symptoms, different subsets of which may occur in different individuals.

pluripotent   A cell's ability to divide to give rise to daughter cells that can specialize in a variety of different ways. Progenitor cells are pluripotent.

point mutation   A single base change in DNA.

polar body   A product of female meiosis that contains little cytoplasm and does not continue to develop into an oocyte.

polar body biopsy   A genetic test performed on a polar body to infer the genotype of the attached oocyte.

polygenic traits   Traits determined by more than one gene.

polymerase chain reaction (PCR)   An amplification technique in which a specific sequence of DNA from a gene of interest is replicated in a test tube to rapidly produce many copies.

polymorphism   A DNA base or sequence at a certain chromosomal locus that varies in at least 1 percent of individuals in a population.

polyploid (cell)   A cell with one or more extra sets of chromosomes.

population   A group of interbreeding individuals.

population bottleneck   Decrease in allele diversity resulting from an event that kills many members of a population, followed by restoration of population numbers.

population genetics   The study of allele frequencies in different groups of individuals.

population study   Comparison of disease incidence in different groups of people.

positional cloning   Identifying a gene by beginning with a phenotype within a large family and narrowing down the segment of a chromosome that includes the gene.

preimplantation genetic diagnosis (PGD)   Removing a cell from an 8-celled embryo and testing it for a disease-causing gene or chromosomal imbalance to decide if the remaining embryo should be implanted in the uterus to continue development.

primary germ layers   The three basic layers of an embryo.

primary immune response   The immune system's response to a first encounter with a foreign antigen.

primary oocyte   A cell in the female that undergoes reduction division.

primary spermatocyte   A cell in the male that undergoes reduction division.

primary (1°) structure   The amino acid sequence of a protein.

primase   The enzyme that builds a short RNA primer at the start of a replicated DNA segment.

primitive streak   A band along the back of a three-week human embryo that forms an axis other structures develop around and that eventually gives rise to the nervous system.

prion   "Proteinaceous infectious particle"—a form of an infectious protein that can cause brain degeneration. Can be inherited or acquired.

progenitor cell   A cell whose descendants can follow any of several developmental pathways.

promoter   A control sequence near the start of a gene.

pronuclei   Packets of DNA in the fertilized ovum.

prophase   The first stage of mitosis or meiosis, when chromatin condenses.

prospective study   A study in which two or more groups are followed into the future.

prostate gland   A gland that contributes secretions to the seminal fluid.

proteasome   A multiprotein structure shaped like a barrel through which misfolded proteins pass and are dismantled.

protein   A type of macromolecule that is the direct product of genetic information; a chain of amino acids.

proteome   The set of proteins that a cell produces.

proto-oncogene   A gene that normally controls the cell cycle. When overexpressed, it functions as an oncogene, causing cancer.

pseudoautosomal region   Genes on the tips of the Y chromosome that have counterparts on the X chromosome.

pseudogene   A gene that does not encode protein, but whose sequence very closely resembles that of a coding gene.

P site   Part of a ribosome that holds a growing amino acid chain.

Punnett square   A diagram used to follow parental gene contributions to offspring.

purine   A type of organic molecule with a two-ring structure, including the nitrogenous bases adenine and guanine.

pyrimidine   A type of organic molecule with a single-ring structure, including the nitrogenous bases cytosine, thymine, and uracil.

 Q

quantitative trait loci   Genes that determine polygenic traits.

quaternary (4°) structure   A protein that has more than one polypeptide subunit.

R

reading frame   The grouping of DNA base triplets encoding an amino acid sequence.

receptor   A structure on a cell, usually a protein, that binds a specific molecule.

recessive   An allele whose expression is masked by another allele.

reciprocal translocation   A chromosome aberration in which two nonhomologous chromosomes exchange parts, conserving genetic balance but rearranging genes.

recombinant   A series of alleles on a chromosome that differs from the series of either parent.

recombinant DNA technology   Transferring genes between species.

reduction division   The first meiotic division, which halves the chromosome number.

relative risk   Probability that an individual from a population will develop a particular condition in comparison to another group, usually the general population.

replacement hypothesis   The theory that Africans replaced Eurasian descendants of *Homo erectus* 200,000 years ago.

replication fork   Locally opened portion of a replicating DNA double helix.

restriction enzyme   An enzyme, derived from bacteria, that cuts DNA at certain sequences.

restriction fragment length polymorphism (RFLP)   Differences in restriction enzyme cutting sites among individuals at the same site among the chromosomes, resulting in different patterns of DNA fragment sizes.

retrovirus   A type of RNA virus that uses reverse transcriptase to produce DNA from viral RNA. This DNA integrates into the host's genome, where it directs reproduction of the virus.

reverse transcriptase   An enzyme that synthesizes a DNA molecule from an RNA molecule.

rhizosecretion   A biotechnology that collects proteins secreted by a plant's roots into a liquid medium.

ribonucleic acid (RNA)   A nucleic acid whose bases are A, C, U, and G.

ribose   A 5-carbon sugar in RNA.

ribosomal RNA (rRNA)   RNA that, with proteins, comprises ribosomes.

ribosome   An organelle consisting of RNA and protein that is a scaffold for protein synthesis.

ribozyme   RNA component of an RNA-protein complex that has enzymatic function.

risk factor   A characteristic associated with increased likelihood of developing a particular medical condition.

RNA   *See* **ribonucleic acid.**

RNA interference   A natural process that destroys specific mRNA molecules using small interfering RNAs that result from transcribing short sequences on both DNA strands.

RNA polymerase (RNAP)   An enzyme that adds RNA nucleotides to a growing RNA chain.

RNA primer   A short sequence of RNA that initiates DNA replication.

Robertsonian translocation   A chromosome aberration in which two short arms of nonhomologous chromosomes break and the long arms fuse, forming one unusual, large chromosome.

S

schizophrenia   Loss of the ability to organize thoughts and perceptions, causing hallucinations and inappropriate behavior.

secondary immune response   The immune system's response to a second or subsequent encounter with a foreign antigen.

secondary oocyte   A cell resulting from meiosis I in the female.

secondary spermatocyte   A cell resulting from meiosis I in the male.

secondary (2°) structure   Folds in a polypeptide caused by attractions between amino acids close together in the primary structure.

segregation   The distribution of alleles of a gene into separate gametes during meiosis. This is Mendel's first law.

semiconservative replication   The synthesis of new DNA in which half of each double helix comes from a preexisting double helix.

seminal fluid   Secretions in which sperm travel.

seminal vesicles   Structures that secrete fructose and prostaglandins into semen.

seminiferous tubules   A network of tubules in the testes where sperm are manufactured.

sex chromosome   A chromosome containing genes that specify sex. A human male has one X and one Y chromosome; a female has two X chromosomes.

sex-influenced trait   Phenotype caused when an allele is recessive in one sex but dominant in the other.

sex-limited trait   A trait that affects a structure or function present in only one sex.

signal transduction   A series of biochemical reactions and interactions that pass incoming information from outside a cell to inside, triggering a cellular response.

single nucleotide polymorphism (SNP)   Single base sites that differ among individuals. A SNP is present in at least 1 percent of a population.

site-directed mutagenesis   Introduction of a base change into a PCR protocol, so that the change is perpetuated.

somatic cell   A nonsex cell, with 23 pairs of chromosomes in humans.

somatic cell nuclear transfer   Transfer of a somatic cell's nucleus from a person with a degenerative illness or injury to an enucleated egg, and growth to the blastocyst stage to obtain inner cell mass cells, which are cultured into embryonic stem (ES) cells. Given appropriate stimulation, the ES cells divide to produce needed cells matched to the nucleus donor.

somatic gene therapy   Genetic alteration of a specific somatic tissue, not transmitted to future generations.

somatic mutation   A mutation occurring only in a subset of somatic (nonsex) cells.

spermatid   The product of meiosis II in the male.

spermatogenesis   Sperm cell development.

spermatogonium   A diploid cell that gives rise to a cell that undergoes meiosis, developing into a sperm.

spermatozoon (sperm)   A mature male reproductive cell (meiotic product).

S phase   The stage of interphase when DNA replicates.

spindle   A structure composed of microtubules that pulls sets of chromosomes apart in a dividing cell.

spontaneous mutation   A genetic change that is a result of mispairing when the replication machinery encounters a base in its rare tautomeric form.

SRY gene   The sex-determining region of the Y, a gene that controls whether the unspecialized embryonic gonad will develop as testis or ovary. If the gene is activated, it becomes a testis; if not, an ovary forms.

stem cells   Cells that give rise to other stem cells that retain the potential to differentiate (specialize) further, as well as to cells that differentiate.

submetacentric   A chromosome in which the centromere establishes a long arm and a short arm.

subtelomeres   The 10,000 or so DNA bases next to the telomeres. They contain short repeats but also protein-encoding genes.

sugar-phosphate backbone   The "rails" of a DNA double helix, consisting of linked, alternating deoxyribose and phosphate groups, oriented opposite one another.

synapsis   The gene-by-gene alignment of homologous chromosomes during prophase I of meiosis.

synonymous codons   DNA triplets that specify the same amino acid.

synteny   The correspondence of genes located on the same chromosome in several species.

T

tandem duplication   A duplicated sequence of DNA located right next to the original sequence on a chromosome.

T cell   A type of lymphocyte that produces cytokines and coordinates the immune response.

telomerase   An enzyme, including a sequence of RNA, that adds DNA to chromosome tips.

telomere   A chromosome tip.

telophase   The stage of mitosis or meiosis when daughter cells separate.

template strand   The DNA strand carrying the information that is transcribed.

teratogen   A substance that causes a birth defect.

tertiary (3°) structure   Folds in a polypeptide caused by interactions between amino acids and water. This draws together amino acids that are far apart in the primary structure.

test cross   Crossing an individual of unknown genotype to an individual who is homozygous recessive for the trait being studied.

testes   Paired sacs that hang outside the male's body that contain the seminiferous tubules, in which sperm develop.

thymine   One of the two pyrimidine bases in DNA.

Ti **plasmid**   A virus that causes tumors in certain plants, used as a vector to create transgenic plants.

totipotent   Ability of a cell (a fertilized ovum or stem cell) to give rise to daughter cells that specialize as any cell type.

transcription   Manufacturing RNA from DNA.

transcription elongation   The process of RNA nucleotides aligning against a template strand of DNA.

transcription factor   A protein that activates the transcription of other genes.

transcription initiation   Joining of transcription factors and RNAP at a promoter.

transcription termination   The ending of transcription that occurs as RNAP encounters a terminator sequence in the DNA template strand.

transdifferentiate   Ability of a cell to become less specialized, then divide to yield daughter cells that specialize into a different cell type.

transfer RNA (tRNA)   A type of RNA that connects mRNA to amino acids during protein synthesis.

transgenic organism   An individual with a genetic modification in every cell.

transition   A point mutation altering a purine to a purine or a pyrimidine to a pyrimidine.

translation   Assembly of an amino acid chain according to the sequence of base triplets in a molecule of mRNA.

translocation   Exchange between nonhomologous chromosomes.

translocation carrier   An individual with exchanged chromosomes, but no signs or symptoms. The person has the usual amount of genetic material, but it is rearranged.

transplantable   The ability of a cancer cell to grow into a tumor if it is transplanted into another individual.

transposon   A gene or DNA segment that moves to another chromosome.

transversion   A point mutation altering a purine to a pyrimidine or vice versa.

trisomy   A human cell with 47 (one extra) chromosomes.

trophoblast   The outermost cells of the preimplantation embryo.

tumor necrosis factor   A cytokine that attacks cancer cells.

tumor suppressor gene   A recessive gene whose normal function is to limit the number of divisions a cell undergoes.

U

ubiquitin   A protein that tags misfolded proteins, targeting them for destruction in a proteasome.

uniparental disomy   Inheriting two copies of the same gene from one parent.

uracil   One of the four types of bases in RNA; a pyrimidine.

urethra   A tube leading from the bladder to the outside of the body.

uterus   A saclike organ in a woman's reproductive tract where embryo and fetus develop.

V

vaccine   An inactivated or partial form of a pathogen that alerts the immune system to produce antibodies when the native pathogen is encountered.

variable regions   The upper parts of antibodies, which differ in amino acid sequence among individuals.

vas deferens   Paired tubes leading from the epididymis to the urethra that deliver sperm.

vesicle   A membrane-bounded, bubblelike structure in a cell.

virus   An infectious particle built of nucleic acid in a protein coat.

W

wild type   The most common phenotype in a population for a particular gene.

X

xenograft   A transplant in which donor and recipient are different species.

X inactivation   The inactivation of one X chromosome in each cell of a female mammal, occurring early in embryonic development.

X inactivation center   A part of the X chromosome that inactivates the chromosome.

X-linked   Genes on an X chromosome.

X-Y homologs   Y-linked genes that are similar to genes on the X chromosome.

Y

Y-linked   Genes on a Y chromosome.

yolk sac   A structure external to the embryo that manufactures blood cells and nourishes the developing embryo.

Z

zygote   A prenatal human from the fertilized ovum stage until formation of the primordial embryo, at about two weeks.

zygote intrafallopian transfer   An assisted reproductive technology in which an ovum fertilized *in vitro* is placed in a woman's fallopian tube.

Credits

Line Art

Chapter 2
Figure 2.25 From Piero Anversa: New England Journal of Medicine, January 1, 2002, © Massachusetts Medical Society, Waltham, MA.

Chapter 6
Box Figure 1, page 114: Courtesy Professor Jennifer A. Marshall-Graves, Australian National University.
Box Figure 3, page 115: Courtesy David Page, Massachusetts Institute of Technology; Howard Hughes Medical Institute Investigator.

Chapter 7
Figure 7.2 Data and print from Gordon Mendenhall, Thomas Mertens, and John Hendrix, "Fingerprint Ridge Court," in *The American Biology Teacher,* vol. 51, no. 4, April 1989, pp. 204–6; **Figure 7.9** From Robert Plomin, et al., "The genetic basis of complex human behaviors," *Science,* vol. 264, 17 June 1994, pp. 1733–39, © 1994 American Association for the Advancement of Science; **Figure 7.10** From The New Yorker Collection 1981 Charles Addams, ©The Cartoon Bank. All Rights Reserved.

Chapter 8
Table 8.1 From Psychiatric Genomics, Inc.
Figure 8.8 ©Robert Gilliam.

Chapter 13
Box Figure 2, page 243: Modified from H. Willard (1998) *Current Opin Genet Dev* 8:219–25; **Figure 13.14** Data reprinted from M. Eisheikh, et al, *Annals of Medicine* 1999, 31:99–105.

Chapter 15
Box Figure 1, page 290: From CDC, *Emerging Infectious Disease,* vol. 4, no. 4, October-December, 1998; **Figure 15.10** Data from Smadar Avigad et al., A single origin of phenylketonuria in Yemenite Jews, *Nature* 344:170, March 8, 1990; **Figure 15.11** From European Working Group on Cystic Fibrosis Genetics: "Gradienyt distribution of the major CF mutation and its associated haplotype", *Human Genetics* 85:436–45, 1990. By permission of Springer Verlag.

Chapter 16
Figure 16.5 From Michael D. Lemonick & A. Dorfman: "The 160,000 year old man," June 23, 2003, *Time Magazine.* **Figure 16.9** From Richard A. Gibbs & Daivd L. Mellon: "Primate shadow play". In *Science,* vol. 299, February 23, 2003.

Chapter 18
Figure 18.8 Adapted from John Goldman and Juania Meb: *New England Journal of Medicine* 344:1084.

Chapter 22
Figure 22.9 Adapted from illustration by MarleneViola. From Ricki Lewis and Barry A. Palevitz, "Genome Economy", *The Scientist* 15(12):21, June 2001. Reprinted by permission. **Figure 22.10** From

Franas Collins et al: "A vision for the future of genomic research." In *Nature* 422:835–847, April 24, 2003.

Photographs

About the Author
Photo by Barry Palevitz.

Brief Contents
Page v top left: ©The McGraw-Hill Companies, Inc./ Bob Coyle, photographer; **p. v middle left:** ©PhotoDics/ Vol. 2; **p. v bottom left:** ©Stephen Simpson/Taxi/Getty Images; p. v top right: ©Peter Dazeley/Stone/Getty Images; **p. v middle right:** ©Brand X/Vol. #X122; **p. v bottom right:** ©Ed Honowitz/Stone/Getty Images.

List of Boxes
Page vi top: Courtesy of Dr. H.F. Willard, Case Western Reserve University.; **p. vi middle:** Courtesy of Lynn Lieberman; **p. vi bottom:** ©Redneck/Getty Images.

Clinical Coverage
Page vii top: ©Dr. Dennis Kunkel/Visuals Unlimited; **p. vii bottom:** ©Grant Faint/Image Bank/Getty Images.

Chapter 1
Opener: ©The McGraw-Hill Companies, Inc./Bop Coyle, photographer; **Figure 1.1a:** ©Susan McCartney/ Photo Researchers; **Figure 1.1b:** ©Doug Pensinger/ Allsport; **Figure 1.3(4):** The National Human Genome Research Institute; **Figure 1.3(5&6):** ©PhotoDisc Website; **Figure 1.3(7):** ©Richard Laird/Getty Images; **Figure 1.4 Chimpanzee:** ©PhotoDisc Website; **Figure 1.4 Fruit fly:** ©David M. Phillips/Photo Researchers; **Figure 1.4 Human:** ©Corbis/R-F Website; **Figure 1.4 Mouse:** ©PhotoDisc/Vol.# 8; **Figure 1.4 Pufferfish:** ©Digital Vision/Getty Images; **Figure 1.4 Sea Squirt:** ©PhotoDisc Website; **Figure 1.4 Yeast:** ©Dr. Stanley Flegler/Visuals Unlimited; **Figure 1.5a:** ©Lester Bergman/ProjectMasters; **Figure 1.5b:** ©Sunstar/Photo Researchers; **Figure 1.6:** Roger Berry, Portrait of a DNA Sequence, 1998, dichroic glass and steel, 18" × 51'. Photo: Joseph Coulombe; **Figure 1.7:** Courtesy of the Massachusetts Historical Society; **Figure 1.8:** ©Jay Sand; **Figure 1.9a:** Courtesy, Thierry LaCombe & Jean Pierre Bruno, I.N.R.A., France; **Figure 1.9b:** ©Alexander Lowry/Photo Researchers; **Figure 1.10a:** ©PhotoDisc Website; **Figure 1.10b:** ©Robert Dowling/Corbis Images; **Figure 1.10c:** ©Porterfield-Chickering/Photo Researchers; **Figure 1.11:** Courtesy Ingo Potrykus, Swiss Federal Institute of Technology; **Figure 1.12:** ©Alexis Rockman, 2000. Courtesy Gorney Bravin + Lee, New York.

Chapter 2
Opener: ©Dr. Dennis Kunkel/Visuals Unlimited; **Figure 2.1a:** ©Muscular Dystrophy Association; **Figure 2.1b:** Courtesy, Cystic Fibrosis Foundation; **Figure 2.1c:** ©Ann States/Corbis Saba; **Figure 2.2:** ©Manfred Kage/Peter Arnold; **Figure 2.3 (bottom):** ©Biophoto Associates/Science Source/Photo Researchers; **Figure 2.3 (left):** ©K.R. Porter/Photo

Researchers; **Figure 2.3 (top):** ©David M. Phillips/The Population Council/Science Source/Photo Researchers; **Figure 2.6:** ©Prof. P. Motta & T. Naguro/SPL/Photo Researchers; **Figure 2.7:** ©D. Friend-D. Fawcett/Visuals Unlimited; **Figure 2.8:** ©Bill Longcore/Photo Researchers; **Figure 2.10:** ©K.G. Murti/Visuals Unlimited; **p. 32:** Courtesy Dr. Brett Casey, Baylor College of Medicine; **Figure 2.13b:** ©Bart's Medical Library/Phototake; **Figure 2.15b:** ©From Dr. A.T. Sumner, "Mammalian Chromosomes from Prophase to Telophase," *Chromosoma,* 100:410–418, 1991. ©Springer-Verlag; **Figure 2.16:** ©Ed Reschke; **Figure 2.18:** From L. Chong, et al. 1995. "A Human Telomeric Protein." *Science,* 270:1663–1667. ©1995 American Association for the Advancement of Science. Photo courtesy, Dr. Titia DeLange; **Figure 2.19 all:** ©Ed Reschke; **Figure 2.24 center & right:** Courtesy of Advanced Cell Technologies, Inc.; **Figure 2.24 left:** ©AP/Wide World Photos.

Chapter 3
Opener: ©The McGraw-Hill Companies, Inc./Barry Barker, photographer; **Figure 3.8:** ©Larry Johnson, Dept. of Veterinary Anatomy and Public Health, Texas A&M University. Originally appeared in *Biology of Reproduction,* 47:1091–1098, 1992; **Figure 3.9b:** ©David M. Phillips/Visuals Unlimited; **Figure 3.9c:** ©Granger Collection; **Figure 3.10:** ©R.J. Blandau; **Figure 3.13b:** ©Francis LeRoy/BioCosmos/SPL/Photo Researchers; **Figure 3.14 left:** ©Petit Format/Nestle/Science Source/Photo Researchers; **Figure 3.14 middle:** ©P.M. Motta & J. Van Blerkom/SPL/Photo Researchers; **Figure 3.14 right:** ©Petit Format/Nestle/Science Source/Photo Researchers; **p. 58:** ©AP/Wide World Photos; **p. 59:** Courtesy UMass Amherst News Office; **Figure 3.17:** ©Steve Wewerka; **Figure 3.18a:** ©Petit Format/Nestle/Photo Researchers; **Figure 3.18b:** ©Carolina Biological Supply Company/Phototake; **Figure 3.18c:** ©Donald Yaeger/Camera M.D. Studios; **Figure 3.19:** ©Richard Nowitz/Phototake; **Figure 3.21b–d:** From Streissguth, A.P., Landesman-Dwyer, S., Martin, J.C., & Smith, D.W. July 1980. "Teratogenic effects of alcohol in human and laboratory animals." *Science,* 209(18):353–361. ©1980 American Association for the Advancement of Science; **Figure 3.22:** ©J.L. Bulcao/Getty Images; **p. 68:** ©Vanessa DeGier, Boston Medical Center.

Chapter 4
Opener: © PhotoDics/Vol. 2; **Figure 4.1:** ©Sands Steven/Corbis Sygma; **Figure 4.15:** ©Nancy Hamilton/Photo Researchers.

Chapter 5
Opener: © Professors P. Motta & T. Naguro/Photo Researchers; **Figure 5.1a:** ©Porterfield-Chickering/ Photo Researchers; **Figure 5.2:** From Genest, Jacques, Jr., Lavoie, Marc-Andre. August 12, 1999. "Images in Clinical Medicine." *New England Journal of Medicine,*

p. 490. ©1999, Massachusetts Medical Society. All Rights Reserved; **Figure 5.5a:** ©North Wind Picture Archives; **p. 99 all:** From G. Pierard, A. Nikkels. April 5, 2001. "A Medical Mystery." *New England Journal of Medicine,* 344: p. 1057. ©2001 Massachusetts Medical Society. All rights reserved.

Chapter 6
Opener: ©Archivo Iconografico, S.A./Corbis Images; **Figure 6.2:** ©Biophoto Associates/Photo Researchers; **p. 114 right:** ©Dr. Walter Just; **p. 114 left:** Photo courtesy of Dr. Jennifer A. Marshall Graves, Comparative Genomic Research Group, Research School of Biological Sciences, The Australian National University; **p. 115 :** Photo by Stanley Rowin; **Figure 6.5:** ©Ward Odenwald, National Institute of Neurological Disease and Stroke; **Figure 6.7:** Courtesy, Dr. Mark A. Crowe; **Figure 6.8:** ©Historical Pictures Service/Stock Montage; **Figure 6.9b:** Courtesy, Richard Alan Lewis M.D., M.S., Baylor College of Medicine; **Figure 6.10a:** From J.M. Cantu et al. 1984. *Human Genetics,* 66:66–70. ©Springer-Verlag, Gmbh & Co. KG. Photo courtesy of Pragna I. Patel, Ph.D/Baylor College of Medicine; **Figure 6.12 a,b:** From Wilson and Foster. 1985. *Williams Textbook of Endocrinol,* 7/e. © W.B. Saunders; **Figure 6.12 c,d:** Courtesy National Jewish Hospital & Research Center; **Figure 6.13a:** ©William E. Ferguson; **Figure 6.13b:** ©Horst Schafer/Peter Arnold; **Figure 6.14 all:** ©Bettmann/Corbis; **Figure 6.16a:** ©The McGraw-Hill Companies, Inc./Carla D. Kipper; **Figure 6.16b:** Courtesy Roxanne De Leon and Angelman Syndrome Foundation; **Figure 6.17a:** Courtesy of Dr. Randy Jirtle, Duke University Medical Center.

Chapter 7
Opener: ©Corbis/R-F Website; **Figure 7.3a:** From Albert & Blakeslee, Corn and Man, *Journal of Heredity,* 1914, Vol. 5, pg. 51. By permission of Oxford University Press.; **Figure 7.3b:** ©Library of Congress; **Figure 7.6:** ©AP/Wide World Photos; **Figure 7.7:** ©Dr. P. Marazzi/Science Photo Library/Photo Researchers; **Figure 7.12:** ©Roche Molecular Systems; **Figure 7.14:** ©David Graham; **Figure 7.15 a,b:** ©John Annerino.

Chapter 8
Opener: ©Digital Vision; **p. 156:** ©Redneck/Getty Images; **Figure 8.2:** ©AP/Wide World Photos; **Figure 8.3:** ©Stanford University Center for Narcolepsy; **Figure 8.6:** PhotoDisc/Vol.#94.

Chapter 9
Opener: ©Stephen Simpson/Taxi/Getty Images; **Figure 9.1:** ©Dr. Gopal Murti/Photo Researchers; **Figure 9.5a:** ©Science Source/Photo Researchers; **Figure 9.5b inset:** From "The Double Helix" by James D. Watson, 1968, Atheneum Press, NY. © Cold Spring Harbor Laboratory Archives; **Figure 9.6:** ©Bettmann/Corbis; **Figure 9.9b:** ©1948 M.C. Escher Foundation/Baarn-Holland, All Rights Reserved.; **p. 174:** ©Stock Montage; **Figure 9.12 bottom:** ©Science VU/Visuals Unlimited; **Figure 9.12 top:** ©1979 Olins and Olins/BPS.

Chapter 10
Opener: ©David Roth/Stone/Getty Images; **Figure 10.5c:** ©Tripos Associates/Peter Arnold; **Figure 10.11:** Courtesy, Alexander Rich; **Figure 10.15a:** ©Kiseleva-Fawcett/Visuals Unlimited; **p. 199:** ©The Nobel Foundation, 1976.

Chapter 11
Opener: ©Leslie Saint-Julien, National Human Genome Research Institute-NIH; **Figure 11.11a:** ©Bristol Biomed Image Archive, University of Bristol. Image by Dr John Eveson.

Chapter 12
Opener: ©Grant Faint/Image Bank/Getty Images; **p. 227:** Courtesy of Lynn Lieberman; **Figure 12.1a:** ©Bill Longcore/Photo Researchers; **Figure 12.1b:** ©Bill Longcore/Photo Researchers; **Figure 12.3:** ©Science Photo Library/Photo Researchers; **p. 225:** Courtesy, Brush Wellman; **p. 225 inset:** Reproduced with permission from Dr. Milton D. Rossman, Hospital of the University of Pennsylvania, Philadelphia, PA; **p. 229 top:** ©David M. Phillips/Visuals Unlimited; **p. 229 all except top:** From R. Simensen, R. Curtis Rogers, "Fragile X Syndrome," *American Family Physician,* 39:186 May 1989. © American Academy of Family Physicians.; **Figure 12.12a:** Courtesy Dr. Alan Lehmann and Dr David Atherton; **Figure 12.12b:** ©Kenneth Greer/Visuals Unlimited.

Chapter 13
Opener: ©Gina Glover/ginaglover.com; **Figure 13.1a:** Courtesy, Colleen Weisz; **Figure 13.1b:** Courtesy Genzyme Corporation; **Figure 13.2:** ©Science VU/Visuals Unlimited; **p. 243:** Courtesy of Dr. H.F. Willard, Case Western Reserve University.; **Figure 13.6d:** Courtesy Genzyme Corporation; **Figure 13.7:** ©GE Medical Systems; **Figure 13.8 b,c:** ©CNRI/Photo Researchers; **Figure 13.9:** ©Courtesy Genzyme Corporation; **Figure 13.11:** Courtesy Dr. Frederick Elder, Dept. of Pediatrics, University of Texas Medical School, Houston.; **p. 256:** Photo taken at the 1999 National Klinefelter Syndrome Conference. Courtesy, Stefan Schwarz; **p. 257:** Photo courtesy of Kathy Naylor; **Figure 13.16b:** Courtesy of Donna Bennett/IDEAS; **Figure 13.18b:** Courtesy Lawrence Livermore National Laboratory; **Figure 13.19 all:** From N.B. Spinner, et al. 1994. *American Journal of Human Genetics,* 55:239, fig. 1, published by the University of Chicago Press, 1994 by The American Society of Human Genetics. All rights reserved.

Chapter 14
Opener: ©Peter Dazeley/Stone/Getty Images; **Figure 14.3:** ©Denise Grady/NYT Pictures; **Figure 14.4a:** ©Paul A. Souders/Corbis Images.

Chapter 15
Opener: ©Corbis/R-F Website; **Figure 15.1:** ©Stapleton Collection/Corbis; **Figure 15.3:** Dr. Victor McKusick/Johns Hopkins University School of Medicine; **Figure 15.5a:** ©Bettmann/Corbis; **Figure 15.5b:** ©Vincent Yu/Wide World Photos; **p. 297 left:** ©Scott Camazine/Photo Researchers; **p. 297 right:** ©Barb Zurawski

Chapter 16
Opener: ©Corbis/R-F Website; **Figure 16.3a:** Michael Hagelberg/Arizona State University Research Publications; **Figure 16.3a:** ©John Reader/SPL/Photo Researchers; **Figure 16.4:** ©Volker Steger/Nordstar-4 Million Years of Man/SPL/Photo Researchers; **Figure 16.6a:** ©Volker Steger/Nordstar/Photo Researchers; **Figure 16.7a:** ©G. Hinter Leitner/Getty Images; **Figure 16.7b:** ©Burt Silverman/Silverman Studios; **Figure 16.8 a&c:** Courtesy, James H. Asher, Jr.; **Figure 16.8b:** ©Vickie Jackson; **Figure 16.11(1):** ©Transparency # 320496, Courtesy Department of Library Services, American Museum of Natural History; **Figure**

16.11(2): ©Zoological Society of London; **p. 317 top left:** ©John Glustina/GIUST/Bruce Coleman; **p. 317 top right:** ©Roland Seitre/Peter Arnold; **p. 317 bottom left:** ©G. C. Kelley/Photo Researchers; **p. 317 bottom right:** ©Tom Ulrich/Visuals Unlimited; **Figure 16.12 a,b:** Courtesy, Dr. H. Hameister; **Figure 16.14 a,b:** From F.R. Goodman and P.J. Scambler. Human Hox Gene Mutations, *Clinical Genetics,* Jan. 2001, page 2, Figures A and E.; **p. 323:** Courtesy of Marie Deatherage.

Chapter 17
Opener: ©Brand X/Vol. #X122; **Figure 17.1:** Courtesy, The Hancock Family; **Figure 17.2a:** ©Barry Dowsett/SPL/Photo Researchers; **Figure 17.3 both:** ©Martin Rotker/Phototake; **Figure 17.5:** ©Manfred Kage/Peter Arnold; **Figure 17.8:** ©Biology Media/Photo Researchers; **Figure 17.12b:** ©Dr. A. Liepins/SPL/Photo Researchers; **Figure 17.15:** ©Courtesy, Dr. Maureen Mayes; **Figure 17.16 bottom:** ©Phil Harrington/Peter Arnold; **Figure 17.16 top:** ©David Scharf/Peter Arnold; **Figure 17.17 a&c:** ©Science VU/Visuals Unlimited; **Figure 17.17b:** ©Hans Gelderblom/Visuals Unlimited.

Chapter 18
Opener: ©Scott Dingman/Taxi/Getty Images; **Figure 18.1:** ©Nancy Kedersha/Immunogen/Photo Researchers; **Figure 18.2:** From: S.A. Armstrong et al. MLL translocations specify a distinct gene expression profile that distinguishes a unique leukemia. *Nature Genetics* Vol. 30 p. 41–47, January 2002; **p. 362:** ©Custom Medical Stock Photo; **p. 364:** Photo courtesy of Patricia Holm; **Figure 18.10 both:** Courtesy, Dr. Tom Mikkelsen; **Figure 18.11 all:** From B. Vogelstein. Sept. 1990. "The Genes That Contribute To Cancer," *Journal of NIH Research,* 2(8):66. Reprinted with permission from Medical Economics Co., Montvale, NJ.; **Figure 18.12 bottom:** ©PhotoDisc/Vol.#19; **Figure 18.12 top:** ©PhotoDisc/Vol.#30.

Chapter 19
Opener: ©Ed Honowitz/Stone/Getty Images; **Figure 19.1:** Photo by Barry Paleritz; **Figure 19.2:** ©Eye of Science/Photo Researchers; **Figure 19.4:** ©SPL/Photo Researchers; **Figure 19.7:** Reprinted with permission from Edvotek, Inc.; **Figure 19.9b:** Courtesy, Calgene Fresh; **Figure 19.12:** Courtesy of Genencor International, Inc.; **p. 383:** ©David Scharf; **Figure 19.14:** From Jacks, Tyler et al. July 1994. *Nature Genetics,* 7:357, fig. 6; **Figure 19.15b:** Courtesy of Calgene Fresh, Inc.

Chapter 20
Opener: ©PhotoDisc Website; **Figure 20.1a:** Reprinted with permission from *The Courier-Journal;* **Figure 20.2a:** ©Courtesy Paul and Migdalia Gelsinger, Photo: Arizona Daily Star; **Figure 20.3a:** Courtesy Ilyce Randell; **Box 20.1 ITOW:** ©Anna Powers; **Figure 20.8:** ©Ann States/Corbis Saba; **Figure 20.10:** Courtesy of Genzyme Genetics.

Chapter 21
Opener: ©PhotoDisc Website; **Figure 21.1:** ©Keri Pickett/Timepix; **Figure 21.2a:** ©Bob Schuchman/Phototake; **Figure 21.2b:** ©Tony Brain/SPL/Photo Researchers; **Figure 21.6c:** Integra. Photo courtesy of Ronald Carson, The Reproductive Science Center of Boston; **Figure 21.4:** ©CNRI/Phototake; **Figure 21.5:** ©Steve Goldstein; **Figure 21.7:** Courtesy, Dr. Anver Kuliev.

Chapter 22
Opener: ©PhotoDisc/Vol. #SS36.

Index

Page numbers followed by an "*f*" indicate figures; numbers followed by a "*t*" indicate tables.